Clinical PET and PET/CT

E. Edmund Kim • Myung-Chul Lee
Tomio Inoue • Wai-Hoi Wong
Editors

Clinical PET and PET/CT

Principles and Applications

Second Edition

Springer

Editors
E. Edmund Kim
Departments of Nuclear Medicine
and Diagnostic Radiology
The University of Texas
Houston, TX, USA

Myung-Chul Lee
Department of Nuclear Medicine
Gachon University School of Medicine
Namdong-Gu, Incheon
Korea, Republic of (South Korea)

Tomio Inoue
Department of Radiology
Yokohama City University
Graduate School of Medicine
Yokohama, Kanagawa
Japan

Wai-Hoi Wong
Department of Experimental Diagnostic
Imaging
The University of Texas
MD Anderson Cancer Center
Houston, TX, USA

ISBN 978-1-4939-3841-4 ISBN 978-1-4419-0802-5 (eBook)
DOI 10.1007/978-1-4419-0802-5
Springer New York Heidelberg Dordrecht London

Printed on acid-free paper

Springer is part of Springer Science+Business Media (www.springer.com)

This book is dedicated to our wives and children.

Preface

Since the first edition of *Clinical PET,* PET/CT has been increasingly utilized as an effective imaging technique for managing patients with tumors, neurodegenerative diseases, and cardiovascular disorders. PET demonstrates the functional processes of metabolic rates, receptor expression, cell-tissue interaction, or events at the molecular level. Many new promising target-specific radioligands have emerged in the clinical research and await its translation for clinical use. CT shows precise localization and characterization of increased tracer uptake and also shows small additional lesions. Reimbursement of high technology imaging cost has led to a growing acceptance of PET/CT in the clinical setting and its full integration into clinical practice.

This second edition has been updated to reflect advances that have occurred since the first edition. Two chapters related to radiation dosimetry in FDG PET and current status of PET/CT have been added to Part I of Basic Principles. The cardiology section in Part II of Clinical Applications has three new chapters dealing with coronary, myocardial, and atherosclerotic diseases. There are five additional new chapters discussing primary unknown tumor, infection and inflammation, PET/CT in radiation treatment, evidence-based PET/CT, and PET/MRI. These advances offer better diagnosis and staging of the diseases, prediction, and evaluation of therapeutic responses as well as risk assessment. Again, this textbook covers the full range of PET and PET/CT applications in oncology, neurology, and cardiology. These chapters were written by experienced experts in the field of nuclear medicine and PET in the United States, Korea, and Japan.

We hope that this new edition will continue to serve as a valuable reference source for both practitioners and trainees in the field of nuclear medicine, radiology, oncology, neurology, and cardiology in utilizing PET and PET/CT in their clinical practice as well as understanding their basic principles.

--E. Edmund Kim, MD

Preface to the 1st Edition

Positron emission tomography (PET) has been around long enough that it is hard to think of it as being anything special. It has been a valuable research tool in academic institutions since the 1970s, but its move into clinical practice in community hospitals has just begun.

Those who are now working with PET, or have made the decision to do so, understand just how different a perspective on disease this modality provides. For most patients in whom it is indicated, PET provides earlier and more sensitive detection. It is special, but not in ways that are immediately evident. It requires a shift in the diagnostic paradigm and adjustments in patient management to capture the advantages of early diagnosis.

Questions remain on how and when payment will be made for PET studies, but as with so much else in medicine, once patients and referring physicians know what PET can do for them, it will not be denied. Given time, it will eventually be documented that PET saves money overall by eliminating unnecessary and futile interventions in patients with advanced disease. That's the power of imaging the body's biochemistry.

The momentum toward the use of PET is expected to grow with the advent of molecular imaging. The sequencing of the genome and proteomes is establishing the fundamental molecular basis of how cells function. Molecules can now be designed to stop the disease or to prevent it from occurring. Imaging of gene expression could eventually provide the basis for developing therapeutic strategies individualized to a patient's genetic characteristics. Biology and genetics have been merged with medicine to produce the new field of molecular medicine which created the need for an imaging technology that looks at the biology of a disease. As drug company research and molecular imaging converge, imaging probes will be used to select patients for treatment with specific drugs.

The main impact of PET on community practice now, and likely for several years to come, is on oncology. Whole-body PET in cancer patients enables clinicians to identify malignant diseases in their early stages, differentiate benign from malignant tumors, examine the entire body for metastases, and determine the effectiveness of cancer therapeutics.

It has been predicted that PET would undergo spectacular growth in the twenty-first century as molecular medicine becomes central to the analysis of disease. The burgeoning world of PET is reflected in recent scientific meetings including those of the Radiological Society of North America (RSNA) and the Society of Nuclear Medicine (SNM).

This book provides comprehensive information on the basic principles and clinical applications of PET. Emphasis is placed on the familiarization of normal distribution, artifacts, and pitfalls of common agents such as fluorodeoxyglucose (FDG) in conjunction with computed tomography (CT), magnetic resonance imaging (MRI), or ultrasound to establish the clinical effectiveness of PET. Practical understanding of updated PET scanners, cyclotron, image process, and quantification is also stressed. This book is therefore divided into two parts: the first part discusses the basic principles of PET, such as instrumentation, image process, fusion, radiopharmaceuticals, radiosynthesis, safety, and economics. The second part discusses the clinical applications of the technique in neurology, cardiology, infection, and oncology.

We hope this book meets the growing needs of diagnostic radiologists, nuclear physicians, and clinicians for understanding the basic principles and clinical applications of PET.

Acknowledgments

I am very appreciative and indebted to all of the contributors for their good work, and also to Mr. Andrew Moyer at Springer in New York for his support and patience during the creation of this book.

E. Edmund Kim, MD
The University of Texas MD Anderson Cancer Center
Houston, TX, USA

Contents

Contributors

Ali Azhadarinia, Ph.D. Houston, TX, USA

Hossain Baghaei, Ph.D. Department of Experimental Diagnostic Imaging, The University of Texas MD Anderson Cancer Center, Houston, TX, USA

Gi-Jeong Cheon, M.D. Molecular Imaging Research Center, Korea Institute of Radiological and Medical Sciences (KIRAMS), Department of Nuclear Medicine, Korea Cancer Center Hospital, Nowon-gu, Seoul, South Korea

Chang Woon Choi, M.D., Ph.D. Research Institute of Radiological & Medical Sciences, Korea Institute of Radiological and Medical Sciences, Seoul, South Korea

Joon Young Choi, M.D., Ph.D. Department of Nuclear Medicine, Samsung Medical Center, Sungkyunkwan University Medical School, Gangnam-gu, Seoul, South Korea

June-Key Chung, M.D., Ph.D. Department of Nuclear Medicine, Seoul National University College of Medicine, Seoul, South Korea

Xiaoyi Duan, M.D. Department of Nuclear Medicine, First Affiliated Hospital, Xian Jiaotong University, College of Medicine, Shaanxi, China

Tetsuya Higuchi, M.D., Ph.D. Department of Nuclear Medicine and Diagnostic Radiology, Gumma University School of Medicine, Maebashi, Japan

Tomio Inoue, M.D., Ph.D. Department of Radiology, Yokohama City University Graduate School of Medicine, Yokohama, Japan

Keon W. Kang, M.D., Ph.D. Department of Nuclear Medicine, Seoul National University College of Medicine, Seoul, South Korea

Won Jun Kang, M.D., Ph.D. Division of Nuclear Medicine, Department of Nuclear Medicine, Yonsei University, Severance Hospital, Seodaemun-gu, Seoul, South Korea

Masashi Kawaguchi Department of Radiology, Yokohama City University Graduate School of Medicine, Yokohama, Japan

Byung-Tae Kim, M.D., Ph.D. Department of Nuclear Medicine, Sungkyunkwan University, School of Medicine Samsung Medical Center, Seoul, South Korea

E. Edmund Kim, M.D., M.S. Departments of Nuclear Medicine and Diagnostic Radiology, The University of Texas MD Anderson Cancer Center and Medical School, Houston, TX, USA

Graduate School of Convergence Science and Technology, Seoul National University, Seoul, South Korea

Sang Eun Kim, M.D., Ph.D. Department of Nuclear Medicine, Seoul National University Bundang Hospital, Seongnam, South Korea

Seok-Ki Kim, M.D. Department of Nuclear Medicine, National Cancer Center, Gyeonggi-do, South Korea

Sung-Eun Kim, M.D., Ph.D. Department of Nuclear Medicine, Korea University College of Medicine, Guro Hospital, Seoul, South Korea

Yu-Kyeong Kim, M.D., Ph.D. Department of Nuclear Medicine, Seoul National University, Bundang Hospital, Gyeonggi-Do, South Korea

Dong Soo Lee, M.D., Ph.D. Department of Nuclear Medicine, Seoul National University College of Medicine, Seoul, South Korea

WCU Department of Molecular Medicine and Biopharmaceutical Sciences, Seoul National University, Seoul, South Korea

Ho-Young Lee, M.D. Department of Nuclear Medicine, Seoul Metropolitan Government-Seoul National University Hospital, Boramae Medical Center, Seoul, South Korea

Jae Sung Lee, Ph.D. Department of Nuclear Medicine, Seoul National University Hospital, Seoul, South Korea

Jong Jin Lee, M.D. Department of Nuclear Medicine, University of Ulsan College of Medicine, Asan Medical Center, Seoul, South Korea

Kyung-Han Lee, M.D., Ph.D. Department of Nuclear Medicine, Samsung Medical Center, Sungkyunkwan University, School of Medicine, Seoul, South Korea

Myung-Chul Lee, M.D., Ph.D. Department of Nuclear Medicine, Gachon University School of Medicine, Incheon, South Korea

Won Woo Lee, M.D. Department of Nuclear Medicine, Seoul National University College of Medicine, Bundang Hospital, Gyeonggi-Do, South Korea

Carlos Gonzàlez Lepera, Ph.D. Department of Experimental Diagnostic Imaging, The University of Texas MD Anderson Cancer Center, Houston, TX, USA

Hongdi Li, Ph.D. Department of Experimental Diagnostic Imaging, The University of Texas MD Anderson Cancer Center, Houston, TX, USA

Sang-Moo Lim, M.D., Ph.D. Department of Nuclear Medicine, Korea Institute of Radiological and Medical Sciences, Seoul, South Korea

Osama Mawlawi, Ph.D. Department of Imaging Physics, The University of Texas MD Anderson Cancer Center, Houston, TX, USA

So Won Oh, M.D. Department of Nuclear Medicine, Seoul Metropolitan Government-Seoul National University Hospital, Boramae Medical Center, Seoul, South Korea

Hidehiko Okazawa, M.D., Ph.D. Division of Biomedical Imaging, The Faculty of Medical Sciences, University of Fukui, Fukui, Japan

Noboru Oriuchi, M.D., Ph.D. Department of Nuclear Medicine and Diagnostic Radiology, Gumma University School of Medicine, Maebashi, Japan

Jin-Chul Paeng, M.D., Ph.D. Department of Nuclear Medicine, Seoul National University Hospital, Seoul, South Korea

Eunkyung (Angela) Park, M.D., Ph.D. Department of Nuclear Medicine, State University of New York at Buffalo, Buffalo, NY, USA

Yale PET Center, Department of Diagnostic Radiology, Yale University School of Medicine, New Haven, CT, USA

Hirofumi Shibata Department of Radiology, Yokohama City University School of Medicine, Yokohama, Japan

I. Hong Shih Department of Experimental Diagnostic Imaging, The University of Texas MD Anderson Cancer Center, Houston, TX, USA

Yoo Sung Song, M.D. Department of Nuclear Medicine, Seoul National University Hospital, Seoul, South Korea

Nobukazu Takahashi, M.D., Ph.D. Department of Radiology, Yokohama City University Graduate School of Medicine, Yokohama, Japan

Ukihide Tateishi, M.D., Ph.D. Department of Radiology, Yokohama City University School of Medicine, Yokohama, Japan

Jorge Uribe, Ph.D. Department of Experimental Diagnostic Imaging, The University of Texas MD Anderson Cancer Center, Houston, TX, USA

Richard Wendt III, Ph.D. Department of Imaging Physics, The University of Texas MD Anderson Cancer Center, Houston, TX, USA

Franklin C.L. Wong, M.D., Ph.D., J.D. Departments of Nuclear Medicine and Neurooncology, The University of Texas MD Anderson Cancer Center, Houston, TX, USA

Wai-Hoi Wong, Ph.D. Department of Experimental Diagnostic Imaging, The University of Texas MD Anderson Cancer Center, Houston, TX, USA

Wai-Hoi Gary Wong, Ph.D. Department of Experimental Diagnostic Imaging, The University of Texas MD Anderson Cancer Center, Houston, TX, USA

David J. Yang, Ph.D. Department of Experimental Diagnostic Imaging, The University of Texas MD Anderson Cancer Center, Houston, TX, USA

Masashi Yukihiro, M.D., Ph.D. Department of Radiology, School of Medicine, Gunma University, Ihara Shizouka, Japan

Part I
Basic Principles

Principles of Positron Emission Tomography Imaging

1

Hossain Baghaei, Wai-Hoi (Gary) Wong, and Hongdi Li

Positron emission tomography (PET) is a noninvasive medical imaging technology that can generate high-resolution images of human and animal physiological functions. It is used for a variety of clinical applications in oncology, neurology, and cardiology, but the principal clinical application of PET is in oncology, where it is used to locate malignant tumors. It can be used not only to detect disease, but also to aid in planning its treatment and monitoring the effectiveness of the treatment. The PET camera is able to detect therapeutic changes earlier than anatomic imaging modalities because the structure being studied must significantly change in size and shape before it is detectable by anatomic imaging devices.

The PET camera measures the distribution of positron-emitting radionuclides (tracers) within an object. Positron-emitting radionuclides are used for imaging because of their unique tomographic capability and the availability of a group of metabolically important radionuclides. The unique tomographic capability comes from the simultaneous emission of two nearly back-to-back 511 keV gamma rays when a positron annihilates with an electron, and from the ability to provide accurate quantitating of tracer uptakes with its attenuation–correction capability. The medical importance of PET imaging derives from the availability of many useful positron-emitting tracers such as isotopes of carbon (^{11}C), nitrogen (^{13}N), and oxygen (^{15}O) which are basic elements of all living organisms and their physiologic processes. Hence, more tissue- and chemistry-specific tracers can be synthesized and injected into humans or animals for studying the physiologic functions of normal or pathologic tissues in vivo. Another important positron-emitting isotope, fluorine (^{18}F), is widely used to make a glucose analog ^{18}F-fluorodeoxyglucose (FDG), which follows the glucose pathway in its transport from plasma to tissue cells. However, unlike glucose, FDG remains trapped in the cell without undergoing further metabolism, which can be used for imaging purposes.

Imaging modalities are commonly categorized as functional or anatomical devices. These two different modalities provide complementary data that can be integrated for the purpose of diagnosis and for planning, performing, and evaluating the effectiveness of therapy. Indeed, the interpretation of nuclear medicine functional images is improved when they are coregistered with anatomical images. For this purpose, the PET camera has been combined with anatomic x-ray computed tomography (CT) to provide CT transmission scans for attenuation correction and for the coregistration of PET and CT data to facilitate the localization of tumors. In recent years, combined PET/CT scanners have been widely

H. Baghaei, Ph.D. (✉) • W.-H.(G). Wong, Ph.D.
H. Li, Ph.D.
Department of Experimental Diagnostic Imaging, The University of Texas MD Anderson Cancer Center, Houston, TX 77030, USA
e-mail: hbaghaei@mdanderson.org; gwong@mdanderson.org; hli@mdanderson.org

E.E. Kim et al. (eds.), *Clinical PET and PET/CT: Principles and Applications*,
DOI 10.1007/978-1-4419-0802-5_1, © Springer Science+Business Media New York 2013

used in both research and clinical applications. Also recently, there have been some efforts to combine PET cameras with magnetic resonance imaging (MRI) scanners. A combined PET/MRI system has several advantages over PET/CT: improved soft-tissue contrast, the possibility of performing truly simultaneous instead of sequential acquisitions, and significant decrease in radiation exposure. However, PET/MRI also has some drawbacks, including longer imaging times, higher costs, larger physical gantry size, gradient coil noise, and attenuation correction of whole-body PET data is expected to be a challenge.

Basic Physics of PET

The atomic nucleus is made up of nucleons: protons and neutrons. The proton has a positive electric charge, and the neutron has no net electric charge. Inside the nucleus, the protons and neutrons are mainly subject to two types of forces: the short-range strong attractive nuclear force that acts between all nucleons to hold them together, and the repulsive electric force that acts between the charged protons. Unstable proton-rich nuclei may transform to a more stable state by reducing their excess positive electric charge. One of the allowed decay processes for a proton-rich nucleus is to have a proton decay into a neutron, a neutrino, and a positively charged particle called positron. Because the mass of a proton is less than that of a neutron, this decay process can take place only inside the nucleus. The neutrino is a particle with no mass and no electric charge that leaves the surrounding tissue without any interaction. The positron (β+) is the antiparticle of the electron (β−) and has the same mass as an electron but with an opposite charge. A proton-rich isotope can be made in an accelerator (e.g., cyclotron) which generates a beam of high energy protons or deuterons to penetrate the target nuclei and implant the target nuclei with more protons [1].

The kinetic energy released in the nucleus decay process is shared between the positron and the neutrino, therefore, the actual energies of the emitted positrons are distributed in a continuous spectrum from almost zero to the full decay energy of the isotope. Table 1.1 shows the average kinetic energy of the emitted positrons for several commonly used radionuclides [2–4]. After a positron is produced, it travels a very short distance (0.2–2 mm for most commonly used tracers) until it loses almost all of its kinetic energy through scattering in the surrounding tissue, and then it combines with an electron in an annihilation process. In this process, both the positron and electron are annihilated and their mass is converted to energy ($E=mc^2$) in the form of a pair of photons. Following the basic laws of physics, the conservation of energy and linear momentum, each gamma ray (photon) has energy of 511 keV, the energy equivalent to the mass of an electron or a positron. The two generated photons are emitted almost back-to-back (180 ± 0.6°), so the net momentum of two gamma rays going in opposite directions is zero, as shown in Fig. 1.1. It is this back-to-back emission of the gamma pair that provides the special tomographic and quantitative imaging properties of positron imaging. The annihilation radiations are detected externally and are used to determine both the quantity and the location of the positron emitter. In addition, PET scanners exploit the back-to-back emission property to "electronically collimate" the photon pairs and determine the path along which the annihilation occurred. Because no physical collimator is required for event localization, the PET camera has a 50–100 times higher sensitivity advantage over single-photon imaging cameras. The lack of a collimator also contributes to higher image resolution.

The emitted positrons travel a short distance before they annihilate and generate the gamma-ray pairs, implying that the site of positron emission

Table 1.1 Physical properties of some common positron-emitting isotopes

Positron isotopes	^{11}C	^{13}N	^{15}O	^{18}F	$^{68}Ga^a$
Half-life (min)	20.4	9.96	2.07	109.7	68.3
Average positron energy (MeV)	0.3	0.4	0.6	0.2	0.7
Average positioning error (mm)	0.28	–	–	0.22	1.35

[a] ^{68}Ga is generated from a $^{68}Ga/^{68}Ge$ generator (the parent ^{68}Ge has a half-life of 275 days)

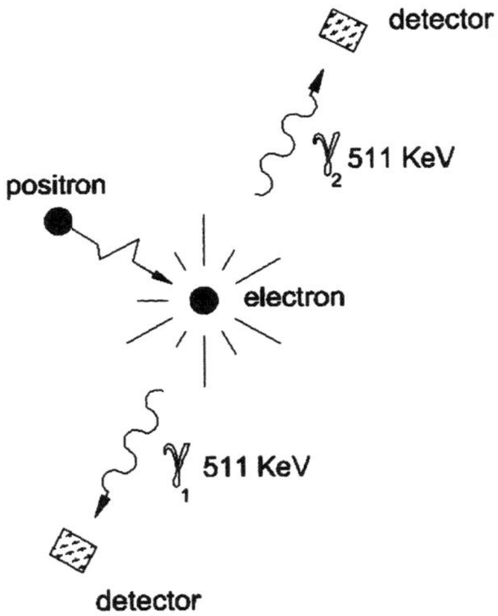

Fig. 1.1 Schematic of positron emission and annihilation with an electron in tissue to generate two gamma rays traveling in opposite direction (180°) which are detected in coincidence by two external scintillation detectors

(the site of the positron-labeled molecule) and the site of generation of two gammas, which are detected by the PET camera, are slightly different. The distance that a positron travels before annihilation, called the "positron range", depends on its initial kinetic energy. The positron range and photon noncolinearity (the fact that the two gamma rays are not exactly back-to-back) cause an uncertainty in positioning the event, and contributes to the fundamental resolution limit of PET imaging (Table 1.1). However, in a conventional PET camera (used for clinical scanning using FDG) the main spatial resolution limitation to PET imaging comes from the size of the individual small crystals used for detection.

Not all the emitted photons in the object (body) reach the surrounding detector system. These photons can either interact with the body tissue or pass through it without interaction. The interactions of photons with the body occur mainly in the form of photoelectric interaction or Compton scattering. The photons involved in photoelectric interaction are completely absorbed and therefore do not reach the detectors. The dominant form of interaction for photons at 511 keV in tissue is Compton scattering, which is caused by the collision of a photon with a loosely bound electron in an outer shell of an atom. When a photon interacts with an electron, it loses some energy and its path is deflected, thereby reducing the number of photons that would otherwise reach the detectors. The loss in photon flux resulting from interactions in a body (or any object) is called attenuation. In PET systems, the probability that the two photons generated in one event (a positron annihilation) "survive" the attenuation in the body is independent of the position of the annihilations along the line joining the two detectors. It is therefore possible to correct for the attenuation effect by performing a transmission scan using an external source.

Coincidence Detection

The PET camera takes advantage of the fact that the two photons generated from the positron annihilation are created simultaneously, and therefore they reject all events that do not satisfy the time–coincidence condition. Two photons are considered to be in coincidence if they are detected within a specific time interval known as the coincidence window, which typically is 6–20 ns. If a detected gamma ray is not accompanied by a second gamma ray within this timing window, the event is discarded. Not every detected coincidence gamma pair necessarily originated from the same annihilation event. Events that are found in coincidence are classified as true coincidences, random coincidences, or scatter coincidences. True events are coincidence events which are originated from the same positron annihilation (Fig. 1.2, event 1). Random (or accidental) events are coincidence events in which two detected photons are originated from two different annihilation events but are found accidentally in coincidence because of the finite size of the coincidence window (Fig. 1.2, event 2). Scatter events are coincidence events that are originated from a single annihilation event, but one or both of the photons are scattered in the object (Fig. 1.2, event 3). The scatter process changes the direction and energy of the photon such that the position information on the event is lost. For many annihilation events, only one of the two photons will be detected, and these events are called

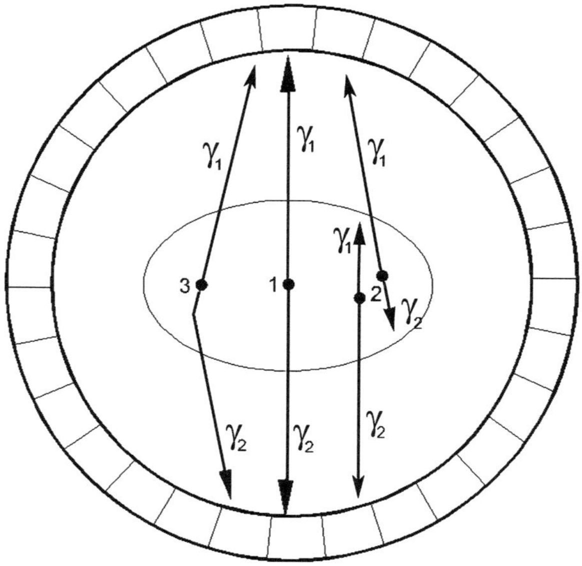

Fig. 1.2 Coincidence events: (1) a true coincidence event, (2) a random coincidence event, and (3) a scatter coincidence event

"singles". There is no way for the detector to determine whether a particular coincidence event is a true, random, or scatter event. The good events are the true events; the other events (random and scatter) should be measured or estimated and removed from the total coincidence events.

In PET measurements, random and scatter events are the sources of background noise. They appear as a general blurring background in the reconstructed image of the tracer distribution, reducing the image quality. The magnitudes of the random and scatter coincidence events depend on the distribution of the tracer activity (inside and outside the field of view [FOV]), the composition of the object under study, and the design of the PET scanner. While true and scatter rates are linearly proportional to the activity concentration, the random rate is proportional to the square of the activity concentration. Thus, the random events could constitute a large fraction of events, especially at high activity levels, and it is important to minimize them. Several techniques are used to reduce the number of random events, including adding lead-tungsten septa between detector rings in multi-ring PET systems and adding endplate shielding to reduce the contribution of activity outside the FOV. In addition, because the random rate is linearly proportional to the coincidence window, minimizing the coincidence window is also important in reducing the number of random events. The random events contribution can be measured directly by a second delayed coincidence window, or it can be estimated from the single rates. Scatter events can also constitute a significant fraction of the events detected by the scanner. However, because scattered photons lose some of their energy, the energy discrimination (energy threshold) can be used to reject a portion of the scatter events. For dedicated PET cameras operating in two-dimensional (2D) mode (with septa between detectors rings), scatter events typically constitute 10–20% of the total counts. In three-dimensional (3D) mode (no septa), scatter events typically constitute 30–60% of the total counts. Scatter events can result in a loss of resolution and an apparent migration of activity from hot to cold regions in images. Scatter correction methods generally fall into two groups: those that estimate the contribution of scatter events by measuring coincidences in one or more energy windows, in addition to the standard photo peak window, and those that model it using complex algorithms and Monte Carlo simulations [5–7]. Scatter correction (in addition to corrections such as attenuation and detector normalization) must be applied when quantitative imaging is required.

Radionuclides

A large number of radionuclides are used in PET imaging. Some of these PET tracer molecules contain isotopes of carbon (^{11}C), nitrogen (^{13}N), and oxygen (^{15}O) that can be used as biologically relevant substances for the human body, while other atoms can be substituted for use as analogs. For example, fluorine (^{18}F) can be substituted for hydrogen in the glucose analog deoxyglucose to form FDG. They usually have very short half-lives ranging from a few minutes to a few hours. The half-lives of the positron isotopes most often used in medical imaging are listed in Table 1.1 [2–4].

Because of the very short half-lives of ^{11}C, ^{13}N, and ^{15}O, they can be used only when a cyclotron is located near the imaging device. In addition, the fast decay of these radionuclides makes them less suitable for low count rate scans. In contrast, ^{18}F has a half-life of about 2 h and can be distributed from a central site with a cyclotron. Although many types of positron-emitting radionuclides have been used to label hundreds of molecules to study basic physiology and disease processes, FDG is used in most clinical applications because every cell uses glucose. FDG, being an analog of glucose, follows the pathway of glucose as it is transported from blood to tissue cells. However, unlike glucose, FDG, which is not a significant substrate for further metabolism, is trapped in cells, and is released slowly.

After the intravenous injection of FDG, patients are usually kept at rest for about 40–60 min to allow for organ uptake of FDG. In the meantime, a large fraction of the free FDG in plasma is cleared because of tissue uptake and because of clearance through the kidneys to the bladder. When FDG is injected into a human, it is distributed to all tissues, but only those tissues metabolizing glucose will take up the FDG. Thus, any metabolically active muscles will show increased uptake relative to the rest of the body. Many malignant tumors also accumulate FDG because of their glycolysis and proliferation rate. Benign tumors usually take up less FDG, and can potentially be distinguished from malignant tumors. Therefore, coincidence detection can also be used to assess the presence of malignancy in patients with known or suspected metastatic disease. In addition, for noninvasive evaluation of cardiac viability and the detection of lesions, FDG imaging with dedicated whole-body PET is a useful technique.

Because the most useful positron isotopes for biologic studies are ^{11}C, ^{13}N, ^{15}O, and ^{18}F, which have only six to nine protons in the nucleus, the electrostatic repulsive force encountered by the accelerated particles (protons/deuterons) on their way to penetrate the nucleus to initiate a nuclear reaction is small. Hence, a small cyclotron that can accelerate protons to the 10–17-MeV range is sufficient to overcome the nuclear electrostatic repulsion force and produce the nuclear reactions for biomedical positron imaging [1]. In recent years, small cyclotrons and chemical synthesis devices have been integrated into one unit to facilitate the synthesis of radiopharmaceuticals for clinical use. Small linear accelerators are also being developed to provide radionuclides.

Image Reconstruction

Tomographic images of the distribution of the positron-emitting radionuclides within the patient are reconstructed based on the assumptions that the annihilation photons are emitted back-to-back (180°), and that the line along which the two photons are detected (i.e., the line that joins the two detectors, also called "line of response") contains the location of the tracer molecule from where the positron originated. Therefore, the sum of all photon pairs emitted along a given direction represents the line integral of positron-emitting activity located on that line (or tube). The set of line integrals having the same angular direction through the tracer distribution comprises a parallel projection of the distribution at that angle. Even though these assumptions are only approximately valid and, therefore, limit the ultimate spatial resolution that can be achieved, for the existing tomographic systems, the limitation in spatial resolution is determined by the detector crystal sizes.

The above assumptions can be applied only to true coincidence events. Therefore, the measured projection data must be corrected for the contribution of random and scatter events. In addition, the effects of attenuation (the fact that some of the photons are absorbed or scattered out of the FOV), detector efficiency, detector geometry, and system dead time must be considered.

From a complete set of line integrals measured at different angular views around the object, the images of positron-emitter distribution, within a slice or volume, can be reconstructed using various techniques. The reconstruction technique most commonly used in PET is the filtered back projection method. If a point in space has a concentration of positron tracer, the emission of coincidence pairs will be uniformly distributed over all angles because the emissions are random, with no preferential direction. If the uniformly distributed detection lines are drawn, a blurred image of the point will emerge. In other words, the parallel projections at each angle are projected back into the image grid, where they are superimposed to form an approximation image of the original object. To obtain a sharper image of the point, the spatial distribution of the coincidence data is filtered numerically before the back projection process. This filtered back projection image reconstruction method is also used in x-ray CT and single photon emission computed tomography (SPECT) cameras [8–11]. Because the object to be imaged can be considered a collection of point sources with different activity levels, an image of the subject can be obtained with coincidence detection data and the filtered back projection reconstruction algorithm. The derivation of filtered back projection is based on noise-free ideal projection data. However, the acquired projection data are noisy, and the filtered back projection technique amplifies this statistical noise. Windowing or reducing the cutoff frequency of the filter could reduce the amount of noise, but it also results in a loss of spatial resolution [12–15]. The most commonly used low-pass windows are the Hann, Hamming, and Butterworth window functions [16, 17].

Conventional multi-ring PET cameras can operate in 2D mode or 3D mode. In 2D mode, tungsten-lead septa separating the detector rings, to reduce single, random, and scatter events. For 2D data, 2D reconstruction algorithms are used, which are fast. Most PET cameras can also operate in 3D mode by removing the septa, and some of the modern cameras do not have septa at all and operate only in 3D mode. A widely used 3D filtered back projection reconstruction algorithm in volume PET imaging is the 3D reprojection (3DRP) algorithm, which is based on an extension of the standard 2D filtered back projection into three dimensions [18]. The 3DRP algorithm incorporates a preliminary step in which projections are partially measured in 3D data acquisition are completed by forward projection of an initial low-statistics image obtained from the completely measured (direct) projections because of the truncated cylindrical geometry of the scanner. The forward-projected sinograms are less noisy than their measured counterparts and show some loss in spatial resolution [19]. Differences between measured sinograms and forward-projected sinograms have a differential effect on the final 3D reconstructed images, because more forward-projected data are proportionally used in the outer planes.

The 3D PET acquisition in comparison with 2D PET acquisition improves the sensitivity of the system and has the potential to reduce the data acquisition time compared with 2D PET. However, because the increase in sensitivity in 3D mode comes at the cost of an increase in random and scatter events, it does not necessarily translate into better image quality, especially for whole-body scans. It has been found that 3D acquisition could have advantages in lesion detection and noise characteristics in imaging of the brain, small patients, and animals, especially at low activity levels [20–23].

Because of large number of lines of response, the 3D image reconstruction is time consuming and much slower than 2D image reconstruction. As an alternative to the full 3D image reconstruction, the 3D projection data can be rebinned (sorted) into a stack of ordinary 2D sinogram data by making certain approximations and then using a 2D reconstruction algorithm; however, rebinning could result in loss of spatial resolution and degrade the image quality. The most widely used rebinning algorithms are the single-slice rebinning (SSRB), multi-slice rebinning (MSRB), and the Fourier rebinning (FORE) algorithms [24–26]. The SSRB algorithm assigns an oblique line of response to the mid-transaxial slice between the two detectors. This is a reasonable approximation when the tracer distribution is concentrated close to the axis of the scanner. In the MSRB method, an oblique line of response contributes to all transaxial slices that it intercepts within the limit of the transverse FOV. In the FORE algorithm, the 2D Fourier transform of each oblique sinogram is taken to produce a set of direct- and cross-plane data. The FORE method is still an approximation; however, it is more accurate than the other two rebinning methods mentioned.

The activity distribution images can be reconstructed from projection data with either analytic techniques (e.g., the 3DRP algorithm) or iterative algorithms. Iterative algorithms progressively improve the estimate of the distribution (image), which, in principle, converges toward a solution that maximizes an objective function. The iterative algorithms can model noise in emission data as well as other physical processes such as attenuation correction, anatomic information, and detector response function and can incorporate them into the reconstruction process to improve image quality. These algorithms are generally more time consuming than filtered back projection methods. The most widely used iterative algorithm is the maximum-likelihood expectation maximization (MLEM) algorithm and its accelerated variant, the ordered subsets expectation maximization (OSEM) method [27, 28]. Iterative reconstruction methods improve the quality of the image, especially by incorporating data corrections and detector spatial response into the reconstruction process [29]. However, MLEM and OSEM have some drawbacks, including a tendency to develop noise artifacts and increasing the number of iterations. To control noise artifacts and drive the image estimate sequence toward a smoother convergence, several methods have been used to regularize the image updating mechanism, including the addition of a smoothing step between iterations, postfiltering, and Bayesian methods [30, 31].

Quality Control and Performance Measurements

Quality Control and Normalization

In PET imaging, standard algorithms for reconstruction of images, such as filtered back projection, require that all lines of response (LORs) have the same sensitivity. However, there are several factors that cause nonuniformity of the response of the detectors. The efficiencies of coincidence detector pairs are inherently nonuniform as a result of the random and systematic variations in efficiencies of individual crystals and the inevitable drift in photomultiplier gains over time. In addition, because of the circular design of PET systems, there are geometric factors that affect the efficiencies of the LORs from the center to the edge of the field of view. Because sinograms are binned as parallel beam, the distance between detector pairs decreases with increasing distance from the center of the field of view, and the exposed face of the crystal decreases. In addition, the angle of incidence of the gamma ray changes. The ability of a scintillation crystal to detect a gamma ray depends not only on the energy of the gamma ray and the size and shape of the crystal, but also on the angle at which the gamma ray hits it.

For multi-ring PET cameras with tens of thousands of crystals, hundreds of photomultipliers (PMTs), and complicated electronics, the quality control measurements to check all detector components at the time of installation and thereafter at regular intervals are critical to ensure that the camera is operating within specifications and to detect changes over time before they become a serious problem. For example, for a scanner using block detectors, where generally a single PMT reads many crystals, the loss of one PMT can disable a large part of the system; even a small gain shift can cause mispositioning of data. Therefore, it is important to develop reproducible quality control procedures to detect problems at an early stage before they affect the image quality, and schedule adjustments or replacement. The quality control procedures should at least check: (1) the shift in PMTs amplification gains and electronics, (2) the stability of the system in terms of the efficiencies of the detectors, and (3) spatial resolution throughout the FOV [32–34]. Currently, performing all of these quality control tests on a daily basis is not practical because of the long data acquisition time. However, performing some of these tests daily, especially the recalibration of PMT gains and checking electronics, is possible with some PET cameras [35, 36].

The stability of the system in terms of detector efficiencies are generally checked by performing a "blank" scan in which a uniform cylindrical phantom, a uniform planar phantom, or attenuation-correction rotating rods are used to illuminate each LOR by the same activity level [32, 34]. The planar source is regarded as the most favorable geometry due to a low level of scattered photons, but it is impractical to implement on a routine basis because it requires measurements at several source positions (e.g., six), extending the data acquisition time. A comparison study has shown that the uniformity obtained from cylinder-derived detector efficiencies is nearly identical to that obtained from planar source-derived efficiencies [37]. In PET imaging, the detection of positron annihilations requires that two gamma rays be detected simultaneously. The ability of a detector pair to detect annihilation on its LOR is proportional to the product of the average detection efficiencies of the individual detectors and a geometric factor. Many PET systems allow angular and axial compression of the data to minimize storage requirements and reconstruction time; in addition, some cameras rotate during data acquisition [38–40]. These features complicate normalization of the detector responses because an individual bin in a sinogram may be the combination of multiple detector pairs. The calibration of LORs referred to as normalization, is important for image reconstruction. The correction factor for each LOR is referred to as the normalization coefficient. After calibration, the individual normalized count rate of all detector pairs should be the same, within the statistical uncertainty, for a uniform source activity.

For modern PET cameras, the number of individual LORs is very high, and acquiring sufficient counts for reasonable statistical accuracy is very time consuming and is not suitable for a daily control check. Usually, normalization coefficients for PET scanners are calculated using a component-based variance reduction method [41, 42]. In this model, normalization coefficients are expressed as the product of intrinsic crystal efficiencies and some geometric factors. These coefficients are not all independent and if the geometric factors are accurately known, the number of unknowns is reduced from the number of LORs to the number of crystals [33, 42]. Because the geometry of the scanner is unlikely to change significantly after initial installation, the geometric correction factors may be calculated or measured using high statistics acquisition that only needed to be acquired occasionally. In recent years, new techniques have been introduced to calculate the crystal efficiency correction factors form a relatively short scan (less than 20 min) of a uniform phantom or even the emission data themselves [43, 44].

Performance Measurements

PET camera performance is generally evaluated with the standard tests established by the National Electrical Manufacturers Association (NEMA) [45–48]. The first PET performance tests were introduced in 1994 and referred to as NEMA NU 2–1994 [45, 46]. In 2001, these tests were updated and the new standard known as NEMA NU 2–2001 [47, 48]. The most significant change in the NU 2–2001 standard, compared with the NU 2–1994 standard, is the replacement of a 19-cm long cylindrical phantom with a 70-cm long cylindrical phantom for some of the tests as discussed below. While the 19-cm long cylindrical phantom can still be used to test the performance of scanners used for brain imaging, the 70-cm long cylindrical phantom is more appropriate for testing cameras used for whole-body studies.

The performance tests are divided into two groups. The first group includes measurements of the basic intrinsic characteristics of the camera such as spatial resolution, sensitivity, scatter fraction, and count rate losses and random coincidences. In general, for a given activity concentration, achieving higher sensitivity and lower random and scattered events is more desirable. The second group includes measurements of the accuracy of corrections for physical effects such as uniformity correction, scatter correction, attenuation correction, and count rate linearity correction. In addition, NEMA NU 2–2001 standard included criteria for evaluating the overall image quality. Only the ^{18}F radioisotope is recommended for these tests.

The spatial resolution is a measure of the camera's ability to distinguish between two points of radioactivity in a reconstructed image, and it is characterized by the width of the image of a point source (point spread function). The width of the point spread function is reported as the full width at half maximum and full width at tenth maximum. It is recommended that a point source of ^{18}F, with dimensions of less than 1 mm in any direction be imaged in air, and resolution be reported for six different locations of the point source. To avoid high count rate problems (dead-time and pile-up effects), the data should be acquired at low count rates. It is also recommended that data be reconstructed with filtered back projection using a ramp filter, with a cutoff at the Nyquist frequency, and the image pixel size should be smaller than one third of the expected resolution.

The sensitivity of a PET scanner represents its ability to detect radiations from annihilation of positrons. In the NEMA NU 2–1994 standard, the sensitivity is suggested to be measured using a standard cylindrical phantom (20 cm diameter, 19 cm long) filled with uniform activity at low concentration, and the rate of coincidence events for a given activity concentration in that phantom be reported. In the more recent NEMA NU 2–2001 standard, it is suggested to use a 70-cm long plastic tube filled with a known amount of radioactivity, which is sufficiently low that counts losses, and random coincidences are negligible. The tubing is encased in metal sleeves of varying thickness and imaged twice: first with tube in the center of the transverse FOV, and then with tube offset radially 10 cm from the transverse FOV.

The intrinsic scatter fraction is a measure of the system sensitivity to scattered events. The scatter fraction is defined as the ratio of scattered events to total events, which are measured at a sufficiently low counting rate so that random coincidences, dead-time effects, and pileup are negligible. Therefore, the total events are the sum of unscattered events (true events) and scattered events. The suggested phantom, based on the NEMA NU 2–20001 standard, for this measurement is a 20-cm diameter solid polyethylene cylinder with an overall length of 70 cm. Activity is placed in a line source (2.3-mm inner diameter) that is threaded through a hole in the cylinder at a radius of 4.5 cm and parallel to the central axis. To measure the scatter fraction for the 3D data, it is suggested to first rebin the 3D data into 2D sinograms using the single-slice rebinning algorithm. The transaxial FOV used for calculation of scatter is limited to 24 cm (4 cm larger than the phantom diameter). The sinogram profile is used to calculate the number of scatter events within the FOV and the number of true coincidences within a 2-cm radius of the source. The scatter within the peak is estimated by assuming a constant background under the peak. The sinogram profile is analyzed as a function of the angle, and the results are averaged. The NEMA NU 2–2001 standard recommends that the scatter fraction for each slice and the average of the slice scatter fraction be reported.

Most PET scans are performed under conditions in which count rate losses, as a result of the dead time, and random coincidences are not negligible. Therefore, it is suggested that the system dead time and random coincidences for a wide range of activity levels be measured. Random coincidences can be determined by delayed coincidence technique or can be estimated from single rates. Dead time is determined from the measured true rate at a given activity level and from the true rate extrapolated from the low count rate data.

The counting rate performance is measured as a function of activity using the same 70-cm polyethylene cylinder and the line source used for the scatter fraction. For this procedure, the line source is filled with a sufficiently high initial activity that allows both the peak true rate and peak noise equivalent count (NEC) rate to be measured. Data are taken until the random coincidences and dead-time losses are negligible. The total counting rate within the 24-cm transverse FOV is determined as the activity decays. The background, resulting from random coincidences and scatter, is estimated and the true events rate is then determined by subtracting the background from the total rate. The total, true, random, scatter, and NEC rates are plotted against the effective activity concentration. From this plot, the peak true counting rate and peak NEC rate should be determined. The NEC rate, which defines an effective true count rate by accounting for additional noise from the random and scatter events, is defined as:

$$R_{NEC} = R_{trues}^2 / (R_{trues} + R_{scatter} + kR_{randoms})$$

where R_{trues} is the true event rate, $R_{scatter}$ is the scatter event rate, $R_{randoms}$ is the random event rate, and $k=2$ if the randoms are measured directly by delayed coincidence technique, and $k=1$ they are estimated (noise free).

The image quality test is designed to produce images simulating those obtained in a whole-body study with both hot and cold lesions. It is suggested that spheres of different diameters placed in a simulated body phantom with nonuniform attenuation be imaged. It is also recommended that activity should be present outside the scanner. To quantitate the image quality, it is suggested that regions of interest on the spheres and throughout the background be drawn and that the coefficient of variations of the means in the background be calculated, along with the contrast recovery coefficient for the hot spheres and cold spheres. The diameters of the region of interest should be equal to the physical inner diameters of the spheres. To assess the accuracy of the corrections for attenuation and scatter, it is suggested that the ratio of the average counts in a region of interest in the lung area and the average counts in the background be calculated.

The Positron Cameras

Any camera that can image a positron-emitting tracer can be called a positron camera. These cameras can range from the simple, less-expensive thallium-doped sodium iodide [NaI(Tl)] gamma cameras to multimillion dollar, multi-ring PET cameras. Positron cameras can be divided into eight groups: (1) NaI(Tl) gamma cameras or SPECT cameras with lead collimators; (2) dual-head rotating NaI(Tl) cameras with modified electronics for coincidence detection and with the lead collimator removed [49]; (3) dedicated NaI(Tl) PET cameras with the detection system in the form of a ring [50, 51]; (4) dedicated multi-ring PET cameras consisting of a large number of small detector elements made from high sensitivity scintillation materials such as bismuth germanate (BGO) [52–55], lutetium oxyorthosilicate (LSO) [56, 57], or lutetium-yttrium oxyorthosilicate (LYSO) [58]; (5) dedicated small animal PET cameras [59–61]; (6) hybrid systems such as SPECT/PET systems, SPECT/CT, PET/CT, and PET/MRI systems [62–64]; (7) PET cameras with time-of-flight (TOF) capability [65]; and (8) positron emission mammography (PEM) dedicated breast cameras [66–68]. Dedicated PET cameras can be further divided into two subgroups: cameras with full detection rings and cameras with partial detection rings. Three basic designs of PET cameras are shown in Fig. 1.3.

Traditionally, gamma cameras have been used only for single photon studies (both planar and tomographic acquisitions), and the imaging of 511-keV photons has been performed with dedicated PET scanners. Despite significant differences between these two modalities, several products have been introduced to fill the gaps between these imaging techniques, including dual-purpose SPECT/PET gamma cameras. The low sensitivity and limited counting rate capability of

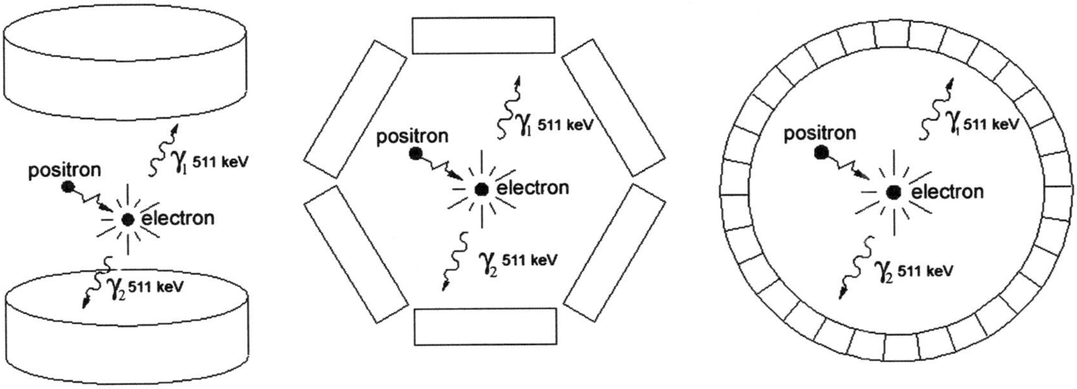

Fig. 1.3 Schematic of three different designs of a PET camera: a dual head single photon emission computed tomography with lead collimators removed and coincidence detection circuit added (*left*), a dedicated positron emission tomography (PET) camera using large NaI(Tl) detectors (*middle*), and a dedicated PET camera using small bismuth germanate detectors (*right*)

gamma camera PET systems are partially offset by the larger FOV. In addition, using thicker NaI(Tl) crystals and removing the collimators also improve the sensitivity of these devices.

NaI(Tl) Gamma Cameras with Lead Collimators

The NaI(Tl) gamma cameras with lead collimators are the least expensive devices for imaging positron-emitting tracer distribution. These cameras also have the lowest detection sensitivity for positron imaging. There are two reasons for their low sensitivity. First, the use of lead collimation to define the direction of the detected gamma ray is very inefficient because the collimator can absorb 95% or higher of the incoming gamma rays. Second, the thin NaI(Tl) detector is optimized for stopping the 140-keV gamma ray for technetium (^{99m}Tc) imaging, and so most of the higher-energy (511-keV) gamma rays from positron annihilation penetrate this thin detector without any interaction (about 70% escape fraction). Therefore, only a small percentage of the positron gamma rays that hit the gamma camera detector are detected. The low-detection efficiency implies that only very large lesions (3 cm) can be detected. This group of cameras may provide a way to take advantage of the more tumor-specific positron tracers, such as breast cancer applications, without incurring the expense of buying and operating a dedicated PET camera [69].

Coincidence Gamma Camera PET Systems

A gamma camera PET system is a modified dual-head rotating NaI(Tl) camera with coincidence electronics added and collimators removed [49]. With added coincidence detection capability, the direction of the two detected gamma rays is defined by two detected locations on opposite sides of the subject, and the inefficient lead collimators are no longer needed. Elimination of the lead collimator increases the detection sensitivity by 20 times or greater over the regular single head gamma cameras. However, the thin NaI(Tl) detector still has low sensitivity for detecting 511-keV gamma rays because the probability of photon interaction (photoelectric and Compton) is approximately 0.3. Therefore, the probability of detecting both photons of positron annihilation for coincidence detection would be approximately 0.09. When compared with a dedicated BGO PET camera, which uses detectors made of BGO scintillation material, the sensitivity of this modified SPECT camera is still 9–10 times lower for identical detection areas. However, the detection sensitivity of this class of camera is a substantial improvement (5–10 times) over dual-head cameras with lead collimators. Studies have shown that this type of camera can detect lesions as small as 1.5–2.0 cm [70, 71]. Hence, this camera type is a better choice than the lead collimator gamma camera for taking advantage of the more tumor-specific positron tracers with a relatively small additional investment.

The removal of the lead collimator, which improves the detection efficiency, leads to new a problem. The head of each gamma camera is basically one large detector, and when a gamma ray is detected, the whole camera head is dead until all the stimulated scintillation light caused by that gamma detection is emitted. If there is a second incoming gamma ray, there will be a pileup of signals in the large detector, resulting in combining the two signals to yield an erroneous energy and position. With the removal of the lead collimator, the flux of gamma rays incident onto the detector causes severe signal pileup in the NaI(Tl) detector, such that the tracer dose injected into the patient must be lowered by roughly 80% compared with the dose used with a dedicated BGO PET camera to minimize the signal pileup artifacts in the image. Hence, the quality of the image is further reduced by the smaller tracer dose in addition to the lower detection efficiency. However, this reduction in injected dose can be improved by some detector signal processing electronic technique such as the high-yield-pileup-event-recovery (HYPER). This technique could eliminate most of the pileup, and recovers the correct energy and position of pileup events, thereby allowing the count rate to be increased by 10 times for NaI(Tl) [72].

Another deficiency of this camera design is that the coincidence detection efficiency in the transaxial FOV is geometrically dependent; the region near the center of rotation has the highest efficiency, and the coincidence efficiency goes to zero at the edge of the camera. Therefore, it is important for this camera type to be larger than the patient FOV to yield usable efficiency at the edge of the field of study. Gamma cameras modified for coincidence PET imaging are no longer manufactured, although some may still be in clinical use.

Dedicated PET Camera with NaI(Tl) Detectors

The dedicated PET camera with a NaI(Tl) detector ring is similar to the dual-head NaI(Tl) gamma camera with coincidence detection electronics. It is a whole-body camera operating in 3D mode and has several planar or curved heads [73]. The heads are configured to form a fixed ring around the patient. Because the camera is designed to be a dedicated PET camera instead of also performing ^{99m}Tc imaging, the thickness of the NaI(Tl) detector is increased (e.g., from 1 cm to 1 in.) to enhance its detection sensitivity. This increased detector thickness contributes to almost fourfold increase in coincidence detection efficiency over a dual-head coincidence camera (with the same active detection area). Furthermore, with the detectors completely surrounding the patient, the detection efficiency is uniform in the transaxial FOV. However, because the detector design is basically that of a gamma camera, the signal pileup can still be a problem if the injected dose of radio tracer is not reduced. Even though these cameras generally use special hardware techniques (e.g., pulse clipping) to shorten signal collection time and to reduce the detector dead time, the injected dose is still needed to be reduced by 60–80% from that used with a dedicated PET using BGO scintillation detectors. The HYPER processing method can also be used in this type of NaI(Tl) PET camera to allow higher dose injection to improve their imaging performance. Although the intrinsic resolution of this camera (about 4.6 mm for curved and 4.9 mm for planar heads) can rival that of the more expensive BGO cameras, the more limited image counts collected causes the practical and clinical image resolution to be lower. Despite the lower production cost of

Table 1.2 Comparison of physical properties of some common scintillator crystals

Crystal	Density (g/cm^3)	Effective atomic number	Attenuation coefficient (cm^{-1})	Light output (NaI(Tl) = 100)	Decay time (ns)
BGO	7.13	75	0.96	15	300
GSO	6.71	59	0.67	41	65
LSO	7.40	65	0.87	75	40
NaI(Tl)	3.67	51	0.35	100	230

this type of dedicated PET cameras, they did not receive wide acceptance used and currently are not manufactured.

Dedicated PET Camera with BGO Detector Rings

The multi-ring PET cameras based on BGO crystals have higher sensitivity and higher spatial resolution than the three previously discussed cameras. These cameras are also the most expensive ($1–2 million). Unlike the three positron camera types discussed previously, which are based on gamma camera technology using a single, large NaI(Tl) detector, the BGO camera uses tens of thousands discrete BGO detectors [52–54]. The discrete BGO detectors are packed into many detector rings circumscribing the patient, eliminating the need to rotate the detection system. The elimination of camera rotation during imaging may be important for imaging tracers that change rapidly with time, such as ^{15}O and ^{13}N with short half-lives. For FDG imaging, camera rotation is not an issue.

The multiplicity of detectors in this kind of camera allows the cameras to operate at much higher count rates, which translates to a higher injected dose to provide a higher quality image. Furthermore, BGO crystals have about two times higher density and about 1.5 times higher atomic number than NaI(Tl) and also have substantially higher detection sensitivity for the higher energy gamma rays generated by positrons annihilation. Hence, the detected counts-per-unit injected dose is also higher with the dedicated PET/BGO than with the other three camera types using NaI(Tl) detectors, enabling this camera to provide further improvement in image quality. Currently, the highest intrinsic spatial resolution of whole-body clinical BGO PET cameras is about 4.5 mm, and for some research-oriented scanners, such as HOTPET [55] and the high-resolution research tomograph (HRRT) [56], it can be better than 3 mm. The practical image resolution could be lower depending on the number of counts collected. For FDG cancer imaging, the smallest detectable lesion size also depends on the ratio of tumor uptake to normal tissue uptake. With current whole-body clinical BGO PET cameras, 6–10 mm tumors are detectable.

Dedicated PET Camera with LSO/LYSO Detector Rings

In recent years, LSO crystals and LYSO crystals have been used extensively in multi-ring PET cameras [57, 58]. Both LSO and LYSO have excellent physical properties, and have high densities and atomic numbers that result in efficient detection of gamma rays. In addition, similar to BGO, they are rugged and nonhygroscopic, which make the detector fabrication less problematic. Table 1.2 compares some of the physical properties of LSO crystals with BGO and NaI(Tl) [74]. LSO and LYSO crystals have some advantages and disadvantages over the BGO crystals. BGO has a slightly higher linear attenuation coefficient and higher probability that the first gamma interaction within the crystal will be a photoelectric interaction, and it is also less expensive. LSO and LYSO have a shorter decay constant, which is good for coincidence timing and handling higher detection rates. In addition, higher light output of the crystals allows the use of smaller, and more, crystals per photomultiplier tube, thereby achieving better spatial resolution. LSO has a low level of natural radioactivity as a result of the presence of ^{176}Lu which generates some undesirable background. This background generates a relatively negligible coincidence background event rate; however, it can have a noticeable effect on the single rate that may be utilized in transmission measurement used for attenuation correction [75].

Dual-Modality PET/CT System

Imaging modalities used in medical imaging are generally differentiated as functional or anatomic devices. These two complementary modalities provide valuable information that can be used for early diagnosis, more accurate tumor detection and localization, and facilitate the planning, performance, and better assessment of patient responses to treatment such as radiation therapy and chemotherapy. In 2000, integrated PET/CT systems capable of providing both functional and anatomic information were introduced and almost all of the systems sold at the present time are PET/CT scanners.

Interpretation of nuclear medicine functional images is improved when they are co-registered with anatomic images, especially in the abdomen, because of the absence of identifiable anatomic structures in PET images. This is achieved either by visual comparison of the two separate datasets or, more effectively, by fusion of images. Until the introduction of combined PET/CT systems, the anatomic and functional images were previously acquired on different and separated scanners, and at different times, and then fused using software tools. However, such procedures were not widely used for studies outside of the brain because of the technical difficulties of implementation on a routine basis. The dual-modality PET/CT systems have overcome some of the difficulties associated with the software approaches by acquiring both anatomic and functional images in a single scanning session. In addition, CT images can provide attenuation correction information and anatomic information to the model-based scatter correction algorithms.

Even with combined PET/CT there are some motions that could affect the accuracy of co-registration of two sets of data. Some of these motions are patient breathing, cardiac motion, and patient movement between the PET and CT studies. Patient motion may be avoidable, but respiratory motion is not and may require some correction by, for example, respiratory gating of PET data [76]. The quality of images will be compromised if co-registration errors occur. Such errors could not only deteriorate the image quality but also lead to wrong anatomic positioning. In a study of patients with lung tumors using a combined PET/CT camera, a maximum 5–6-mm misalignment of the PET and CT images for tumors in the anterior region of the lungs was observed; however, such mismatch did not affect the diagnostic accuracy of the fused image [77]. In another study, it was found that the accuracy of PET/CT image co-registration for lung lesions is better in patients who underwent CT scanning during normal expiration than that in patients who performed shallow breathing during CT scanning, and it is better in the upper and central parts of the lung [78]. In another study of lesion mislocalization on PET/CT studies, it was found that when CT data of 300 patients that were scanned were used for both fusion and for attenuation correction, 2% (six patients) had lesion mislocalization, likely resulting from respiratory motion differences between PET and CT [79].

Time-of-Flight PET Camera

The concept of utilizing TOF information to further improve PET scanner performance is not new and was first proposed in the early stages of PET camera development [80–82]. The early TOF PET cameras were developed in the 1980s using fast barium fluoride (BaF2) or cesium fluoride (CsF) scintillators [83, 84]. However, it was soon found that scanners made with these scintillators could not match the spatial resolution and sensitivity of non-TOF PET cameras using BGO scintillators. BaF2 and CsF scintillators had very good timing resolution but low stopping power, compared with BGO, and low light output that limits the detector design choices for light sharing and decoding crystals.

The availability of new scintillation crystals such as LSO and LYSO [85–88] that combine fast timing decay with high light output and high stopping power and improvements in performance and reliability of fast PMTs in combination with improvements in high-speed electronics made it practical to develop the new generation of TOF PET scanners. In addition, progress in image reconstruction, especially in iterative reconstruction methods, further improved PET images by including TOF and other physical effects in the system model [89–94].

A non-TOF PET scanner could detect coincidence photons of an annihilated positron and record the corresponding line of response between the two detector crystals, but the actual location of the annihilation along the line of response would not be measured. However, in a TOF PET system in where the difference in the arrival time of the two coincidence photons is also measured, it is possible to localize the event within a small range along the line of response. In principle, reconstruction would be unnecessary with perfect TOF information, as the location of each positron annihilation would be identified on the basis of time difference information. However, because of imperfect timing resolution of the scanners, the TOF information is used to improve the image reconstruction by localizing the coincidence along the line connecting the detectors. The distance that a given event is projected along the LOR is defined by an uncertainty (Δx) that with good timing resolution, can be much smaller than the diameter of the patient (D), over which counts would be distributed equally in the forward and back projection steps of non-TOF reconstruction.

TOF has the potential to improve the accuracy of a lesion uptake measurement through better signal localization and reduced noise propagation. The effective sensitivity gain, thus the reduction of noise, for a uniform distribution is estimated to be proportional to $D/\Delta x$, where $\Delta x = c.\ \Delta t/2$ when c is the speed of light and Δt is the timing resolution of the system [95]. For two uniform distributions with diameters of 20 and 35 cm, for a scanner with a timing resolution of 600 ps the calculated sensitivity gains are estimated to be 2.2 and 3.9, respectively. For 300 ps timing resolution, the sensitivity gains will be 4.4 and 7.8, respectively. The uniform distribution with a diameter of 20 cm can represent a thin patient and the 35-cm distribution can represent a heavy patient [96]. Therefore, TOF PET is particularly [95] suitable for whole-body imaging because the improvement in image quality is expected to increase with the size of the patient. For heavy patients where the attenuation effect and scatter contribution are bigger issues, the improvement in the image quality is especially more important.

The initial results of the TOF PET scanners have shown improved performance over non-TOF scanners. Philips has developed a PET/CT system with TOF capability (Gemini TF PET/CT) based on LYSO with an intrinsic spatial resolution of about 4.8 mm [65]. This fully 3D scanner has a coincidence timing resolution of 585 ps when measured with a point source in air. However, there is a count-rate effect on the timing resolution that causes it to degrade to about 650–700 ps for typical clinical count rates [95]. A scanner from Siemens based on LSO with added TOF features has been reported [96]. However, because this system was not initially designed for TOF, it had a timing resolution of 1.2 ns and the impact on clinical studies has been modest. Recently, Siemens announced a new PET/CT system (Biograph mCT) with TOF capability that claims it could further improve the signal-to-noise ratio by a factor of 4. GE has also announced a new PET/CT scanner (Discovery PET/CT 690) with TOF capability.

Dedicated Breast PET Camera

Breast cancer is the most common cancer and the second leading cause of cancer death in women in the United States. For 2009, the American Cancer Society had predicted that approximately

192,370 women in the United States would be found to have invasive breast cancer and about 40,170 women would die from the cancer [97]. Breast cancer mortality rates have been dropping in recent years as a result of improved screening and treatment methods and also because more women are being screened [98]. Despite advances in the last decade, diagnosis of cancer, especially for small tumors, and monitoring therapy response remain a challenge.

Currently, mammography is the most widely used imaging method for breast cancer screening. The sensitivity of screening mammography for breast cancer detection is about 85% that decreases to 68% for dense breasts [99]. In addition, mammography is limited in the accurate differentiation between benign and malignant tumors. Therefore, other imaging methods such as PET scanning, are needed to improve breast cancer detection. The PET ability to detect metabolic changes in body tissues is the main advantage of PET over mammography. Additionally, PET imaging is not affected by dense breast or silicone implants, making PET effective for screening high-risk young women, older women with hormone replacement therapy, and those with implants [100–102]. In addition, PET has superiority over conventional imaging in detecting distant metastases and recurrent disease and in monitoring therapy response [103, 104].

Despite the powerful molecular imaging nature of PET, the current whole-body PET cameras have critical limitations for breast cancer imaging because: (1) the spatial resolution and sensitivity of current whole-body PET cameras practically limit the detection of breast lesions to relatively large lesion (>1 cm) and high FDG uptakes, (2) a typical clinical PET/CT camera is large and expensive, and (3) a typical clinical PET/CT is designed primarily for whole-body cancer staging; therefore, with detectors too far from the breast, the patient body attenuates higher than 80% of the breast signal, and the low signal detection efficiency requires a long imaging time (10–15 min). These limitations prevent the widespread use of conventional whole-body PET for breast cancer. A recent comparison of the whole-body mode and breast mode of a transformable full-ring PET camera with spatial resolution of better than 3 mm, using small phantom lesions of 4–7 mm inserted into a breast phantom attached to a torso phantom, has shown significant improvement in lesion detection in breast mode that demonstrated the advantage of dedicated breast PET scanners [105].

In recent years, several partial-ring dedicated breast PET scanners, commonly referred to as PEM, are being developed to improve the cost effectiveness for detecting breast cancers [106–115]. These PEM scanners have special geometries that are different from the conventional circular design of whole-body PET scanners and, compared with whole-body PET, they can have greater sensitivity for detecting breast cancers. A PEM system with high resolution, high sensitivity, and low cost could improve early detection of small tumors to improve survivability and breast conservation.

The most popular PEM design is the dual planar geometry with or without rotating capability around the patient's breast. Rotation allows obtaining complete angular sampling that has the potential to improve breast imaging over PEM with stationary dual planar detector by reducing blurring, especially normal to the detector. This dual planar design is easier to construct than the full-ring camera and has greater flexibility in positioning the object in the FOV. The stationary dual planar cameras are generally designed to image the compressed breast in the projection mode similar to x-ray mammography instead of the tomography mode. This geometry also allows performing of needle biopsy while a patient is in the scanner, and has the ability to acquire the PET image in conjunction with a mammography unit. The planes are arranged in close proximity to the patient, which leads to a higher sensitivity then clinical PET scanners and reduced attenuation of photons traveling through the patient chest wall. More recently, there have been proposed scanner designs with depth-of-interaction (DOI) measurement capability [116, 142–144]. The DOI capability allows for maintaining of the high spatial resolution throughout the FOV of the small diameter scanners.

Future Developments in PET

Recent trends in the development of positron cameras have been concentrated on several issues: (1) lowering the production cost of the cameras, (2) combining the functional and anatomic modalities, (3) adding TOF capability and improving timing resolution, (4) adding DOI capability and improving spatial resolution, and (5) improving image reconstruction.

For current PET cameras, with pixilated crystals, the detection system often accounts for greater than 50% of the total production cost. Hence, some of the development efforts have concentrated on lowering the detection system cost. A PET detector design has been introduced based on a photomultiplier-quadrant sharing technique to substantially reduce detector cost by reducing the number of photomultipliers [117, 118]. Two research cameras with transformable geometry based on this design have been constructed and have achieved a spatial resolution of better than 3 mm [55, 118]. Another way for reducing detector cost has been to build partially populated detector rings and rotate them during the scan. In the 1990s, a rotating BGO multi-ring PET camera was built with two thirds of the detectors removed from the ring so that only two opposing sectors of the detection system remained [39]. This reduced the camera cost by 50%, but it also reduced the camera sensitivity by approximately 66% for smaller objects and 80% for large objects. The partial-ring PET systems have not received much acceptance except for use in PEM cameras.

Integrated PET and CT (PET/CT) systems, capable of acquiring data by both devices and displaying the fused image, have been commercially available since the early 2000s and have shown some improvement over PET alone. A comparable PET/MRI system that could acquire and fuse PET and MRI scans is not currently commercially available. However, there are some experimental units that can acquire both scans simultaneously and clinical units are under development [119–121]. The goal is that, by fusion of the metabolic information obtained by PET scans with the MRI scan, the specificity of MRI will be increased. MRI has a high sensitivity for identifying tissue abnormalities but not high specificity.

Additional ongoing research is aimed at improving the spatial resolution and sensitivity of PET cameras. Using smaller (narrower) and shorter crystals could potentially improve spatial resolution of the system. However, there is a tradeoff between sensitivity and spatial resolution. Increasing crystal length to achieve higher sensitivity leads to deterioration of spatial resolution, especially of the center of the camera because of the increased probability of detecting a gamma photon that has penetrated through more than one crystal. There have been many scanner designs with DOI measurement capability [122, 123, 142–144]. The DOI capability allows maintaining of the high spatial resolution throughout the FOV, which is more important for scanners with small diameters such as dedicated animal cameras, dedicated breast cameras, and dedicated brain cameras.

Another recent development has been the addition of a TOF capability to PET cameras. Several TOF cameras have been introduced based on new LSO and LYSO crystals. However, the timing resolution of these systems currently is not optimized (more than 600 ns). The next step is to further improve the timing resolution.

A major improvement in PET image reconstruction was achieved with the introduction of iterative reconstruction in the 1990s. Originally, reconstruction was performed in 2D and the sinograms were corrected prior to image reconstruction for such effects as attenuation, detector normalization, random, and scatter. The correction of sinograms is not desirable because of the distortion of the Poisson nature of the data and the production of less ideal images. With the increased speed and memory of computers it became possible to perform fully 3D reconstruction and incorporate some of the corrections, including normalization and attenuation, into the system probability matrix and some of the corrections, including scatter and random corrections, into the forward projected sinograms. Currently, the incorporation of the spatial response of the detector system, and TOF information into the reconstruction process are promising to further improve the image quality [93, 94].

Quantitation and Parametric Imaging

In PET imaging the tracer uptake and dynamic in principle can be accurately qualified from the image data because of PET attenuation-correction capability. This information can help to expand the observer's ability in interpreting images. PET imaging with FDG, the most clinically useful cancer imaging tracer today, can benefit from using quantitative measures of uptake to determine the likelihood that a tumor is malignant, from its level of metabolic activity, and to assess tumor response to therapy.

There are several ways to approach quantitation, from visual assessment to complex kinetic analysis, with dynamic data acquisition and blood sampling [124–141]. In clinical practice, the simplest and the main tool for image interpretation is visual inspection of images. A slightly better method is graded visual assessment where the abnormality is classified relative to normal structures on a 5–10 point scale using pseudo-color representation of the tissue uptake. Tumor to normal tissue activity ratio is the next level of quantitation. It requires attenuation-corrected images, but no other calibration. This approach is more objective but has significant limitations. Values derived depend on placement of regions of interest (ROIs), definition of normal tissue, reconstruction algorithm, image resolution, and whether maximum or average counts are used. The tumor to normal ratio method can be useful but should be implemented with explicit attention to these factors.

The most widely used quantitative method for assessing FDG uptake is the standardized uptake value (SUV), which estimates fractional FDG uptake by tumor [125, 126]. This measure is also referred to as the dose uptake ratio, or differential uptake ratio (DUR). SUV is often used as a measure to characterize the malignancy versus benignancy of lesions. The SUV can be defined as the tissue concentration of tracer as measured by a PET camera divided by the activity injected divided by body weight,

$$\text{SUV} = [\text{tissue activity in } \mu\text{Ci / gr}] / [\text{injected dose in } \mu\text{Ci per gr body weight}].$$

Many physiologic and technical factors affect the outcome of the SUV [125]. The use of SUV requires, in addition to data correction, that the administered dose be accurately determined, corrected for residual activity in syringe and tubing, and the dose must be decay-corrected to the time of imaging. In addition, patient preparation methods, scanner performance, image reconstruction algorithms, and data analysis tools can also affect the outcome of the SUV. Because manufacturers are using different acquisition protocols, image reconstruction algorithms, and data analysis tools, the comparison and exchange of SUV results between varying centers is not an easy task.

Currently, there is no NEMA standard procedure for measuring SUV; however, several recommendations and guidelines have been proposed with the aim of minimizing the variability of SUVs across different institutes and studies [125, 127]. For FDG, the tissue activity used is generally the tracer uptake between 30–60 min after injection. However, to achieve a model independent assessment of glucose metabolism, SUV should be measured after FDG tissue concentration has reached a plateau. There is much variability in this measurement depending on the exact implementation in each clinical site. To minimize variability for comparison purposes, all the studies at the same site should follow the same quality control parameters, such as the waiting period after injection, the duration of imaging, and fasting protocols. To further minimize variability, plasma glucose level correction [128, 129] should also be applied:

$$\mathrm{SUV}(\text{corrected}) = \mathrm{SUV} \times [\text{plasma glucose} / 100]$$

In addition, there should be a body fat correction term [130, 131] to account for the reduced uptake of FDG in body fat. The SUV can be extracted either as the peak value in an ROI or displaying the SUV pixel-by-pixel as a pseudocolor-quantitation SUV image.

The SUV quantitation is not as accurate as the compartmental analysis, but is easy to implement and requires no blood sampling, which may be more practical in a clinical environment. There are more reliable, but also more complex, quantitation methods including simplified kinetic analysis, Patlak graphical analysis, and kinetic analysis with parameter optimization; however, because of practical constraints, these methods are usually not used except in research studies.

With tracer transport modeling and multiple scans over a time period (dynamic imaging), functional parameters can be quantified. Some common physiologic parameters generated by PET are blood flow [132–134], metabolic rates [135], blood volume [136, 137], and receptor densities. These quantified parameters may be more useful than a simple tracer uptake image. For example, a region with a high relative uptake of FDG may be either an area of high blood volume/perfusion, especially if the images are taken immediately after injection, or an area of high glucose metabolism; quantified parameters of glucose metabolic rate and blood space would differentiate such an important ambiguity. The quantitation can be carried out in two different ways, depending on the complexity of the tracer transport model and the quality of the raw image data: (1) if the model is complex, involving many parameters coupled with noisy image data, it would be better to draw an ROI on the image data, e.g., on a suspected tumor site, and compute the average functional parameters within the region; and (2) if the model is simple (1–2 parameters) and the image quality is high, it may be more useful to generate a parametric image set that is equivalent to perform an ROI parametric calculation on a pixel-by-pixel basis for the whole image set. A set of parametric images displaying the metabolic rate distribution and the blood volume distribution separately can be more useful clinically for cancer detection and treatment monitoring. Quantitation is especially useful for accurately monitoring the efficacy of therapy if a similar quantitation is performed before treatment.

Tracer modeling and parametric quantitation techniques for FDG have been studied extensively with different degrees of refinement and simplification, resulting in a compromise between practicality and accuracy [135, 138]. Most FDG methods are based on the three compartment models as shown in Fig. 1.4. The physiologic parameters to be deduced are the rate constants k_1, k_2, k_3, and k_4 (Fig. 1.4). k_1 and k_2 are the rate of FDG transport from plasma into tissue and from tissue back into plasma, k_3 is the rate of FDG phosphorylation, and k_4 the rate of FDG dephosphorylation. One way to find the rate constants of a lesion is by drawing an ROI on the image set and extracting the time-activity data within the ROI. The ROI time-activity data are then combined with the time-activity data of the blood plasma tracer activity levels as inputs to a curve-fitting computer program for the three-compartment model. The curve-fitting program would output the rate constants [139]. This procedure generates the average rate constants in the ROI instead of a set of parametric images of the rate constants. Conceptually, the same method can be applied pixel-by-pixel to generate a set of parametric images of the rate constants. However, such an image processing procedure requires the image quality of the original uptake data to be very high so that the statistical errors for all the pixels are small. Furthermore, the curve-fitting time for all the image pixels may be impractically lengthy compared with the present computing technology.

A more practical method of generating an FDG metabolic image is based on the unidirectional flow model [136, 137], also called the Patlak plot method, which is basically a three-compartment model, as shown in Fig. 1.4, except that k_4 is assumed to be insignificantly small. A negligible k_4 implies that there is no leakage of

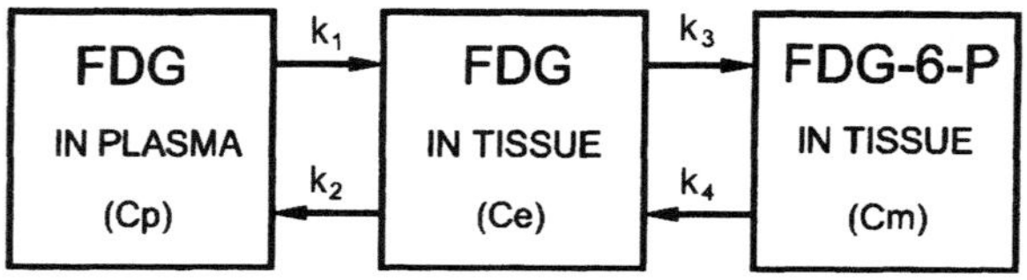

Fig. 1.4 The ^{18}F-fluorodeoxyglucose three-compartment system consisting of reaction in blood, tissue, and product in tissue

the tracer from the trapped cell space. This simplifies the model from four parameters (k_1, k_2, k_3, and k_4) to two parameters (Ki and Vd), where Ki is the macro metabolic rate constant and Vd is the blood distribution volume and vascular space. Mathematically, the macro metabolic rate constant Ki of the tissue-bound compartment is equivalent to $k_1\, k_3/[k_2+k_3]$ in the three-compartment model. This method is computationally fast and less demanding on the quality of the raw image data. However, even this simplified method still requires the measurement of the tracer input function, the blood time-activity curve. Parametric imaging methods require the measurement of the tracer input function. The extraction of 30 blood samples over the imaging period and the effort to measure the blood activity information of these samples are rather demanding, especially for clinical studies. As PET imaging moves into clinics, many different ways of reducing the amount of blood sampling have been proposed, but the most accurate and simple way is with the use of an automated blood sampling system [140, 141].

References

1. Fowler JS, Wolf AP. Positron emitter-labeled compounds: priorities and problems. In: Phelps M, Mazziotta J, Schelbert H, editors. Positron emission tomography and autoradiography: principles and applications for the brain and heart. New York: Raven; 1986. p. 391–450.
2. Derenzo SE. Precision measurement of annihilation point spread distributions for medically important positron emitters. Proceedings of the 5th International Conference on Positron Annihilation, Sendai, Japan; 1979. p. 819–24.
3. Phelps ME, Mazziotta JC, Schelbert HR, editors. Positron emission tomography and autoradiography principles and applications for the brain and heart. New York: Raven; 1986.
4. Sorenson JA, Phelps ME. Physics in nuclear medicine. 2nd ed. Philadelphia: W.B. Saunders Company; 1987.
5. King MA, Hademenos G, Glick SJ. A dual photopeak window method for scatter correction. J Nucl Med. 1992;33:605–12.
6. Bentourkia M, Msaki P, Cadorette J, Lecomte R. Assessment of scatter components in high-resolution PET: correction by nonstationary convolution subtraction. J Nucl Med. 1995;36:121–30.
7. Watson CC, Newport D, Casey ME, et al. Evaluation of simulation-based scatter correction for 3-D PET cardiac imaging. J Nucl Med. 1997;44:90–7.
8. Defrise M, Kinahan PE. Data acquisition and image reconstruction for 3D PET. In: Bendriem B, Twonsend DW, editors. The theory and practice of 3D PET. Dordrecht/Boston: Kluwer; 1998. p. 11–50.
9. Brooks RA, DiChiro G. Theory of image reconstruction in computed tomography. Radiology. 1975; 117:561–72.
10. Brownell GL, Burnham CA, Chesler CA, et al. Transverse section imaging of radionuclide distribution in heart, lung and brain. In: Ter-Pogossian MM, Phelps ME, Brownell GL, editors. Reconstruction tomography in diagnostic radiology and nuclear medicine. Baltimore: University Park Press; 1977. p. 293–307.
11. Shepp LA, Logan BF. The fourier reconstruction of a head section. IEEE Trans Nucl Sci. 1974; NS-21:21–43.
12. Gilland DR, Tsui BMW, McCartney WH, et al. Determination of the optimum filter function for SPECT imaging. J Nucl Med. 1988;29:643–50.
13. Beis JS, Celler A, Barney JS. An automatic method to determine cutoff frequency based on image power spectrum. IEEE Trans Nucl Sci. 1995;42:2250–4.
14. Farquhar TH, Chatziioannou A, Chinn G, et al. An investigation of filter choice for filtered back-projection reconstruction in PET. IEEE Trans Nucl Sci. 1998;45:1133–7.
15. Baghaei H, Wong WH, Li H, et al. Evaluation of the effect of filter apodization for volume PET imaging using the 3-D RP algorithm. IEEE Trans Nucl Sci. 2003;50:3–8.
16. Chesler DA, Riederer SJ. Ripple suppression during reconstruction in transverse tomography. Phys Med Biol. 1995;20:632–6.

17. Baghaei H, Wong W-H, Li H, Uribe J, Wang Y, Aykac M, Liu Y, Xing T. Evaluation of the effect of filter apodization for volume PET imaging using the 3-D RP algorithm. IEEE Trans Nucl Sci. 2003; 50 I:3–8.
18. Kinahan PE, Rogers JG. Analytic 3D image reconstruction using all detected events. IEEE Trans Nucl Sci. 1989;46:964–8.
19. Cherry SR, Dahlbom M, Hoffman EJ. Evaluation of a 3D reconstruction algorithm for multi-slice PET scanners. Phys Med Biol. 1992;37:779–90.
20. Kadrmas DJ, Christian PE, Wollenweber SD, et al. Comparative evaluation of 2D and 3D lesion detectability on a full-ring BGO PET scanner. J Nucl Med. 2002;43(5):56.
21. Pajevic S, Dauve-Witherspoon ME, Bacharach SL, Carson RE. Noise characteristics of 3-D and 2-D PET images. IEEE Trans Med Imag. 1998;17:9–23.
22. Baily DL, Jones T, Spinks TJ, Gilardi MC, Townsend DW. Noise equivalent count measurements in a neuro-PET scanner with retractable septa. IEEE Trans Med Imag. 1991;10:256–60.
23. Stearns CW, Cherry SR, Thompson CJ. NECR analysis of 3D brain PET scanner designs. IEEE Trans Nucl Sci. 1994;42:1075–9.
24. Daube-Witherspoon ME, Muehllehner G. Treatment of axial data in three-dimensional PET. J Nucl Med. 1997;28:1717–24.
25. Lewitt RM, Muehllehner G, Karp JS. Three-dimensional reconstruction for PET by multi-slice rebinning and axial image filtering. Phys Med Biol. 1994;39:321–39.
26. Defrise M, Kinahan PE, Townsend DW, Michel C, Sibomana M, Newport DF. Exact and approximation rebinning algorithms for 3-D PET data. IEEE Trans Nucl Sci. 1997;16:145–58.
27. Shepp LA, Vardi Y. Maximum likelihood reconstruction for emission tomography. IEEE Trans Med Imag. 1982;MI-1:113–22.
28. Hudson HM, Larkin RS. Accelerated image reconstruction using ordered subsets of projection data. IEEE Trans Nucl Sci. 1994;13:601–9.
29. Panin VY, Kehren F, Michel C, Casey M. Fully 3-D PET reconstruction with system matrix derived from point source measurements. IEEE Trans Med Imag. 2006;25(7):907–21.
30. Jacobson M, Levkovitz R, Ben-Tal A, et al. Enhanced 3D PET OSEM reconstruction using inter-update Metz filtering. Phys Med Biol. 2000;45:2417–39.
31. Herbert TJ, Leahy RM. A generalized EM algorithm for 3-D Bayesian reconstruction from Poisson data using Gibs priors. IEEE Trans Med Imag. 1989; 8:194–202.
32. Daghighian F, Hoffman EJ, Huang SC. Quality control in PET systems employing 2-D modular detectors. IEEE Trans Nucl Sci. 1989;36:1034–7.
33. Hoffman EJ, Guerrero TM, Germano G, et al. PET system calibrations and corrections for quanitative and spatially accurate images. IEEE Trans Nucl Sci. 1989;36:1108–12.
34. Defrise M, Townsend DW, Bailey D, et al. A normalization technique for 3D PET data. Phys Med Biol. 1991;36:939–52.
35. Li H, Liu Y, Xing T, Wang Y, Uribe J, Baghaei H, Xie S, Ramirez R, Wong W-H. An instantaneous photomultiplier gain calibration method for PET or gamma camera detectors using a LED network. IEEE Trans Nucl Sci. 2005;52:1295–9.
36. Knoess C, Gremillion T, Schmand M, et al. Development of a daily quality check procedure for the high-resolution research tomograph (HRRT) using natural LSO background radioactivity. IEEE Trans Nucl Sci. 2002;49:2074–8.
37. Oakes TR, Sossi V, Ruth TJ. Normalization in 3D PET: comparison of detector efficiencies obtained from uniform planar and cylindrical sources. IEEE 1997 Nuclear Science Symposium. 1997;2:1625–9.
38. Adam LE, Zaers J, Ostertag H, et al. Performance evaluation of the whole-body PET scanner ECAT EXACT HR+following the IEC standard. IEEE Trans Nucl Sci. 1997;44:1172–9.
39. Townsend DW, Wensveen M, Byars LG, et al. A rotating PET camera using BGO block detectors: design, performance and applications. J Nucl Med. 1993;34:1367–993.
40. Baghaei H, Wong W-H, Uribe J, et al. Correction factors for a high resolution variable field of view PET. J Nucl Med. 2000;40:279.
41. Casey ME, Gadagkar H, Newport D. A component based method for normalisation in volume PET. Proceedings of the 3rd International Meeting on Fully Three-Dimensional Image Reconstruction in Radiology and Nuclear Medicine. Aix-les-Bains; 1995. p. 67–71.
42. Badawi RD, Lodge MA, Marsden PK. Algorithms for calculating detector efficiency normalization coefficients for true coincidences in 3D PET. Phys Med Biol. 1998;43:189–205.
43. Baghaei H, Li H, Wang Y, Zhang Y, Kim S, Ramirez R, Liu J, Liu S, Wong W-H. A new component-based normalization method for PET cameras. J Nucl Med. 2007;48(Suppl 2):432.
44. Zhang Y, Li H, Baghaei H, Liu J, Liu S, Ramirez R, An S, Wong C, Wong W. A new self-normalization for PET cameras. J Nucl Med. 2008;49(Suppl 1):64.
45. National Electrical Manufacturers Association. NEMA standards publication NU 2–1994: performance measurements of positron emission tomographs. Washington, DC: National Electrical Manufacturers Association; 1994.
46. Karp JS, Daube-Witherspoon ME, Hoffman EJ, et al. Performance standards in positron emission tomography. J Nucl Med. 1991;32:2342–50.
47. National Electrical Manufacturers Association. NEMA standards publication NU 2–2001: performance measurements of positron emission tomographs. Rosslyn: National Electrical Manufacturers Association; 2001.
48. Daube-Witherspoon ME, Karp JS, Casey ME, et al. PET performance measurements using the NEMA NU 2–2001 standard. J Nucl Med. 2002;43:1398–409.

49. Patton JA, Turkington TG. Coincidence imaging with a dual-head scintillation camera. J Nucl Med. 1999;40:432–41.
50. Karp JS, Muehllehner G, Mankoff D, et al. Continuous-slice PENN-PET: a positron tomograph with volume imaging capability. J Nucl Med. 1990;31:617–27.
51. Adam LE, Karp JS, Daube-witherspoon ME, et al. Performance of a whole-body PET scanner using curve-plate NaI(Tl) detectors. J Nucl Med. 2001; 42:1821–30.
52. Brix G, Zaers J, Adam LE, et al. Performance evaluation of a whole-body PET scanner using the NEMA protocol. National Electrical Manufacturers Association. J Nucl Med. 1997;38:1614–23.
53. DeGrado T, Turkington T, Williams J, Stearns C, Hoffman J. Performance characteristics of a whole-body PET scanner. J Nucl Med. 1994;35: 1398–406.
54. Lewellen TK, Kohlmyer SG, Miyaoka RS, et al. Investigation of the performance of the general electric ADVANCE positron emission tomograph in 3D mode. IEEE Trans Nucl Sci. 1996;43:2199–206.
55. Li H, Wong W-H, Baghaei H, Uribe J, Wang Y, Zhang Y, Kim S, Ramirez R, Liu J, Liu S. The engineering and initial results of a transformable low-cost high-resolution PET camera. IEEE Trans Nucl Sci. 2007;54:1583–8.
56. Eriksson L, Wienhard K, Eriksson K, et al. The ECAT HRRT: NEMA NEC evaluation of the HRRT system, the new high-resolution research tomograph. IEEE Trans Nucl Sci. 2002;49:2085–8.
57. Jakoby BW, Bercier Y, Watson CC, Bendriem B, Townsend DW. Performance characteristics of a new LSO PET/CT scanner with extended axial field-of-view and PSF reconstruction. IEEE Trans Nucl Sci. 2009;56:633–9.
58. Kemp BJ, Kim C, Williams JJ, Ganin A, Lowe VJ. NEMA NU 2–2001 performance measurements of an LYSO-based PET/CT system in 2D and 3D acquisition modes. J Nucl Med. 2006;47:1960–7.
59. Chatziioannou AF, Cherry SR, Shao Y, et al. Performance evaluation of microPET: a high-resolution lutetium oxyorthosilicate PET scanner for animal imaging. J Nucl Med. 1999;40:1164–75.
60. Baghaei H, Wong W-H, Zhang Y, Li H, Ramirez R, Kim S, Liu J, Liu S, Wang Y. Monte Carlo simulation of a high resolution and high sensitivity small animal PET camera using GATE/GEANT. IEEE Trans Nucl Sci. 2007;54(5):1568–73.
61. Bao Q, Newport D, Chen M, Stout DB, Chatziioannou AF. Performance evaluation of the inveon dedicated PET preclinical tomograph based on the NEMA NU-4 standards. J Nucl Med. 2009;50:401–8.
62. Jones WF, Casey ME, van Lingen A, et al. LSO PET/SPECT spatial resolution: critical on-line DOI rebinning methods and results. IEEE Nuclear Science Symposium Conference Record. 2000;3:16/54–58.
63. Beyer T, Townsend DW, Brun T, et al. A combined PET/CT scanner for clinical oncology. J Nucl Med. 2000;41:1369–79.
64. Pichler BJ, Judenhofer MS, Catana C, et al. Performance test of an LSO-APD detector in a 7-T MRI scanner for simultaneous PET/MRI. J Nucl Med. 2006;47:639–47.
65. Surti S, Kuhn A, Werner ME, Perkins AE, Kolthammer J, Karp JS. Performance of Philips Gemini TF PET/CT scanner with special consideration for its time-of-flight imaging capabilities. J Nucl Med. 2007;48(3):471–80.
66. Murthy K, Aznar M, Thompson CJ, et al. Results of preliminary clinical trials of the positron emission mammography system PEM-I: a dedicated breast imaging system producing glucose metabolic images using FDG. J Nucl Med. 2000;41:1851–8.
67. Ramirez RA, Zhang Y, Liu S, Li H, Baghaei H, An S, Wang C, Jan M-L, Wong W-H. A lower-cost high-resolution LYSO detector development for positron emission mammography (PEM). IEEE Trans Nucl Sci. 2009;56(5):71–7.
68. Bowen SL, Wu Y, Chaudhari AJ, et al. Initial characterization of a dedicated breast PET/CT scanner during human imaging. J Nucl Med. 2009;50:1401–8.
69. Holle LH, Trampert L, Lung-Kurt S, et al. Investigations of breast tumors with fluorine-18-fluorodeoxyglucose and SPECT. J Nucl Med. 1996;36:615–22.
70. Yutani K, Tatsumi M, Shiba E, et al. Comparison of dual-head coincidence gamma camera FDG imaging with FDG PET in detection of breast cancer and axillary lymph node metastasis. J Nucl Med. 1999;40:1003–8.
71. Gerbaudo VH, Sugarbaker DJ, Britz-Cunningham S, et al. Assessment of malignant pleural mesothelioma with 18F-FDG dual-head gamma-camera coincidence imaging: comparison with histopathology. J Nucl Med. 2002;43:1144–9.
72. Wong WH, Li H, Uribe J, Baghaei H, Wang Y, Yokoyam S. Feasibility of a high speed gamma camera design using the high-yield-pileup-event-recovery (HYPER) method. J Nucl Med. 2001;42:624–32.
73. Adam LE, Karp JS, Daube-Witherspoon ME, Smith RJ. Performance of a whole-body PET scanner using curve-plate NaI(Tl) detectors. J Nucl Med. 2001; 42:1821–30.
74. Melcher CL. Scintillation crystals for PET. J Nucl Med. 2000;41:1051–5.
75. Huber S, Moses WW, Jones WF, Watson CC. Effect of ^{176}Lu background on singles transmission for LSO-based PET cameras. Phys Med Biol. 2002; 47:3535–41.
76. Nehmeh S, Erdi Y, Ling C, et al. Effect of respiratory gating on reducing lung motion artifacts in PET imaging of lung cancer. Med Phys. 2002;29: 366–71.
77. Townsend DW. A combined PET/CT scanner: the choices. J Nucl Med. 2001;42:533–4.
78. Goerres GW, Kamel E, Seifert B, et al. Accuracy of image coregistration of pulmonary lesions in patients with non-small cell lung cancer using an integrated PET/CT system. J Nucl Med. 2002;43:1469–75.

79. Osman MM, Cohade C, Nakamoto Y, et al. Clinically significant inaccurate localization of lesions with PET/CT: frequency in 300 patients. J Nucl Med. 2003;44:240–3.
80. Mullani NA, Markham J, Ter-Pogossian MM. Feasibility of time-of-flight reconstruction in positron emission tomography. J Nucl Med. 1980;21:1095–7.
81. Budinger TF. Time-of-flight positron emission tomography: status relative to conventional PET. J Nucl Med. 1983;24:73–8.
82. Wong WH, Mullani NA, Philippe EA, et al. Performance-characteristics of the University-of-Texas TOFPET-I PET camera. J Nucl Med. 1984; 25(Suppl):46–7.
83. Laval M, Moszynski M, Allemand R, Cormoreche E, Guinet P, Odru R, Vacher J. Barium Fluoride inorganic scintillator for subnanosecond timing. Nucl Instrum Methods Phys Res. 1983;206(1–2):169–76.
84. Allemand R, Gresset C, Vacher J. Potential advantages of a cesium fluoride scintillator for a time-of-flight positron camera. J Nucl Med. 1980;21(2): 153–5.
85. van Eijk CWE. Inorganic scintillators in medical imaging. Phys Med Biol. 2002;47:R85–106.
86. Moses WW, Derenzo SE. Prospects for time-of-flight PET using LSO scintillator. IEEE Trans Nucl Sci. 1999;46(3):474–8.
87. Moses WW. Current trends in scintillator detectors and materials. Nucl Instrum Methods A. 2002;487: 123–8.
88. Surti S, Karp JS, Muehllehner G, Raby PS. Investigation of lanthanum scintillators for 3-D PET. IEEE Trans Nucl Sci. 2003;50(3):348–54.
89. Tomitani T. Image-reconstruction and noise evaluation in photon time-of-flight assisted positron emission tomography. IEEE Trans Nucl Sci. 1981;28(9): 4582–9.
90. Snyder DL, Politte DG. Image reconstruction from list-mode data in an emission tomography system having time-of-flight measurements. IEEE Trans Nucl Sci. 1983;30(3):1843–9.
91. Parra L, Barrett HH. List-mode likelihood: EM algorithm and image quality estimation demonstrated on 2-D PET. IEEE Trans Med Imag. 1998;17(2): 228–35.
92. Reader AJ, Erlandsson K, Flower MA, Ott RJ. Fast accurate iterative reconstruction for low-statistics positron volume imaging. Phys Med Biol. 1998;43(4):835–46.
93. Groiselle CJ, Glick SJ. 3D PET list-mode iterative reconstruction using time-of-flight information. Proceedings of IEEE Nuclear Science Symposium and Medical Imaging Conference; 2004 Oct; Rome; 2004; vol. 4, p. 2633–8.
94. Matej S, Surti S, Jayanthi S, Daube-Witherspoon ME, Lewitt RM, Karp JS. Efficient 3-D TOF PET reconstruction using view-grouped histo-images: DIRECT-direct image reconstruction for TOF. IEEE Trans Med Imag. 2009;28(5):739–51.
95. Karp JS, Surti S, Daube-Witherspoon ME, Muehllehner G. Benefit of time-of-flight in PET: experimental and clinical results. J Nucl Med. 2008;49(3):462–70.
96. Conti M, Bendriem B, Casey M, Chen M, Kehren F, Michel C, Panin V. First experimental results of time-of-flight reconstruction on an LSO PET scanner. Phys Med Biol. 2005;50(19):4507–26.
97. American Cancer Society: http://www.cancer.org. Cancer facts and figures 2009.
98. Tabar L, Yen M-F, Vitak H-HTCB, Smith RA, Duffy SW. Mammography service screening and mortality in breast cancer patients: 20-year follow-up before and after introduction of screening. Lancet. 2003;361:1405–10.
99. Berm RF, Schoonjans JM, Kieper DA, Majewski S, Goodman S, Civelek C. High-resolution scintimmography: a pilot study. J Nucl Med. 2002; 43(7):909–15.
100. Hodgson NC, Gulenchyn KY. Is there a role for positron emission tomography in breast cancer staging? J Clin Oncol. 2008;26(5):712–20.
101. Avril N, Rosé CA, Schelling M, Dose J, Kuhn W, Bense S, Weber W, Ziegler S, Graeff H, Schwaiger M. Breast imaging with positron emission tomography and fluorine-18 fluorodeoxyglucose: use and limitations. J Clin Oncol. 2000;18(20):3495–502.
102. Quon A, Gambhir S. FDG-PET and beyond: molecular breast cancer. J Clin Oncol. 2005;23(8): 1664–73.
103. Jadvar H, Alavi A, Gambhir SS. 18F-FDG uptake in lung, breast, and colon cancers: molecular biology correlates and disease characterization. J Nucl Med. 2009;50(11):1820–7.
104. Fuster D, Duch J, Paredes P, Velasco M, Muñoz M, Santamaría G, Fontanillas M, Pons F. Preoperative staging of large primary breast cancer with [18F]fluorodeoxyglucose positron emission tomography/computed tomography compared with conventional imaging procedures. J Clin Oncol. 2008;26(29):4746–51.
105. Baghaei H, Li H, Zhang Y, Ramirez RA, Wang C, An S, Liu S, Wong W-H. A breast phantom lesion study with the high resolution transformable HOTPET camera. IEEE Trans Nucl Sci. 2010;57: 2504–09.
106. Thompson CJ, Murthy K, Picard Y, Weinberg IN, Mako R. Positron emission mammography (PEM): a promising technique for detecting breast-cancer. IEEE Trans Nucl Sci. 1995;42:1012–7.
107. Murthy K, Aznar M, Thompson CJ, Loutfi A, Lisbona R, Gagnon JH. Results of preliminary clinical trials of the positron emission mammography system PEM-I: a dedicated breast imaging system producing glucose metabolic image using. J Nucl Med. 2000;41(11):1851–8.
108. Zhang N, Thompson CJ, Cayouette F, Jolly D, Kecani S. A prototype modular detector design for high resolution positron emission mammography imaging. IEEE Trans Nucl Sci. 2003;50(5):1624–9.

109. Doshi NK, Shao YP, Silverman RW, Cherry SR. Design and evaluation of an LSO PET detector for breast cancer imaging. Med Phys. 2000;27:1535–43.
110. Raylman RR, Majewski S, Wojcik R, Weisenberger AG, Kross B, Popov V, Bishop HA. The potential role of positron emission mammography for detection of breast cancer: a phantom study. Med Phys. 2000;27:1943–54.
111. Raylman RR, Majewski S, Weisenberger AG, Popov V, Wojcik R, Kross B, Schreiman JS, Bishop HA. Positron emission mammography-guided breast biopsy. J Nucl Med. 2001;42:960–6.
112. Raylman RR, Majewski S, Weisenberger A, Popov V, Kross B, Wojcik R. Pixelated NaI(Tl) arrays for use in positron emission mammography (PEM). J Nucl Med. 2002;43:11.
113. Wang G-C, Huber JS, Moses WW, Qi J, Choong W-S. Characterization of the LBNL PEM camera. IEEE Trans Nucl Sci. 2006;53(3):1129–35.
114. Abreu MC, Aguiar JD, Almeida FG, et al. Design and evaluation of the clear-PEM scanner for positron emission mammography. IEEE Trans Nucl Sci. 2006;53(1):2621–7.
115. Levin CS, Foudray AMK, Habte F. Impact of high energy resolution detectors on the performance of a PET system dedicated to breast cancer imaging. Phys Med. 2006;21:28–34.
116. Yang YF, Dokhale PA, Silverman RW, Shah KS, McClish MA, Farrell R, Entine G, Cherry SR. Depth of interaction resolution measurements for a high resolution PET detector using position sensitive avalanche photodiodes. Phys Med Biol. 2006;51:2131–42.
117. Wong W-H, Uribe J, Hicks K, Zambelli M. A 2-dimensional detector decoding study on BGO arrays with quadrant sharing photomultipliers. IEEE Trans Nucl Sci. 1994;41:1453–7.
118. Uribe J, Baghaei H, Li H, et al. Basic imaging characteristics of a variable field of view PET camera using quadrant sharing detector design. IEEE Trans Nucl Sci. 1999;46:491–7.
119. Catana C, Wu Y, Judenhofer MS, Qi J, Pichler BJ, Cherry S. Simultaneous acquisition of multislice PET and MR images: initial results with a MR-compatible PET scanner. J Nucl Med. 2006;47:1968–76.
120. Judenhofer MS, Catana C, Swann BK, et al. PET/MR images acquired with a compact MR-compatible PET detector in a 7-T magnet. Radiology. 2007;244:807–14.
121. Schlemmer HP, Pichler B, Schmand M, et al. Simultaneous MR/PET imaging of the human brain: feasibility study. Radiology. 2008;248:1028–35.
122. Yongfeng Y, Yibao W, Cherry SR. Investigation of depth of interaction encoding for a pixelated LSO array with a single multi-channel PMT. IEEE Trans Nucl Sci. 2009;56:2594–9.
123. Chaudhari AJ, Yang Y, Farrell R, Dokhale PA, Shah KS, Cherry SR, Badawi RD. PSPMT/APD hybrid DOI detectors for the PET component of a dedicated breast PET/CT system: a feasibility study. IEEE Trans Nucl Sci. 2008;55:853–61.
124. Graham MM, Peterson LM, Hayward RM. Comparison of simplified quantitative analyses of FDG uptake. Nucl Med Biol. 2000;27:647–55.
125. Boellaard R. Standards for PET image acquisition and quantitative data analysis. J Nucl Med. 2009; 50(Suppl 5):11s–20.
126. Hamberg LM, Hunter GJ, Alpert NM, et al. The dose uptake ratio as an index of glucose metabolism: useful parameter or oversimplification? J Nucl Med. 1994;35:1308–12.
127. Fletcher JW, Djulbegovic B, Soares HP, et al. Recommendations on the use of 18F-FDG PET in oncology. J Nucl Med. 2008;49:480–508.
128. Lindholm P, Minn H, Leskinen-Kallio S, et al. Influence of the blood glucose concentration on FDG uptake in cancer – a PET study. J Nucl Med. 1993;34:1–6.
129. Langen K-J, Braun U, Kops ER, et al. The influence of plasma glucose levels on fluorine-18-fluorodeoxyglucose uptake in bronchial carcinomas. J Nucl Med. 1993;34:355–9.
130. Zasadny KR, Wahl RL. Standardized uptake values of normal tissues at PET with 2-[fluorine-18-]-fluoro-2-deoxy-D-glucose: variations with body weight and a method for correction. Radiology. 1993;189:847–50.
131. Kim CK, Gupta NC, Chandramouli B, Alavi A. Standardized uptake values of FDG: body surface area correction is preferable to body weight correction. J Nucl Med. 1994;35:164–7.
132. Frackowiak RSJ, Lenzi G-L, Jones T, Heather JD. Quantitative measurement of emission tomography: theory, procedure and normal values. J Comput Assist Tomogr. 1980;4:727–36.
133. Huang S-C, Carson RE, Hoffman EJ, et al. Quantitative measurement of local cerebral blood flow in humans by positron computed tomography and 15O-water. J Cerb Blood Flow Metab. 1983; 3:141–53.
134. Ruotsalainen U, Raitakari M, Nuutila P, et al. Quantitative blood flow measurement of skeletal muscle using oxygen-15-water and PET. J Nucl Med. 1997;38:314–9.
135. Phelps ME, Huang SC, Hoffman EJ, et al. Tomographic measurements of local cerebral glucose metabolic rate in humans with [18F]2-fluro-2-deoxy-D-glucose: validation of method. Ann Neurol. 1979;6:371–88.
136. Patlak C, Blasberg R, Fenstermacher J. Graphical evaluation of blood-to-brain transfer constants from multiple-time uptake data. J Cereb Blood Flow Metab. 1983;3:1–7.
137. Gjedde A. Calculation of cerebral glucose phosphorylation from brain uptake of glucose analogs in vivo: a re-examination. Brain Res Rev. 1982;4:237–74.
138. Sokoloff L, Reivich M, Kennedy C, et al. The (14C)-deozyglucose method for the measurement of

local cerebral glucose utilization: theory, procedure and normal values in the conscious and anesthetized albino rat. J Neurochem. 1977;28:897–916.

139. Carson RE. Parameter estimation in positron emission tomography. In: Phelps M, Mazziotta J, Schelbert H, editors. Positron emission tomography and autoradiography: principles and applications for the brain and heart. New York: Raven; 1986. p. 347–90.
140. Hutchins GD, Hichwa RD, Koeppe RA. A continuous flow input function detector for H215O blood flow studies in positron emission tomography. IEEE Trans Nucl Sci. 1986;NS-33:546–9.
141. Eriksson L, Holte S, Bohm C, et al. Automated blood sampling systems for positron emission tomography. IEEE Trans Nucl Sci. 1988;Ns-35: 703–7.
142. Tsuda T, Murayama H, Kitamura K, Inadama N, Yamaya T, Yoshida E, Nishikido F, Hamamoto M, Kawai H, Ono Y. Performance evaluation of a subset of a four-layer LSO detector for a small animal DOI PET scanner: jPET-RD. IEEE Trans Nucl Sci. 2006;53:35–9.
143. Knoess C, Lenox R, Vollmar M, Casey S, Fluegge M, Lammertsma G, et al. Evaluation of the depth of interaction (DOI) for the high resolution research tomograph (HRRT): a comparison between scanners with and without DOI. IEEE NSS-MIC Conference Record; 2002. p. M10–49.
144. Inadama N, Murayama H, Watanabe M, Omura T, Yamashita T, Kawai H, Orita N, Tsuda T. Performance of 256ch flat panel PS-PMT with small crystals for a DOI PET detector. IEEE Trans Nucl Sci. 2005; 52:15–20.

Production of Isotopes

2

Carlos González Lepera and Wai-Hoi Wong

The rapid development and increasing interest in the use of metabolic imaging techniques has created a steady demand for on-site or regional production of radioisotopes. This chapter presents some basic concepts associated with radioisotope production, in particular, those aspects related to cyclotron production of positron-emitting radionuclide.

Concepts

Nuclear Reactions

The force experienced between two charged particles is expressed by Coulomb's law according to the relation (we have omitted some constant factors from the equations to simplify their expression):

$$F(r) = Q_1 Q_2 / r^2 \qquad (2.1)$$

The potential associated with Coulomb's force described in Eq. 2.1 is

$$V(r) = Q_1 / r \qquad (2.2)$$

where Q_1 and Q_2 are the electric charges of particles 1 and 2, respectively, and r is the distance between them. In the case of atomic nuclei this potential barrier can be represented as in Fig. 2.1, where the potential energy of the particles inside the nucleus (radius R) U_0, is assumed to be much lower than the barrier height B, that is $U_0 \ll B$. Experimental evidence strongly supports this assumption.

In a simplified picture to describe a nuclear reaction, an incoming positively charged projectile (proton or deuteron) needs to surmount this repulsive positively charged barrier presented by the target nucleus. In other words, the projectile must approach the target nucleus at a minimum distance of the order of the nuclear radius for a nuclear reaction to occur. This minimum energy is therefore

$$E_B = Z_1 Z_2 e^2 / R \qquad (2.3)$$

with $Q_1 = Z_1 e$, $Q_2 = Z_2 e$, and where Z_1 and Z_2 are the atomic number of projectile and target, respectively, e is the electron charge, and R is the nuclear radius. For protons incident on carbon this value is $E_B = 2.3$ MeV, and for aluminum $E_B = 4.4$ MeV. From Eq. 2.3, a higher projectile energy is needed to penetrate the nucleus of a heavier target to produce a nuclear reaction.

The so-called compound nucleus model for nuclear reactions was first proposed by Bohr in 1936. It assumes that when a target T is bombarded by an incident nuclear particle i, the two may combine to form a compound nucleus $(T+i)$. This new compound nucleus possesses an excitation energy directly related to the incident

C.G. Lepera, Ph.D. (✉) • W.-H. Wong, Ph.D.
Department of Experimental Diagnostic Imaging, The University of Texas MD Anderson Cancer Center, 1515 Holcombe Blvd, Box 0059, Houston, TX 77030, USA
e-mail: cegonzalez1@mdanderson.org; gwong@mdanderson.org

E.E. Kim et al. (eds.), *Clinical PET and PET/CT: Principles and Applications*,
DOI 10.1007/978-1-4419-0802-5_2,

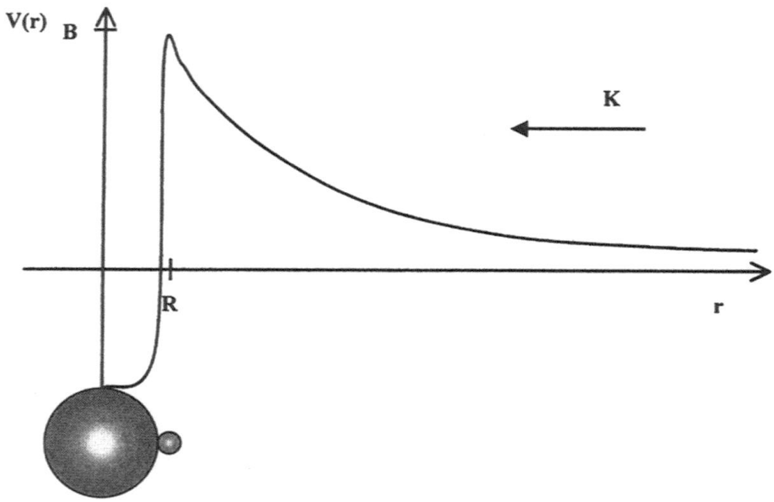

Fig. 2.1 Coulomb potential $V(r)$ between two charged nuclides as a function of their distance r. The barrier height B represents the minimum energy that the projectile has to carry to penetrate the target when it reaches the target outer radius R. A projectile with kinetic energy K as shown would not be able to penetrate the target nucleus

projectile energy. The identity of the incoming particle is lost, and the total energy of the excited compound nucleus is shared in a complicated manner by all the nucleons. The same compound nucleus in the same excited state can also be formed starting from a different combination of projectile/target; that is, it is possible to have $(T+i)=(T'+i')$. The properties of the compound nucleus are independent of the reaction. As an example, the compound nucleus $^{30}Zn^{64}$ can be formed according to the following scheme:

Cross Section for Nuclear Reactions

The cross section for production of a certain final nuclear product reaction channel can be expressed as the probability of formation of the compound nucleus (intermediate state) times the probability of decaying into that channel. It is expressed in units of area ($1\ \text{mbarn}=10^{-3}\ \text{b}=10^{-27}\ \text{cm}^2$). It can be interpreted as the *effective surface per nucleus presented by the target to the incoming projectile.* Due to quantum mechanical effects,

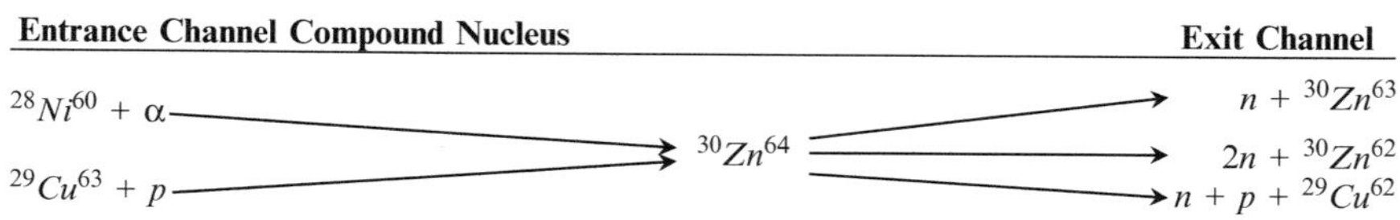

the cross section for production of the compound nucleus is nonzero even for incident projectile energies lower than the Coulomb barrier. Figures 2.2, 2.3, 2.4, and 2.5 present experimental cross sections for the production of some short-lived radioisotopes (^{11}C, ^{13}N, ^{15}O, ^{18}F).

Particle Accelerators

The force experienced by a particle with electric charge q in the presence of an electromagnetic field is described by the Lorentz force according to

$$\vec{F}=q(\vec{E}+\vec{v}\times\vec{B}) \tag{2.4}$$

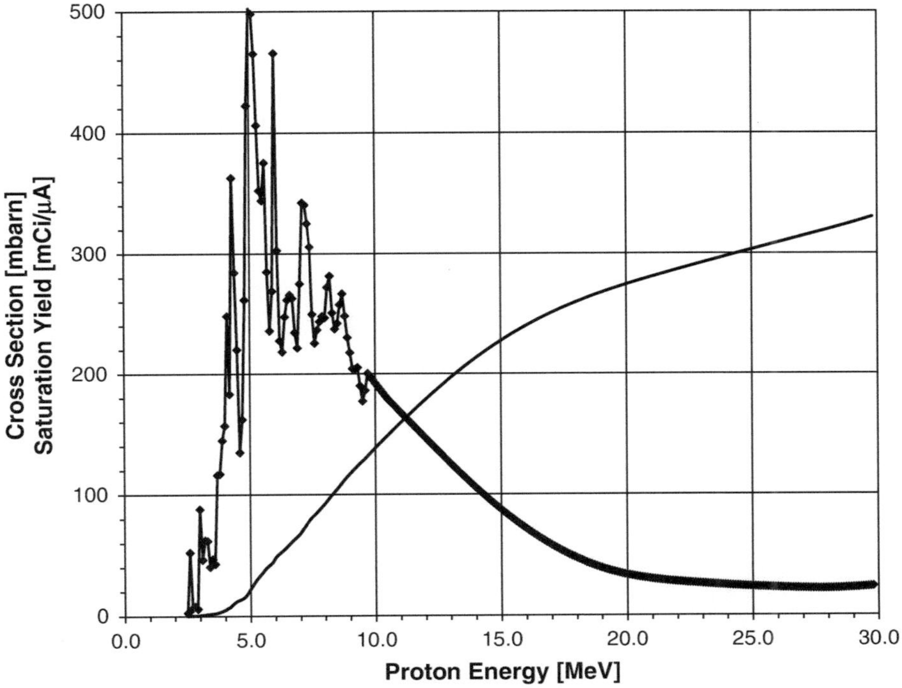

Fig. 2.2 Experimental cross section and theoretical saturation activity shown as a continuous line (Eq. 2.19) for the reaction $^{18}O(p,n)^{18}F$

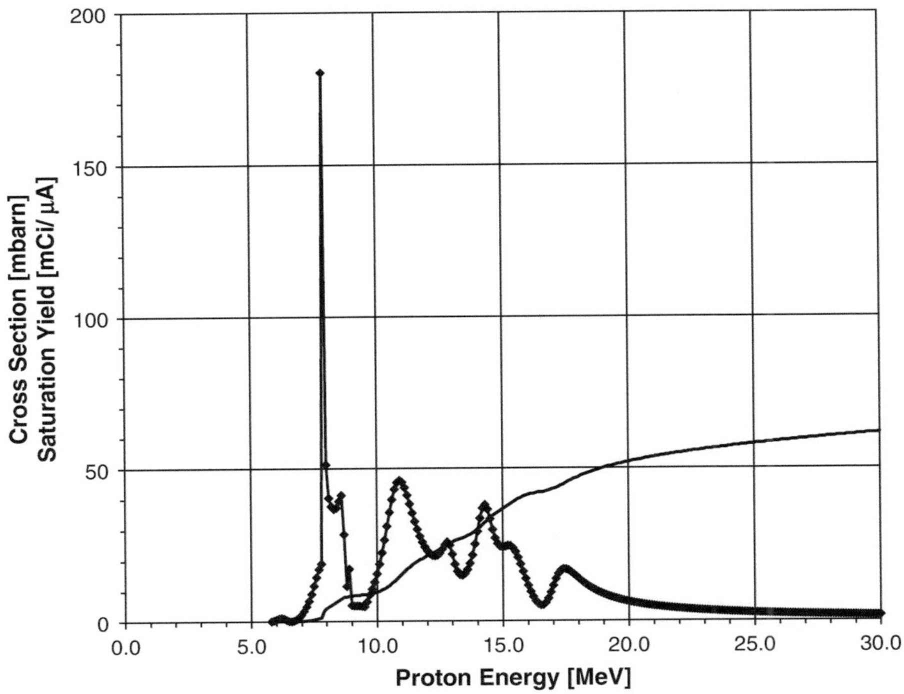

Fig. 2.3 Experimental cross section and theoretical saturation activity shown as a continuous line (Eq. 2.19) for the reaction $^{16}O(p,\alpha)^{13}N$

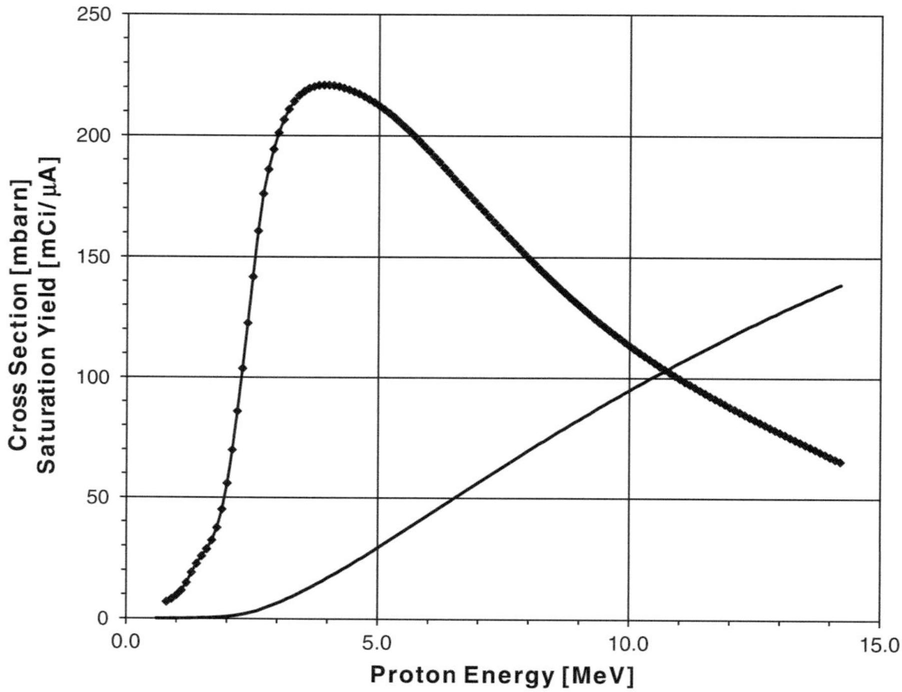

Fig. 2.4 Experimental cross section and theoretical saturation activity shown as a continuous line (Eq. 2.19) for the $^{14}N(d,n)^{15}O$ reaction

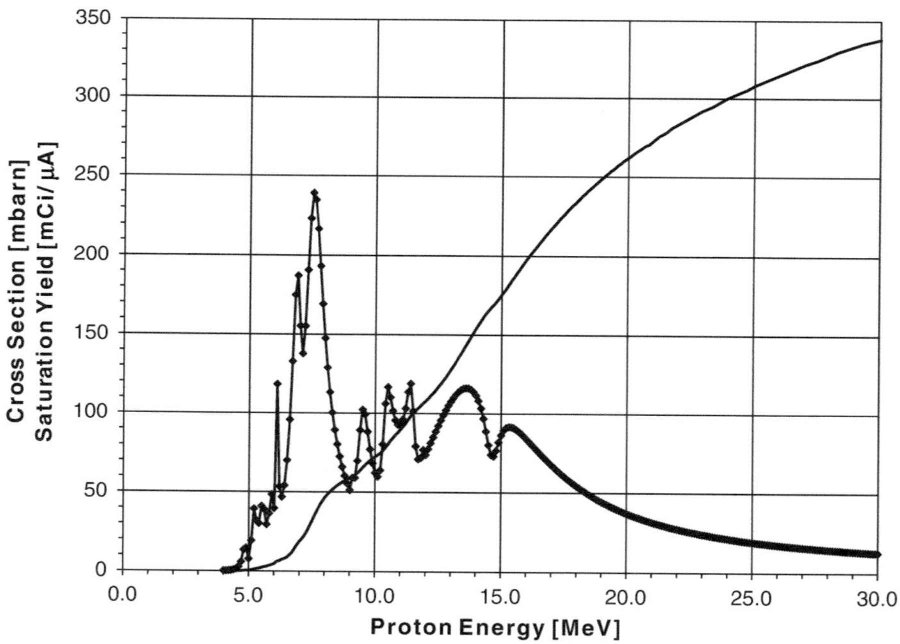

Fig. 2.5 Experimental cross section arid theoretical saturation activity shown as a continuous line (Eq. 2.19) for the $^{14}N(p,\alpha)^{11}C$ reaction

Where $\vec{E}$ is the electric field, $\vec{B}$ is the magnetic field, and $\vec{v}$ is the particle velocity. The vectorial nature of Eq. 2.4 requires intensity and spatial orientation to be considered for the magnitudes involved. The second term within the parentheses, defined as $\vec{v}\times\vec{B}=|v||B|\sin(v\angle B)$, shows that the magnetic field affects only the velocity component perpendicular to it. The electric field $\vec{E}$ is described as the difference in electric potential V per unit distance (gradient).

In the absence of magnetic fields, a particle exposed to a potential difference V will be accelerated to a final energy given by

$$E = E_0 + qV \tag{2.5}$$

where E_0 is the initial energy (not to be confused with electric field E). Equation 2.5 represents the basic accelerating mechanism behind any particle accelerator.

Static and alternating electric fields, from a few volts up to tens of megavolts (MV), are currently used for charged particle acceleration. For example, on an early Van de Graaff accelerator, an ion source is located inside a high-voltage terminal. Ions produced at this high voltage potential are accelerated toward ground potential, where the target is located. The acceleration takes place in an evacuated tube to avoid collisions between the ions and the air molecules. Maximum attainable voltage at the terminal is limited by practical considerations, and is close to 25 MV for state-of-the-art, large installations.

From Eq. 2.4 it follows that an alternative method to increase the ion's final energy, for a given potential difference, is to increase the ion's charge state (higher q). To take advantage of this mechanism, Van de Graaff accelerators have been modified to operate in tandem geometry. In this mode, the high-voltage terminal (dome) is kept at a positive potential respect to ground. Negative ions are produced instead, at the ion source outside the accelerator, and injected into the accelerator tube. The negative ions are attracted, and hence accelerated by the positive dome. After acceleration toward the positive dome, electrons are stripped off the negative ions by collisions with gas molecules or a micron-thin carbon foil. Projectiles thus converted into positive ions are accelerated by repulsion again toward ground potential (target). This configuration is very effective in achieving higher energies, especially for heavy ions, because the final energy is a function of the ion final charge state. For protons, the maximum attainable energy can be only twice the value of the dome potential. Another limitation of the tandem configuration is that not all species can be produced as negative ions in usable amounts.

Alternating electric fields are also utilized for charged particle acceleration. In this way, extremely high energies have been achieved. Again, positive ions are produced and accelerated toward a series of electrodes where an alternating electric field is applied. When the ions exit the first electrode, the electric field has already changed polarity, further accelerating the ions. Bunches of ions are then accelerated in this fashion. These linear structures, commonly known as linear accelerators, which are up to several kilometers in length, have successfully been used to accelerate ions to velocities approaching the speed of light. The applied electric fields amount to several hundred kilovolts at frequencies from tens of Hz to GHz.

The Cyclotron

First conceived by Lawrence in 1929, and successfully demonstrated in 1930 with important contributions from Livingston, the cyclotron was and still is one of the primary sources for medical radioisotope production. According to Eq. 2.4, in the presence of a magnetic field the total force experienced by the charged particle will have an additional component perpendicular to the plane defined by the particle velocity and magnetic field, thereby restraining the moving particles into circular orbits. These types of accelerators are known as *circular accelerators* (betatron, cyclotron, synchrotron), due to the approximately circular orbits described by the particles.

The introduction of negative ion cyclotrons over the past two decades has significantly improved exit projectile flux, which increases the amount of radioisotope produced. The main components of the cyclotron are the following:

1. Vacuum chamber: To minimize collisions between ions and air molecules and thus minimize beam loss, the acceleration process takes place in areas where air density has been reduced to approximately 10^{-9} times that of atmospheric pressure. A short aluminum cylinder provides an airtight seal between the magnet polar pieces. Vacuum pumps remove the air from this chamber.
2. Ion source: Positive ions are typically produced by collisions between gas molecules (hydrogen in the case of protons) and accelerated electrons emitted from a cathode. Source geometry and applied electric fields facilitate the extraction of produced ions into the main accelerating field. Negative ions are created by exposing desired gas molecules to an intense plasma discharge and again using favorable geometries and electric and magnetic fields to extract hydrogen (or deuterium) atoms that have an extra electron attached.
3. Magnet: A strong (~1.5 T) magnetic field is applied across the magnet pole pieces defining the vacuum region. The effect of the magnetic field on the ion trajectories is to maintain them in circular orbits and to constrain the orbits near a plane perpendicular to the applied magnetic field as determined by Eq. 2.4.
4. Radiofrequency field: Ions are extracted from the source and injected into the vacuum chamber by a high-voltage alternating electric field applied to the accelerating structures, also known as *dees* because of the original shape proposed by Lawrence. While inside these hollow structures, ions continue to travel in an approximately circular orbit. When the ions reach the transition region between dees, the electric field has reversed polarity so that the distal dee has a higher potential than the proximal dee to accelerate the particles in the transitional gap. The particles are not accelerated inside the dees. Tens of kiloelectron volts (keV) are gained during each transition. As the ion energy increases, its orbital radius becomes larger. Near the outer radius, where the magnetic field sharply decreases, ions have reached their maximum energy.
5. Extraction: When the ions reach the outer region of the vacuum chamber, the extraction mechanism varies depending on the polarity of the ions as injected from the ion source. In the case of positive ions, a negative voltage is applied to a plate placed around the outer radius, pulling the positive ions from the trapping magnetic field and directing them to proper targets or through a beam line for further transport. During this process, between 10% and 50% of the beam is lost. When negatively charged ions are accelerated, a thin foil, typically a few micrometers-thick carbon, is placed on the ions' path. At several million electron volt (MeV) energies, the beam will traverse the foil with insignificant energy loss. Electrons from the negative ions are lost by interaction (stripping) with the solid foil, thereby converting them into positive ions. This sudden reversal of charge polarity reverses the Lorentz force direction (see Eq. 2.4) and the ions are pushed out of the machine by the same magnetic field that was keeping them inside. Extraction efficiencies close to 100% are currently achieved using this mechanism.
6. Targets: Although the main purpose of the cyclotron is to accelerate a particle beam to fairly high energies, targets for radioisotope production should be considered an integral part of the machine. Liquid, gas, or solid targets for production of radioisotopes need to be tailored to the particular characteristics of a given cyclotron to optimize use of beam energy, intensity, and profile. They can be located in close proximity to the cyclotron, or the beam can be transported through evacuated tubes (beam lines) under the guidance of focusing magnets (quadrupoles) to a distal location or a different room.

Cyclotrons for medical radioisotope production are commercially available from several manufacturers (Table 2.1). Typical beam energies ranging from 8 or 9 MeV up to 30 MeV are considered standard. Single-energy proton-only machines are widely used for production of positron emission tomography (PET) tracers. The energy range

Table 2.1 Commercially available cyclotrons

Manufacturer	Model	Energy	Standard features	Options
CTI molecular imaging Knoxville, TN (www.ctimi.com)	RDS 111	11-MeV protons	50-μA beam single port	RDS Eclipse; higher beam current and higher yield; 18 F targets
			40-μA per target in dual-port mode (80-μA total); self-shielded	
EBCO technologies Richmond, BC, Canada (www.ebcotech.com)	TR13-19	13–19-MeV protons	100-μA protons; dual-port irradiations; fix energy or field upgradable to 19 MeV	Vault or self-shielded; 9-MeV deuterons on TR-19; 300-μA protons; multiple beam lines on one or both ports
GE medical systems (www.gemedicalsystems.com)	PETtrace MINItrace	16.5-MeV protons 8.4-MeV deuterons; 9.6-MeV protons	75-μA protons; six ports for targets Self-shielded	Vault or self-shielded Dual-port irradiations
IBA Louvain-la-Neuve, Belgium (www.iba.be)	CYCLONE 10/5	10-MeV protons 5-MeV deuterons	60-μA protons 35-μA deuterons	Dual-port irradiations standard on both models; multiple beam lines on one or both ports
	CYCLONE 18/9	18-MeV protons; 5-MeV deuterons	80-μA protons 35-μA deuterons	

Stated machine characteristics were extracted from brochures and/or Web sites provided by manufacturers. For latest features, contact cyclotron manufacturers between 8 and 19 MeV can supply most PET radioisotopes. Cyclotrons with energies of 30 MeV and higher can also be used for production of single photon emission computed tomography (SPECT) tracers (Tl 201, Ga 67, In 111, etc.). The other parameter defining radioisotope production rate is the available beam current from the machine. The higher the beam current tolerated by the target, the higher the amount of isotope that can be expected from a production run.

Production of PET Isotopes

Radioisotopes for PET

The physical properties of the four radioisotopes most widely used for PET studies are given in Table 2.2. These "organic" radioisotopes are particularly well suited for labeling biomolecules. Their short half-life provides the benefit of fast clearing from the patient's body, but it requires the on-site or nearby production of the radioisotope. Another important advantage of these radioisotopes is their high branching ratio for positron emission. The number of potentially useful positron emitters is certainly not limited to those included in Table 2.2. Several others have been successfully used for PET studies. Depending on the desired radioisotope, a combination of highly enriched target material or higher cyclotron energy or both may be necessary.

Production Cross Section

The concept of *cross section* for some event (σ_A) can be defined as the effective area per target atom presented to the projectile. Consider a target with area *S*, thickness Δx (small), and containing *N* atoms per unit volume. The probability (P_A) for a projectile to interact with a target atom producing an event (*A*) is given by the ratio of effective to total area:

$$P_A = n\sigma_A / S = N\Delta x\sigma_A \qquad (2.6)$$

where $n = NS\Delta x$ is the total number of target atoms

If the beam has a current density $J = I / S$, where *I* is the beam current, the average number of events (*A*) per unit time is given by

$$JSP_A = Jn\sigma_A \qquad (2.7)$$

Equation 2.7 is valid only for single charged projectiles. Because we are dealing with a number of events, the important quantity is the actual number of incident projectiles and not their charge state. For projectiles with charge state different from unity, for example; α particles, Eq. 2.7 needs to be divided by the projectile charge state.

Radioactive Decay

The total number of atoms $A(t)$ at time *t* remaining from the radioactive decay of A_0 atoms at time to, is

$$A(t) = A_0 e^{-\lambda(t-to)} \qquad (2.8)$$

where λ is the radioactive decay rate and $T = \ln 2/\lambda = 0.693/\lambda$ is the half-life of the radionuclide.

The total radioactive decay rate at any time is equal to the product of the total number of atoms *A* times the probability for radioactive decay λ_A, i.e., $A\lambda_A$.

Differential Equation for a Daughter Product

The radioactive decay of a nuclide A into a nuclide B, which is also radioactive, can be represented by

$$A \xrightarrow{\lambda_A} B \xrightarrow{\lambda_B} C$$

At any time, the activity of A is $A\lambda_A$ and of B is $B\lambda_B$. The rate of change dB/dt in the number of atoms of type B is then equal to the balance between supply as a result of the decay of A minus the rate of loss of B through its own decay:

$$\frac{dB}{dt} = A\lambda_A - B\lambda_B \qquad (2.9)$$

Table 2.2 Characteristics of commonly used PET isotopes

Isotope	Half-life (min)	Mode of decay (%)	End-point energy of β^+ groups (keV)	Maximum β^+ range in water (mm)	Principal nuclear reactions (energy range MeV)
^{11}C	20.3	β^+ (99.8), EC (0.2)	960	4.1	$^{14}N(p,\alpha)^{11}C$ (15–4)
^{13}N	9.96	β^+ (100)	1,190	5.1	$^{16}O(p,\alpha)^{13}N$ (20–5)
^{15}O	2.03	β^+ (99.9), EC (0.1)	1,723	7.3	$^{14}N(d,n)^{15}O$ (6–0)
					$^{15}N(p,n)^{15}O$ (15–5)
^{18}F	109.7	β^+ (96.9), EC (3.1)	635	2.4	$^{18}O(p,n)^{18}F$ (18–3)
					$^{20}Ne(d,\alpha)^{18}F$ (30–0)

EC electron capture

Replacing the number of atoms of type A at any given time using Eq. 2.9, we have

$$\frac{dB}{dt} = A_0\lambda_A e^{-\lambda_A t} - B\lambda_B \tag{2.10}$$

and solving the differential equation we obtain

$$B = A_0 \frac{\lambda_A}{\lambda_B - \lambda_A}\left(e^{-\lambda_A t} - e^{-\lambda_B t}\right) \tag{2.11}$$

The activity of B is $B\lambda_B$ or

$$B\lambda_B = A_0\lambda_A \frac{\lambda_B}{\lambda_B - \lambda_A}\left(e^{-\lambda_A t} - e^{-\lambda_B t}\right) \tag{2.12}$$

and since the activity of A at time *t* is $A\lambda_A = A_0\lambda_A e^{-\lambda_A t}$, we can replace into Eq. 2.12 to obtain

$$B\lambda_B = (A\lambda_A)\frac{\lambda_B}{\lambda_B - \lambda_A}\left(1 - e^{-(\lambda_B - \lambda_A)t}\right) \tag{2.13}$$

Production Yield

The process of radioisotope production by nuclear bombardment is mathematically analogous to the process of radioactive decay into a daughter product. The number of target atoms that are exposed to the beam during irradiation can be called A_0. The probability of transforming one of the atoms into nuclei B per unit of time can be called λ_A. Then, $A_0\lambda_A$ is the rate at which new atoms of B are produced. The target is equivalent to a radionuclide with activity $A_0\lambda_A$ producing the radioactive substance B. The probability λ_A is very small, but the product $A_0\lambda_A$ can be significant because A_0 is very large and can be taken as constant during irradiation ($A \equiv A_0$). Assuming that $\lambda_A << \lambda_B$, Eq. 2.13 can be approximated by

$$B\lambda_B = A\lambda_A(1 - e^{-\lambda_B t}) \tag{2.14}$$

The net activity accumulated during time *t* is therefore

$$B\lambda_B = A_0\lambda_A(1 - e^{-\lambda_B t}) \tag{2.15}$$

The interaction rate per unit of time λ_A can be calculated as the product of the current *I* of incident projectiles and the cross section, summed over the projectile trajectory, that is,

$$\lambda_A = I\int_{x_1}^{x_2} \sigma(x)dx \tag{2.16}$$

and by replacing $dx = \frac{dE}{(dE/dX)}$ and $\sigma(x) \equiv \sigma(E)$ we obtain

$$\lambda_A = I\int_{E_i}^{E_{Th}} \frac{\sigma(E)}{(dE/dX)}dE \tag{2.17}$$

where E_i is the incident projectile energy, E_{Th} is the threshold energy for the given nuclear reaction, $\sigma(E)$ is the cross section, and dE/dx is the projectile energy loss per unit of path length. Both magnitudes, $\sigma(E)$ and dE/dx, are experimentally obtained and readily available from the literature.

Rewriting Eq. 2.16 in a more practical way, we obtain

$$B\lambda_B = \frac{N_A\rho}{M} I(1 - e^{-\lambda_B t})\int_{E_i}^{E_{Th}} \frac{\sigma(E)}{(dE/dX)}dE \tag{2.18}$$

with $A_0 = \frac{N_A \rho}{M}$, and N_A the Avogadro's number, M the atomic mass, and ρ the target density.

Equation 2.18 contains all of the information necessary to calculate production yield for a given radioisotope. The number of new radioactive atoms being produced is proportional to the integral term, while the buildup of activity is described by the term inside the parentheses, which is a function of decay rate as well as the duration of irradiation. The exponential nature of the term within parentheses shows that 50% of the maximum attainable activity is produced in one half-life of the isotope. Extending irradiation through another half-life produces only an extra 25%.

The terms in Eq. 2.18 that are independent of beam current and irradiation time describe a quantity commonly known as *saturation activity:*

$$S_a = \frac{N_A \rho}{M} \cdot \int_{E_i}^{E_{Th}} \frac{\sigma(E)}{(dE/dX)} dE \qquad (2.19)$$

This magnitude is a function of projectile incident energy and is usually expressed in units of [mCi/μA]. It includes all of the necessary information to calculate production yields for any given projectile/target combination. Another commonly used magnitude that describes the production process is the *yield (Y),* representing the slope at the origin from Eq. 2.18 and is defined as

$$Y = S_a \cdot \lambda_B \qquad (2.20)$$

Production of Radiopharmaceuticals

The higher resolution and sensitivity provided by PET as compared to SPECT as a consequence of the colinearity of the two 511-keV photons after an annihilation event are not the only advantageous characteristics of the technique. The short half-life of the radioisotopes being used results in lower overall radiation doses to the patient. Simultaneously, it allows the use of labeled drugs in concentrations so small so as not to overwhelm the biologic systems or compete with the normal metabolic function while remaining well below any toxic levels. As an example, a typical 15-mCi dose of ^{13}N-labeled ammonia routinely used for myocardial perfusion studies represents 13 pg of product, many orders of magnitude below what is considered a permissible safety level.

Since the introduction of PET as a research and clinical tool, ^{18}F has been the radioisotope most widely used because of its practical half-life of nearly 2 hours as compared to other tracers with half-lives of just a few minutes. The reaction of choice for the production of ^{18}F during the early stages of development was ^{20}Ne(d,α) ^{18}F. After the introduction of the no-carrier added synthesis for 2-[^{18}F]-Fluoro-2-Deoxy-D-Glucose (FDG) in the mid 1980s by Hamacher et al. [1] , the production of ^{18}F using the reaction ^{18}O(p,n)^{18}F with highly enriched ^{18}O-water targets became the method of choice. Furthermore, it permitted proton-only machines with energies as low as 10 MeV to produce considerable amounts of ^{18}F. This rapid and highly efficient conversion method motivated equipment manufacturers to offer remote and automated equipment for the synthesis of FDG. Second- or even third-generation synthesis boxes can produce single, double, or up to four batches of FDG with a single setup. Decay-corrected radiochemical yields (conversion efficiency from ^{18}F into FDG) as high as 75–80% are routinely achieved. Preventive maintenance programs combined with proper personnel training have improved equipment reliability to better than 98%. Some FDG production equipment permits, through software reconfiguration, modification of the system to process other compounds.

^{15}O demands that the location of the camera facility be not more than a few hundred meters from the production facility. Proton-only machines require use of the enriched isotope ^{15}N as target material through the ^{15}N(p,n)^{15}O reaction. Given the high cost of the starting material, provisions to recover the enriched isotope should be implemented, if not supplied, by the cyclotron manufacturer. Facilities where deuterons are available can take advantage of the ^{14}N(d,n)^{15}O reaction without recycling the target. Rapid processing of the radioisotope transforms the target product into ^{15}O-water, ^{15}O-O_2, or $C^{15}O$ depending on the application.

Production of ^{13}N and simultaneous conversion to ^{13}N-ammonia is commonly achieved inside the target followed by a quick and efficient purification step through a disposable cartridge to remove potential contaminants (mainly traces of ^{18}F and metal ions from the target foil). Use of this tracer is limited to in-house production or distribution from a production facility within a relatively short distance.

Large amounts of C11 can be produced even with modest energy cyclotrons through the $^{14}N(p,\alpha)^{11}C$ reaction. Several commercial units permit rapid and efficient methylation of the target product (typically in the form of $^{11}CO_2$) as the precursor step for the radiolabeling of any number of compounds.

In general, a good number of other PET tracers can also be produced using enriched target materials at the low-energy end of commercial cyclotrons, with the option of in some cases using natural targets as the cyclotron energy is increased or when deuterons are available. Depending on the specific program requirements for one or several radioisotopes, a detailed analysis of different production routes, cost analysis of recovery processes in the case of enriched target materials, and an analysis of potential by-product impurities should be conducted prior to deciding on a particular cyclotron.

Facility Design

During planning and design of a particular facility, local and federal regulations for production of radiopharmaceuticals should be considered to ensure compliance and also to minimize the risk of potentially expensive upgrades or retrofit of the facility at a later time. Furthermore, current Good Manufacturing Practice guidelines and regulations should be firmly implemented together with a strong training and enforcement program to assure product safety and quality as well as adherence to the ALARA (as low as reasonably achievable) concept to minimize radiation exposure to production personnel and the public in general. Cyclotron manufacturers provide assistance with facility design and planning, but their responsibility is typically limited to issues related to machine installation and commissioning. In the case of self-shielded cyclotrons, radiation levels outside the shields and within some distance as promised by the manufacturer should be incorporated as part of the machine acceptance criteria. This acceptance test should be conducted at maximum machine output during irradiation conditions that maximize production of γ-rays and neutrons.

A health or medical physicist or other qualified professional should be consulted during design stages to address whether (or not) to install the cyclotron in a vault to evaluate the overall radiation shielding issues of fire and air conditioning, ventilation, air flow patterns, and exhaust monitoring. Personnel access and circulation through restricted areas should also be considered. Most facilities have adopted the criteria of keeping the vault or room where the cyclotron is located at negative pressure relative to the room where radioisotope processing occurs. The isotope production room, where the hot cells are typically installed, is also kept at negative pressure from the surrounding area for radiation safety reasons.

Reference

1. Hamacher K, Coenen HH, Stöcklin G. Efficient stereospecific synthesis of no-carrier-added 2-[^{18}F]-fluoro-2-deoxy-D-glucose using aminopolyether supported nucleophilic substitution. J Nucl Med. 1986;27:235–8.

From PET to PET/CT

3

Osama Mawlawi, Richard Wendt III, and Wai-Hoi Gary Wong

Preamble

In the decade since the previous edition of this chapter was written, positron emission tomography (PET) and more recently PET/computed tomography (CT), has continued to grow in prominence within the field of nuclear medicine imaging. Surveys conducted by the market research firm IVM (Greenbelt, MD) show an average annual increase of 10.4% in the number of PET and PET/CT studies performed between 2005 and 2008 [1]. The trend, however, has seen a decline in more recent years. The advantages of PET/CT over dedicated PET imaging (described below) have also drastically changed the characteristics of the scanner models that are available from manufacturers. As of the middle of the first decade of 2000, none of the three principal manufacturers of PET scanners (GE Healthcare, Siemens Medical Solutions, and Philips Medical Systems), still offered a dedicated PET system; only hybrid PET/CT systems were being manufactured.

As we predicted in the first publication of this book chapter, the majority of PET/CT disadvantages – high density media such as intravenous or oral contrast, mismatch between PET and CT as a result of respiratory motion, and truncation resulting from differences in the size of the field of view between PET and CT – have been mitigated through the development of hardware and software solutions. A brief description of these solutions is provided under the "Challenges of PET/CT Imaging" subsection.

The advances in PET/CT imaging that have occurred since the first publication of this book chapter have resulted in a dramatic improvement in PET image quality. Examples of these advances include: higher sensitivity through the use of 3D imaging and longer axial fields of view (FOVs), accurate modeling of the imaging chain in fully 3D iterative reconstruction techniques, higher light output and shorter decay time with new detectors, higher image contrast with time of flight imaging, and finally richer image fusion through the emergence of PET/magnetic resonance imaging (MRI) as a new hybrid modality. A description of each of these advances is included in the section "Recent Advances in PET Imaging."

Finally, the section titled "PET/CT Scanner Designs" has been updated to include the current commercially available systems from the three main manufacturers of PET/CT systems.

O. Mawlawi, Ph.D. (✉) • R. Wendt III, Ph.D.
Department of Imaging Physics, The University of Texas MD Anderson Cancer Center, Houston, TX 77030, USA
e-mail: omawlawi@mdanderson.org; rwendt@mdanderson.org

W.-H.G. Wong, Ph.D.
Department of Experimental Diagnostic Imaging, The University of Texas MD Anderson Cancer Center, Houston, TX 77030, USA
e-mail: gwong@mdanderson.org

E.E. Kim et al. (eds.), *Clinical PET and PET/CT: Principles and Applications*,
DOI 10.1007/978-1-4419-0802-5_3, © Springer Science+Business Media New York 2013

Introduction

In the past decade PET has emerged as a unique imaging modality with applications in cardiology, neurology, oncology, and psychiatry. It is unique among medical imaging methods in its ability to produce accurately quantifiable images of physiologic information, whereas other imaging techniques excel in their depiction of anatomic structures or their ability to image rapidly moving structures. The quantitative advantage of PET, coupled with the extended PET reimbursement by the major insurance carriers in the United States for a range of PET oncology studies, has further fueled the rapid increase in the clinical demand for this imaging modality. In this regard, research groups and industry have striven to optimize this imaging technique. One of the most recent developments in PET imaging has been the introduction of a combined PET/CT scanner. This chapter presents the reasons for this development. It discusses the advantages and artifacts presented by such imaging systems, the impact of PET/CT on patient management, and its applications in other areas such as radiation treatment planning.

PET Imaging and Its Disadvantages

PET is a noninvasive, diagnostic imaging technique for measuring the Accumulation of radiotracer in the human body. The majority of PET imaging has been performed in the field of oncology, where a whole-body PET scan using the radiolabeled glucose analog fluorodeoxyglucose (FDG) plays an important role in the diagnosis and management of cancer. FDG accumulation detected by PET has been shown to be a reliable method for accessing the glucose metabolic rate of human cells [2, 3]. Given that many malignant cells exhibit elevated glucose metabolism [4], FDG-PET has been used in the primary staging and therapeutic monitoring of cancer. The high sensitivity, specificity, and accuracy of FDG-PET in detecting cancer in different regions of the body have been the driving forces behind its widening use [5, 6]. PET imaging however suffers from several drawbacks such as: 1) high noise content in attenuation correction factors, 2) long scan duration, and 3) lack of anatomical landmarks. These drawbacks are further described in the next sections and are the main motivation for the development of PET/CT systems.

Transmission Scan and Attenuation Correction

In a whole-body FDG scan, the patient receives the radiopharmaceutical as an intravenous injection and then rests quietly for about one hour while the FDG distributes within the body. Following this waiting period, the patient is moved to the scanner and lies supine on the patient couch. The patient is then positioned within the field of view of the scanner and the imaging session is initiated. A PET scan is composed of an emission scan and a transmission scan. The emission scan is used to depict the distribution of the radiopharmaceutical in the body (Fig. 3.1a), while the transmission scan is used for attenuation correction of the emission data. In ordinary PET, patient attenuation is measured by rotating radioactive sources around the patient while the detectors that surround the patient collect the transmitted annihilation photons – hence the term *transmission scan*. The transmission scan is used to compute a map representing the linear attenuation coefficients of different tissue types at the corresponding anatomic locations in a manner similar to x-ray CT but with poorer image resolution and quality (Fig. 3.1b). Multiplying the emission scan by the attenuation correction map generates the final, corrected PET image (Fig. 3.1c). Accurate attenuation correction is a major advantage of PET over other nuclear medicine imaging techniques. Corrected PET images depict an accurate distribution of the injected activity with minimal distortion in the shape, size, and location of a lesion. The value of

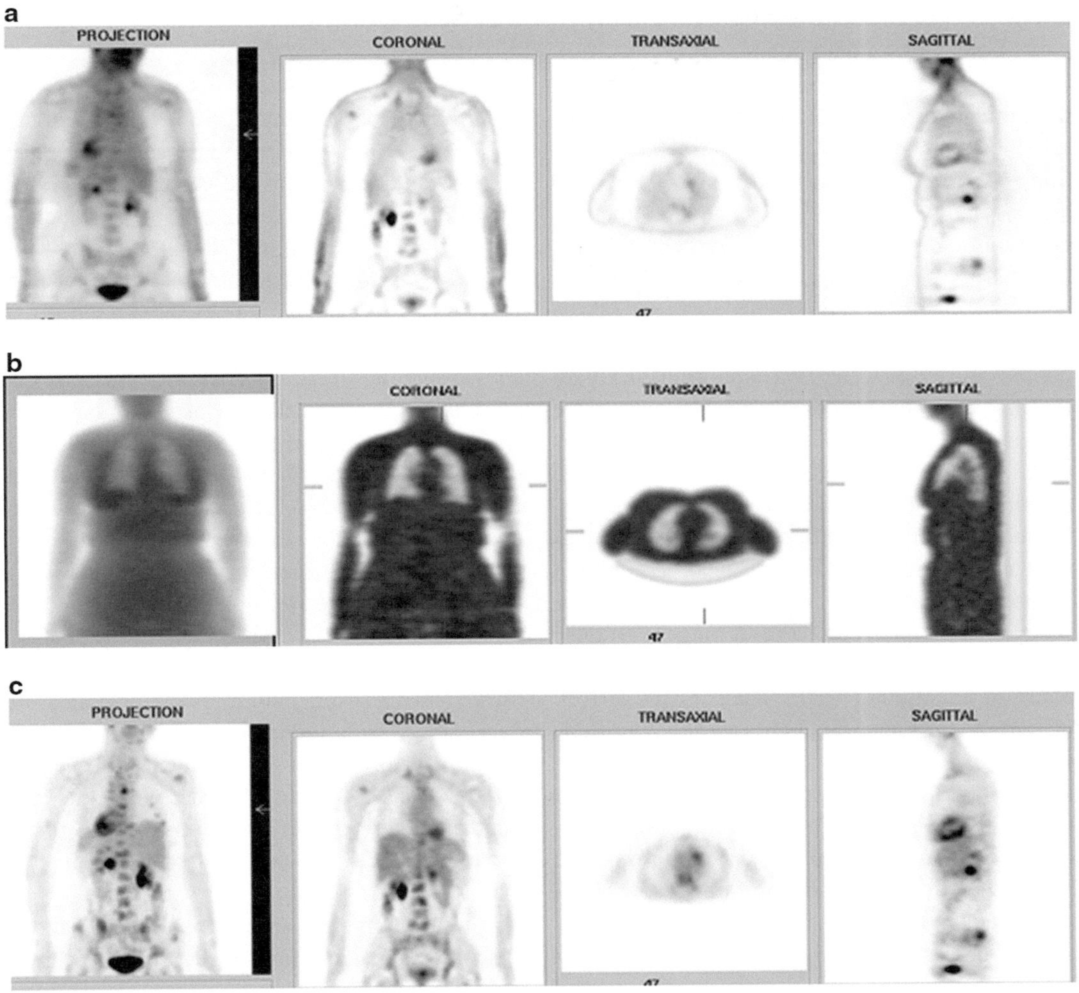

Fig. 3.1 (**a**) Nonattenuation corrected PET images; (**b**) reconstructed attenuation PET images; (**c**) attenuation corrected PET images

attenuation correction is further increased when it can be performed reliably and accurately with minimal inconvenience to the patient [7].

Historically, transmission scans have been obtained before the acquisition of the emission data. The time that it takes for the FDG to distribute in the patient (about an hour), and the requirement for exactly the same patient positioning for the acquisition of both the emission and the transmission data necessitated that the emission and transmission data be acquired consecutively without any time lapse. However, this produces transmission scans that are inherently contaminated by emission data. Such cross talk results in underestimated attenuation coefficients that can lead to inaccurate quantification of PET images [8]. Additionally, transmission scans using a rotating radioactive source are noisy as a result of the low gamma-ray flux of the radioactive source. The noisy data result in noisy attenuation coefficients. The propagation of that noise into the final, corrected image decreases the apparent lesion contrast and reduces the detectability of small lesions in the final image.

Several techniques have been proposed and implemented in routine clinical settings to correct these transmission scanning drawbacks [9]. For emission contamination, transmission windowing and/or transmission image segmentation are in use currently. Windowing restricts the accepted coincident events only to those compatible with the instantaneous location of the radioactive source as it is rotating around the patient and rejects the emission data in which the line of response could not physically have included the transmission source, which reduces much of the emission contamination in the acquired transmission data. Transmission segmentation, on the other hand, restricts the reconstructed transmission scan to a predefined number of tissue types (typically air, water, bone) that are based on a preset range of attenuation values. Each segment is then filled with a constant attenuation value that is characteristic of that tissue type [10, 11]. Transmission segmentation also significantly reduces the noise in the attenuation correction, thereby yielding a higher signal-to-noise ratio in the final, corrected images. Although these techniques have minimized the effects of emission contamination and noise, transmission segmentation results in an attenuation map composed of only the predetermined tissue types. Segmented transmission scans ignore the intermediate tissue densities in the patient [11], such as when a segment or voxel contains more than one tissue type. Noise in the transmission scan can also be reduced by acquiring transmission data for a longer period of time or by using higher radioactivity transmission sources. Both of these techniques, however, have drawbacks. A longer transmission scan time results in a higher probability of patient motion during the scanning session which reduces the spatial accuracy of the transmission image, and increases the inconvenience to the patient. A higher radioactivity source on the other hand, results in larger detector dead time and less accuracy in determining the attenuation factors.

PET Scan Duration

The acquisition of a transmission and emission scan to generate a corrected PET image requires a relatively long imaging session, particularly when whole-body scans are performed. Because the axial field of view of current PET scanners is only 15–17 cm, several pairs of emission and transmission scans (typically 5–7 in number) are needed to cover the whole height of a patient to obtain a whole body scan. Clinical studies have shown that the optimum scan duration per axial field of view (often called a "bed position") is in the range of 3–5 min for the acquisition of the emission data and 2–3 min for the acquisition of the transmission data. The ranges reflect differences among scanners and the effect of the girth of the patient. This translates into a total scanning time of 25–60 min (of which 10–20 min is for transmission data), during which the patient should remain motionless to minimize the mismatch between the emission and transmission data, as well as to reduce image blurring. Such a scanning paradigm is inconvenient and uncomfortable for the patient. Furthermore, the PET scanner could output more (i.e., scan more patients in a day) if each patient's examination took less time.

The challenge lies in the compromise among the competing demands of increasing the accuracy of attenuation correction by, lowering the noise propagated into the final image by this process, minimizing the mismatch between the true and measured attenuation maps, and minimizing the scanning time for maximum patient throughput. Ideally, attenuation correction would add little to the overall scanning time, giving it a negligible effect on patient throughput, and there would be essentially no noise and no segmentation errors propagated into the final attenuation-corrected image. These requirements, contrasted with the current state of attenuation correction, have led some clinics to skip transmission scanning altogether and to rely on images that have not been corrected for attenuation for their clinical evaluation of patients. The benefit of eliminating the lengthy transmission scan is argued to by far outweigh the gain from accurate depiction of activity concentration [12, 13]. However, the clinical importance of quantitative PET, especially with accurate mapping to the patient's anatomy, as described in this book, would contradict this argument and bolster the case for attenuation correction for the sake of good care of the patient.

Image Registration and Fusion

Following the acquisition, attenuation correction, and reconstruction of PET data, the images are displayed for clinical evaluation. Regions of interest are usually drawn around areas of relatively high activity concentration, and an outcome measure such as the standardized uptake value (SUV) is reported. A major difficulty for the precise interpretation of PET scans is the absence of anatomic structures. PET images are characterized by lower resolution and are imprecise in their anatomic localization of foci of abnormal uptake. The accurate anatomic localization of a lesion coupled with its activity concentration can be important information that can be used in the diagnosis, staging, and treatment of patients. The usefulness of fusing functional PET data with anatomic information from CT or MRI has been recognized in oncology [14–17]. It has been shown that the visual correlation of PET with CT can improve the accuracy of interpretation over that using PET alone [18]. Traditionally, image registration and fusion have been performed through the use of computer algorithms. Before the advent of the hybrid PET/CT scanner, two image sets acquired from two different imaging modalities at two different times would be analyzed by the registration algorithms, and a mathematical transformation that would align one image set with the other would be generated. One of the major difficulties with the registration of images acquired at different times, and perhaps for different primary purposes, is the different patient positioning between the two image sets. Although this difficulty is minimal when registering images of rigid bodies such as the brain [19], its effect on aligning whole-body images, wherein the internal organs are nonstationary and deformable, has resulted in less satisfactory registrations. For whole-body images, nonlinear image warping algorithms are needed; however, these algorithms require additional time to compute and are not always successful at aligning the two images, making their use less attractive in routine clinical PET imaging. Mental registration between PET and CT/MR images is usually performed by image readers. Such mental image registrations have, in the past, met the needs of experienced readers.

Advantages of PET/CT

To further improve PET imaging, the combined PET/CT scanner has been developed. CT measures the photon attenuation of the object being imaged, albeit at different electromagnetic energies than that used in PET. Mapping the CT attenuation coefficients corresponding to the different tissue types obtained at the CT equivalent energy to that of PET (511 keV) generates an attenuation correction map without the need to acquire a separate transmission scan [20]. CT images that have been acquired following FDG injection are less contaminated by emission data than are the source-based transmission scans described above. This is because of the large difference in flux (i.e., photons per second) between the CT x-rays and the emission gamma rays. In addition, CT images are characterized by shorter acquisition time and lower noise content than transmission images. This latter characteristic is dependent on the x-ray current setting of the CT scanner. The brief duration of CT scans occupies a small fraction of the overall time to scan a patient. Shortening the time that a patient must hold motionless reduces the discomfort of the examination for a patient and lessens the likelihood that a patient will move. Finally, CT images provide high-resolution anatomic information, which, when combined with PET images, can improve diagnostic accuracy and patient management [21–26].

Patient scheduling and radiation treatment planning are additional areas that benefit from PET/CT. Most patients who are scheduled for a

PET scan also receive a diagnostic CT scan prior to or after their PET imaging session [27]. These separate scans could be performed on the same PET/CT scanner in one extended session, thus facilitating patient scheduling and eliminating the need for transportation of the patient from one imaging suite to another. Patient waiting time would be reduced and throughput would improve. For radiation treatment planning, it has been shown that incorporating PET data into treatment planning along with CT has the potential to improve the accuracy of delineating the primary target volume [28–30]. Obtaining the PET and the CT data as a registered dataset greatly facilitates using the PET data in planning the treatment.

Challenges of PET/CT Imaging

Although combining a PET and a CT scanner has many advantages, this hybrid imaging system also presents a new set of difficulties, most of which are in regard to the use of CT for attenuation correction of the PET data. One of the major areas of difficulty is the presence of dense material such as dental fillings, metallic prostheses, and contrast agents within the field of view of the CT image. In the case of dental fillings and metallic prostheses, the resulting CT images are characterized by pronounced streaking artifacts as a result of the very high attenuation values. These artifacts are propagated into the PET image upon mapping the CT attenuation values to those corresponding to PET at 511 keV [31]. The propagated artifacts are manifested as high attenuation correction factors, which result in an artifactual increase in the apparent tracer concentration in the PET image [32]. For contrast agents, whether oral (barium sulfate) or intravenous (iodine), the overestimation of the attenuation correction factor presents an even more complicated challenge because the overestimation is dependent on the concentration of the administered contrast agent. The concentration of contrast agents in the body is not a fixed amount, but varies depending on several factors such as patient size, clearance, blood flow, and most importantly, the interval of time between the administration of the contrast agent and the acquisition of the CT. It has been shown that both oral and intravascular contrast agents affect the quantitative and qualitative accuracy of PET images depending on the contrast concentration [33–37].

In the case of contrast media, whether oral or intravenous, these effects have been minimized on current PET/CT scanners through the use of modified transformations from CT numbers to PET attenuation values. Figure 3.2 shows the standard bilinear transformation used to map CT numbers to PET attenuation values. The same graph also shows other transformations for different CT kVp settings that are used when an oral or intravenous contrast agent is present in the CT image. At the onset of a PET/CT scan, the operator of the scanner presses a button to indicate whether the patient has oral or intravenous contrast. This in turn selects the appropriate transformation based on the CT kVp setting and reduces any artificial increase in PET attenuation coefficients because of a corresponding increase in CT number. PET/CT scanners from all manufacturers are currently equipped with a similar approach to minimize the effect of oral or intravenous contrast. Extending this technique to handle the effects of other high-Z materials is an ongoing endeavor.

Another complication of replacing the transmission scan with a CT scan is the attenuation artifact induced by the patient respiration. The CT scans are characterized by short duration and may be acquired during any phase of the patient's respiratory cycle. The PET scans, on the other hand, require longer imaging times and therefore are acquired over multiple respiratory cycles. Thus, images from the two scanning modalities might show discrepancies in the anatomic locations of various organs. This is particularly evident in the areas that are the most affected by respiration such as the dome of the liver and the base of the lungs. Because the CT images are used for attenuation correction of the PET emission data, the mismatch between the two image sets results in large quantitative and qualitative errors in the corrected PET images [38–41]. It has been shown, however, that by acquiring the

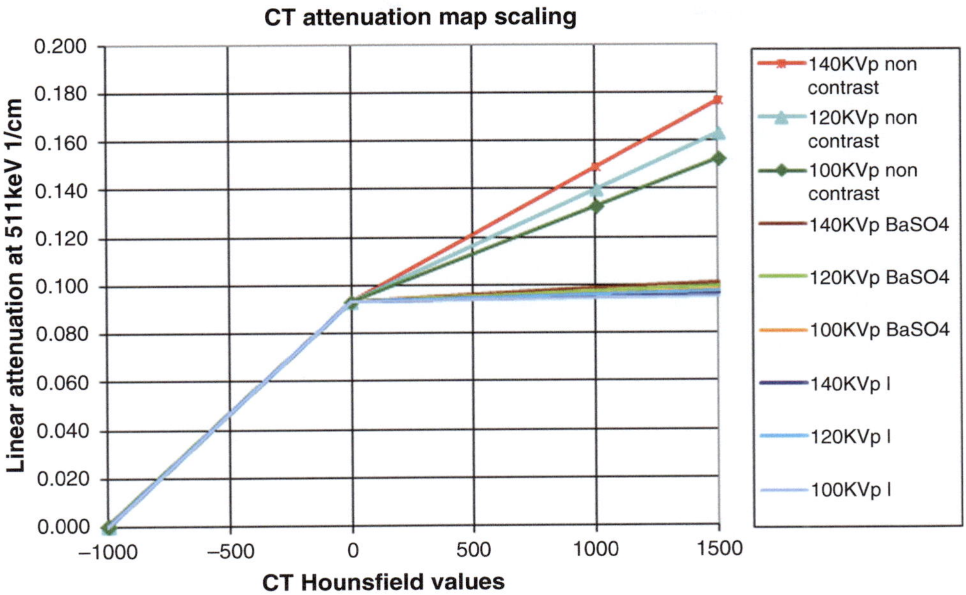

Fig. 3.2 Bilinear transformation to map CT numbers to PET attenuation coefficients at different x-ray tube energies. The graph also shows other transformations that are used when oral or intravenous contrast is used

CT when the patient holds his or her breath at normal expiration, or while the patient breathes shallowly, the CT images best align with the PET images, thereby largely reducing the magnitude of the mismatch effect [39, 42]. Alternatively, computing an average CT scan from multiple CT scans that have been acquired at different phases of the respiratory cycle can be used to mimic the average position captured during PET imaging [43, 44]. Respiratory motion is currently an active research topic in PET/CT imaging particularly because of its effects on radiation treatment planning. By accurately tracking the extent and trajectory of respiratory motion, the treatment plan can be improved by conforming the radiation field to the underlying tumor motion while sparing healthy tissues.

In addition to the mismatch between PET and CT, respiratory motion also blurs the PET image which reduces the measured activity concentration in areas of interest that are moving, such as lung tumors. Both of these effects have prompted manufacturers to develop motion tracking and suppression techniques that are collectively referred to as four-dimensional (4D) PET/CT. With 4D PET/CT, the acquired PET data are divided into multiple bins (usually 6–10 bins) depending on the phase or amplitude of the breathing cycle. Similarly, CT images are generated at the same temporal points as those at which the PET images were constructed. Each CT image is then used to properly attenuate its corresponding PET image. The resultant PET/CT image sets are then registered to one another and summed to generate a single PET/CT image set that is devoid of motion and mismatch artifacts. To track the breathing motion, several devices are now available from PET/CT manufacturers. The devices depend on either video cameras (such as the real-time position management system by Varian) or respiratory bellows (such as those from Anzai Medical Systems) to track and record a patient's breathing cycle. The complete set of software and hardware components necessary to acquire and process 4D PET/CT data is now available from all PET/CT manufacturers on different scanner models and can be purchased as an option on these systems.

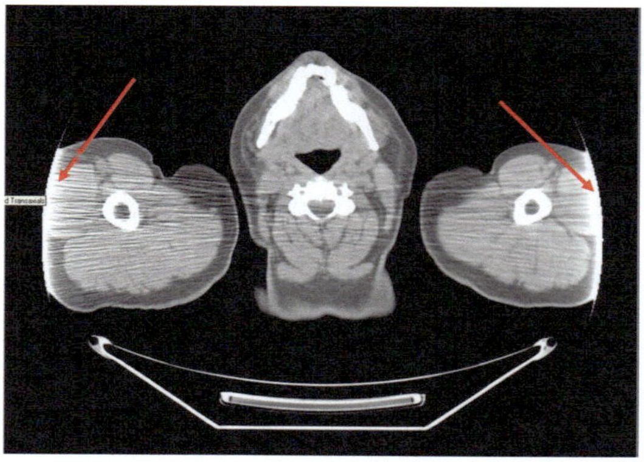

Fig. 3.3 A CT scan of a 145-kg man imaged with arms up. *Arrows* show truncation artifacts

Another technical problem that is encountered in PET/CT imaging is the difference in the size of the FOV of the CT and PET scanners, resulting in so-called truncation artifacts. Truncation artifact encompasses two forms of error. The first is encountered when imaging a large patient whose cross section extends beyond the FOV of the CT scan (typically a diameter of 50 cm), thus producing severe truncation at the edges of the reconstructed CT images (Fig. 3.3). The second is a result of missing attenuation data resulting from the difference in the FOV size between the PET (typically having an FOV with a diameter of 70 cm) and CT images. The first error is manifested as streaking artifacts at the edge of the CT image, thus causing an artificial overestimation of the attenuation coefficients used in PET as well as degrading the quality of the CT image. The second error results in uncorrected PET data around the periphery of the PET FOV. The two errors have been shown to affect the quantitative and qualitative accuracy of PET images [45, 46]. One way of minimizing these errors is by scanning the patient, in both the CT and PET positions, with the arms raised above the head, thereby reducing the cross-sectional dimension of the patient. This scanning position, however, is very uncomfortable for most patients and increases the likelihood of involuntary movement during the relatively long PET imaging session. Furthermore, scanning patients with their arms up strains the shoulder muscles, which might alter the accumulation of FDG in this region.

Another approach which is currently implemented on all commercially available PET/CT scanners, is to artificially increase the CT reconstructed FOV to match that of the PET. This process can be achieved in different ways, one of which is based on the assumption that the total attenuation per projection is the same independent of the angle at which it was acquired. That is, if all of the attenuation values are summed, that total should be the same regardless of the angle of the projection, as if the CT scanner measured just one huge voxel. Using this assumption, the missing attenuation from truncated projections can be estimated from projections that do not suffer from truncation. This process will result in artificially generated CT attenuation values in areas of the image where such values were not previously recorded. The accuracy of these generated values largely depends on the underlying estimation process. However, because in the majority of the cases the truncated areas are soft tissue, the estimation process results in relatively little error in CT attenuation values. Different proprietary names are given to this process by manufacturers, such as WideView or AC Plus. The scanner operator should preselect the extended FOV option during image reconstruction to ensure that there is no truncation between the PET and CT.

Recent Advances in PET/CT Imaging

Several advances in PET/CT imaging have been achieved since the first edition of this book chapter. PET image quality has improved dramatically, particularly with regard to image resolution, sensitivity, and signal-to-noise ratio. A description of each of the principle means by which the field has advanced to its current state follows.

3D Imaging and Increased Scanner Sensitivity

PET is intrinsically a three-dimensional (3D) imaging modality, replacing physical collimation required for single photon imaging with electronic collimation. Historically, most PET imaging was performed in two-dimensional (2D) mode, wherein lead septa were placed between the planes of detector elements primarily to reduce scattering photons from being detected. The result was better reconstructed image quality than was possible in the absence of the septa. 2D imaging was also preferred over 3D imaging because of the complexity of 3D image reconstruction algorithms, even though 2D imaging requires more administered activity to obtain adequate count rates, and 3D has roughly a five-fold greater sensitivity. This situation changed in the middle of the first decade of 2000 with the development of new scatter correction techniques and faster and more efficient 3D reconstruction algorithms. Those advances allowed 3D imaging to become the predominant mode of PET data acquisition. The advancement has convinced the manufacturers of PET/CT scanners to abandon 2D imaging altogether. Today, none of the manufacturers of PET/CT scanners are designing new systems that are capable of 2D imaging.

More recently, and in an effort to further increase scanner sensitivity, some manufacturers have increased the axial FOV of the PET system. PET scanners have historically had axial FOV extents of about 15–16 cm, as they were primarily used for brain imaging. Oncologic applications, requiring whole-body imaging, dominate the current demand for PET cameras and thus the value of a longer axial FOV is greater. Today, two of the three major manufacturers provide PET scanners with axial FOV extents longer than 16 cm. All scanners from Philips have axial FOVs of 18 cm. Siemens offers an option called True V on their scanners that extends the axial FOV from 16.2 cm to 21.6 cm, which improves the sensitivity of the scanner by approximately 80% as well as enabling the acquisition of a whole-body scan to be accomplished with fewer bed positions, and hence, shorter time period.

Iterative Reconstruction Algorithms

Originally, PET images were reconstructed using filtered back projection (FBP) techniques similar to single-photon and CT imaging. With the adoption of 3D imaging, FBP was extended to 3D with the work of Kinahan and Rogers [47] and the introduction of the reprojection algorithm. Statistically based expectation maximization iterative reconstruction techniques were developed for 2D PET image reconstruction and improved the reconstructed image quality compared with that from FBP. These reconstruction algorithms, however, only gained wider acceptance in clinical practice with the introduction of their accelerated version known as ordered subset expectation maximixation (OSEM), which was introduced by Hudson and Larkin in 1994. One of the advantages of the iterative reconstruction techniques is their ability to model various aspects of the imaging chain (such as attenuation, scatter, and normalization) during the reconstruction process. This in turn improves the quality of the reconstructed image while maintaining the Poisson nature of its counting statistics in the reconstructed image. More recently a fully 3D version of the OSEM iterative reconstruction algorithm that incorporates corrections for randoms events, scatter events, and attenuation has been developed [48, 49]. In 2006, this algorithm was improved by including corrections for the detector spatial response function resulting in a nearly constant resolution across the transverse FOV of the PET scanner [50]. The point spread function (PSF) of a PET scanner varies within the FOV. Photons emanating from the center of the FOV are normally incident upon the detectors. The obliquity of the path of the annihilation photons with respect to the detector elements is greater when the origin of the photons is closer to the periphery of the FOV. By measuring this variability and then modeling the PSF, improved and nearly uniform spatial resolution can be achieved throughout the FOV. Different forms of this algorithm are now provided by all manufacturers on their respective PET/CT scanners under different proprietary names such as HD or Sharp IR.

Time-of-Flight Imaging

The availability of fast scintillators with high-stopping power such as cerium-doped lutetium oxyorthosilicate (LSO) (or other lutetium-based detectors such as LYSO) has revived interest in the decades-old concept of time-of-flight (TOF) PET [51, 52]. TOF imaging requires the measurement of the difference between the detection times of the two annihilation photons from the annihilation event – hence the need for fast detectors. The difference in detection time is used to calculate the location of the annihilation event along the line of response (LOR) path. This process improves upon conventional PET imaging (non-TOF) where the location of an annihilation event is not known and hence is placed with equal probability anywhere along the LOR during image reconstruction. Unfortunately, the accuracy by which the arrival time of photons can be detected is on the order of several hundred picoseconds, which translates into a spatial uncertainty of approximately 10 cm in the location of the annihilation event. Even though there is still appreciable uncertainty in the location of the event, with this improved information the TOF reconstruction algorithms can significantly improve the reconstructed image. This improvement in image quality is manifest as an increase in the signal-to-noise ratio (SNR) that is proportional to the square root of D/d where D is the diameter of the activity distribution (i.e., of the object being scanned) and d is the spatial uncertainty. Current commercially available PET/CT scanners with TOF capability are equipped with timing resolution that can identify the location of an annihilation event to within 7–10 cm of spatial uncertainty in the scanner's FOV. For a 40-cm diameter uniform distribution of radioactivity (equivalent to an adult patient cross section), the increase in SNR is on the order of 2–2.3. As the TOF resolution improves, the spatial uncertainty decreases and the SNR increases by a larger factor. Furthermore, as the cross section of the object being imaged increases, the improvement in SNR also increases by a large factor. This is a particularly large advantage in image quality for large patients because conventional imaging of this patient population yields inferior quality because of low counting rates, or requires long scanning sessions at the expense of patient comfort.

Currently, all manufacturers of PET/CT scanners have systems with TOF capabilities. Philips was the first manufacturer to provide such a system in 2007 with the introduction of the Gemini Trueflight TF. Siemens and GE then followed suit with the introduction of the Biograph mCT and GE 690, respectively.

PET/MRI

Although this chapter carries PET/CT in its title, a brief description of PET/MRI is necessary to provide a complete picture of the status of hybrid PET systems. In as much as separately acquired CT images were fused with PET studies, separately acquired MRI data have also been fused with PET. The results have been enticing. Since the introduction of PET/CT imaging and its widespread use by the medical imaging community, manufacturers as well as physicians and scientists started thinking about replacing CT with MRI for a PET/MRI hybrid system. The attraction of such a combined system is based upon the high tissue contrast and nonionizing radiation of MRI as compared with CT imaging. PET/MRI has the further advantage of simultaneous acquisition of the two modalities as compared with the contemporaneous, but sequential imaging process in PET/CT. The latter advantage has specific utility for brain imaging when conducting challenge studies where the stimuli and processes being studied are dynamic. On the other hand, the technical challenges of PET/MRI include the lack of photon attenuation information with which to correct the PET data, nonuniformity of the MRI FOV, truncation artifacts resulting from differences in the FOV size between PET and MRI, susceptibility artifacts in MRI, detecting photons in the presence of a strong magnetic field, and most importantly, a clinical application that specifically would benefit from a hybrid PET/MRI as opposed to PET/CT. This last challenge is of particular importance when keeping in mind that PET/CT imaging is mainly used for oncologic whole-body imaging where simultaneous data acquisition might not be of great advantage. Notwithstanding, both Siemens and Philips have introduced hybrid PET/MRI systems that are commercially available. The Siemens system, named mMR, is a true simultaneous PET/MRI device whereby the PET scanner is integrated within the MRI FOV. To actualize this system, Siemens had to utilize new PET detectors, which are based on avalanche photo diodes that are immune to the effects of magnetic fields. These detectors, however, are not capable of highly precise timing resolution and therefore the mMR system from Siemens is not capable of TOF imaging. Still, this device is the first true PET/MRI system available on the market that is capable of simultaneously acquiring PET and MR images. The system uses advanced MRI acquisition techniques to help in segmenting the MR images into different tissue types that are later transformed into PET attenuation coefficients for attenuation correction.

The system from Philips on the other hand, is based on contemporaneous acquisition of PET and MRI data similar to the PET/CT design. In this system, the two gantries (PET and MRI) are physically separated from one another by about 4.5 m to minimize the effects of the MRI magnetic field on the PET detectors. Additional PET detector magnetic shielding has also been designed to further reduce the magnetic field effects. A patient couch is installed between the two gantries and is designed to move the patient from one scanner to the other while allowing the patient to remain still in the frame of reference of the couch. The minimized effects of the magnetic field on the PET detectors allows Philips to still offer this scanner with TOF capabilities, which is an advantage over the Siemens design. However, the large distance between the two gantries requires room space that is much larger than that needed for a standard PET/CT. The entire PET/MRI room must be shielded to exclude radiofrequency interference as well as to attenuate ionizing radiation.

Currently, GE Healthcare does not offer a PET/MRI system. Their solution to PET/MRI is to provide a transporter that moves the patient between a dedicated PET/CT and an MRI system. The transporter helps keep the patient in the same orientation during the imaging processes of both PET/CT and MRI, thereby ensuring good image registration without the need to rely on deformable registration algorithms that would be necessary if the patient were to walk from one scanner to the other. The transporter has a pallet that can dock onto the PET/CT and MRI systems without having to move the patient on its couch. During imaging, the patient lies on the pallet and is later transported to the other scanner. One advantage of this approach is that patient utilization of the two scanners is maximized as one scanner need not be idle while the other scanner is being used, which is the case in the Philips design. At the time of this writing, GE Healthcare indicated that they are working on a new simultaneous PET/MRI system that will be available in the next 1–2 years.

The remainder of this chapter discusses the design specifications of PET/CT scanners in general, and of those that are commercially available in particular.

PET/CT Scanner Design

PET/CT scanners are composed of a PET scanner attached to a CT scanner back-to-back with coaxial bores. The combined structure (except for scanner designs from Philips medical systems) is housed in a single gantry. The CT scanner is usually in the front, and the PET device is located behind the CT. The centers of the two tomographs are separated by 60–70 cm axially to allow space for the CT and PET electronics and to minimize cross talk between the CT and PET detectors. This distance is also important to minimize the temperature variations – critical for the stability of the PET detectors – inside the gantry as a result of turning the CT x-ray tube on and off. The patient couch is located in front of the scanner and is used to advance the patient from the CT to the PET FOV. Because the center of the two tomographs is separated by a large distance, the whole patient couch assembly is translated in the axial direction rather than just translating the patient pallet. This is done to minimize the deflection of the pallet because of patient weight as it is extending from the CT to the PET FOV.

Depending on the manufacturer, the individual CT and PET scanner designs can vary considerably. All CT scanners are now multi-slice systems with helical or axial imaging capabilities, and with different rotation speeds, whereas the PET scanners are capable of only 3D imaging, with bismuth germinate (BGO), LSO, or other lutetium-based detectors such as LYSO, and have a different number of slices per axial FOV. The functionality of PET/CT scanners, however, is the same regardless of manufacturer. Typically, a CT localizer (sometimes called a scout view or a topogram) is acquired to ensure proper patient positioning. This is followed by the CT scan, which is used to generate anatomic images and attenuation maps. At the end of the CT scan, the patient couch assembly is advanced from the CT to the PET FOV, where the PET acquisition is initiated. Following the data acquisition and reconstruction, the PET and CT images can be displayed side by side or fused together. The acquisition of PET data followed by CT is also possible on the systems of all manufacturers. Sophisticated image processing algorithms allow the PET and CT data to be displayed at the same anatomic location even though the PET and CT slices have different thicknesses.

The first prototype PET/CT scanner was developed by David Townsend at the University of Pittsburgh in joint collaboration with CTI Inc. (Knoxville, TN). The initial design work began with a grant from the National Cancer Institute in 1995, and the prototype became operational in 1998. The prototype PET/CT scanner was based on a spiral CT scanner, the single-slice Somatom AR.SP (Siemens; Iselin, NJ), mated to a rotating partial-ring positron emission tomograph, the emission computed axial tomography, advanced rotating tomograph scanner. Both the PET and CT components were mounted on the same assembly with the PET components on the reverse side of the rotating support of the CT scanner. Both scanners were housed inside a single gantry with the centers of the two tomographs offset by 60 cm in the axial direction, allowing a dual-modality examination range of only 100 cm. The design specifics and the first PET/CT images produced on this prototype scanner can be found elsewhere [53]. The widespread recognition of the importance of imaging anatomy and function together, led by the studies performed on this prototype PET/CT scanner, created a demand for combined PET/CT scanners for imaging cancer in the medical community and stimulated intense commercial activity.

Currently there are three main manufacturers of PET/CT scanners: GE Healthcare, Siemens Medical Solutions, and Philips Medical Systems. Each manufacturer has three scanner models categorized in three tier levels – entry, intermediate, and advanced. GE offers the Optima 560, Discovery 600, and Discovery 690, respectively. Siemens offers the Biograph TruePoint, Biograph mCT 20 Excel, and Biograph mCT, respectively. Philips offers the Gemini TF PET/CT, the Gemini TF Big Bore PET/CT, and the Ingenuity TG PET/CT, respectively.

GE Healthcare PET/CT Scanners

Optima 560

The Optima 560 is the entry level PET/CT scanner from GE Healthcare. The major design considerations of this scanner are the following: (1) 3D-only system, which is a departure from the offering GE used to have on their previous scanners that were capable of both 2D and 3D imaging. (2) The PET system is based on BGO detectors. (3) It has 12,288 detector elements of $4.7 \times 6.3 \times 30$ mm arranged in four rings of 6×8 detectors. (4) PET axial FOV of 15.7 cm resulting in 47 slices each with a 3.27-mm thickness. (5) A transaxial FOV and a patient port of 70 cm. (6) The CT component comes in 8 and 16 slices with the smallest slice thicknesses equal to 1.25 and 0.625 mm, respectively. (7) Rotation as fast as 0.5 s per revolution. (8) The x-ray tube has a maximum power of 53 kW. (9) The maximum current output at 120 kV is 440 mA. (10) The weight of the scanner, including the couch, is 5,200 kg, and its dimensions are 225 cm (W), 146 cm (D), and 193 cm (H). Performance characteristics of the optima 560 PET/CT can be found elsewhere [54].

Discovery 600

The Discovery 600 is the intermediate PET/CT offering from GE Healthcare. This system is similar to the Optima 560 except that it has additional capabilities particularly related to motion compensation techniques. The system has the same PET and CT detector design and configuration and is provided in only 8- and 16-slice CT versions. Additional capabilities of the Discovery 600 are related to the performance characteristics of the PET system resulting in higher sensitivity (9.1 vs. 6.5 cps/kBq) and peak noise equivalent count rate (NECR) performance (76 vs. 54 kcps) when compared with the Optima 560. These are probably achieved by allowing larger coincidence acceptance angles in the axial direction. The Discovery 600 scanner also comes with the ability to reduce the nonstationary resolution behavior of PET scanners along the transverse FOV by modeling the PSF during the image reconstruction process. The system also has the option to allow data acquisition in list mode. The list mode gives the user a greater flexibility in designing protocols to evaluate image quality with different scan times. The Discovery 600 system is configured with an adaptive statistical iterative reconstruction engine for CT data, which allows dose reduction while maintaining the quality of the CT images. The system has the same dimensions as the Optima 560 scanner and the performance characteristics of the PET scanner can be found elsewhere [55].

Discovery 690

The Discovery 690 is the premium PET/CT scanner from GE Healthcare. This system has the same capabilities as the Discovery 600 scanner with the following two major differences: (1) LYSO detectors, and (2) TOF imaging capabilities. The LYSO detector elements are slightly smaller in size than their BGO counterparts with sizes equal to 4.2×6.3×25 mm arranged in the same manner as in the Discovery 600 and the Optima 560 systems. This configuration results in a total of 13,824 detector elements in the scanner. Because of the difference in detector material (LYSO vs. BGO) the PET performance characteristics of this system are different than the Discovery 600 and the Optima 560. The system sensitivity is 7.0 kcps/kBq while the peak NECR is 130 kcps. The lower energy window setting on this system is similar to all other systems from GE Healthcare and is equal to 425 keV. The overall PET performance characteristics of this system can be found elsewhere [56]. This system is offered with two versions of CT scanners; 16 and 64 slices. The latter is known as volume CT because of its relatively large axial extent of 4 cm.

Siemens Medical Solutions PET/CT Scanners

Biograph TruePoint

The Biograph TruePoint is the entry PET/CT scanner from Siemens Medical Solutions. The major design considerations of this scanner are the following: (1) 3D only PET data acquisition. This is a continuation of the trend that Siemens started in the past with scanners that are septaless and hence only allow 3D imaging. (2) 24,336 LSO detectors arranged in blocks of 13×13 detector elements of 4×4×20 mm. (3) PET axial FOV of 16.2 cm resulting in 81 slices of 2-mm thickness. (4) A transaxial FOV and a patient port of 70 and 60.5 cm, respectively. (5) The CT component previously came in four different versions allowing for 6, 16, 40 and 64 slices per tube rotation. Now this system is only available with a 16-slice CT scanner. (6) Maximum tube rotation times of 0.6–0.33 s per revolution depending on the CT option purchased. (7) The x-ray tube has a maximum power ranging from 50 to

80 kW also depending on the CT version used. (8) The weight of the scanner ranges from 3,200 to 3,980 kg, also depending on the CT version used. The scanner dimensions are 239 cm (W), 156 cm (D), and 202 cm (H). One upgrade option that is available on this system is an extended axial FOV from 16.2 to 21.6 cm (which Siemens refers to as the True V option). This option drastically improves the overall sensitivity performance of the scanner and represents the largest axial extent of any PET/CT scanner on the market. The other upgrade option is modeling the PSF during the PET image reconstruction, which Siemens refers to as the HD option. This improves the transverse resolution across the FOV. In addition, the scanner has motion management capabilities (both respiratory and cardiac). The performance characteristics of the Biograph scanner with and without the True V option can be found elsewhere [57].

Biograph mCT 20 Excel

The Biograph mCT 20 Excel is the intermediate PET/CT system from Siemens Medical Solutions. This system is similar to the TruePoint scanner except for a few additional software and hardware options. First, the CT portion comes in only a 20-slice CT version. The PET component, on the other hand, has TOF imaging capabilities and respiratory motion management. The combination of TOF and HD imaging (see above) is known as the Ultra HD option by Siemens. The patient port was increased from 70 to 78 cm and the transverse FOV was increased to 70 cm to match the size from other manufacturers. The sensitivity and peak NECR of this system have been optimized and improved over the TruePoint system and are equal to 5.3 cps/kBq and 100 kcps/kBq/cc, respectively. The same parameters of the TruePoint system are 4.2 cps/kBq and 96 kcps/kBq/cc. All measurements are based on a lower energy threshold of 435 keV. This system does not come with the option of extended axial FOV (True V) like the TruePoint system. The performance characteristics of this scanner can be found elsewhere [58].

Biograph mCT

The Biograph mCT is the top of the line PET/CT scanner from Siemens Medical Solutions. It combines the flexibility of other scanners by Siemens with respect to different CT slice options, TOF, and motion mitigation options for PET. The system has the same design features as the mCT 20 Excel with respect to patient port and transaxial FOV size. CT slice options available on this system are 40, 64 and 128. For the 128-slice option, the x-ray tube is rated at 100 kW. This system also comes with a True V option and has list mode imaging capabilities. This last feature (list mode), which allows greater flexibility for rebinning the acquired data, is only available on this scanner from Siemens. The performance characteristics of this scanner with and without True V option can be found elsewhere [59].

Philips Medical Systems PET/CT Scanners

The Philips Medical Systems PET/CT scanners are all based on an open design which is a departure from the standard integrated PET and CT systems within a single gantry (Fig. 3.4). The open design has a 30-cm gap between the PET and CT scanners. This distance can be further increased to 88 cm if needed. This design feature maximizes patient acceptance and comfort and allows easy access to the patient during the time of examinations. Philips Medical Systems was the first manufacturer to introduce a TOF PET/CT system to the market. In this regard, all PET/CT scanner models from Philips are TOF-capable and have a timing resolution of 495 ps. The "TF" in the name of all their scanner models captures this capability.

Gemini TF

The Gemini TF is the entry-level PET/CT system from Philips Medical Systems. Other design features of the Gemini TF system include: (1) 3D only imaging capabilities. (2) 28,336 LYSO

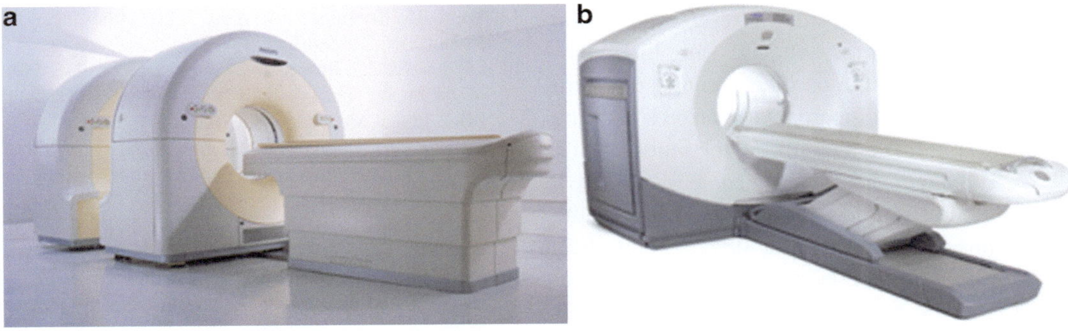

Fig. 3.4 Open PET/CT scanner design from Philips Medical Systems (**a**) compared with a conventional closed system (**b**). The conventional design shown is for the GE Healthcare Discovery 600

detector elements of 4×4×22 mm arranged in a continuous pixilated array. (3) PET axial FOV of 18 cm resulting in 91 slices of 2-mm thickness. This is the largest standard axial FOV extent on a commercial PET/CT scanner excluding the True V option from Siemens. (4) A transaxial FOV and a patient port of 67.6 and 70 cm, respectively. (5) The CT component comes in 16- and 64-slice options with the thinnest slices being 0.6 and 0.5 mm, respectively. (6) Rotation times of 0.4 s per revolution for both CT options. (7) Maximum x-ray tube output of 60 kW. (8) Maximum current of 500 mA. (9) The weight of the Gemini TF including the couch is 4,140 kg for the 16-slice CT option and 4,200 kg for the 64-slice option. The scanner dimensions are 225 cm (W), 549 cm (D), and 213 cm (H). Although this is an entry-level system, the Gemini TF has several options allowing it to compete with the highest tier PET/CT systems. Options available for this system are: Motion mitigation techniques and list mode acquisition. The sensitivity of the system is 7.1 cps/kBq while the peak NECR is 110 kcps/kBq measured at a lower energy discriminator of 440 keV. The performance characteristics of the Gemini TF scanner can be found elsewhere [60].

Gemini TF Big Bore

The Gemini TF Big Bore system is identical to the Gemini TF except that the patient port has been widened to 85 cm. This system is specifically designed to accommodate radiation oncology patients who need to be positioned in specific orientations to accommodate treatment plans. To allow for the enlarged patient port, the manufacturer needed to redesign some of the external shielding of the scanner and thus slightly modified the system performance. The system sensitivity of the big bore scanner is 6.6 cps/kBq while the peak NECR is 90 kcps/kBq when both are measured at a lower energy discriminator of 460 keV. The scanner dimensions and weight are slightly different than the Gemini TF. The CT scanner on this model comes only with 16 slices. All other features and performance characteristics are similar to the Gemini TF.

Ingenuity TF

The Ingenuity TF scanner is the high-end PET/CT scanner from Philips Medical Systems. The PET system design and performance characteristics of this scanner are identical to those of the Gemini TF. The CT components, however, are different. The Ingenuity TF has a CT scanner that is based on the Ingenuity platform, which is capable of acquiring 128 slices per rotation compared with the 16- or 64-slice options of the Brilliance CT platform available on the Gemini scanner. The 128 slices are achieved through wobbling the x-ray focal spot during data acquisition or what Philips refers to as the Ingenuity data acquisition and sampling technique. The x-ray tube on the Ingenuity platform is rated at 80 kW compared with the 60 kW of the Brilliance platform. In addition, the Ingenuity TF PET/CT system has optimized CT and PET reconstruction engines that allow reducing the patient dose without affecting image quality (CT optimization), as well as reducing the reconstruction time of the TOF data (PET optimization). All other features and performance characteristics are similar to the Gemini TF.

References

1. IMV Medical Information Division. PET market summary report. http://www.imvinfo.com/index.aspx?sec=pet&sub=dis&itemid=200076. 2008.
2. Phelps ME, Huang SC, Hoffman EL, et al. Tomographic measurement of local cerebral glucose rate in humans with (F-18)2-fluoro-2-deoxy-D-glucose: validation of method. Ann Neurol. 1979;6(5):371–88.
3. Huang SC, Phelps ME, Hoffman EJ, et al. Noninvasive determination of local cerebral metabolic rate of glucose in man. Am J Physiol. 1980;238(1):E69–82.
4. Smith TA. FDG uptake, tumor characteristics and response to therapy: a review. Nucl Med Commun. 1988;19(2):97–105.
5. Delbeke D. Oncological applications of FDG-PET imaging: brain tumors, colorectal cancer, lymphoma and melanoma. J Nucl Med. 1999;40(4):591–603.
6. Gambhir SS, Czernin J, Schwimmer J, et al. A tabulated summary of the FDG-PET literature. J Nucl Med. 2001;42(5):1S–93.
7. Bailey DL. Transmission scanning in emission tomography. Eur J Nucl Med. 1998;25:774–87.
8. Zaidi H, Hasegawa B. Determination of the attenuation map in emission tomography. J Nucl Med. 2003;44(2):291–315.
9. Meikle SR, Dahlbom M, Cherry SR. Attenuation correction using count-limited transmission data in positron emission tomography. J Nucl Med. 1993;34:143–50.
10. Xu M, Cutler P, Luk W. An adaptive local threshold segmented attenuation correction method for whole-body PET imaging. IEEE Trans Nucl Sci. 1996; 43:331–6.
11. Bettinardi V, Pagani E, Gilardi M. An automatic classification technique for attenuation correction in positron emission tomography. Eur J Nucl Med. 1999;26:447–58.
12. Bengel FM, Ziegler SI, Avril N, et al. Whole-body positron emission tomography in clinical oncology: comparison between attenuation corrected and uncorrected images. Eur J Nucl Med. 1997;24:1091–8.
13. Wahl RL. To AC or not to AC: that is the question. J Nucl Med. 1999;40:2025–8.
14. Diederichs CG. Prospective comparison of FDG-PET of pancreatic tumors with high end spiral CT and MRI. J Nucl Med. 1998;39(5):81.
15. Eubank WB, Mankoff DA, Schmeidl UP. Imaging of oncologic patients: benefit of combined CT and FDG-PET in the diagnosis of malignancy. Am J Roentgenol. 1998;171:1103–10.
16. Wahl RL, Quint LE, Greenough RL, et al. Staging of mediastinal non-small cell lung cancer with FDG-PET, CT and fusion images: preliminary prospective evaluation. Radiology. 1994;191(2):371–7.
17. Wahl RL, Quint LE, Cieslak RD, et al. "Anatometabolic" tumor imaging: fusion of FDG-PET with CT or MRI to localize foci of increased activity. J Nucl Med. 1993;34(7):1190–7.
18. Vanteenkiste JF, Stroobants SG, Dupont PJ, et al. FDG-PET scan in potentially operable non-small cell lung cancer: Do anatometabolic PET-CT fusion images improve the localization of regional lymph node metastases? The Leuven Lung Cancer Group. Eur J Nucl Med. 1998;25(11):1495–501.
19. Woods RP, Cherry SR, Mazziotta JC. Rapid automated algorithm for aligning and reslicing PET images. J Comput Assist Tomogr. 1992;16(4):620–33.
20. Kinahan PE, Townsend DW, Beyer T, et al. Attenuation correction for a combined 3D PET/CT scanner. Med Phys. 1998;25:2046–53.
21. Hany TF, Steinert HC, Goerres GW, et al. PET diagnostic accuracy: improvement with in-line PET-CT system: initial results. Radiology. 2002;225(2):575–81.
22. Israel O, Mor M, Gaitini D, et al. Combined functional and structural evaluation of cancer patients with a hybrid camera-based PET/CT system using F-18-FDG. J Nucl Med. 2002;43(9):1129–36.
23. Cohade C, Osman M, Leal J, et al. Direct comparison of FDG-PET arid PET-CT imaging in colorectal cancer. J Nucl Med. 2002;43(Suppl 5):78.
24. Freudenberg LS, Antoch G, Mueller SP, et al. Preliminary results of whole-body FDG-PET/CT in lymphoma. J Nucl Med. 2002;43(Suppl 5):106.
25. Yeung HW, Schoder H, Larson SM. Utility of PET/CT for assessing equivocal PET lesions in oncology: initial experience. J Nucl Med. 2002;43 (Suppl 5):115.
26. Bar-Shalom R, Keidar Z, Guralnik L, et al. Added value of fused PET/CT imaging with FDG in diagnostic imaging and management of cancer patients. J Nucl Med. 2002;43(Suppl 5):117.
27. Mah K, Caldwell CB, Ung YE, et al. The impact of 18F-FDG-PET on target and critical organs in CT-based treatment planning of patients with poorly defined non-small-cell lung carcinoma: a prospective study. Int J Radiat Oncol Biol Phys. 2002;52(2):339–50.
28. Erdi YE, Rosenzweig K, Erdi AK, et al. Radiotherapy treatment planning for patients with non-small-cell lung cancer using positron emission tomography (PET). Radiother Oncol. 2002;62:51–60.

29. Mutic S, Grigsby PW, Low DA, et al. PET-guided three-dimensional treatment planning of intracavitary gynecologic implants. Int J Radiat Oncol Biol Phys. 2002;52(4):1104–10.
30. Dizendorf E, Ciernik IF, Baumert B, et al. Impact of integrated PET CT scanning on external beam radiation treatment planning. J Nucl Med. 2002;43 (Suppl 5):118.
31. Goerres GW, Hany TF, Kamel E, et al. Head and neck imaging with PET and PET/CT: artifacts from dental metallic implants. Eur J Nucl Med Mol Imag. 2002;29(3):367–70.
32. Goerres GW, Ziegler SI, Burger C, et al. Artifacts at PET and PET/CT caused by metallic hip prosthetic material. Radiology. 2003;226(2):577–84.
33. Antoch G, Freudenberg LS, Egelhof T, et al. Focal tracer uptake: a potential artifact in contrast-enhanced dual-modality PET/CT scans. J Nucl Med. 2002;10: 1339–42.
34. Dizendorf EV, Treyer V, von Schulthess GK, et al. Application of oral contrast media in coregistered positron emission tomography-CT. AJR. 2002;179(2): 477–81.
35. Cohade C, Osman M, Nakamoto Y, et al. Initial experience with oral contrast in PET/CT: phantom and clinical studies. J Nucl Med. 2003;44(3):412–6.
36. Arttoch G, Freudenberg LS, Stattaus J, et al. A whole-body positron emission tomography-CT: optimized CT using oral and IV contrast materials. AJR. 2002;179(6):1555–60.
37. Mawlawi O, Macapinlac H, Erasmus J, et al. Transformation of CT numbers to PET attenuation factors in the presence of iodinated IV contrast. Eur J Nucl Med Mol Imag. 2002;29:S108.
38. Goerres GW, Burger C, Kamel E, et al. Respiration-induced attenuation artifact at PET/CT: technical considerations. Radiology. 2003;226(3):906–10.
39. Goerres GW, Kamel E, Heidelberg TNH, et al. PET-CT image co-registration in the thorax: influence of respiration. Eur J Nucl Med Mol Imag. 2002; 29(3):351–60.
40. Blodgett T, Beyer T, Antoch G, et al. The effect of respiratory motion on PET/CT image quality. J Nucl Med. 2002;43(Suppl 5):209.
41. Chin BB, Nakamoto Y, Kraitchman DL, et al. Quantitative differences in F-18 FDG uptake due to respiratory motion in PET CT: attenuation correction using CT in end inspiration and end expiration versus Ge-68 correction. J Nucl Med. 2002;43(Suppl 5):210.
42. Goerres GW, Kamel E, Seifert B, et al. Accuracy of image coregistration of pulmonary lesions in patients with non-small cell lung cancer using an integrated PET/CT system. J Nucl Med. 2002; 43(11):1469–75.
43. Pan T, Mawlawi O, Nehmeh SA, et al. Attenuation correction of PET images with respiration-averaged CT images in PET/CT. J Nucl Med. 2005;46(9):1481–7.
44. Pan T, Mawlawi O, Luo D, et al. Attenuation correction of PET cardiac data with low-dose average CT in PET/CT. Med Phys. 2006;33:3931–8.
45. Carney J, Townsend DW, Kinahan PE, et al. CT-based attenuation correction: the effects of imaging with the arms in the field of view. J Nucl Med. 2001;42 (Suppl 5):211.
46. Cody D, Mawlawi O, Forster K. Preliminary study of CT transmission truncation and beam hardening artifacts on quantitative PET activity. Semin Nucl Med (accepted abstract). J Nucl Med 2003;44(Suppl 5):273.
47. Kinahan PE, Rogers JG. Analytic 3d image-reconstruction using all detected events. IEEE Trans Nucl Sci. 1989;36(1):964–8.
48. Comtat C, Bataille F, Michel C, et al. OSEM-3D reconstruction strategies for the ECAT HRRT. IEEE Nuclear Science Symposium Conference Record 2004; vol 6, p. 3492–6.
49. Liu X, Comtat C, Michel C, et al. Comparison of 3-D reconstruction with 3D-OSEM and with FORE+OSEM for PET. IEEE Trans Med Imag. 2001;20(8):804–14.
50. Panin VY, Kehren F, Michel C, et al. Fully 3-D PET reconstruction with system matrix derived from point source measurements. IEEE Trans Med Imag. 2006;25(7):907–21.
51. Mullani N, Wang W, Hartz P, et al. Sensitivity improvement of TOFPET by the utilization of the inter-slice coincidences. IEEE Trans Nucl Sci. 1982;29(1):479–83.
52. Budinger TF. Time-of-flight positron emission tomography: status relative to conventional PET. J Nucl Med. 1983;24:73–8.
53. Beyer T, Townsend DW, Brun T, et al. A combined PET/CT scanner for clinical oncology. J Nucl Med. 2000;41(8):1369–79.
54. GE Optima PET/CT 560 data sheet, 2011.
55. De Ponti E, Morzenti S, Guerra L, et al. Performance measurements for the PET/CT Discovery-600 using NEMA NU 2–2007 standards. Med Phys. 2011;38(2):968–74.
56. Kemp B, Williams J, Ruter R, et al. Performance measurements of a whole body PET/CT system with time-of-flight capability. J Nucl Med. 2009;50(Suppl 2):1546P.
57. Jakoby BW, Bercier Y, Watson CC, et al. Performance characteristics of a new LSO PET/CT scanner with extended axial field-of-view and PSF reconstruction. IEEE Trans Nucl Sci. 2009;56(3):633–9.
58. Siemens Biograph mCT 20 Excel data sheet, 2011.
59. Jakoby BW, Bercier Y, Conti M, et al. Performance investigation of a time-of-flight PET/CT scanner. IEEE Nuclear Science Symposium Conference Record 2008; Dresden, Germany p. 3738–43.
60. Surti S, Kuhn A, Werner ME, et al. Performance of Philips Gemini TF PET/CT scanner with special consideration for its time-of-flight imaging capabilities. J Nucl Med. 2007;48(3):471–80.

Radiopharmaceuticals

4

David J. Yang, Tomio Inoue, and E. Edmund Kim

Radiolabeled Ligands

Several imaging modalities including computed tomography (CT), magnetic resonance imaging (MRI), ultrasound, optical imaging, and gamma scintigraphy have been used to diagnose cancer. Although CT and MRI provide considerable anatomic information about the location and the extent of tumors, they do not adequately differentiate residual or recurrent tumors from edema, radiation necrosis, or gliosis. Ultrasound images provide information about local and regional morphology with blood flow. Although optical imaging showed promising results, its ability to detect deep tissue penetration was not well demonstrated. Radionuclide imaging modalities such as positron emission tomography (PET) and single photon emission computed tomography (SPECT) are diagnostic cross-sectional imaging techniques that map the location and concentration of radionuclide-labeled compounds [1–3]. Beyond showing precisely where a tumor is and its size, shape, and viability, PET and SPECT are making it possible to "see" the molecular makeup of the tumor and its metabolic activity. Whereas PET and SPECT can provide a very accurate picture of metabolically active areas, their ability to show anatomic features is limited. As a result, new imaging modalities have begun to combine PET and SPECT images with CT scans for treatment planning. PET/CT and SPECT/CT scanners combine anatomic and functional images taken during a single procedure, without having to reposition the patient between scans. To improve the diagnosis, prognosis, planning, and monitoring of cancer treatment, characterization of tumor tissue is extensively determined by development of more tumor-specific pharmaceuticals. Radiolabeled ligands as well as radiolabeled antibodies have opened a new era in scintigraphic detection of tumors and have undergone extensive preclinical development and evaluation.

Glucose Transport

^{18}F-fluorodeoxyglucose (FDG) PET has been used to diagnose and stage tumors [4–14], myocardial

D.J. Yang, Ph.D. (✉)
Department of Experimental Diagnostic Imaging, The University of Texas MD Anderson Cancer Center, Houston, TX 77030, USA
e-mail: dyang@mdanderson.org

T. Inoue, M.D., Ph.D.
Department of Radiology, Yokohama City University Graduate School of Medicine, Yokohama 236-0004, Japan
e-mail: tomioi@yokohama-cu.ac.jp

E.E. Kim, M.D., M.S.
Departments of Nuclear Medicine and Diagnostic Radiology, The University of Texas MD Anderson Cancer Center and Medical School, Houston, TX 77030, USA

Graduate School of Convergence Science and Technology, Seoul National University, Seoul, South Korea
e-mail: ekim@mdanderson.org

E.E. Kim et al. (eds.), *Clinical PET and PET/CT: Principles and Applications*,
DOI 10.1007/978-1-4419-0802-5_4, © Springer Science+Business Media New York 2013

infarction [15], and neurologic disease [16, 17]. 2-Deoxy-2-[^{18}F]fluoro-D-glucose was developed in 1976 for the specific purpose of mapping brain glucose metabolism in living humans. After the first synthesis of ^{18}F-FDG via an electrophilic fluorination with ^{18}F gas, small-volume enriched water targets were developed that made it possible to produce large quantities of [^{18}F]fluoride ion via the high yield ^{18}O(p,n)^{18}F reaction. This was followed by a major milestone, the development of a nucleophilic fluorination method that produced [^{18}F]-FDG in very high yields. These advances and the remarkable properties of ^{18}F-FDG have largely overcome the limitations of the 110-min half-life of ^{18}F. Although tumor metabolic imaging using [^{18}F]-FDG has been studied in the past two decades, its clinical application is still hampered by its limitations, such as differentiation of infection and tumor recurrence, and differentiation of low-grade and high-grade tumors [18]. To improve the diagnosis, prognosis, planning, monitoring, and predicting results of the cancer treatment, several other PET imaging agents are used to characterize tumor targets.

Amino Acid Transport

^{11}C-methionine is useful for metabolic imaging of tumors by PET [19]; however, it has too many metabolic pathways that make it difficult to obtain a rate constant [20, 21]. Because of its short half-life, it is also difficult to image tumors with slow uptake. To overcome these drawbacks, L-α-methyltyrosine (L-AmT) has been investigated in nuclear medicine, not only because of its biologic importance in the synthesis of protein or thyroid hormone, but also because of its involvement in dopamine or tyramine neurotransmitters [22]. Its analog, ^{123}I-α-methyltyrosine, has also been used for SPECT studies on brain and pancreatic tumors [23–25]. High accumulation of ^{123}I-α-methyltyrosine (I-LAmT) in tumors were reported. PET examination with ^{124}I-labeled α-methyltyrosine has been carried out in patients with brain tumors [25]. L-^{18}F-α-methyltyrosine (L-^{18}FAmT) was also developed. L-^{18}FAmT was synthesized by reacting L-AmT with $CH_3COO^{18}F$. A similar technique has been used to synthesize ^{18}F-labeled metatyrosine [26]. An electrophilic reactant, $CH_3COO^{18}F$, reacts with L-AmT to give a meta-oriented position on the benzene ring. L-^{18}FAmT is quite stable in vivo compared with 2-^{18}F-fluorotyrosioe [27, 28] or ^{11}C-tyrosine, which produce too many metabolites, thus making it difficult to obtain quantitative analysis [29, 30]. Although the radiochemical yield of L-^{18}FAmT was $20.3 \pm 5.1\%$ ($n = 5$) based on the radioactivity trapped in the reaction vessel, the radiochemistry purification using preparative high-performance liquid chromatography (HPLC) is time consuming. For instance, ^{19}F-nuclear magnetic resonance (NMR) analysis gave two isomer spectra of L-^{19}FAmT with chemical shifts of −57.5 and −61.0 using trifluoroacetic acid as an internal standard [31]. These two isomer product ratios are 1 to 5.6, which corresponds to 2-L-^{19}FAmT and 3-L-^{19}FAmT, respectively. These assignments were based on the isomer of ^{19}F-meta-tyrosine spectra reported by Dejesus et al. [31]. Recently, a rapid synthesis with high yield of O-2-^{18}F-fluoroethyltyrosine was developed [32–34]. Because introducing a methyl group in the α position could slow down the protein incorporation process, ^{18}F-fluoropropyl-AmT (L-^{18}FPAmT) was developed using a similar technique. The synthetic scheme is shown in Fig. 4.1. Both L-^{18}FamT and L-^{18}FPAmT are discussed in this chapter.

Markers of Estrogen Receptor Tissue

The presence of sex hormone receptors in both primary and secondary breast tumors is an important indicator for both prognosis and choice of therapy for the disease [35]. Currently, receptors are determined by in vitro analysis of biopsy specimens and the use of antiestrogens. Tamoxifen is the therapy of choice for estrogen receptor-positive (ER+) tumors. The detection and measurement of ER+ tumors by the use of a radiolabeled ligand should provide a useful tool for the detection of primary and secondary tumors, as it may assist in selecting and following the most favorable therapy, as well as predicting

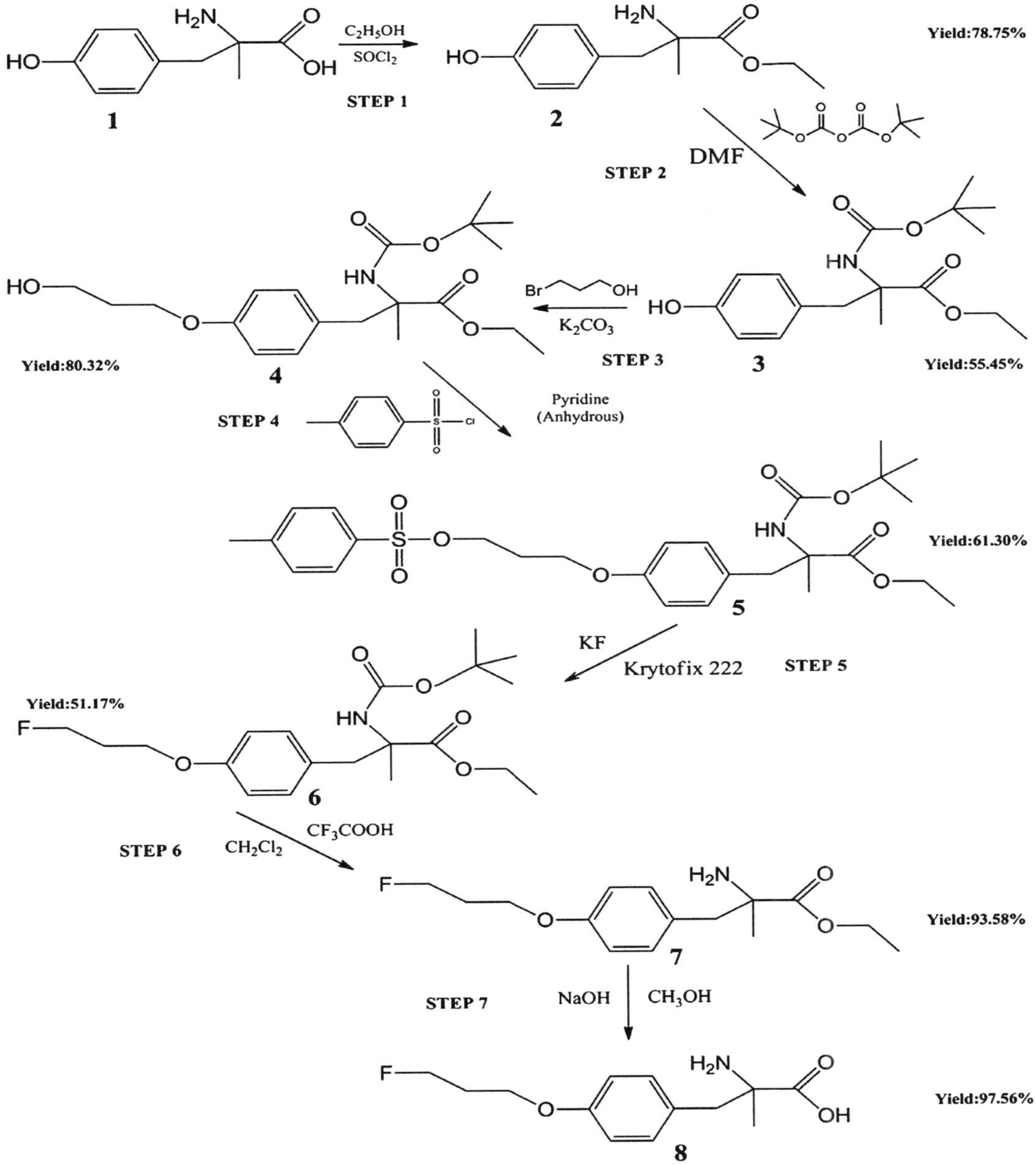

Fig. 4.1 Synthesis of ^{18}F-fluoropropyl-α-methyltyrosine

its outcome. To this end a number of variations of substituted estradiols have been prepared containing the radioisotope fluorine in the 16 position [36–38]. These compounds have been relatively successful in detecting ER-rich tissue in vivo, but their ability to provide quantitative information on receptor concentration in either animal models or humans has been less clearly demonstrated.

Tamoxifen therapy results are positive in 30% of unselected patients with breast cancer. A response rate of 50–60% was obtained in patients with ER+tumors [39]. Patients with metastatic cancer who do respond to the treatment have a response duration of 10–18 months and prolonged survival [40]. A radiolabeled tamoxifen ligand would be useful in diagnosing diseases that produce high levels of ERs, such as ovarian cancer, endometriosis, uterine carcinoma, and meningioma. Our rationale is that if the binding of the ligands with tumors can be detected with PET or SPECT, then such ligands may predict the response to anticancer agents' therapy for cancer. Radiolabeled tamoxifen would also be useful in investigating tamoxifen's mechanisms of action because it would provide more accurate information about the effectiveness of antiestrogen (tamoxifen) therapy.

Markers of Tumor Hypoxia

Misonidazole (MISO) is a hypoxic cell sensitizer, and labeling MISO with different halogenated radioisotopes (e.g., fluorine-18 or iodine-131) could be useful for differentiating a hypoxic but metabolically active tumor from a well-oxygenated active tumor by PET or planar scintigraphy [41–46]. [^{18}F] Fluoromisonidazole (FMISO) has been used to assess the hypoxic component in brain ischemia, myocardial infarction, and various tumors [47–52]. Moreover, the assessment of tumor hypoxia with labeled MISO prior to radiation therapy would provide a rational means of selecting patients for treatment with radiosensitizing or bioreductive drugs (e.g., mitomycin C). Such selection of patients would permit more accurate evaluation because the use of these modalities could be limited to patients with hypoxic tumors. It is also possible to select proper modalities of radiotherapy (neutron versus photon) by correlating labeled MISO results with tumor response.

It has been reported that MISO produced peripheral sensory neuropathy at the dose level required for radiosensitization [53, 54]. Thus, we have developed new MISO analogs by adding one hydroxymethyl group to MISO. This new ligand (halogenated erythronitroimidazoles; ETNIM) is more hydrophilic than FMISO. We used autoradiograms and radionuclide imaging techniques to demonstrate the potential application of FMISO and fluoro-ETNIM (FETNIM) to diagnose tumor hypoxia.

Markers of Lipid Metabolism

An elevated level of phosphatidylcholine has been found in tumors. It is the most abundant phospholipid in the cell membranes of all eukaryotic cells and provides a potential target for tumor imaging. This elevation is thought to be the result of increased uptake of choline, a precursor of the biosynthesis of phosphatidylcholine. Malignant tumors show a high proliferation and increased metabolism of cell membrane components that will lead to an increased uptake of choline [55]. Thus, [^{11}C]choline can be used as a PET marker for imaging cell membrane proliferation in prostate cancer [56], brain tumors [57], and many other types of tumors [58] that lack the urinary radioactivity seen with ^{18}F-FDG [56, 59]. [^{18}F] Fluorocholine and fluorine-18-labeled choline analogs also have been developed as new and promising oncologic PET tracers for prostate cancer and breast cancer [60–62].

Markers of Tumor Cell Proliferation

Noninvasive imaging assessment of tumor cell proliferation could be helpful in the evaluation of tumor growth potential and the degree of malignancy, and in the early assessment of treatment response prior to changes in tumor size. Radiolabeled nucleoside/nucleotide analogs should provide proliferative imaging information of primary and secondary tumors [28–32]. They may also assist in selecting and following the most favorable choice of nucleoside/nucleotide therapy and in following its outcome. Our rationale is that if the binding of nucleoside/nucleotide to tumor cell DNA/RNA can be detected with PET, then such a nucleoside/nucleotide analog may be useful in evaluating the response of nucleoside/nucleotide (e.g., 5-fluorouracil, 5-fluorodeoxyuridine, 5-bromodeoxyuridine, cytidine, cytarabine) therapy for tumors. Thus, for DNA/RNA markers, ^{18}F-fluoroadenosine, ^{18}F-fluorothymidine, and fluoro-^{11}C-methyl-arabinofuranosyluracil were developed. These ligands are intended to improve the understanding of the biologic behavior of malignant tumors, which should lead to better prognostic evaluation, treatment follow-up, and patient management.

Gene Expression Markers

Radiolabeled pyrimidine and purine probes for imaging herpes simplex virus type 1 thymidine kinase (HSV-1-*tk*) expression and other reporter genes by PET have been developed. For example, pyrimidine nucleoside (e.g., FIAU, 2′-fluoro-2′-deoxy-5-iodo-1-β-D-ribo-furanosyl-uracil [FIRU], 2′-fluoro-2′-5-methyl-1-β-D-arabinofuranosyl-uracil [FMAU] 2′-fluoro-2′-deoxy-5-iodovinyl-1-β-D-ribofuranosyl-uracil [IVFRU] and acycloguanosine [9-[(2-hydroxy-1-(hydroxymethyl) ethoxy)methyl]-guanine (GCV) and 9-[4-hydroxy-3-(hydroxymethyl)butyl]guanine (PCV)) [63–68] and other ^{18}F-labeled acycloguanosine analogs, such as 8-fluoro-9-[(2-hydroxy-1-(hydroxymethyl) ethoxy)methyl]guanine (FGCV) [65, 66], 8-fluoro-9-[4-hydroxy-3-(hydroxymethyl)butyl]guanine (FPCV) [67, 68], 9-[3-fluoro-1-hydroxy-2-propoxymethyl]guanine (FHPG) [69, 70], and 9-[4-fluoro-3-(hydroxymethyl)butyl]guanine (FHBG) [71], have been developed as reporter substrates for imaging wild type and mutant [67] HSV-1-*tk* expression. Recently, imaging, pharmacokinetics, and dosimetry of ^{18}F-FHBG were reported in healthy volunteers as a first step to imaging HSV-1-*tk* reporter expression in clinical gene therapy trials [72]. The difficulty with these probes is that HSV-1-*tk* enzyme expression depends on HSV-1-*tk* gene transduction with adenoviral vectors. The level of HSV-1-*tk* enzyme expression is likely to be different in the different transduced cells and tissues; thus, the application of the HSV-1-*tk* probe is limited. Understanding of tumor proliferative activity could aid in the selection of optimal therapy by estimating patient prognosis and selecting the proper management.

Synthetic Materials and Methods for PET Agents

Glucose Transport

A major advance in the synthesis of ^{18}F-FDG from [^{18}F]fluoride was made using kryptofix to increase the reactivity of [^{18}F]fluoride. Kryptofix masks the potassium ions, which are the counter ions of the [^{18}F]fluoride. The reaction of [^{18}F]fluoride with 1,3,4,6-tetra-O-acetyl-2-O-trifluoromethanesulfonyl-B-D-marmopyranase to give 1,3,4,6-tetra-O-acetyl-2-[^{18}F]fluoro-B-D-glycopyranase results in a 95% incorporation of ^{18}F, and the overall synthesis, including purification, proceeds to give approximately a 60% yield. The synthesis involves two steps: displacement with [^{18}F]fluoride and deprotection with HCl.

Amino Acid Transport

A nucleophilic reactant K^{18}F reacts with L-tosylpropyl-AmT to yield ^{18}F-fluoropropyl-AmT (FPAMT, 40–50%). The synthetic scheme is shown in Fig. 4.1.

Markers of Estrogen Receptor Tissue

Using clomiphene, a three-step process to hydroxytamoxifen, tosyl tamoxifen, and halogenated tamoxifen was developed [73, 74]. Eight *cis* and *trans* isomers of halogenated tamoxifen analogs were then prepared. In testing these two conformational isomers, we compared their killing power on human breast tumor cells as well as their binding power. Under our approved investigation of new drugs (IND number 40,589) from the Food and Drug Administration (FDA), we have assessed ER+breast tumors in 10 patients using ^{18}F-FTX (2–12 mCi IV). In a typical study, a patient is positioned supine in the scanner so that the detector rings span the entire breast. A 20-min attenuation scan is performed with a 4-mCi [68] Ge-ring source prior to administering ^{18}F-FTX. After each patient receives ^{18}F-FTX, six consecutive 20-min scans are taken. Serial transaxial images are obtained using the scanner (Posicam 6.5, Positron Corp., Houston, TX), which has a field of view of 42 cm on the transverse plane and 12 cm on the coronal plane. The axial resolution in the reconstructed plane is 1.2 cm. Twenty-one transaxial slices separated by 5.2 mm are reconstructed. Visual inspection as well as semiquantitative evaluation using standard uptake value (SUV, the activity in tumor/injected dose × body weight) was used. Before PET scanning, the position of breast tumors is determined by contrast-enhanced CT (High Speed Advantages, General Electric Co., Milwaukee, WI) or MRI using the 1.5-T scanner (GE Medical System, Milwaukee, WI). Eight of ten patients received tamoxifen therapy after the PET study. The response to tamoxifen therapy was evaluated after 6 months.

Markers of Tumor Hypoxia

Synthesis of [^{18}F]FMISO and [^{18}F]FETNIM

Aliquots containing 500–800 mCi of ^{18}F activity after 1-h beam time (18 μA current) were collected. The irradiated water was combined with kryptofix-2,2,2 (26 mg) and anhydrous potassium carbonate (4.6 mg), heated under reduced pressure to remove ^{18}O water, and dried by azeotropic distillation with acetonitrile (3 × 1.5 mL). The tosyl analog of 2-nitroimidazole (20 mg) was dissolved in acetonitrile (1.5 mL), added to the kryptofix-fluoride complex, and then warmed at 95°C for 7 min [42, 52]. After cooling, the reaction mixture was passed through a silica gel Sep-Pak column (Whatman Inc., Clifton, NJ) and eluted with ether (2 × 2.5 mL). The solvent was evaporated and the resulting mixture hydrolyzed with 2 N HCl (1 mL) at 105°C for 7 min. The mixture was cooled under N_2 and neutralized with 2 N NaOH (0.8 mL) and 1 N $NaHCO_3$ (1 mL). The mixture was passed through a short alumina column, a C-18 Sep-Pak column, and a 0.22-μm millipore filter, followed by eluting 6 mL of 10% ethanol/saline. A yield of 80–100 mCi of pure product was isolated (25–40% yield, decay corrected) with the end of bombardment (EOB) at 60 min. HPLC was done on a C-18 ODS-120 T column, 4.6 × 25 mm, with water/acetonitrile, (80/20), using a flow rate of 1 mL/min. The no-carrier-added product corresponded to the retention time (6.12 min) of the unlabeled FMISO under similar conditions. The radiochemical purity was greater than 99%. There were no other impurities under the ultraviolet (UV) ray detector (310 nm). A radio-TLC scanner (Bioscan, Washington, DC) showed a retardation factor of 0.6 for FMISO using a 5 × 20 cm silica gel plate (Whatman, Inc., Clifton, NJ), eluted with chloroform/methanol (7:3), which corresponds to the unlabeled FMISO. In addition, kryptofix-2,2,2 was not visualized (developed in the iodine chamber) on the silica-gel-coated plate using 0.1% (v/v) triethylamine in methanol as art eluent. The specific activity of [^{18}F]FMISO and [^{18}F]FETNIM determined were 1 Ci/μmol based on UV and radioactivity detection of a sample of known mass and radioactivity.

PET Imaging of Head and Neck Tumor Hypoxia Using [18F]FMISO

Under our approved IND number 43,997 from the FDA, we have completed three studies using [^{18}F]FMISO. In a typical study, a patient is positioned supine in the scanner so that the detector rings span the entire head and neck. A 20-min attenuation scan is performed with a 4 mCi [68] Ge-ring source prior to administering [^{18}F]FMISO. After each patient receives 10 mCi of [^{18}F]FMISO, six consecutive 20-min scans are taken. Serial transaxial images are performed using the scanner (Posicam 6.5, Positron Corp., Houston, TX), which has a field of view of 42 cm on the transverse plane and 12 cm on the coronal plane. The axial resolution in the reconstructed plane is 1.2 cm. Twenty-one transaxial slices separated by 5.2 mm are reconstructed and displayed in SUV, which measures the ratio of tissue [^{18}F]FMISO uptake to that of whole-body uptake (normalized for body weight and injected dose) for each scan. Before PET scanning, the position of head and neck tumors is also determined by contrast-enhanced CT (High Speed Advantages, GE Medical System, Milwaukee, WI).

Autoradiographic Studies of Misonidazole Analogs in Tumor-Bearing Rats

After receiving [^{18}F]FMISO (1–1.5 mCi IV), female Fischer 344 breast tumor-bearing rats and Lewis lung tumor-bearing mice (3/ligand) were euthanized at 1 h. The rodent body was fixed in a carboxymethyl cellulose (4%) block. The frozen body in the block was mounted to a cryostat microtome (LKB, Ijamsville, MD), and 100-ttm coronal sections were made. The section was freeze-dried and then placed on x-ray film (X-Omat AR, Kodak, Rochester, NY) for 24 h.

Polar Graphic Oxygen Needle Probe Measurements

To confirm hypoxic tumors detected by imaging, intratumoral pO_2 measurements were performed using the Eppendorf computed histographic system. Twenty to 25 pO_2 measurements along each of two to three linear tracks were performed at 0.4-mm intervals on each tumor (40–75 measurements total). Tumor pO_2 measurements were made on three tumor-bearing rats and three rabbits. Using an on-line computer system, the pO_2 measurements of each track were expressed as absolute values relative to the location of the measuring point along the track, and as the relative frequencies within a pO_2 histogram between 0 and 100 mmHg with a class width of 2.5 mm.

Markers of Lipid Metabolism

After ^{11}C-carbon dioxide production in a cyclotron and the subsequent ^{11}C-methyl-iodide synthesis, methyl-^{11}C-choline was synthesized by the reaction of ^{11}C-methyl-iodide with "neat" dimethylaminoethanol at 120°C for 5 min. Purification was achieved by evaporation of the reactants followed by passage of the aqueous solution of the product through a cation-exchange resin cartridge. The time required for overall chemical processing, excluding the cyclotron operation, was 15 min. Radiochemical yield was >98%. Radiochemical purity was >98%. Chemical purity was >90% (dimethylaminoethanol was the only possible impurity). Specific radioactivity of the product was >133 GBqb/μmol. PET was performed on cancer patients from the level of the pelvis to the lower abdomen. After transmission scanning, 370 MBq ^{11}C-choline was injected intravenously. The emission scan was performed 5–15 min postinjection. Finally, PET images were displayed so that each pixel was painted by a specified color representing the degree of SUV. The ^{11}C-choline image was compared with the ^{18}F-FDG image obtained from the same patient.

No-carrier-added [^{18}F]fluoroethyl choline [^{18}F] FECh was synthesized by two-step reactions: first, tetrabutylammonium (TBA) ^{18}F-fluoride was reacted with 1,2-bis(tosyloxy)ethane to yield 2-^{18}F-fluoroethyl tosylate; second, 2-^{18}F-fluoroethyl tosylate was reacted with *N,N*-dimethylethanolamine to yield ^{18}F-FECh, which was then purified by chromatography. An automated apparatus was constructed for preparation of the ^{18}F-FECh injection solution. In vitro experiments were performed to examine the uptake of ^{18}F-FECh in Ehrlich ascites tumor cells, and the metabolites were analyzed by solvent extraction followed by various kinds of chromatography. Clinical studies of ^{18}F-FECh PET were performed on patients with untreated primary prostate cancer, and the data were compared with those of ^{11}C-choline PET on the same patients.

Markers of Tumor Cell Proliferation

Using ^{18}F-Fluoro-2′-Deoxyadenosine [9-(2′-Deoxy-2′-Fluoro-b-D-Arabinofuranosyl)Adenine](FAD)

2′-O-p-toluenesulfonyladenosine (100 mg, 0.238 mmol) was derivatized along with N^6, O-3′, and O-5′ acetylated analogs by dissolving in tetrahydrofuran (5 mL) and acetic anhydride (2 mL), along with pyridine (2 mL) [75, 76]. The reaction was stirred overnight. The solvent, excess of pyridine, and unreacted acetic anhydride were removed by evaporation, and the residue was chromatographed on silica gel (with ethyl acetate as eluent). Aliquots containing 20–40 mCi of [18F]fluoride were combined with kryptofix-2,2,2 and anhydrous potassium carbonate and heated to remove $[^{18}O]H_2O$. The triacetylated tosyl analog of adenosine was dissolved in acetonitrile, added to the kryptofix-fluoride (fluorine-18) complex, and then heated at 95°C for 10 min. After cooling, the reaction mixture was passed through a silica-gel–packed column (SPE, 500 mg) and eluted with acetonitrile (ACN, 2 mL). After solvent evaporation, the acetyl groups were deprotected with 2 N HCl (1 mL) at 105°C for 10 min. The product was neutralized with 2 N NaOH (0.8 mL) and 1 N $NaHCO_3$ (1 mL). The product was then eluted through a reverse phase C-18 column (Sep-Pak Cartridge, Waters, Milford, MD) and a 0.22-mm filter, followed by saline (3 mL).

Markers of Gene Expression

Using a known procedure, di-tritylated tosylbutylguanine (TsHBG) was synthesized. Mass spectrum and NMR spectrum were determined. Under similar conditions for the synthesis of ^{18}F-fluorinated adenosine, ^{18}F-FHBG was synthesized. A C-18 reverse-phase Sep-Pak was used to purify the compound.

Results of Synthesis for PET Agents

The overall synthesis of ^{18}F-FDG including purification proceeds to result in approximately a 60% yield after displacement with [^{18}F]fluoride and deprotection with HCl. The simplest method to remove kryptofix is the incorporation of a short cation exchange resin in the synthesis system so that the hydrolysate (HCl) passes through the cartridge before final purification; 2-deoxy-2-chloro-D-glucose (ClDG) was identified as an impurity with less than 100 μg during chromatographic determination of the specific activity of ^{18}F-FDG preparations from the nucleophilic route.

Amino Acid Transport

Proton NMR spectrum of L-tosylpropylAmT is shown in Fig. 4.2. Figures 4.3 and 4.4 show HPLC and radio-TLC analysis of [^{18}F]FPAMT. There was a similarity in cellular uptake both in vitro (Fig. 4.5) and in vivo (Fig. 4.6) between [^{18}F]FPAMT and [^{18}F]FDG. Due to a zwitterion, there was much less uptake in brain compared to [^{18}F]FDG. Clinical images indicated that low-grade brain tumor could be imaged with [^{18}F]FPAMT.

Markers of Estrogen Receptor Tissues

Using MCF-7 cells incubated for 72 h, we observed that the eight new compounds were superior in killing power compared with tamoxifen; for example, the bromo had almost 25 times the killing power of tamoxifen [77, 78]. By using pig uterine cytosol, we noted that halogenated tamoxifen had a better binding affinity than tamoxifen itself. Bromotamoxifen was 150 times better than tamoxifen, and fluorotamoxifen had a binding power 30 times that of tamoxifen.

Of these eight different agents, we pursued fluorotamoxifen for its killing and binding power and were interested in using this technology as a PET imaging agent. Using the PET camera, the uterus of a pig was defined. We then administered the fluorotamoxifen and noted a configuration that was much like what we saw in the anatomic specimen, with the uterus and the fallopian-tube–ovarian complex. From the cross-sectional configuration it appears that fluorotamoxifen can be used as an imaging agent as well. By administering tamoxifen, or diethylstilbestrol (DES), the uptake in the target organ could be blocked [79]. As a breast tumor model, we used a rat with deposition of ER+ tumor cells (NF 13762 cell line) in the flank. In utilizing fluorotamoxifen, we observed uptake within the uterus as well as in the tumor in the flank, which suggests we have a fluorinated

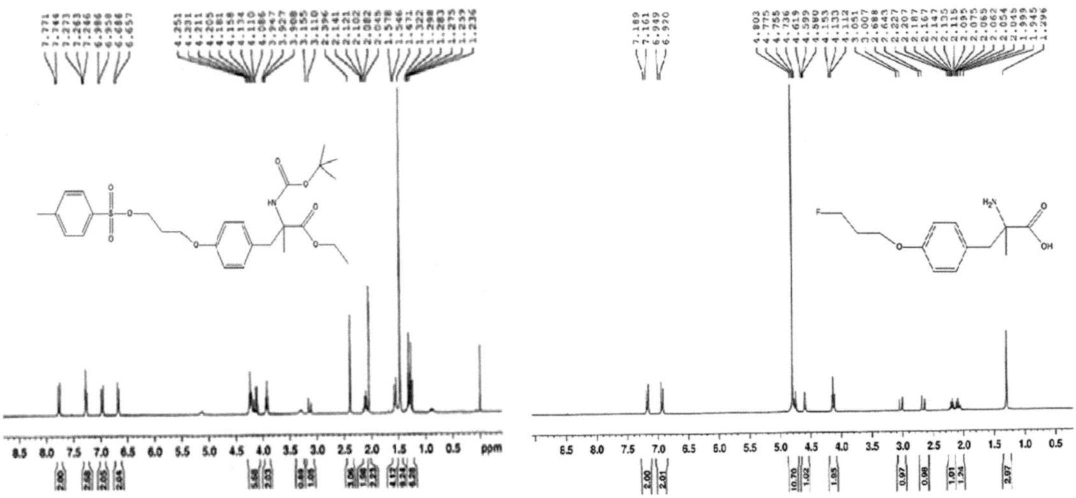

Fig. 4.2 ^{1}H-NMR of N-BOC-tosylpropyl-α-methyltyrosine methyl ester

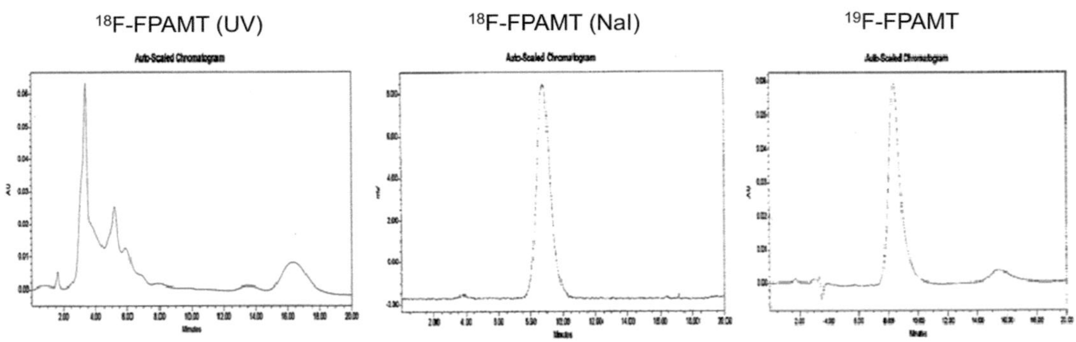

Fig. 4.3 High-performance liquid chromatography (HPLC) analysis of ^{18}F-FPAMT (*left*: radioactive, *right*: ultraviolet [UV])

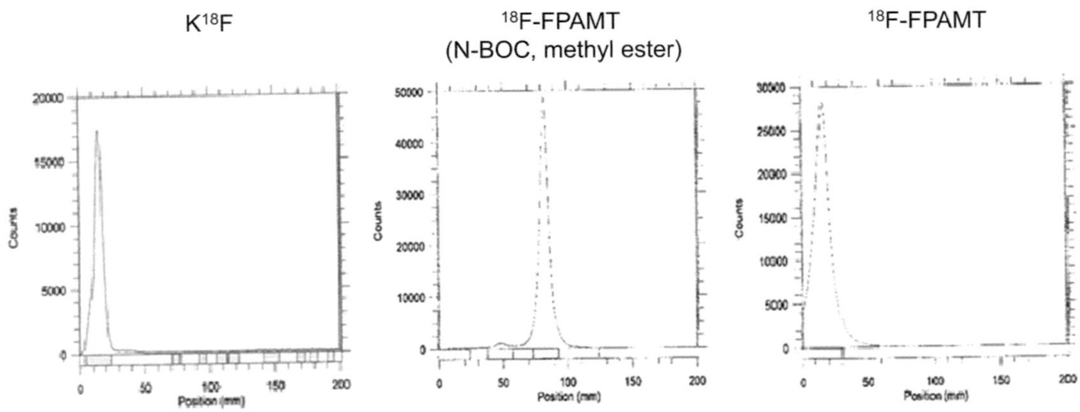

Fig. 4.4 Radio-TLC analysis of ^{18}F-FPAMT

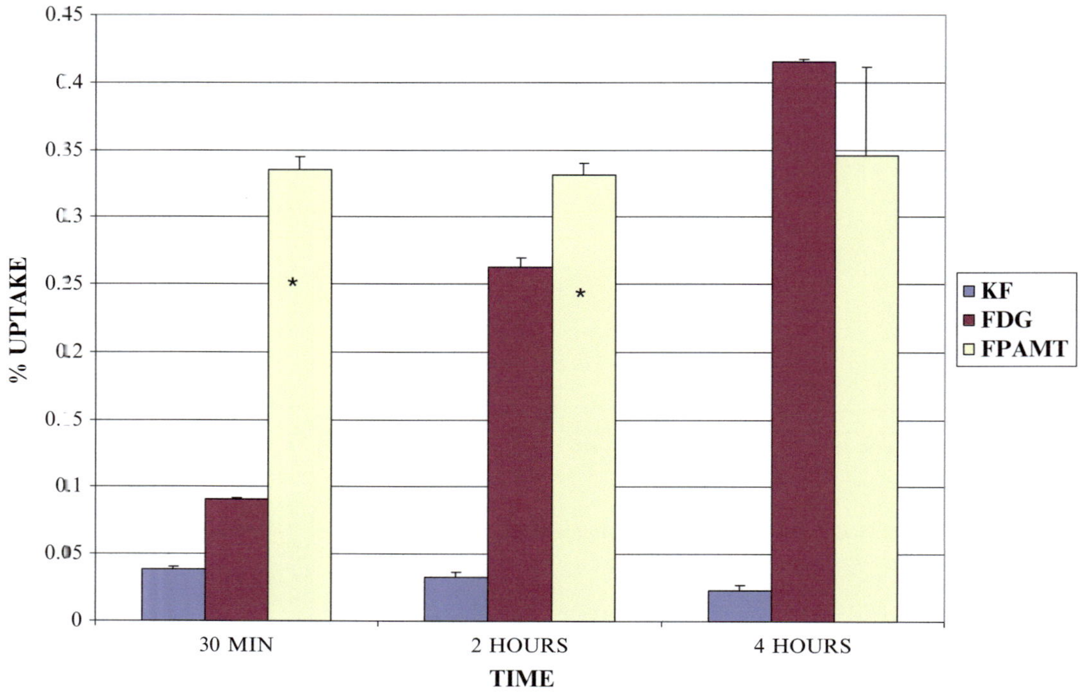

Fig. 4.5 Cellular uptake of ^{18}F-FDG and ^{18}F-FPAMT in breast cancer cell line

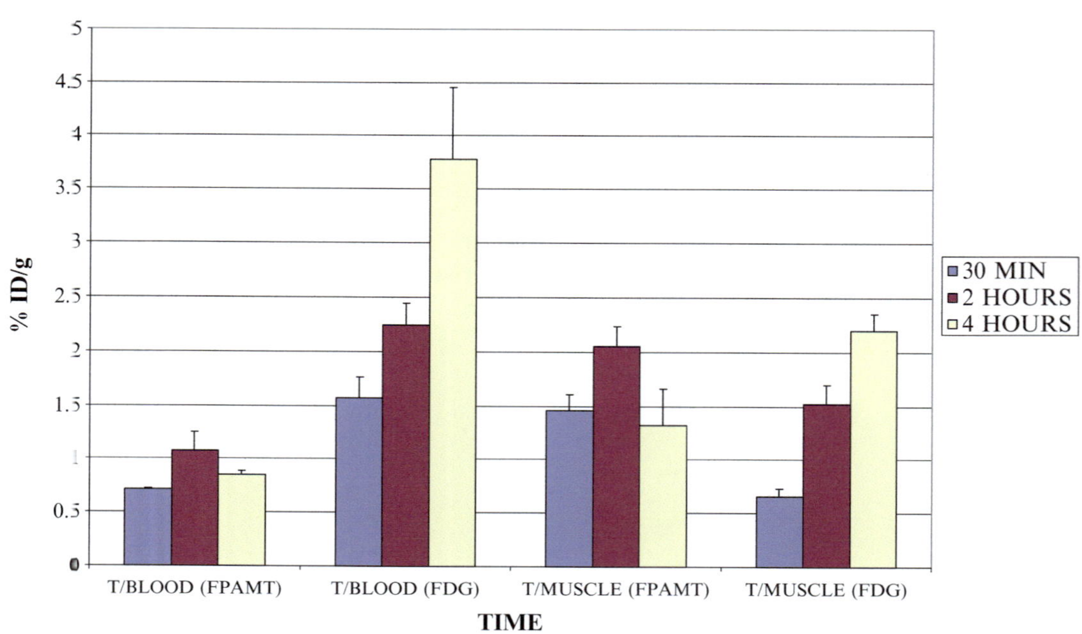

Fig. 4.6 Tumor-to-tissue count density ratios of ^{18}F-FDG and ^{18}F-FPAMT in breast tumor-bearing rats

Table 4.1 PET results of diagnostic accuracy

	Sensitivity	Specificity
C-11 choline	67% (18/27 lesions)	95% (53/56 lesions)
FDG	48% (13/27 lesions)	100% (56/56 lesions)

tamoxifen that can readily visualize ER sites, even in the implanted neoplasm. In studying the distribution, we noted fairly good uptake in the tumor, brain, and liver. We found fairly good biodistribution in the uterus/blood count ratio. The count ratio was 13.5, and the uterine uptake could be blocked somewhat by any of the estrogens or by tamoxifen itself. Fluorotamoxifen can be prepared as an analog of tamoxifen itself with high specific activity, and it can image ER+ sites in the animal models and in humans [80, 81]. In addition, such ligands might help in determining the causes of occasional failure of tamoxifen therapy when biopsy indicators are ER+.

To date we have used an ^{18}F-labeled tamoxifen ligand (2–12 mCi IV) to image 10 patients with ER+ breast tumors (IND number 40,589) by PET. We found that it is possible to visualize both primary and metastatic breast tumors by their uptake of the radiolabeled tamoxifen ligand. Of the ten patients, three had tumors that showed good uptake of the radiolabeled ligand and positive responses to tamoxifen therapy [82, 83]. However, we observed high uptake in the liver and lung, which affected the imaging and created difficulty in interpretation of tumors near those organs. Others have also reported that liver and lung tamoxifen uptake levels can remain high between 3 and 14 days of therapy.

Markers of Tumor Hypoxia

Autoradiographs of ^{18}F-FMISO showed that tumor necrotic region could be differentiated. Clinical PET studies showed that the tumors could be well visualized on ^{18}F-FMISO and ^{18}F-FETNIM tests. The tumor oxygen tension was 3–6 mm Hg as compared with the normal, 30–40 mm Hg.

Marker of Lipid Metabolism

Imaging of prostate cancer and its local metastasis was difficult when ^{18}F-FDG was used because within the pelvis, the areas of high uptake were concealed by the overwhelmingly abundant radioactivity in urine (in ureters and bladder). By contrast, it was easy when ^{11}C-choline was used because the urinary activity was negligible and tumor uptake was marked. The radioactivity concentration of ^{11}C-choline in prostate cancer and metastatic sites was at an SUV of more than 3 in most cases. The SUV of ^{18}F-FDG was considerably lower than that of ^{11}C-choline. The sensitivity and specificity of ^{18}F-FDG and ^{11}C-choline are shown in Table 4.1. ^{18}F-FECh was prepared in high yield and purity. The in vitro experiment revealed that ^{18}F-FECh was incorporated into tumor cells by active transport, then phosphorylated (yielding phosphoryl^{18}F-FECh) in the cells, and finally integrated into phospholipids. The clinical PET studies showed marked uptake of ^{18}F-FECh in prostate cancer [60, 61]. A dynamic PET study on one patient revealed that the blood level of ^{18}F-FECh decreased rapidly (in 1 min), the prostate cancer level became almost maximal in a short period (1.5 min) and remained constant for a long period of time (60 min), and the urinary radioactivity became prominent after a short time lag (5 min). Static PET studies conducted under bladder irrigation showed no difference between ^{18}F-FECh uptake and ^{11}C-choline uptake in prostate cancer. However, ^{18}F-FECh gave a slightly higher spatial resolution of the image, which was attributed to the shorter positron range of ^{18}F. The synthesis of ^{18}F-FECh was easy and reliable. ^{18}F-FECh PET was very effective in detecting prostate cancer in patients.

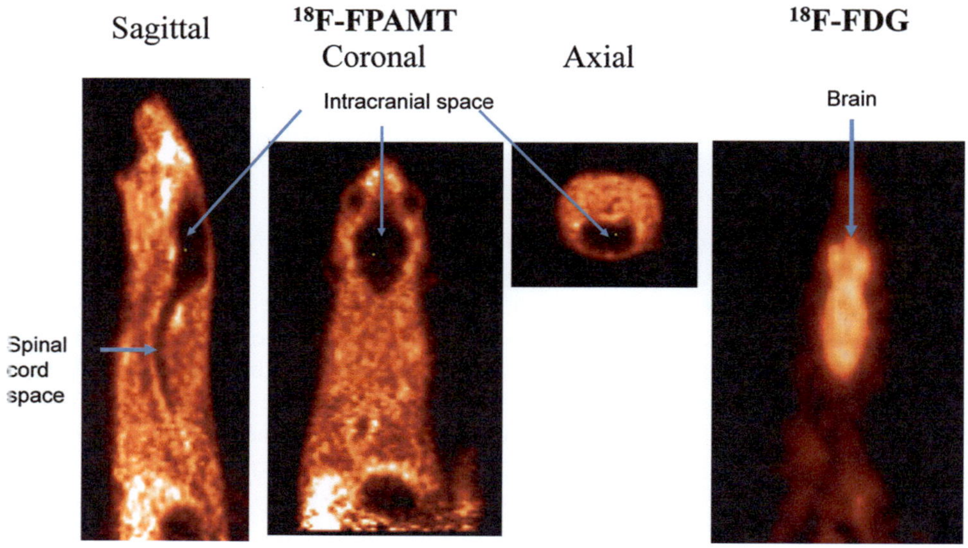

Fig. 4.7 Structure of ^{18}F-fluorinated adenosine

Fig. 4.8 Structure of ^{18}F-fluorinated fluoroethyl uracil

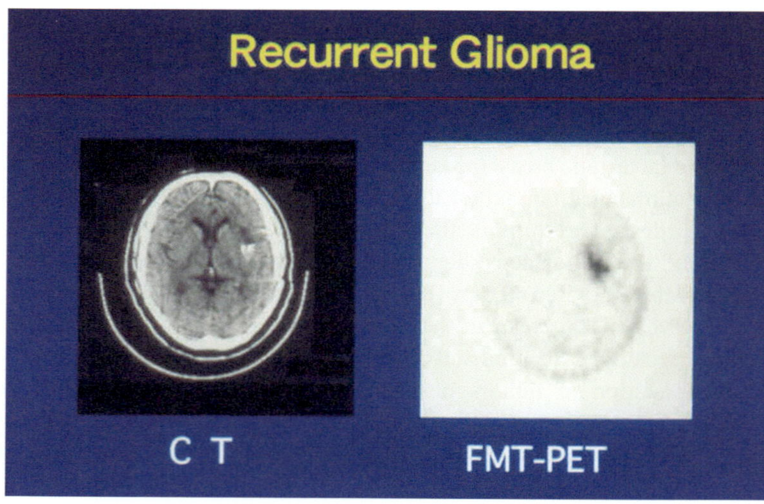

Markers of Tumor Cell Proliferation

The radioactivity of the final product (structure shown in Fig. 4.7 was 7–15 mCi, 50–60%, decay corrected) with the end of bombardment at 70 min. Under similar condition, ^{18}F-fluorinated uracil (structure shown in Fig. 4.8) was synthesized. An autoradiogram showed that the tumor could be visualized with ^{18}F-fluorinated uracil.

Markers of Gene Expression

Using a known procedure, di-tritylated tosylpenclovir (TsHBG) was synthesized. Mass spectrum and NMR spectrum are shown in Figures 4.9 and 4.10. Under similar condition for the synthesis of ^{18}F-fluorinated adenosine, ^{18}F-FHBG was synthesized. A C-18 reverse phase Sep-Pak was used to purify the compound. The radiochemical yield of

Fig. 4.9 Mass spectrometry of di-tritylated tosylpenciclovir

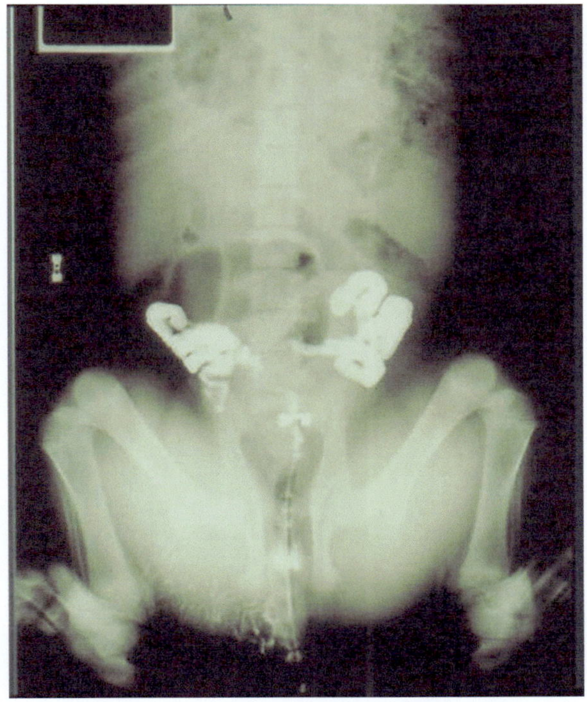

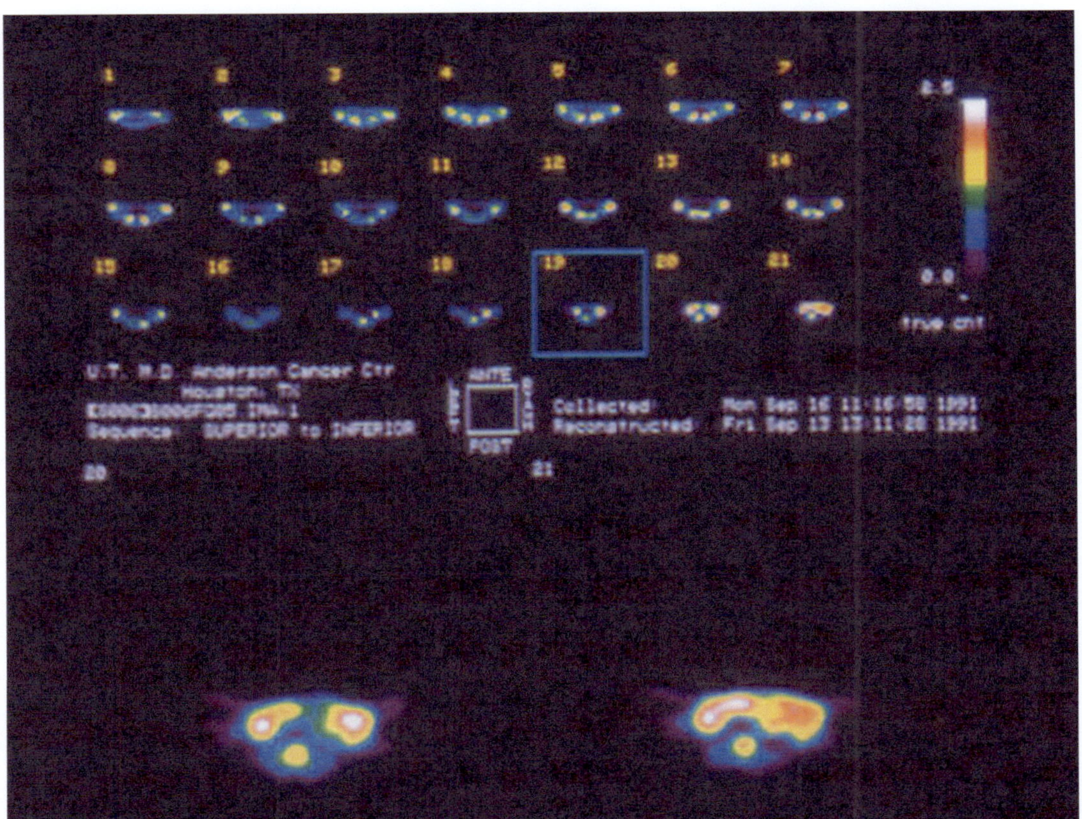

Fig. 4.10 ^{19}F-nuclear magnetic resonance of tosyl chloride and di-tritylated tosylpenciclovir

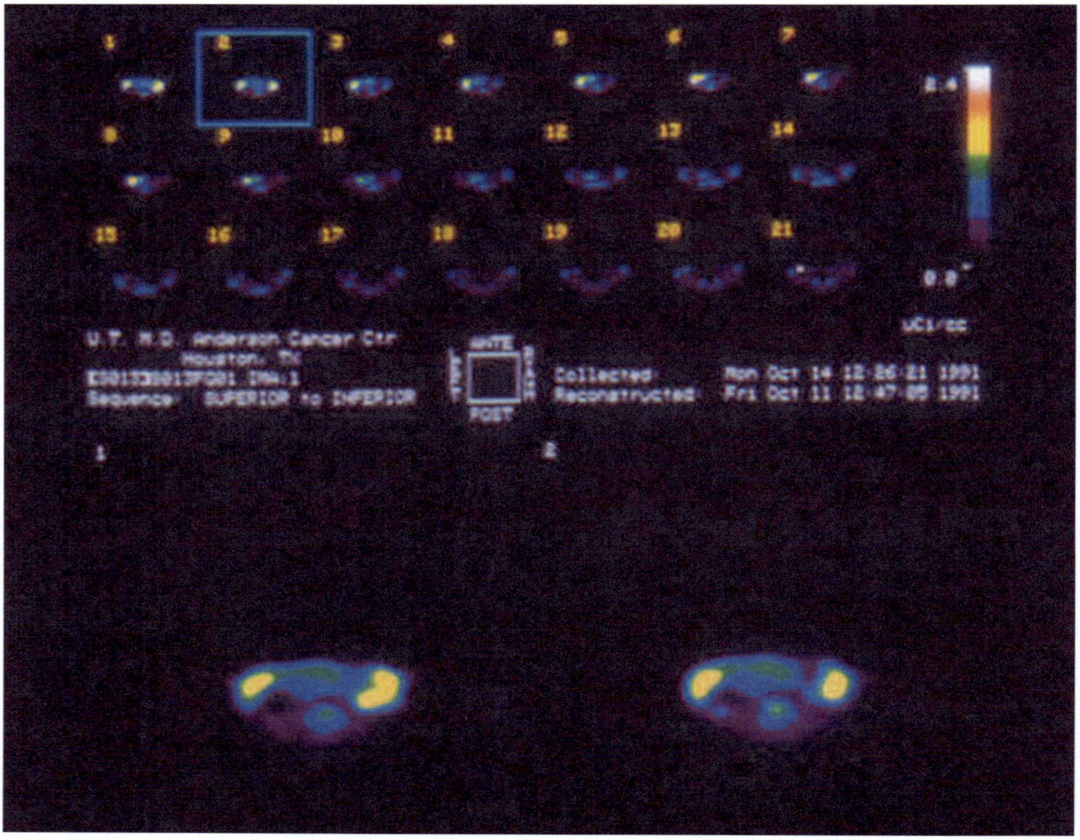

Fig. 4.11 Radiosynthesis of ^{18}F-FHBG

^{18}F-FHBG was 10–15% (decay corrected), with the end of bombardment at 90 min. Radio-TLC is shown in Fig. 4.11.

Discussion

Placing an iodine atom or a fluorine atom on the aromatic ring of tamoxifen has been previously reported [84, 85]. These analogs produced either low affinities for estrogen receptors or low specific activities, neither suitable for imaging estrogen responsive tissues. When ^{11}C-labeled tamoxifen was synthesized, the specific activity was also low [86]. Placing a chlorine atom on the aliphatic side chain of tamoxifen produced a higher affinity than that of tamoxifen [87]. However, this compound is not suitable for imaging purposes because there is no existing cyclotron-produced isotope for chlorine. Previous studies by our group indicate that replacing a chlorine with a halomethyl group develops a higher binding affinity for tamoxifen.

At present, 10 patients with ER+ breast tumors (IND number 40,589) using ^{18}F-labeled tamoxifen ligand (2–12 mCi IV) were imaged by PET. Both primary and metastatic breast tumors could be diagnosed by ^{18}F-labeled tamoxifen ligands. Three lesions in three patients were considered to be truly negative for breast cancer on the basis of biopsy specimens and/or clinical course. Five of seven patients (71.4%) and 16 of 20 lesions (80%) were interpreted to be truly positive for breast cancer. The mean SUV of the radiotracer in tumor was 2.8 on delayed images. There was no significant correlation between the SUV of [^{18}F]fluorotamoxifen in the lesion and the ER concentration in primary or metastatic lesions. Eight of ten patients received tamoxifen therapy after the PET study. Three patients who had a good response to tamoxifen therapy showed an SUV of [^{18}F]fluorotamoxifen of more than 2.4 in the tumor, whereas four of five patients who had a poor response to tamoxifen therapy showed an SUV of [^{18}F]fluorotamoxifen of less than 2.0 in the lesion. PET imaging using [^{18}F]fluorotamoxifen as the radiotracer provides useful information in predicting the effect of tamoxifen therapy in patients with recurrent or metastatic ER+ breast cancer. Results from the present study also indicate that radioiodinated and indium-labeled tamoxifen analogs are feasible to diagnose ER+ lesions.

The key to the development of ^{18}F-FMISO is to prepare (2′-nitro-1′-imidazolyl)-2-O-acetyl-3-O-tosylpropanol precursor. This intermediate could be prepared easily by treatment of 2-acetyl-1,3-ditosyl glycerol and 2-nitroimidazole as described previously. Both labeled compounds produced sufficient radioactivity and high radiochemical purity. Others have used ^{18}F-epifluorohydrin with 2-nitroimidazole or 1,3-ditosyl-O-tetrahydropyran to react with 2-nitroimidazole, followed by ^{18}F-displacement. These reactions take longer synthetic steps, have a longer reaction time, or provide lower radiochemical yield. Numerous in vitro and in vivo experiments have shown that cells irradiated under low oxygen tensions are more resistant to the lethal effects of low linear energy transfer (LET) ionized radiation compared with cells irradiated under "normal" oxygen tensions. Our clinical trial with PET demonstrated that ^{18}F-FMISO is capable of providing functional images of tumor hypoxia. Autoradiographs of all four analogs showed that tumor hypoxia could be easily demonstrated in rodents. Tumor oxygen tension was determined to be 3.2–6.0 mm Hg, whereas normal muscle tissue had 30–40 mm Hg.

Because tumor uptake of ^{11}C-choline is higher than that of ^{18}F-FDG (i.e., synovial sarcoma), and shorter imaging time is required for ^{11}C-choline, ^{11}C-choline appeared to be a promising PET tracer. There was no effect on tumor uptake in patients with diabetes mellitus. ^{11}C-choline is feasible for detecting intrapelvic lesions because of low urinary excretion. ^{18}F-fluorinated choline revealed in vitro phosphorylation was similar to that of choline. The PET images of a patient with recurrent prostate cancer showed uptake of ^{18}F-fluorinated choline in the prostatic bed and in metastases to lymph nodes. ^{18}F-fluorinated choline PET showed uptake in malignancies in a patient with metastatic breast cancer. PET revealed ^{18}F-fluorinated choline uptake in biopsy-proven recurrent brain tumor with little confounding uptake by normal brain tissues. The ^{18}F-fluorinated choline may serve as a probe of choline uptake and phosphorylation in cancer cells. Preliminary PET studies on patients with prostate cancer, breast cancer, or brain tumor support further studies to evaluate the usefulness of fluorocholin (FCH) as an oncologic probe.

To enhance the biologic activity and increase chemical or metabolic stability, fluorine substitution at the C2′ position of the sugar moiety (arabino configuration) has been widely investigated in drug research [88–90]. [^{18}F]FAD is structurally closer to 2′-deoxyadenosine due to the similarity in the van der Waals radii between the C-H bond and C-halogen bond. Deep-seated tumors in blood-rich organs may require significantly higher ratios for assessment of proliferation. Tumor-to-muscle ratios of [^{18}F]FAD at 2 and 4 h postinjection were 5.2 and 14.3, respectively. Tumor-to-blood ratios at the same time intervals were 2.8 and 5.3, respectively. These data were considered to be acceptable as a tumor imaging agent. Although many other radiopharmaceuticals could be used for assessment of tumor proliferation or metabolic activity, the choice should be determined not only by the biologic behavior of radiopharmaceuticals, but also by their ease of preparation, as well as by the logistics of imaging.

Although we have synthesized FHBG, we have not conducted preclinical studies. Results from other studies showed that FHBG is a promising PET gene expression probe. For instance, Inubushi et al. [91] showed that HSV-1-*sr39tk* reporter gene expression can be monitored with ^{18}F-FHBG and micro-PET in rat myocardium quantitatively and serially with high detection sensitivity. Cardiac PET reporter gene imaging offers the potential of monitoring the expression of therapeutic genes in cardiac gene therapy. Tjuvajev et al. [92] also concluded that the in vitro and in vivo results (including the PET images) show that FIAU is a substantially more efficient probe than FHBG or FHPG for imaging HSV1-*tk* expression, with greater sensitivity and contrast as well as lower levels of abdominal background radioactivity at 2 and 24 h. Alauddin et al. [71] concluded that ^{18}F-FHBG may yield high-contrast PET images of HSV-*tk* expression in tumors. Thus, it is a very promising radiotracer for monitoring of gene therapy of cancer with PET.

Acknowledgments The animal research reported here is supported by a Cancer Center Core grant, NIH-NCI CA-16672.

References

1. Bar-Shalom R, Valdivia AY, Blaufox MD. PET imaging in oncology. Semin Nucl Med. 2000;30:150–85.
2. Plowman PN, Saunders CA, Maisey M. On the usefulness of brain PET scanning to the paediatric neuro-oncologist. Br J Neurosurg. 1997;11:525–32.
3. Weber WA, Avril N, Schwaiger M. Relevance of positron emission tomography (PET) in oncology. Strahlenther Onkol. 1999;175:356.
4. Lau CL, Harpole DH, Patz E. Staging techniques for lung cancer. Chest Surg Clin North Am. 2000;10(4):781–801.
5. Schulte M, Brecht-Krauss D, Heymer B, et al. Grading of tumors and tumor like lesions of bone: evaluation by FDG PET. J Nucl Med. 2000;41(10):1695–701.
6. Yutani K, Shiba E, Kusuoka H, et al. Comparison of FDG-PET with MIBI-SPECT in the detection of breast cancer and axillary lymph node metastasis. J Comput Assist Tomogr. 2000;24(2):274–80.
7. Franzius C, Sciuk J, Daldrup-Link HE, et al. FDG-PET for detection of osseous metastases from malignant primary bone tumors: comparison with bone scintigraphy. Eur J Nucl Med. 2000;27(9):1305–11.
8. Folpe AL, Lyles RH, Sprouse JT, et al. (F-18) fluorodeoxyglucose positron emission tomography as a predictor of pathologic grade and other prognostic variables in bone and soft tissue sarcoma. Clin Cancer Res. 2000;6(4):1279–87.
9. Meyer PT, Spetzger U, Mueller HD, et al. High F-18 FDG uptake in a low-grade supratentorial ganglioma: a positron emission tomography case report. Clin Nucl Med. 2000;25(9):694–7.
10. Franzius C, Sciuk J, Brinkschmidt C, et al. Evaluation of chemotherapy response in primary bone tumors with F-18 FDG positron emission tomography compared with histologically assessed tumor necrosis. Clin Nucl Med. 2000;25(11):874–81.
11. Carretta A, Landoni C, Melloni G, et al. 18-FDG positron emission tomography in the evaluation of malignant pleural diseases – a pilot study. Eur J Cardiothorac Surg. 2000;17(4):377–83.
12. Torre W, Garcia-Velloso MJ, Galbis J, et al. FDG-PET detection of primary lung cancer in a patient with an isolated cerebral metastasis. J Cardiovasc Surg. 2000;41(3):503–5.
13. Brunelle F. Noninvasive diagnosis of brain tumors in children. Childs Nerv Syst. 2000;16(10–11):731–4.
14. Mankoff DA, Dehdashti F, Shields AF. Characterizing tumors using metabolic imaging: PET imaging of cellular proliferation and steroid receptors. Neoplasia. 2000;2:71.
15. Fitzgerald J, Parker JA, Danias PG. F-18 fluorodeoxyglucose SPECT for assessment of myocardial viability. J Nucl Cardiol. 2000;7(4):382–7.
16. Schwarz A, Kuwert T. Nuclear medicine diagnosis in diseases of the central nervous system. Radiology. 2000;40(10):858–62.
17. Roelcke U, Leenders KL. PET in neuro-oncology. J Cancer Res Clin Oncol. 2001;127(1):2–8.
18. Brock CS, Meikle SR, Price P. Does ^{18}F-fluorodeoxyglucose metabolic imaging of tumors benefit oncology? Eur J Nucl Med. 1997;24:691–705.
19. Syrota A, Comar D, Cerf M, et al. [^{11}]C-methionine pancreatic scanning with positron emission computed tomography. J Nucl Med. 1979;20:778–81.
20. Syrota A, Duquesnoy N, Dasaf A, et al. The role of positron emission tomography in the detection of pancreatic disease. Radiology. 1982;143:249–53.
21. Kubota K, Yamada K, Fukuda H, et al. Tumor detection with carbon-11 labeled amino acid. Eur J Nucl Med. 1984;9:136–40.
22. Hagenfeldt L, Venizelos N, Bjerkenstedt L, et al. Decreased tyrosine transport in fibroblasts from schizophrenic patients. Life Sci. 1987;41:2749–57.
23. Tisljar U, Kloster G, Stocklin G. Accumulation of radioiodinated L-alpha-methyltyrosine in pancreas of mice: concise communication. J Nucl Med. 1979;20:973–6.
24. Kloss G, Leven M. Accumulation of radioiodinated tyrosine derivatives in the adrenal medulla and in melanomas. Eur J Nucl Med. 1979;4:179–86.
25. Langen KJ, Coenen HH, Roosen N, et al. SPECT studies of brain tumors with L-3-[^{123}I]-Iodo-alpha-methyl tyrosine: comparison with PET, ^{124}IMT and first clinical results. J Nucl Med. 1990;31:281–6.

26. Tomiyoshi K, Hirano T, Inoue T, et al. Positron emission tomography for evaluation of dopaminergic function using a neurotransmitter analog L-^{18}F-m-tyrosine in monkey brain. Bioimages. 1996;4(1):1–7.
27. Wienhard K, Herholz K, Coenen HH, et al. Increased amino acid transport into brain tumors measured by PET of L-(2-^{18}F)fluorotyrosine. J Nucl Med. 1991; 32:1338–46.
28. Coenen HH, Kling P, Stocklin G, et al. Metabolism of L2-^{18}F-fluorotyrosine, new PET tracer for protein synthesis. J Nucl Med. 1989;301:367–1372.
29. Ishiwata K, Valvurg W, Elsigna PH, et al. Metabolic studies with L-^{11}C-tyrosine for the investigation of a kinetic model of measuring protein synthesis rate with PET. J Nucl Med. 1988;29:524–9.
30. Bolster JM, Valburg W, Paans AMJ, et al. Carbon-11 labeled tyrosine to study tumor metabolism by positron emission tomography (PET). Eur J Nucl Med. 1986;12:321–4.
31. Dejesus OT, Sunderland JJ, Nicles R, et al. Synthesis of radiofluorinated analogs of m-tyrosine as potential L-dopatracers via direct reaction with acetylhypofluorite. Appl Radiat Isot. 1990;41(5):433–7.
32. Tang G, Wang M, Tang X, et al. Pharmacokinetics and radiation dosimetry estimation of O-(2-[18 F]fluoroethyl)-L-tyrosine as oncologic PET tracer. Appl Radiat Isot. 2003;58(2):219–25.
33. Hamacher K, Coenen HH. Efficient routine production of the ^{18}F-labelled amino acid O-2-^{18}F fluoroethyl-L-tyrosine. Appl Radiat Isot. 2002;57(6):853–6.
34. Rau FC, Weber WA, Wester HJ, et al. O-(2-[(18)F] Fluoroethyl)-L-tyrosine (FET): a tracer for differentiation of tumour from inflammation in murine lymph nodes. Eur J Nucl Med Mol Imaging. 2002;29(8): 1039–46.
35. Fernandez MD, Burn JI, Sauven PD, et al. Activated estrogen receptors in breast cancer and response to endocrine therapy. Eur J Cancer Clin Oncol. 1984;20:41–6.
36. McGuire AH, Dehdashti F, Siegel BA, et al. Positron tomographic assessment of 16-alpha-[^{18}F]fluoro-17-beta-estradiol uptake in metastatic breast carcinoma. J Nucl Med. 1991;32:1526–31.
37. McManaway ME, Jagoda EM, Kasid A, et al. [^{125}I]17-beta-iodovinyl-11-beta-methoxyestradiol: interaction in vivo with ERS in hormone independent MCF-7 human breast cancer transfected with V-ras H oncogene. Cancer Res. 1987;47:2945–8.
38. Jagoda EM, Gibson RE, Goodgold H, et al. [^{125}I]17-Iodovinyl-11-beta-methoxyestradiol: in vivo and in vitro properties of a high affinity estrogen-receptor radiopharmaceutical. J Nucl Med. 1984;25:472–7.
39. Hamm JT, Allegra JC. Hormonal therapy for cancer. In: Witts RE, editor. Manual of oncologic therapeutics. New York: Lippincott; 1991. p. 122–6.
40. Wittliff JL. Steroid-hormone receptor in breast cancer. Cancer Res. 1984;53:630–43.
41. Rasey JS, Nelson NJ, Chin L, et al. Characterization of the binding of labeled fluoromisonidazole in cells in vitro. Radiat Res. 1990;122:301–8.
42. Cherif A, Yang DJ, Tansey W, et al. Synthesis of [^{18}F]fluoromisonidazole. Pharm Res. 1994;11:466–9.
43. Hwang DR, Dence CS, Bonasera TA, et al. No-carrier-added synthesis of 3-[^{18}F]fluoro-1-(2-nitro-1-imidazolyl)-2-propanol. A potential PET agent for detecting hypoxic but viable tissues. Int J Radiat Appl Instrum A. 1989;40:117–26.
44. Jerabeck PA, Patrick TB, Kilbourn D, et al. Synthesis and biodistribution of ^{18}F-labeled fluoronitroimidazoles: potential in vivo markers of hypoxic tissue. Appl Radiat Isot. 1986;37:599–605.
45. Parliament MB, Chapman JD, Urtasun RC, et al. Noninvasive assessment of tumor hypoxia with ^{123}I-iodoazomycin arabinoside: preliminary report of a clinical study. Br J Cancer. 1992;65:90–5.
46. Valk PET, Mathis CA, Prados MD, et al. Hypoxia in human gliomas: demonstration by PET with [^{18}F]fluoromisonidazole. J Nucl Med. 1992;33:2133–7.
47. Martin GV, Caldwell JH, Rasey JS, et al. Enhanced binding of the hypoxic cell marker [^{18}F]fluoromisonidazole in ischemic myocardium. Nucl Med. 1989;30:194–201.
48. Martin GV, Cardwell JH, Graham MM, et al. Nonivasive detection of hypoxic myocardium using [^{18}F]fluoromisonidazole and PET. J Nucl Med. 1992;33:2202–8.
49. Yeh SH, Liu RS, Hu HH, et al. Ischemic penumbra in acute stroke: demonstration by PET with fluorine-18 fluoromisonidazole. J Nucl Med. 1994;35(5):205. abst.
50. Yeh SH, Liu RS, Wu LC, et al. Fluorine-18 fluoromisonidazole tumour to muscle retention ratio for the detection of hypoxia in nasopharyngeal carcinoma. Eur J Nucl Med. 1996;23(10):1378–83.
51. Liu RS, Yeh SH, Chang CP, et al. Detection of odontogenic infections by [F-18]fluoromisonidazole. J Nucl Med. 1994;35(5):113. abst.
52. Yang DJ, Wallace S, Cherif A, et al. Development of F-18-labeled fluoroerythronitroimidazole as a PET agent for imaging tumor hypoxia. Radiology. 1995;194:795–800.
53. Cherif A, Wallace S, Yang DJ, et al. Development of new markers for hypoxic cells: [^{131}I]iodomisonidazole and [^{131}I]iodoerythronitroimidazole. J Drug Target. 1996;4(1):31–9.
54. Inoue T, Yang DJ, Wallace S, et al. Evaluation of [^{131}I] iodoerythronitroimidazole as a predictor for the radiosensitizing effect. Anticancer Drugs. 1996;7(8): 858–65.
55. Podo F. Tumor phospholipid metabolism. NMR Biomed. 1999;12:413–39.
56. Hara T, Kosaka N, Kishi H. PET imaging of prostate cancer using carbon-11-choline. J Nucl Med. 1998; 39:990–5.
57. Hara T, Kosaka N, Shinoura N, et al. PET imaging of brain tumor with [methyl-^{11}C]choline. J Nucl Med. 1997;38:842–7.
58. Hara T, Kosaka N, Kishi H, et al. Imaging of brain tumor, lung cancer, esophagus cancer, colon cancer, prostate cancer, and bladder cancer with [C-11]choline. J Nucl Med. 1997;38:250P.

59. Kotzerke J, Prang J, Neumaier B, et al. Experience with carbon-11 choline positron emission tomography in prostate carcinoma. Eur J Nucl Med. 2000;27:1415–9.
60. DeGrado TR, Baldwin SW, Wang S, et al. Synthesis and evaluation of (18)F-labeled choline analogs as oncologic PET tracers. J Nucl Med. 2001;42(12): 1805–14.
61. Price DT, Coleman RE, Liao RP, et al. Comparison of [^{18}F]fluorocholine and [^{18}F]fluorodeoxyglucose for positron emission tomography of androgen dependent and androgen independent prostate cancer. J Urol. 2002;168(1):273–80.
62. DeGrado TR, Reiman RE, Price DT, et al. Pharmacokinetics and radiation dosimetry of 18 F-fluorocholine. J Nucl Med. 2002;43(1):92–6.
63. Haberkorn U, Khazaie K, Morr I, et al. Ganciclovir uptake in human mammary carcinoma cells expressing herpes simplex virus thymidine kinase. Nucl Med Biol. 1998;25:367–73.
64. Gambhir SS, Barrio JR, Wu L, et al. Imaging of adenoviral-directed herpes simplex virus type 1 thymidine kinase reporter gene expression in mice with radiolabeled ganciclovir. J Nucl Med. 1998;39: 2003–11.
65. Gambhir SS, Barrio JR, Phelps ME, et al. Imaging adenoviral-directed reporter gene expression in living animals with positron emission tomography. Proc Natl Acad Sci USA. 1999;96:2333–8.
66. Namavari M, Barrio JR, Toyokuni T, et al. Synthesis of 8-[^{18}F]fluoroguanine derivatives: in vivo probes for imaging gene expression with positron emission tomography. Nucl Med Biol. 2000;27:157–62.
67. Gambhir SS, Bauer E, Black ME, et al. A mutant herpes simplex virus type 1 thymidine kinase reporter gene shows improved sensitivity for imaging reporter gene expression with positron emission tomography. Proc Natl Acad Sci USA. 2000;97:2785–90.
68. Iyer M, Barrio JR, Namavari M, et al. 8-[^{18}F] Fluoropenciclovir: an improved reporter probe for imaging HSV1-tk reporter gene expression in vivo using PET. J Nucl Med. 2001;42:96–105.
69. Alauddin MM, Conti PS, Mazza SM, et al. 9-[(3-[^{18}F]-Fluoro-1-hydroxy-2-propoxy)methyl]guanine ([^{18}F]-FHPG): a potential imaging agent of viral infection and gene therapy using PET. Nucl Med Biol. 1996;23:787–92.
70. Alauddin MM, Shahinian A, Kundu RK, et al. Evaluation of 9-[(3-^{18}F- fluoro-1-hydroxy-2-propoxy) methyl]guanine ([^{18}F]-FHPG) in vitro and in vivo as a probe for PET imaging of gene incorporation and expression in tumors. Nucl Med Biol. 1999;26:371–6.
71. Alauddin MM, Conti PS. Synthesis and preliminary evaluation of 9-(4-[^{18}F]-fluoro-3-hydroxymethylbutyl) guanine ([^{18}F]FHBG): a new potential imaging agent for viral infection and gene therapy using PET. Nucl Med Biol. 1998;25:175–80.
72. Yaghoubi S, Barrio JR, Dahlbom M, et al. Human pharmacokinetic and dosimetry studies of [^{18}F]FHBG: a reporter probe for imaging herpes simplex virus type-1 thymidine kinase reporter gene expression. J Nucl Med. 2001;42:1225–34.
73. Yang DJ, Cherif A, Tansey W, et al. N, N-diethylfluoromethyltamoxifen: synthesis assignment of ^{1}H and ^{13}C spectra and receptor assay. Eur J Med Chem. 1992;27:919–24.
74. Yang D, Tewson T, Tansey W, et al. Halogenated analogs of tamoxifen: synthesis, receptor assay and inhibition of MCF7 cells. J Pharm Sci. 1992;81: 622–5.
75. Kim CG, Yang DJ, Kim EE, et al. Assessment of tumor cell proliferation using [^{18}F]fluorodeoxyadenosine and [^{18}F]fluoroethyluracil. J Pharm Sci. 1996;85(3):339–44.
76. Cherif A, Yang DJ, Tansey W, et al. Radiosynthesis and biodistribution studies of [F-18]fluoroadenosine and [I-131]-5-iodo-2′-O-methyl-uridine for the assessment of tumor proliferation rate. Pharm Res. 1995;12(9):128.
77. Yang D, Wallace S. High affinity tamoxifen derivatives and uses thereof. U.S. Patent no 5,192,525; 1993.
78. Yang D, Wallace S, Wright KC, et al. Imaging of estrogen receptors with PET using ^{18}F-fluoro analogue of tamoxifen. Radiology. 1992;182:185–6.
79. Yang DJ, Kuang L-R, Cherif A, et al. Synthesis of ^{18}F-alanine and ^{18}F-tamoxifen for breast tumor imaging. J Drug Target. 1993;1:259–67.
80. Yang DJ, Li C, Kuang L-R, et al. Imaging, biodistribution and therapy potential of halogenated tamoxifen analogues. Life Sci. 1994;55(1):53–67.
81. Yang DJ, Wallace S. High affinity halogenated tamoxifen derivatives and uses thereof. U.S. Patent no 5,219,548; 1993.
82. Inoue T, Kim EE, Wallace S, et al. Positron emission tomography using [^{18}F]fluorotamoxifen to evaluate therapeutic responses in patients with breast cancer: preliminary study. Cancer Biother Radiopharm. 1996;11(4):235–45.
83. Inoue T, Kim EE, Wallace S, et al. Preliminary study of cardiac accumulation of F-18 fluorotamoxifen in patients with breast cancer. Clin Imaging. 1997;21(5): 332–6.
84. Hanson RN, Seitz DE. Tissue distribution of the radiolabeled antiestrogen [^{125}I]iodotamoxifen. Int J Nucl Med Biol. 1982;9:105–7.
85. Ram S, Spicer LD. Radioiodination of tamoxifen. J Label Compd Radiopharm. 1989;27:661–8.
86. Kangas L, Nieminen A-L, Blanco G, et al. A new triphenylethylene, FC-1157a, antitumor effects. Cancer Chemother Pharmacol. 1986;17:109–13.
87. Kallio S, Kangas L, Blanco G, et al. A new triphenylethylene, FC-1157a, hormonal effects. Cancer Chemother Pharmacol. 1986;17:103–8.
88. Kawai G, Yamamoto Y, Kamimura T, et al. Conformational rigidity of specific pyrimidine residues in tRNA arises from posttranscriptional modifications that enhance steric interaction between the base and the 2′-hydroxyl group. Biochemistry. 1992;31:1040–5.

89. Uesugi S, Kaneyasu T, Ikehara M. Synthesis and properties of ApU analogues containing 2′-halo-2′-deoxyadenosine. Effect of 2′ substituents on oligonucleotide conformation. Biochemistry. 1982;21:5870–7.
90. Ikehara M, Miki H. Studies of nucleosides and nucleotides. Cyclonucleosides. Synthesis and properties of 2′-halogeno-2′-deoxyadenosines. Chem Pharm Bull. 1978;26:2449–53.
91. Inubushi M, Wu JC, Gambhir SS, et al. Positron-emission tomography reporter gene expression imaging in rat myocardium. Circulation. 2003;107(2):326–32.
92. Tjuvajev JG, Doubrovin M, Akhurst T, et al. Comparison of radiolabeled nucleoside probes (FIAU, FHBG, and FHPG) for PET imaging of HSV1-tk gene expression. J Nucl Med. 2002;43(8):1072–83.

Automated Synthesis of Radiopharmaceuticals

5

David J. Yang, I. Hong Shih, and E. Edmund Kim

Importance of Nuclear Molecular Imaging in Oncology

Drug discovery is accelerating as a result of mapping of molecular targets and the rapid synthesis of high-throughput in vitro testing of compounds in their early stage of the drug development process. The development of radiolabeled biochemical compounds, understanding molecular pathways and imaging devices to detect the radioactivity by external imaging has expanded the use of nuclear molecular imaging studies in drug development. Nuclear molecular imaging modalities, positron emission tomography (PET), and single photon emission computed tomography (SPECT), are in vivo imaging methods that use gamma radiotracers to track biochemical processes in humans and animals. The cyclotron-produced positron emitters commonly used to label compounds are ^{11}C(t ½=20.4 min); ^{18}F(t½=110 min); ^{13}N(t½=10 min), ^{15}O (t ½=2.0 min), ^{124}I (t ½=4.18 days), ^{61}Cu (t ½=3.3 h), ^{62}Cu (t ½=10 min), ^{64}Cu (t ½ =12.7 h), and ^{68}Ga (t ½=68 min). The commonly used SPECT radioisotopes are ^{131}I (t ½=7 days), ^{123}I (t ½=13 h), ^{111}In (t ½=67 h), ^{201}Tl (t ½=3.038 days), ^{67}Ga (t ½=3.26 days), and ^{99m}Tc (t ½=6 h). Among non-generator-produced isotopes, ^{18}F and ^{123}I are the most suitable for the preparation of a more complex chemistry and for a longer observation period in biologic experiments.

PET and SPECT map the location and concentration of radionuclide-labeled compounds [1–3]. At present, PET and SPECT gamma cameras are hybrid with CT to enhance their sensitivity to quantify drug properties in vivo in real-time dynamic events. PET/CT and SPECT/CT are better than PET and SPECT alone because multiple slices by CT and serial images by PET and SPECT provide better delineation in tumor volumes. In addition, combining the anatomic and morphologic location from CT, such as SPECT/CT and PET/CT, provides the capability to accurately evaluate post-therapy anatomic alteration. PET/CT and SPECT/CT agents show high specific activities because they are made through a nuclear transformation and use carrier free forms of isotopes. Moreover, PET/CT and SPECT/CT chelator-based agents do not produce detectable pharmacologic effects but provide important information regarding the characterization of varieties diseases, such as vascular angiogenesis [4–6], hypoxia [7–9], apoptosis [10, 11], cellular signaling and transcriptional activity

D.J. Yang, Ph.D. • I.H. Shih
Department of Experimental Diagnostic Imaging, The University of Texas MD Anderson Cancer Center, Houston, TX 77030, USA
e-mail: dyang@mdanderson.org

E.E. Kim, M.D., M.S. (✉)
Departments of Nuclear Medicine and Diagnostic Radiology, The University of Texas M.D. Anderson Cancer Center and Medical School, Houston, TX 77030, USA

Graduate School of Convergence Science and Technology, Seoul National University, Seoul, South Korea
e-mail: ekim@mdanderson.org

E.E. Kim et al. (eds.), *Clinical PET and PET/CT: Principles and Applications*, DOI 10.1007/978-1-4419-0802-5_5, © Springer Science+Business Media New York 2013

[12–14]. PET/CT and SPECT/CT may assist in the determination of optimal therapeutic dosing, differential diagnosis between inflammation/infection and recurrence, sensitivity or resistance to treatment response, grading of tumors, and the prediction of treatment response by selecting patients who may or may not respond to therapy. On the other hand, CT, MRI, and sonography are prognostic tools because they do not provide cellular target information, thus, assessment of the effectiveness of cancer therapy is not optimal.

Regulatory Requirements for Radiopharmaceuticals Production

There are two classes of radiopharmaceuticals. The first class is the chelator-based radiopharmaceuticals. In this class, included are drug substance (pro-drug) and drug product (end product). Food and Drug Administration (FDA)-certified generator-produced isotopes are readily available for drug product. The second class belongs to non-FDA certified isotopes such as short-lived PET or SPECT isotopes. The preparation and quality control of PET and SPECT cyclotron-produced radiopharmaceuticals present a challenge. Radiopharmaceutical chemistry requires handling of radioactive exposure, fast reaction times, ease of synthesis, and reproducible results. Automated synthesis provides a solution to overcome these obstacles. The FDA guidance document entitled "PET Drug Products—Current Good Manufacturing Practice (cGMP)" mandates requirements regarding safety, identity, strength, quality, and purity of radiopharmaceuticals and establishes cGMP requirements in conjunction with the United States Pharmacopeia (USP) general chapter on compounding PET radiopharmaceuticals (USP 26–823) [15]. cGMP requirements cover (1) Personnel and resources; (2) Quality control systems; (3) Facilities and equipment; (4) Control of components, in-process materials and finished products; (5) Production and process controls; (6) Laboratory controls; (7) Acceptance criteria; (8) Labeling and packaging controls; (9) Distribution controls; (10) Complaint handling; and (11) Recordkeeping. cGMP must be implemented to ensure that the requirements for safety and quality control of PET drugs meet quality standards. The documents emphasize the importance of validation and quality control of the final drug product. To fulfill the requirement of cGMP radiopharmaceuticals, automated devices are needed.

Regulatory Requirements for Automated Devices

Regulatory guidelines for the design and operation of automated radiochemical synthesizers are outlined in general chapter 1015 of the USP. These devices are regulated as drug manufacturing equipment for the most part, rather than as traditional medical devices. Manufacturers of automated devices can file a Type II Drug Master File (DMF) for radiopharmaceutical synthesis with the FDA. The DMF should contain specific performance, qualification, and functionality of the synthesizer and provide support to the Chemistry, Manufacturing and Controls (CMC) section of an investigational new drug (IND). Users of the automated synthesizers can then reference the DMF for use in future IND applications and new drug applications to make and distribute PET radiotracers in the United States. It should be noted that prior to development of a new synthesizer for commercial use, the regulatory pathway should be clearly defined to reduce cost and time to reach a market.

Requirement of Radiotracers Beyond FDG in Oncology

The metabolic activity of tumor cells, as qualitatively measured by FDG PET has been linked to both an increase in the amount of glucose membrane transporters and an increase in the activity of the principal enzymes controlling the glycolytic pathways. FDG is complementary to CT and MRI, and allows detection of unsuspected distant metastases. Though FDG PET is concordant with the findings of CT and MRI in diagnosing various tumors, FDG also has its drawbacks. FDG utilizes two main glucose transporters and hexokinase phosphorylated processes, but is trapped in cell cytosol for tumor imaging [16–18]. FDG exhibits poor differentiation between inflammation/infection and tumor recurrence as a result of its high uptake in granulocytes and macrophages [19]. FDG has poor contrast in brain tumors because of the high uptake of glucose in normal brain tissue [20]. Because of high brain uptake and poor specificity and poor specificity, FDG does not provide the selection of patients for therapeutic response. Therefore, it is amenable to develop an alternative radiotracer for better differential diagnosis and responsiveness in cancers.

Radiotracers Beyond FDG from Existing Automated Devices

Radiosynthesis of PET and SPECT must be rapid because of the higher risk of radiation exposure during radiosynthesis. An automated apparatus is needed to assure production efficiency and minimize the radiation exposure by PET and SPECT isotopes. ^{18}F-fluorodeoxyglucose (^{18}F-FDG) has been widely used in various PET centers. In cancer patients, ^{18}F-FDG uptake in tumors is increased as a result of the faster glycolysis of tumor cells. At present, there are commercially available boxes built by General Electric (GE), Siemens, Sumitomo, Bioscan, EBCO, and other private developers. They are suitable for the production of ^{18}F-FDG, fluorine-18-L-dihydroxyphenylalanine (^{18}F-DOPA), [^{18}F]fluorothymidine, [^{18}F]α-methyltyrosine, [^{11}C]choline, [^{13}N]NH_3, and [^{15}O]H_2O, but not for the preparation of other compounds or for research purposes. Each box is aimed at its high and reliable output, ease of use, and compliance with pharmaceutical practices. For instance, the GE TRACERlabM$_x$ produces FDG ready for quality control with high yield and high purity. The easy-to-use, disposable sterilized cassettes allow for multiple, back-to-back production runs, with easy setup and high FDG yield in a disposable, fluid pathway design are the focus. Synthesis time of FDG is 25 min with production yield (not corrected for decay) 60%. Radiochemical yield (corrected for decay) is typically 70%. Another TRACERlabF$_x$DOPA by GE is fully automated for ^{18}F-DOPA production from [^{18}F] F_2. Purification of ^{18}F-DOPA is achieved by an integrated preparative high-performance liquid chromatography (HPLC) system. TRACER labF$_x$DOPA box is aimed for easy to operate and compatible with the GE PET trace F_2 target system, making the training of staff in doing this usually difficult synthesis fast and economical. Synthesis time of ^{18}F-DOPA is 40 min with production yield (not corrected for decay) 20%. Radiochemical yield (corrected for decay) is typically 25%. GE TRACERlabF$_x$F-N is an automated versatile synthesizer for easy and efficient production of [^{18}F] tracers via nucleophilic substitution with [^{18}F]fluoride trapped from [^{18}O] water. Purification is achieved by an integrated, preparative HPLC system. Through application software, all process steps are easily programmed to produce the required tracers such as [^{18}F]fluoro-6-thia-heptadecanoic acid for anaerobic metabolism and cardiac ischemia, [^{18}F]fluoromisonidazole for tissue hypoxia, [^{18}F]methylbenperidol for dopaminergic D2-receptors, [^{18}F]fluoroestradiol for estrogen receptors, [^{18}F]altanserine for serotonergic S2 receptor, and [^{18}F]FLT (fluoro-L-thymidine) for cell proliferation.

GE TRACERlabF$_x$F-E is an automated, versatile synthesizer for easy and efficient production of general ^{18}F tracers via electrophilic substitution with [^{18}F]fluorine in the form of F_2. Purification is achieved by an integrated, preparative HPLC system. Through application software, all process steps are easily programmed to efficiently produce the required tracers. Examples of [^{18}F] tracers are [^{18}F]-DOPA for dopamine synthesis, [^{18}F]fluoro-L-m-tyrosine for dopamine conversion, [^{18}F]fluoro-L-tyrosine for protein synthesis and amino acid transport, [^{18}F]fluorouracil for RNA assessment. TRACERlabF$_x$C is an automated versatile synthesizer for easy and efficient production of ^{11}C-labeled tracers, mainly through methylation reactions with [^{11}C]methyliodide. Purification is achieved by an integrated preparative HPLC system. Through the application software, all process steps are easily programmed to produce the required tracers. In 2007, GE launched a second-generation module called FASTlab™. FASTlab™ is an automated PET radiochemistry synthesis platform features a single-use cassette system that accommodates different chemistries to facilitate the production of multiple fluoride-based PET tracers such as FLT—ensuring the capacity to always keep ahead of future molecular imaging applications. According to the GE Web site, this module has 70% typical uncorrected yield for FDG synthesis (81% corrected yield), independent of starting activity (for FDG, up to 15 Ci starting activity) about 15% additional FDG doses than the TRACERlabM_x. An integrated cassette preloaded with reagents that simply snaps into place is provided. This module features a short synthesis time (< 23 min for FDG) and short and simple set up (< 1 min).

Bioscan (Washington, D.C.) offers the AutoLoop ^{11}C-Methylation System, which uses the "Loop" technique. This requires no heating or cooling to improve system reliability. Sumitomo installed the first in-house cyclotron for PET diagnosis in 1979. Since then, Sumitomo has developed cyclotron technologies for PET, and a large number of studies have accumulated, some of which are listed in the reference list. Sumitomo has the majority of the market in Japan. The remarkable technology, for which Sumitomo is highly reputed, is not limited to cyclotrons, but also to radiochemistry production systems such as FDG synthesis modules. Featuring disposable kits that fit easily onto the unit's front panel, the Coincidence unit reduces preparation time and cleaning requirements to a minimum. The kit and reagent set contain everything for one production run, and low residual activity allows the user to replace the kit and begin a new synthesis immediately. Operator intervention is minimized, as a self-diagnostic routine is performed automatically and all cartridges are conditioned during the synthesis. The synthesis unit is controlled by a dedicated industrial programmable logic controller interfaced with a graphic menu-driven program on a personal computer (PC). All relevant parameters are displayed and recorded. The operator is informed when the FDG synthesis is complete, and the final product can be delivered to a remote location. The Coincidence synthesizer allows the recovery of [^{15}O] water, the most expensive raw material in the process, and has built-in radiation detectors. The FDG Module by EBCO design is less complicated, more reliable, easier to operate, and less expensive than other FDG modules available in the market place. The module has a 95% reliability and > 90% reproducibility rate from run to run.

Automated Radiotracer Production Apparatus

The Automated Radiotracer Production Apparatus (STAR) system (shown in Fig. 5.1) consists of an apparatus and a computer unit. The apparatus has two parts. The first part is designed to adapt to a cyclotron, either to produce Na^{18}F or depressurize during ^{18}F transfer. The second part uses 32 valves as well as other fittings and is housed in the lead-shielded hot cell. Two ^{18}C silica Sep-Pak columns and one alumina Sep-Pak column are first washed with 10 mL of 95% ethanol and then with 20 mL of water. The ^{18}C silica column between the vessels (tube 1 to tube 2) is left wet. The remaining two columns are forced with air until dry, and hen 10 mg of ion exchange resin AG1-X8 in the $^{-}$OH form is added to the column connected to the ^{18}F target system. In addition to the main unit, a vacuum pump is used to generate sufficient vacuum for waste collection and venting; a +24 V DC power supply is used to supply electric current to drive the valves. The same power supply is used to drive the carousel motor. A PC (Pentium) hosting two 24-channel parallel I/O cards is used to operate the relays via software. The software is a simple Microsoft Windows graphic user-interface that allows the operator to turn individual solenoid valves on and off by clicking graphic buttons.

The electrical system is located above the fluid system to prevent a potential electrical hazard resulting from fluid leakage. Three modules on each side, each corresponding to a product stage, are mounted on cards that can easily slide in and out of the chassis for servicing and replacement. A printed circuit board backplane used to connect

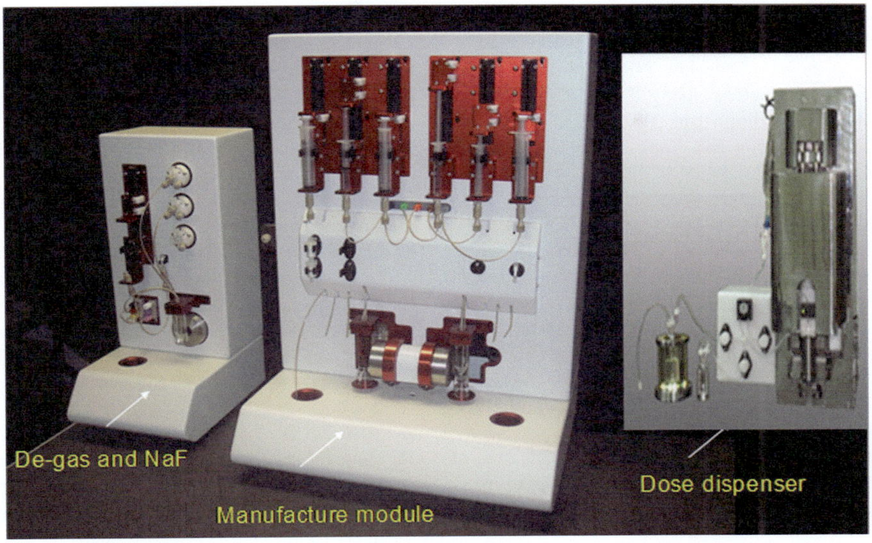

Fig. 5.1 Automated Radiotracer Production Apparatus (STAR) module for automated radiochemistry

the solenoid valves on each module to the relay circuits reduces the amount of point-to-point wiring, and therefore reduces the overall bulk. The motorized test tube carousel is used to eliminate the need to manually insert individual test tubes into the heater for heating. An infrared spot heater is used for rapid, focused heating via a side opening. The front cover is used to expose the apparatus for visibility, and the use of high-density valve packaging permits the unit to be portable. The drug product can connect to a dispenser for final drug product formulation. Using this module, synthesis of 3-[^{18}F]Fluoropropyl-hydroxytrptophan ([^{18}F]FHTP) using ^{18}F/kryptofix preparation (routine procedure) for molecular imaging of neuroendocrine disease was achieved. The final products were sterile with radiochemical yield 38% (decay corrected) and purities > 95% [21].

In summary, specific cGMP-compliant production standards and controls are necessary to ensure the safety and quality of PET drugs. Furthermore, scaling up manual synthesis for clinical imaging is challenging for multiple reasons: (1) Each batch of radiopharmaceutical usually leads to only a single administration; (2) Batch-to-batch reproducibility is required to demonstrate suitable radiochemical yield, radiochemical purity, and other quality control analysis; (3) Synthesis time must be fast when dealing with radionuclides with a short half-life; and (4) Synthesis must be arranged to maintain radiation exposures to ALARA (as low as reasonably achievable). As a result of these challenges, automated systems have been utilized as an avenue for broader development and clinical use of functional PET tracers. Automated systems can be placed in shielded hot cells and operated remotely to significantly reduce personnel exposure during synthesis. Furthermore, an automated synthesizer is often more reproducible and efficient than manual methods, reducing production time and variability between batches. With its reproducibility and cGMP it is assured that it should be able to speed radiopharmaceutical approval from bench to clinic.

References

1. Buerkle A, Weber WA. Imaging of tumor glucose utilization with positron emission tomography. Cancer Metastasis Rev. 2008;27(4):545–54.
2. Delbeke D, Coleman RE, Guiberteau MJ, et al. Procedure guideline for tumor imaging with 18F-FDG PET/CT. J Nucl Med. 2006;47(5):885–95.

3. Strauss LG, Conti PS. The application of PET in clinical oncology. J Nucl Med. 1991;32:623–48.
4. Yang DJ, Kim KD, Schechter NR, et al. Assessment of antiangiogenic effect using ^{99m}Tc-EC-endostatin. Cancer Biother Radiopharm. 2002;17:233–45.
5. Schechter NR, Wendt RE, Yang DJ, et al. Radiation dosimetry of ^{99m}Tc-labeled C225 in patients with squamous cell carcinoma of the head and neck. J Nucl Med. 2004;45(10):1683–7.
6. Gong J, Yang DJ, Kohanim S, Humphreys R, et al. Novel *in vivo* imaging demonstrates upregulation of death receptors by paclitaxel and correlates with enhanced antitumor effects of receptor agonist antibodies. Mol Cancer Ther. 2006;5(12):2991–3000.
7. Yang DJ, Ilgan S, Higuchi T, et al. Noninvasive assessment of tumor hypoxia with ^{99m}Tc-labeled metronidazole. Pharm Res. 1999;16(5):743–50.
8. Song HC, Bom HS, Cho KH, et al. Prognostication of recovery in patients with acute ischemic stroke using brain spect with ^{99m}Tc-metronidazole. Stroke. 2003; 34:982–6.
9. Ito M, Yang DJ, Mawlawi O, et al. PET and planar imaging of tumor hypoxia with labeled metronidazole. Acad Radiol. 2006;13(5):598–609.
10. Kurihara H, Yang DJ, Cristofanilli M, et al. Imaging and dosimetry of 99mTC EC annexin V: preliminary clinical study targeting apoptosis in breast tumors. Appl Radiat Isot. 2008;66:1175–82.
11. Vriens PW, Blankenberg FG, Stoot JH, et al. The use of technetium ^{99m}Tc annexin V for in vivo imaging of apoptosis during cardiac allograft rejection. J Thorac Cardiovasc Surg. 1998;116:844–53.
12. Yang DJ, Ozaki K, Oh C-S, et al. ^{99m}Tc-EC-guanine: synthesis, biodistribution and tumor imaging in animals. Pharm Res. 2005;22(9):1471–9.
13. Takahashi N, Yang DJ, Kohanim S, et al. Targeted functional imaging of estrogen receptors with ^{99m}Tc-GAP-EDL. Eur J Nucl Med Mol Imaging. 2007;34:354–62.
14. Wu JY, Yang DJ, Angelo LS, et al. Molecular imaging of Bcr-Abl phosphokinase in a xenograft model. Mol Cancer Ther. 2009;8(3):703–10.
15. US Pharmacopeia <823>. Radiopharmaceuticals for positron emission tomography-compounding; 2003.
16. Delappe E, Dunphy M. ^{18}F-2-deoxy-D-glucose positron emission tomography-computed tomography in lung cancer. Semin Roentgenol. 2011;46(3):208–23.
17. Khan N, Islam MM, Mahmood S, et al. 18 F-fluorodeoxyglucose uptake in tumor. Mymen-singh Med J. 2011;20(2):332–42.
18. Fang J, Luo XM, Yao HT, et al. Expression of glucose transporter-1, hypoxia-inducible factor-1α, phosphatidylinositol 3-kinase and protein kinase B (Akt) in relation to [(18)F]fluorodeoxyglucose uptake in nasopharyngeal diffuse large B-cell lymphoma: a case report and literature review. J Int Med Res. 2010;38(6):2160–8.
19. Chang JM, Lee HJ, Goo JM, et al. False positive and false negative FDG-PET scans in various thoracic diseases. Korean J Radiol. 2006;7(1):57–69.
20. Rosenbaum SJ, Lind T, Antoch G. False-positive FDG PET uptake–the role of PET/CT. Eur Radiol. 2006; 16(5):1054–65.
21. Yang DJ, Tzen K, Oh CS, et al. Development of F-18-FHTP for imaging neuroendocrine tumors. J Nucl Med. 2007;48(2):305P.

Cost Analysis and Effectiveness of PET and PET/CT

6

E. Edmund Kim and Franklin C.L. Wong

Positron emission tomography (PET) has been used for almost 37 years to quantify normal physiology and metabolism, to characterize disease, and to evaluate the changes resulting from disease processes. The data that have been developed from these research applications have led to the clinical applications. Clinical PET is one of the many uses of PET, including clinical care, and it is reimbursed by insurance companies. Clinical PET became a reality only after widespread reimbursement became available for the procedure. Rapid growth in the utilization of PET is directly related to changes in radiopharmaceutical regulation and reimbursement. In the Food and Drug Administration (FDA) Modernization and Accountability Act passed by Congress in 1997, it was stated that PET radiopharmaceuticals have the equivalence of FDA approval until a new process for regulating PET radiopharmaceuticals is developed. In 1998, the Health Care Financing Administration (HCFA) began covering fluorodeoxyglucose (FDG) PET for the evaluation of solitary pulmonary nodules, initial staging of lung cancer, detection of recurrent colorectal cancer with rising carcinoembryonic antigens, staging of lymphoma, and detection of recurrent malignant melanoma. The HCFA-approved indications were paid using G codes, and hospital outpatients have been reimbursed using the Ambulatory Payment Classification (APC). The PET imaging devices, both dedicated and hybrid systems, have also been covered [1]. The growing recognition of the cost effectiveness of FDG PET in cancer management has made oncology the focus for most clinical PET studies [2].

The coverage or payment for the treatment of breast cancer and Alzheimer's disease as well as myocardial viability has been recently approved. The revenue generated by PET is now a substantial portion of the total nuclear medicine department income. With the expanded coverage by Medicare of PET in oncology and cardiology, the trend of clinical PET applications seems to be toward continued growth [3]. However, the survival of PET centers may be affected by the potential decrement in reimbursement and by competition for patients from nearby PET centers. The short age of human resources may be another challenge in the future, and the reimbursement for tracers other than ^{18}F and ^{82}Rb may be necessary for further growth in clinical PET.

E.E. Kim, M.D., M.S. (✉)
Departments of Nuclear Medicine and Diagnostic Radiology, The University of Texas MD Anderson Cancer Center and Medical School, Houston, TX 77030, USA

Graduate School of Convergence Science and Technology, Seoul National University, Seoul, South Korea
e-mail: ekim@mdanderson.org

F.C.L. Wong, M.D., Ph.D., J.D.
Departments of Nuclear Medicine and Neurooncology, The University of Texas MD Anderson Cancer Center, Houston, TX 77030, USA
e-mail: fwong@mdanderson.org

E.E. Kim et al. (eds.), *Clinical PET and PET/CT: Principles and Applications*,
DOI 10.1007/978-1-4419-0802-5_6, © Springer Science+Business Media New York 2013

PET Facility

To ensure a financially successful PET center, whether hospital based or in a private practice, several steps should be followed in the initial planning and developing of the facility. A mission statement should be created to define the type of facility and its goals, which can be clinically based or research oriented, or a combination of both. The decision-making process for purchasing a PET scanner is very complicated, entailing choice of equipment, potential clinical use in the service area, physician knowledge, and FDG availability. The equipment options are dedicated PET scanners with or without a cyclotron, a coincidence camera-based PET, and a mobile PET service. There are multiple camera options with varied capabilities and differences in purchasing and operating costs. The least costly venture with the lowest financial risk is either a mobile PET service or a dual-head coincidence camera for both FDG and general nuclear imaging. The most costly and financially risky venture is a dedicated PET scanner with a cyclotron, which costs as much as $5 million. The operating cost of the cyclotron increases the operating cost of the facility by as much as one half million dollars per year. The physical location of the facility should meet federal, state, and city requirements.

The purchase of the equipment should include having the vendor as a continuous resource because the vendor's support is critical for a new technology. The following programs also should be included: initial and ongoing technician training, preceptorship and over-read programs for physicians, assistance of reimbursement, and a marketing program (speakers, materials, and a resource library). Minimum space planning should include estimations for the cyclotron room (500 sq. ft.), the heat exchanger room (150 sq. ft.), the hot/cold pharmacy laboratory (800 sq. ft.), the clinical laboratory (450 sq. ft.), the imaging suite (400 sq. ft.), the equipment control areas (100 sq. ft.), the patient preparation rooms (125 sq. ft.), and specialized support areas [4]. The cyclotron room must be capable of supporting at least 120,000 lbs for cyclotron and ancillary shielding. Adequate bench space, atmospheric exhaust hoods to hold up to 1,500 lbs, and laminar exhaust hoods should be included in the design of the pharmacy facility. Hot cells are priced at approximately $70,000 each, and remote manipulators are usually priced at $25,000 per arm. The cost of computer-assisted robotic systems for radiochemical synthesis is approximately $100,000, and the cost of automated synthesis modules for ^{18}F products are approximately $55,000 each. Specific equipment includes high-pressure liquid chromatography ($75,000), gas chromatography ($25,000), radionuclide dose calibrators, flammable safety storage cabinets, incubation ovens, and glassware. In the clinical laboratory, a glucose analyzer, a blood gas analyzer, microfuges, and a sampling device are needed for assaying blood samples. Patient preparation rooms should be configured conveniently with the imaging suite, and should be of adequate size with a nurse call system as well as a sound- and light-controlled environment.

Feasibility Study

To prepare a feasibility study of the PET operation, information should be gathered about the number of prospective referring physicians, the physicians' clinical awareness of PET, the reimbursement by third party carriers, the competition in the service area, and the commercial availability of FDG. The list of physicians to be interviewed include medical, surgical, and radiation oncologists; neurologists and neurosurgeons; and cardiologists and radiologists. Patient demographics are important if non-reimbursed procedures will constitute a significant portion of the work. Before interviewing the physicians, a matrix should be prepared that lists the local and national insurance carriers and their PET policy by covered clinical indications. After the interviews are completed, the potential number of requested scans can be estimated, and the potential financial success of the project may be computed. Total revenue (number of scans × $2,000 per scan) minus bad debt (25% of revenue) yields the net revenue. Expenses include costs of equipment leasing, facility (utilities and insurance, maintenance, radiopharmaceuticals, and supplies), and staffing (technicians, a secretary, and their benefits). There are three options for purchasing equipment: direct purchase, direct financed lease/bank debt, and operating lease. Most manufacturers have capital finance companies that can assist in the financing of the equipment. To review the ability to collect fees for the studies completed, a review must be undertaken of existing practices by the payers (Medicare and private insurers), to gather information related to covered indications, preauthorization, precertification, and payment for services.

Financial Decision and Marketing

The most common business structure is for the hospital or private practice to purchase the equipment. In a fee-for-service contract, the hospital enters into an agreement with a company, usually a mobile provider. The hospital is responsible for the purchase of the radiopharmaceuticals and related supplies. The joint venture structure has been very effective in the PET market for both scanners and cyclotrons. The FDG vendors develop a distribution network to provide other sites with FDG by either ground or air transport. The price of FDG is approximately $800 per 10 mCi and is often negotiable. Projected financial stability both on a cash and accrual basis should be maintained. There should be enough funds to carry the PET center during the start-up phase and during difficult periods for collecting accounts receivable. The marketing plan is as critical as the financial analysis. Education is the key to developing a successful marketing program. A series of grand rounds or lectures for a broad overview of PET and its clinical uses should be set up. A general brochure and scientific articles on PET as well as information for the patients also should be sent to the physicians.

Computed tomography (CT) and PET are clinically useful in the staging of non–small-cell lung cancer because it reduces unnecessary surgeries [5]. It also has been shown to be economical, with a savings of $1,154 per patient [5]. It saves significantly more by not pursuing biopsy in patients with positive CT and PET results. Significant additional savings would result if PET was used to rule out surgical candidates based on the detection of distant metastases. Compared with optimized Ga-67 single photon emission computed tomography, FDG PET achieves a higher detection rate and more accurate staging in patients with high-risk melanoma and can also detect synchronous or metachronous primary malignancies more sensitively [6]. This incremental information can alter management in approximately 10% of patients at only marginally higher cost, providing a cost-effective alternative. The entire community, including the general population, insurance providers, and the administration of the hospital, in addition to physicians, needs to be educated on all aspects of PET. The newest and fastest growing source for consumers is the Internet. A public relations company places articles about PET, such as features and patient stories, in newspapers, magazines, and on television and radio.

Cost Analysis and Effectiveness of PET and PET/CT

PET centers may be set up and operated in many different ways. Various configurations of equipment, staffing, and supplies may be combined to develop a fully functioning PET program.

The cost of developing a comprehensive PET center ranges from $5 million to $7 million as an investment for the equipment and facilities, with projected operating expenses ranging from $2 million to $2.5 million per year [7]. The cyclotron could serve the needs of multiple PET scanners in a region, and dual-use coincidence or hybrid scanners to image positron-emitting radiopharmaceuticals and traditional nuclear compounds cost less than dedicated PET scanners. Sharing operating resources between PET and other services in the hospital, developing below-market leasing rates, and securing endowment funds to cover part of the operating costs are some of many ways to reduce costs. Developing the clinical demand for more than one scanner is another way to expand revenues. The impact of the concept of radiopharmaceutical distribution is best depicted by the difference in radiopharmaceutical cost per patient.

Medicare coverage has been expanded to broadly include the use of PET in almost all cancer types. Cost analyses are important tools used by business leaders and administrators, and cost studies provide data that are useful in pricing services and benchmarking operations. Given that reimbursement levels in the public sector are fixed, it is critical to understand the net margin per study at a level of demand. Business risk is generally thought to be a function of several factors, including operating leverage (fixed or variable costs), revenue diversification, competition, and market potential. These risks are quantified somewhat by the analysis of diagnostic sensitivity.

The cost effectiveness of the diagnostic strategy must take into account not only the monetary costs of the diagnostic tests, but also the downstream effects that the test has on both the cost of medical management and the patient's clinical outcome with or without the test. Clinical utility or effectiveness is defined in terms of patient life expectancy, and the cost is defined in terms of dollars of medical expenditure. Optimization of cost effectiveness as defined by these terms is chosen to ensure an algorithm in which the costs are minimized without any decrease in patient life expectancy. The potential cost effectiveness of using FDG PET in the management of non–small-cell lung cancer through rigorous decision tree analysis has been reported [5]. It has been shown that a CT+PET strategy is more economical and has a marginal increase in patient life expectancy as compared with the conventional strategy of staging patients with CT alone. PET/CT usually enhances the diagnostic specificity rather than sensitivity compared with PET alone.

References

1. Coleman RE, Tesar R, Phelps M. HCFA and expanded coverage of PET. J Nucl Med. 1999;42:11–2N.
2. Coleman RE. PET in lung cancer. J Nucl Med. 1999;40:814–20.
3. Wong CO, Hill J. A review of trends and demands for PET imaging; one community hospital's experience. J Nucl Med. 2001;42:21–4N.
4. Chilton HM. Planning and financing a PET center. J Nucl Med. 1991;32:35–8N.
5. Gambhir SS, Hoh CK, Phelps ME, et al. Decision tree sensitivity analysis for cost-effectiveness of FDG-PET in the staging and management of non-small cell lung carcinoma. J Nucl Med. 1996;37:1428–36.
6. Kalff V, Hicks RJ, Ware RE, et al. Evaluation of high-risk melanoma: comparison of F-18 FDG PET and high dose Ga-67 SPECT. Eur J Nucl Med. 2002;29:506–15.
7. Keppler JS, Conti PS. A cost analysis of positron emission tomography. AJR. 2001;177:31–40.

Technical Principles, Radiation Safety, and Image Interpretation

7

E. Edmund Kim and Franklin C.L. Wong

The role of positron emission tomography (PET) in clinical practice is increasing. Clinical decisions based on PET studies are changing patient management by adding functional information to that obtained from conventional morphologic modalities. Focal areas of abnormally increased fluorodeoxyglucose (FDG) uptake are considered suspicious for malignant disease, as metabolic changes often precede the anatomic changes associated with disease. Disease management depends on the tumor type, extent and aggressiveness of the lesion, and on local and distant metastases. Whole-body FDG PET is becoming a standard procedure for the imaging of cancer, and FDG PET can play a significant role in establishing therapeutic response.

There is difficulty in interpreting FDG PET scans, particularly of the neck and abdomen, because of the absence of identifiable anatomic structures. The low contrast and resolution in the PET scan is insufficient for precise anatomic structures and anatomic localization of abnormal uptake. A combined PET/CT scanner successfully acquires co-registered anatomic and functional images in a single scanning session. Technical factors must be considered when evaluating organ function because they may introduce artifacts and findings that are, in reality, normal variants. These include the time between injection and scanning, the dose administered, filtering and processing steps, test-retest variability, and the type of scanner. Patient preparation, with good instructions and a questionnaire, is vitally important for proper PET scanning.

Radiopharmaceutical, Dosimetry, and Instrument

2-F-18-fluoro-2-deoxy-D-glucose (^{18}F-FDG), 5–20 mCi, is administered intravenously (IV) through an intracatheter (23–25 gauge) or butterfly needle and flushed with 10–20 cc of normal saline. The IV system should then be removed and a residual activity should be checked. If whole-body imaging will be performed in addition to the brain study, then 15–20 mCi of ^{18}F-FDG should be given. If three-dimensional (3D) imaging is necessary, a lower dose of ^{18}F-FDG should be given so that the ratio between true and random activity remains in an ideal range.

The bladder wall is the critical organ and receives 3.15 rad per 5 mCi ^{18}F-FDG. Radiation

E.E. Kim, M.D., M.S. (✉)
Departments of Nuclear Medicine and Diagnostic Radiology, The University of Texas MD Anderson Cancer Center and Medical School, Houston, TX 77030, USA

Graduate School of Convergence Science and Technology, Seoul National University, Seoul, South Korea
e-mail: ekim@mdanderson.org

F.C.L. Wong, M.D., Ph.D., J.D.
Departments of Nuclear Medicine and Neurooncology, The University of Texas MD Anderson Cancer Center, Houston, TX 77030, USA
e-mail: fwong@mdanderson.org

E.E. Kim et al. (eds.), *Clinical PET and PET/CT: Principles and Applications*, DOI 10.1007/978-1-4419-0802-5_7, © Springer Science+Business Media New York 2013

dose estimates for the bladder, heart, and brain are 1.10, 2.20, and 1.20 rad per 5 mCi ^{18}F-FDG, respectively.

The Siemens Medical System CTI ECAT HR+ dedicated full-ring PET scanner and the GE Medical Systems Discovery LS PET/CT system are commonly utilized equipment.

General Procedure

1. Patient checks in at the reception area.
2. Nurse confirms the chart and required paperwork.
3. Nurse reviews and answers any of the patient's questions regarding the procedure, and ensures that all of the required preparation before the examination has been performed.
4. Patient can change into a hospital gown or simply remove all metal objects, prostheses, etc.
5. Nurse should alert the technologist or physician if there is reason to believe that the patient cannot tolerate the procedure.
6. Patient's height and weight should be measured.
7. Patient's blood sugar levels should be measured and recorded with a glucometer. If the patient's blood sugar level exceeds 200 mg/dL, the nurse should notify the technologist or physician.
8. Patients should answer questionnaire, and female patients should sign the consent form.
9. Nurses should then begin a 20- to 23-gauge intracatheter or butterfly.
10. The prepared dose of radiopharmaceutical should be checked out from the radiopharmacy.
11. The dose of 5–20 mCi of ^{18}F-FDG and flush with 10–20 cc of normal saline should be given to the patient. The syringe should be checked to determine the residual, which should be documented.
12. Patient waits comfortably in the holding area for 30–45 min postinjection.
13. The patient should be positioned in the scanner supine with the head toward the gantry. The head should be secured to limit patient movement.
14. Set up the protocol (energy window centered at 511 keV) with lower level discriminator of 350 and upper level discriminator of 650, and assure that the correct time of injection, dose administered, and patient height and weight are entered for the procedure.
15. Perform scanning of the patient, taking care to ensure correct positioning.
16. If no transmission scan is needed because emission and normative data will be used to calculate attenuation, the study may be stopped after completion of the emission scan.
17. Upon completion of scanning, the patient may change back into their clothes and wait for the images to be reviewed before leaving. The gown or scrubs used should be placed in the linen bag to ensure there is no radiation contamination from urine.

Protocol for Whole-Body PET Using 18F-FDG

Procedure

1. Set up the protocol. Ensure that the patient's height is represented in the database of the patient. Also, ensure that the correct time of injection, dose administered minus residual, and patient weight are entered for the procedure.
   - Use 2D, seven planes of overlap, or 3D, 15 planes of overlap whole-body imaging.
   - Check the number of bed positions based on the height of the patient.
2. Position the patient from the orbits to 2 cm below the pubic symphysis. The first bed position should be over the pelvis to avoid artifacts in the retrovesical region from later accumulation of radioactive urine in the bladder.
3. Data acquisition of PET/CT. A combined PET/CT system (Discovery LS, GE Medical Systems, Waukesha, WI) is able to obtain CT images and PET data of the same patient in one session (Fig. 7.1). A GE Advance Nxi PET scanner and a multidetector-row helical CT (LightSpeed Plus) are integrated into this

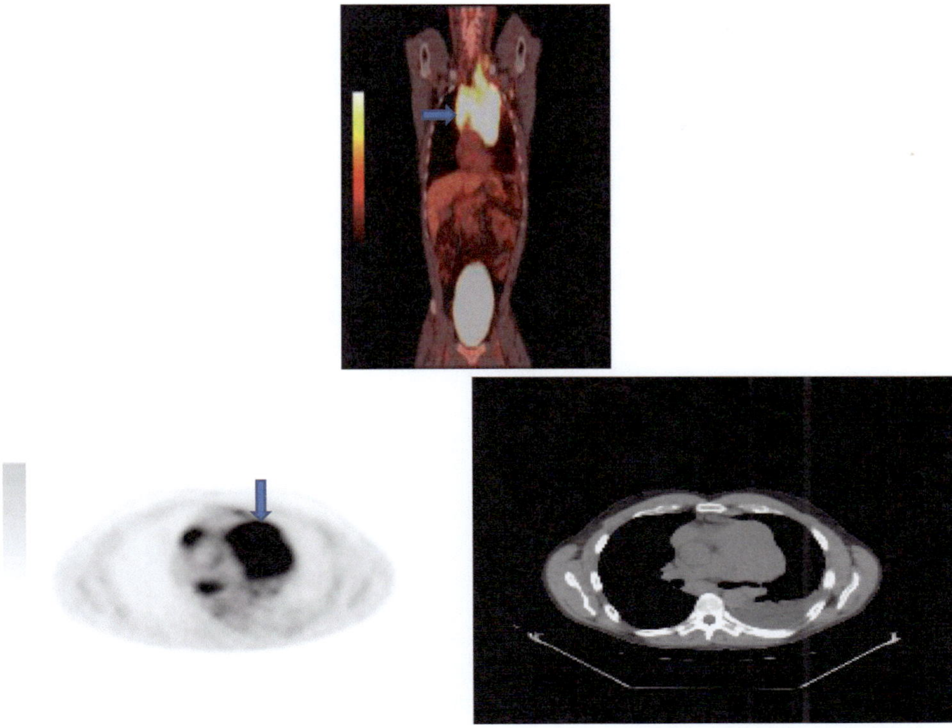

Fig. 7.1 Selected coronal PET/CT image (*top*) of the axial body with ^{18}F FDG shows a large focal area of markedly increased activity in the upper mediastinum (*arrow*) extending into left supraclavicular lymphatic chain. Selected axial PET image of the upper chest (*left lower*) shows a large focal area of markedly increased activity in the anterior mediastinum (*arrow*) as well as preaortic and right paraesophageal lymphatic chains. Axial noncontrast CT image (*right lower*) of upper chest at the same level shows ill-defined masses corresponding to increased activities. Diagnosis was Hodgkins' disease

dedicated system. The table excursion permits scanning of six continuous PET sections covering 867 mm, which gives adequate coverage from head to pelvic floor in all patients. The PET and CT datasets are acquired on two independent computer consoles that are connected by an interface to transfer CT data to the PET scanner. For viewing of the images, the PET and CT datasets are transferred to an independent, personal computer-based workstation by DICOM transfer. All viewing of co-registered images is performed with dedicated software (eNTEGRA, ELGEMS, Haifa, Israel). While PET images are acquired during free breathing and each image is acquired over multiple respiratory cycles, CT scans are acquired during shallow breathing.

The patients are fasted for at least 4 h prior to the intravenous administration of 10 mCi (370 MBq) of FDG. Forty-five minutes postinjection, the combined examination begins. CT data are acquired first. The patient is positioned on the table in a head-first, supine position. The arms of the patient are placed in an elevated position above the head to reduce beam-hardening artifacts. However, in patients unable to maintain this position, arms are positioned in front of the abdomen. For the CT data acquisition, the following parameters are used: tube rotation time 0.5 s/evolution; 140 kV; 80 mA; 22.5 mm/rotation; slice pitch 6 (high-speed mode); reconstructed slice thickness 5 mm; scan length 867 mm; acquisition time 22.5 s per CT scan. No intravenous or oral contrast agents are used.

After the CT data acquisition is completed, the tabletop is automatically advanced into the PET gantry, and acquisition of PET emission data is started at the level of the pelvic floor. Six incremental table positions are obtained with minimal overlap, thereby covering 867 mm of table travel. For each position, 35 2D non-attenuations–corrected scans are obtained simultaneously over a 5-min period. No transmission scans are obtained because CT data are used for transmission correction. Transaxial, attenuation-corrected slices are reconstructed using iterative reconstruction. Image reconstruction matrix is 128×128 with a transaxial field of view (FOV) of 49.7×49.7 cm.

4. Image analysis of PET/CT: Clinical preimaging data are available for reviewers. This information includes location of primary tumor, suspicion of local recurrence, and/or metastases. Image interpretation is performed without any objective measurements regarding FDG uptake. However, the images are consistently windowed so that brain FDG activity is in the over range and the lower window level is close to zero. On a grading scale from 0 to 4, activity comparable with brain was 4; between brain and liver, 3; liver, 2; and below liver, 1. Lesions are called positive only if they had FDG uptake of at least level 3 in PET, while in PET/CT small lesions noted on CT such as multiple intrapulmonary lesions are called positive even in the face of negative PET.

For lesion-based image analysis, the following three categories are evaluated if applicable: recurrence of primary, metastases, and second primary tumor. Because localization of the lesion is crucial for staging, all lesions are assigned to an anatomic region. Therefore, the full evaluation of a dataset includes status as well as location of recurrence, number and location of regional and distant metastases, and possible number and location of second primary tumors.

Protocol for PET Using 15O Water or Gases and 11C Methionine

1. ^{15}O water is used to measure blood flow. PET data can be acquired in 3D mode with a model-based correction applying to account for 35% of 3D scatter fraction. Images are reconstructed with a Harming filter (cutoff Nyquist). For each ^{15}O water study, 15–20 mCi are injected in 5 mL saline as a rapid bolus using an automated injector with simultaneous sampling of arterial blood and 4-min gynamic PET scan (23 frames; 10×3 s, 3×10 s, 4×15 s, and 6×20 s). The arterial blood data (input function) are collected over 4 min. Blood is drawn at a 6-mL/min rate and radioactive events are detected. Eight sequential PET scans are obtained at 20-min intervals. The data are analyzed using the tissue compartment model.
2. ^{15}O gases are used to measure blood flow and volume as well as oxygen extraction and metabolism. ^{15}O gases, O_2, CO_2, and CO, are administered sequentially in one session to provide three separate datasets.

The ^{15}O O_2 and ^{15}O CO_2 gases are delivered continuously at flows of 10 mCi/min at 80 mL/min, and 5 mCi/min at 60 mL/min, respectively during the study period. Labeled gases are mixed with 200 mL/min of medical air, and are supplied to the patient through a plastic face mask. Once inhalation of the labeled gas is initiated, equilibrium will be established over a 12-min period, followed by scans with 1.5–2.5 million for each ^{15}O O_2 image and 2–4 million ^{15}O for each CO_2 image. ^{15}O CO is administered at 80 mCi at 100 mL/min for 4 min. The ^{15}O CO supply is then discontinued, and following a 1-min equilibrium period, images can be obtained with 300,000–500,000 true coincidences. Blood samples are obtained from an arterial line for the measurement of blood gases throughout the studies.

The oxygen analysis program generates maps for the functional parameters for each anatomic plane as a composite dataset. The oxygen extraction fraction and metabolic rate are corrected for blood volume.

3. ^{11}C-Methionine PET. ^{11}C-methionine is another tracer for PET that can be used to assess metabolic demand for amino acids in cancer cells. Methionine PET has been useful in the differential diagnosis of benign and malignant lesions in the brain and lungs. Patients fast for at least 6 h before the PET

scan. A transmission scan is acquired for 20 min using a rotating ^{68}Ge source, and the total counts per slice are more than seven million. Emission scans are obtained over a 15-min scanning period, 20–30 min after intravenous injection of 10 mCi ^{11}C-methionine, with more than three million counts per slice. Image reconstruction in a 128 × 128 matrix using measured attenuation correction is performed using a Shepp and Logan filter.

Common Questions Asked by Patients and Answers

What Is PET?

PET is a technology that combines the fields of medicine, computer science, chemistry, physics, and physiology to study the function of organs such as the heart, brain, and bone. It is different from conventional imaging equipment such as radiography, CT, sonography, and MRI, in that PET images contain information about how tissues function. The other imaging modalities show what the tissues look like.

What Does a PET Scanner Look Like?

The PET scanner is similar in shape to a CT or MRI scanner; however, a PET scanner makes no noise. The bed on the scanner moves during the examination so that each area of the body can be imaged.

What Can I Expect?

- You will be asked questions about your illness.
- Your blood glucose (sugar) levels will be checked.
- A small IV tube will be placed into your arm to administer a very small quantity of a radioactive material. This allows for the PET scanner to "see" where sugar metabolizes in your body.
- Because the injection you will receive is radioactive and because it is important that you are relaxed and quiet after the injection, family members are not allowed in the area while you are in the PET suite.
- Depending on the type of PET scan that you are receiving, you may be given a medicine called Lasix through the same IV line that the radioactive sugar was injected. Lasix is a diuretic that will stimulate you to urinate.
- Again, depending on the type of PET scan, you might need to have a tube, also known as a Foley catheter, placed in your bladder. This is done so that the scanner can "see" the area surrounding your bladder.
- After the injection, you will need to rest quietly until it is time for your scan. Again, the amount of quiet time depends on the study, but be prepared to wait for between 45 and 90 min.
- During the scan, you will lie on your back on a table.
- The amount of time the scan takes depends on how tall you are and why you are having the test.
- When the examination is over, the data will be processed and the results will be reported to your physician the following day.

Can I Eat?

No. We cannot emphasize this enough. If you eat within 6 h of your test, there is an exceptionally high chance that your examination will be canceled. The reason for this is that the scan relies on how your body absorbs sugar, and if you have eaten, your body is saturated with sugar and the medication we give will not distribute properly.

If your PET scan is scheduled in the morning, you must only drink water. No caffeine or sugar products may be consumed. If your scan is later in the afternoon, do not eat for at least 6 h before your test. You may take all of your medications. If the medication needs to be taken with food, we will contact your physician and give you further instructions.

How Long Does the Test Take?

Overall, you should allow approximately 3 h for your test. The preparation for the scan takes about 45 min. The procedure typically takes a little over an hour. However, the physician may want to obtain additional images.

Is PET Safe?

PET is a noninvasive technique that provides maximum information to your physicians with minimal radiation exposure. The radiotracers remain in the body for only short periods of time and have no known side effects.

Questionnaire for Patients

Table 7.1 is an example of a questionnaire given to patients.

Worksheet for PET

Table 7.2 is an example of a worksheet for staff.

Checklist for Female Patients

Table 7.3 is an example of a checklist for female patients.

Radiation Safety

Gamma quanta and radiographs are ionizing radiations that produce various biological effects in tissues. The energy doses delivered to patients in PET/CT are far below the 0.5 Gy threshold dose. Radiation exposure in CT may occur to organs located directly in the path of the X-ray beam or may result from the scattering of radiation inside or outside the body. The energy dose in CT depends on the current–time product (mAs), the kilovoltage (kv), and scanner-specific features. The dose is also indirectly affected by parameters such as slice thickness, object thickness, pitch factor, scan time, rotational speed, and FOV. The effective dose is the sum of the energy doses accumulated in an organ exposed to x-rays and gamma rays multiplied by tissue-weighting factors specific to that organ.

The properties of both gamma rays and x-rays must be accounted for in the radiation protection of technical staffs involved in PET/CT examinations. The half-value layer for lead shielding (the thickness of lead needed to reduce radiation intensity by one half) is 0.1 mm for x-rays (150 kv) and 4.5 mm for gamma rays (511 kev). The lead aprons used for the protection of diagnostic x-rays are of no practical value because of the penetrating power of gamma rays.

Interpretation of PET/CT

PET/CT is a combination of two highly specialized examinations, and thus each procedure must be evaluated individually to interpret all the findings correctly. PET, with its sensitive detection of metabolically active foci, can draw attention to even very subtle morphologic changes. However, this must not lead to a failure to evaluate the CT results with diagnostic intent based on classic analytical criteria. In general, FDG PET is a very sensitive but less specific modality. Therefore, an approach to optimal interpretation is to maximize specificity by correlations with clinical data and morphologic imaging. For typical PET scans, three sets of data are provided. The nonattenuation and attenuation-corrected images are typically reconstructed in axial, sagittal, and coronal planes. Findings on all datasets should be closely correlated. Errors caused by attenuation correction may lead to an apparent decrease in metabolic activity. Lowering the arms during the acquisition will usually cause artifacts of attenuation correction, especially about the shoulder girdle but also in the chest. PET has decreased sensitivity but increased specificity in small lesions while PET has increased sensitivity but possibly decreased specificity in larger lesions. A low level of metabolic activity does not always exclude a tumor.

Table 7.1 Questionnaire

Patient Name ________	Patient ID ________		
Weight ____lb ______kg	Height ________cm		
Blood sugar level mg/dL: (1)____ (2) ____	(3) ____		
1. Have you been fasting?	Yes	No	Comment: ________
2. Are you hydrated?	Yes	No	
3. Surgical history ________			
4. Where are your incision sites? ________			
5. Have you had any biopsies recently?	Yes	No	If yes, where? ________
6. Have you had chemotherapy?	Yes	No	If yes, when? ________
7. Have you had radiation therapy?	Yes	No	If yes, when? ________
8. Do you have an ostomy site?	Yes	No	If yes, where? ________
9. Do you have a catheter (CVC or porta-cath) placed?	Yes	No	
If yes, where? ________ when? ________			
10. Do you have any metal objects or prostheses on?	Yes	No	
11. Do you have a pacemaker?	Yes	No	
12. Have you had any of the following:			
Inflammation	Yes	No	If yes, when? ________
Recent injury	Yes	No	If yes, when? ________
Infection (sinus, throat, bladder, etc.)	Yes	No	If yes, when? ________
13. Are you positive for any of the following inflammatory diseases?			
Tuberculosis	Yes	No	
Rheumatoid arthritis	Yes	No	
Toxoplasmosis	Yes	No	
14. Were you instructed not to eat 6 h prior to the study?	Yes	No	
15. Were you instructed to drink 6–8 glasses of water?	Yes	No	
16. Are you aware that the study takes approximately 3 h to complete?	Yes	No	
17. Were you told that family members are not allowed into the PET suite?	Yes	No	
18. Do you have any questions or issues?			
If so, what were they? ________			
Scheduled ________	Time		
Scheduled ________	AM/PM		
Patient information completed by: ________			

Table 7.2 Worksheet

1. General Information

Patient Name ______________________________

Medical Record Number (MRN) ______________ Height______________

Outpatient [ ] Inpatient [ ] (room #_________) DOB______________

Weight _________

Male [ ] Female [ ] (Pregnant? Yes [ ] No [ ])

Translation services required? No [ ] Yes [ ] language:______________

Contact numbers:

Home______________________ Work______________________

(Local/cell)______________________

Requesting physician______________________________

2. Patient instructions

   a. Is the patient a diabetic? Yes [ ] No [ ]
      If yes, what was the last reading? ___________<200? Yes [ ] No [ ]
      Note: If the patient's glucose level is 200 or higher, contact the nuclear medicine special procedures physician
   b. Is the patient able to lie on his/her back for over an hour? Yes [ ] No [ ]
      Note: If the patient is unable to lie on his/her back for that amount of time, he/she may wish to contact his/her physician for a dose of pain medication.
   c. Is the patient claustrophobic? Yes [ ] No [ ]
      Has the patient ever had a problem having with MRI or CT? Yes [ ] No [ ]
      Note: If the patient answers yes to either of these questions, refer this case to a
      PET nurse to evaluate for conscious sedation.
   d. Has the patient had radiation therapy? Yes [ ] No [ ]
      (If yes, is the patient currently undergoing treatment, or when was the radiation therapy completed? ______________)
   e. Is the patient receiving chemotherapy? Yes [ ] No [ ]
      (If yes, include list of medications in the next question.)
   f. Has the patient had a previous PET/gallium scan? Yes [ ] No [ ]
      If answer is yes, date:____________
      List medications (name, dosage, and frequency) that the patient is taking.

g.	Was the patient instructed not to eat 6 h prior to the study?	Yes [ ]	No [ ]
h.	Was the patient instructed to drink 6–8 glasses of water?	Yes [ ]	No [ ]
i.	Is the patient aware the study takes approximately 3 h to complete?	Yes [ ]	No [ ]
j.	Was the patient told that family members are not allowed into the PET suite?	Yes [ ]	No [ ]
k.	Did the patient have any questions or issues?	Yes [ ]	No [ ]

If so, what were they?

____

Scheduled________________________________ Time

Scheduled________________________________ AM/PM

Patient information completed by: ______________________

Table 7.3 Checklist for female patients

1. Have you passed menopause:	Yes	No
If your answer is yes, go to question 6. If your answer is no, please answer all of the following questions.		
2. Are you pregnant or do you believe you might be pregnant?	Yes	No
3. How many days has it been since the beginning of your last menstrual cycle? _____		
4. Are you practicing any form of birth control?	Yes	No
5. Are you nursing a baby?	Yes	No
6. Are you currently taking any hormones?	Yes	No
7. Do you have young children at home?	Yes	No
8. Have you had surgery on your breasts? Implants, reconstruction?	Yes	No
9. Do you understand the above questions?	Yes	No
10. Do you have any questions about using radioactive substances or about the questions above that you would like to discuss with a physician?	Yes	No

Because PET is performed during free breathing whereas CT may be acquired during a breath-hold, inaccurate localization of lesions may result. The head and breast may be changed in position between CT and PET examinations.

A hypermetabolic lesion does not always signify malignancy. It is associated with reconstruction artifacts, metallic implants, barium-based contrast media, certain benign tumors, inflammations, and brown fat. For oncologic patients, it is important to report standard uptake values of index lesions. The impression should state clearly any potential limitations of PET for the specific disease process, and the relevance of PET findings should be stated explicitly. A uniform color scale should be used for evaluating maximum intensity projection and sectional images. Inverted gray and yellow-red scales have proved effective in practice.

Normal and Variable Patterns in PET

8

Ho-Young Lee, Myung-Chul Lee,
and E. Edmund Kim

Introduction

The clinical applications and investigations of positron emission tomography (PET) have recently been increasing. The majority of the clinical PET studies and the use of ^{18}F-fluoro-2-deoxyglucose (FDG) are related to oncology, but the uptake of this radiopharmaceutical is not specific to malignant tissue. There are several physiologic uptakes and artifacts which make it difficult to evaluate or detect malignant tissue. It is important to be aware of normal variants and benign diseases that may mimic more serious pathology. Uptake of FDG in a number of sites may be variable and may normally be seen in the skeletal muscle after exercise or under tension, in the myocardium, in parts of the gastrointestinal tract, especially the stomach and cecum, and in the urinary tract. Some causes of increased physiologic uptake are avoidable, and measures can be taken to minimize accumulation [1].

In certain clinical situations, the lack of specificity of ^{18}F-FDG uptake has led to the applications of L-[methyl-C-11] methionine. Because of the short half-life of C-11, use of this radiopharmaceutical is limited to those PET scanners that are not far from a cyclotron. However, C-11 methionine has now become one of the most commonly used radiopharmaceuticals in clinical PET [2].

PET Imaging with 18F-FDG

A. Uptake mechanism

18F-FDG is an analog of glucose that is an energy substrate of metabolism [3]. Although tumors show increased glycolysis compared with normal tissues, the uptake of 18F-FDG is not specific to malignant tissue. 18F-FDG is transported into tumor cells by glucose transporter membrane proteins (Glut-1 to Glut-5). In particular, the expression of Glut-1 is increased in many tumors. After being transported into the cell, 18F-FDG is converted to 18F-FDG-6-phosphate by hexokinase.

H.-Y. Lee, M.D. (✉)
Department of Nuclear Medicine, Seoul Metropolitan Government-Seoul National University Hospital, Boramae Medical Center,
Seoul 156-707, South Korea
e-mail: md1004_2000@yahoo.co.kr

M.-C. Lee, M.D., Ph.D.
Department of Nuclear Medicine, Gachon University School of Medicine, 1198 Guwol-dong,
Namdong-Gu, Incheon 405, South Korea
e-mail: mclee@gilhospital.com

E.E. Kim, M.D., M.S.
Departments of Nuclear Medicine and Diagnostic Radiology, The University of Texas MD Anderson Cancer Center and Medical School,
Houston, TX 77030, USA

Graduate School of Convergence Science and Technology, Seoul National University,
Seoul, South Korea
e-mail: ekim@mdanderson.org

E.E. Kim et al. (eds.), *Clinical PET and PET/CT: Principles and Applications*,
DOI 10.1007/978-1-4419-0802-5_8, © Springer Science+Business Media New York 2013

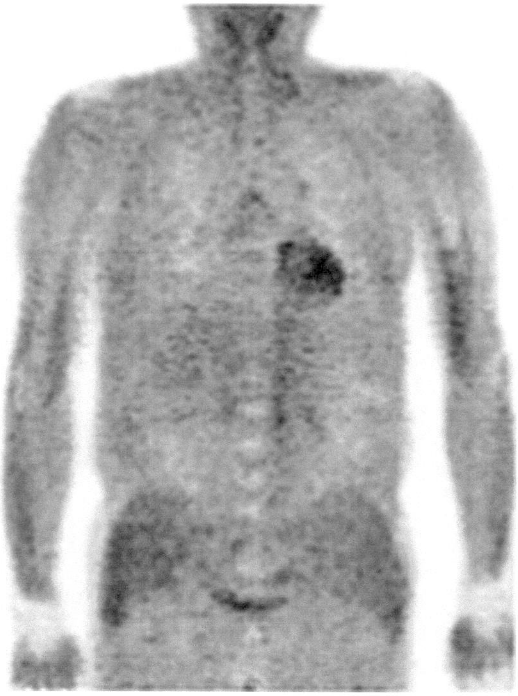

Fig. 8.1 Coronal 18F-FDG PET images of patient after meal. Note significantly decreased activities in liver, spleen, etc., which have normal FDG uptake. In contrast to liver, the muscle activities are increased

Following that, it does not enter further enzymatic metabolic process. Because of its negative charge, it remains trapped in tissue. Glucose-6-phosphatase mediated dephosphorylation of the 18F-FDG-6-phosphate. It occurs slowly in myocardium, brain. Many tumors have low concentrations of that enzyme, and hence the accumulation of 18F-FDG-6-phosphate is proportional to the rate of glycolysis. Conversely, tissues such as the liver, kidney, intestine, and resting skeletal muscle with high glucose-6-phosphatase activity may show lower activity.

Tumor uptake of 18F-FDG is poor in acute hyperglycemia as a result of competition between 18F-FDG and glucose. To optimize the accumulation in tumors, patients are usually fasted for 4–6 h prior to scanning. Hyperglycemia after meals reduce uptake in tumor and normal uptake in the liver, spleen, etc., and increased uptake in muscle (Fig. 8.1). Fortunately it appears that chronic hyperglycemia, as seen in diabetic patients, only minimally reduces tumor uptake, but that insulin-induced hypoglycemia may actually impair tumor identification by reducing tumor uptake and increasing background muscle activity.

It has also been noted that the hypoxia in tumors may increase the accumulation of 18F-FDG and also probably occurs through the activation of the anaerobic glycolytic pathway.

B. Normal physiologic distribution of ^{18}F-FDG
In the abdomen, low-grade accumulation of FDG is usually seen in the liver and the spleen. Small and large bowel activity may be variable, and unlike glucose, ^{18}F-FDG is excreted in the urine, leading to variable appearance in the urinary tract.

Skeletal muscle at rest usually shows low-grade uptake of ^{18}F-FDG but active skeletal muscle, after exercise, shows increased accumulation. Low-grade FDG uptake in muscles is part of the normal biodistribution pattern [4]. When this uptake is symmetric and corresponds to the location of a specific group of muscles, it is easily recognized.

Myocardial uptake of ^{18}F-FDG is also very variable [4,5]. Normal myocardial metabolism depends on free fatty acids and glucose. Optimal uptake of ^{18}F-FDG in myocardial metabolic studies can be encouraged by the administration of oral glucose to increase glucose metabolism with or without insulin to enhance the myocardial uptake of glucose, and hence ^{18}F-FDG. A hyperinsulinemic euglycemic clamping technique may further improve myocardial ^{18}F-FDG uptake but is technically more difficult. This allows maximal insulin administration without rendering patients hypoglycemic. An alternative method to encourage glucose metabolism in the myocardium is to reduce circulating free fatty acids pharmacologically. Improved cardiac uptake after administration of oral nicotinic acid derivatives has been reported. This will be a simple and safe intervention which may also be effective in diabetic patients.

The brain typically shows high uptake of ^{18}F-FDG in the cortex, basal ganglia, and thalamus but a generalized reduction in cortical activity may be seen with sedative and general anesthetic drugs which may be required for uncooperative patients and children. This may limit the sensitivity for the detection of areas of hypometabolism. There is a general decline in metabolic activity in the frontal and somatosensory areas with normal aging [6].

C. Physiologic variants that may mimic pathology

1. Skeletal muscle

At rest, skeletal muscle does not show significant accumulation of ^{18}F-FDG, but after exercise or if contraction takes place during the uptake period after ^{18}F-FDG injection, there is an increased uptake in active skeletal muscle.

This relates to increased aerobic glycolysis of active muscle tissue.

Increased aerobic glycolysis of active skeletal muscle such as paraspinal, posterior cervical, or trapezius muscle may lead to increased accumulation of ^{18}F-FDG after exercise or as a result of tension, and is one of the most common causes of interpretative problems. Symmetric FDG uptake in the shoulder, neck, and thoracic spine region is possibly related to activated brown fatty tissue in underweight patients during increased sympathetic nerve activity as a result of cold stress [7]. Laryngeal muscle activity may be related to speech, and swallowing may cause hyoid and tongue base activities. Hyperventilation may create a diaphragmatic uptake. Exercise should be prohibited on the day of scanning to minimize muscle uptake, and benzodiazepines may be used to abolish the characteristic paraspinal and posterior cervical muscle uptakes often seen in tense patients. Even with these precautions, skeletal muscle activity may still be seen. Anxiety-related increased muscular tension may cause symmetric or asymmetric uptake in neck and paravertebral muscles.

Problems may also result from involuntary muscle spasm such as that seen with torticollis, which can lead to asymmetric, unilateral uptake in the sternocleidomastoid muscle, and that may either mimic or obscure the pathology in the neck. Accurate interpretation of asymmetric muscle activity in the neck, shoulder, or arm is at times difficult [8]. Trauma and inflammation may also cause an enhanced skeletal muscle activity.

2. Gastrointestinal system

A number of regions in the gastrointestinal system may show uptake of ^{18}F-FDG. This may be partly because of smooth muscle activity, although it has been shown that gastrointestinal uptake of ^{18}F-FDG in rats may be reduced either by bowel lavage or by use of antimicrobials, suggesting an alternative mechanism such as smooth muscle peristalsis [9]. In humans, ^{18}F-FDG activity is most noticeable in the large bowel and to a lesser extent in the stomach and small intestine. Low-to-moderate stomach wall activity, particularly fundal activity, is commonly noted and may be mistaken for a tumor mass. Sagittal slices may be helpful in defining the oblique position of the stomach as it passes caudally. Marked activity may on occasion be seen in the cecum and sigmoid/rectum, leading to difficulties in interpretation when assessing local recurrence of large bowel tumors.

Lymphoid tissues may also demonstrate the significant uptake of ^{18}F-FDG, and the normal appearance of the tonsils and adenoids (which may be particularly marked in children) would be recognized [5]. After radiotherapy or surgery, pharyngeal lymphoid activity may become asymmetric, making it more difficult to differentiate from physiologic activity. It is also possible that cecal activity, which is often seen as the normal variant, may be because of lymphoid tissue that is present in this region [1].

Apart from excreted ^{18}F-FDG through the urinary system, which could be seen

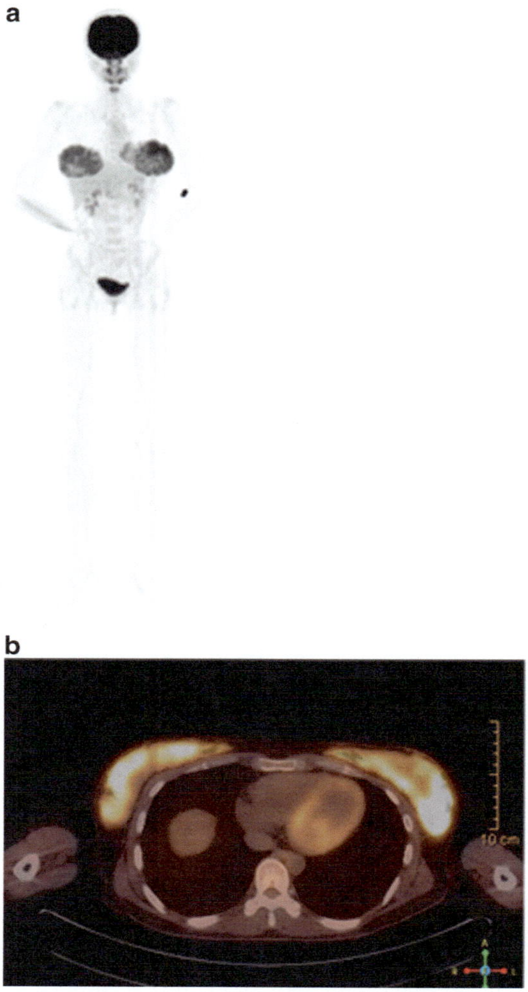

Fig. 8.2 Coronal ^{18}F-FDG PET image of nursing female. Note intense increased uptake of FDG in bilateral breast

anywhere within the urinary tract, prior knowledge of any urinary diversion procedure may be helpful to avoid errors in interpretation. An ileal conduit or other urinary intestinal diversions may produce unusual images unless the alteration in anatomy is appreciated.

3. Urinary tract

   Unlike glucose, FDG is not totally reabsorbed in the renal tubules [1]. Significant and variable urinary activity is seen in all patients. Renal collecting system activity is easily recognized but may limit the use of FDG in the investigation of tumors in the urinary tract. If there is significant hold up in the renal collecting system of an obstructed kidney, reconstruction artifacts may interfere with visualization of the upper abdomen. Imaging may be improved in a nonobstructed but dilated system by keeping the patients well-hydrated, and by administrating diuretics.

4. Reticuloendothelial system

   Hepatic and splenic activities on attenuation-corrected images are slightly nonuniform, and thus small metastatic lesions are very difficult to be identified.

   Hepatic activity on uncorrected images is similar to lung uptakes with slightly increased activity in the periphery. There is no gallbladder activity.

   Bone marrow and thymus harbor many white cells which are known to take up ^{18}F-FDG. When these cells are activated by the growth factors or cytokine therapy, the activities in the bone marrow and spleen are markedly increased. Increased marrow activity is also seen in patients with acute infection resulting from increased production of white cells [10].

5. Miscellaneous variants

   On occasion, skin contamination from urinary activity may be limited at the superficial areas which are usually easily recognized as such. Breast uptake may be variable, and focal increased uptake may be seen at the nipple. Asymmetric uptake may be noted in a woman who fed her baby on one side. Thymic activity may be seen in children or late teens with an inverted V shape [1].

6. Other variants

   Intense breast tissue uptake of ^{18}F-FDG is noted in breast-feeding women (Fig. 8.2). Glandular breast tissue often demonstrates moderate uptake of ^{18}F-FDG in premenopausal women. After menopause there is little breast activity, but women on estrogen for hormone replacement therapy (HRT) may also show an enhanced uptake. The symmetric nature would suggest taking HRT but there is the potential for lesions to be obscured by this physiologic activity.

D. Artifacts

If attenuation correction is not performed on whole-body PET imaging, it may lead to higher apparent activity in superficial structures such as the skin, which may obscure lesions (e.g., cutaneous melanoma metastases). A common artifact resulting from this phenomenon is caused by the axillary skin fold, where a double layer of skin may mimic focal lymphadenopathy on coronal sections. The linear distribution of activity on axial or sagittal planes would help to prevent a misinterpretation.

Artifacts caused by prostheses are usually readily recognizable. Photon-deficient areas may result from metallic hip prostheses, breast prostheses, implants, medallions, and coins and keys in pockets, etc. Ring artifacts may occur if there is a misregistration between transmission and emission data (e.g., due to slight patient movement), and are especially apparent at borders where there are sudden large changes in activity (e.g., at a metal prosthesis).

Patient movement may compromise image quality. In brain imaging, splitting the study into a number of time frames may be helpful so that if movement occurs in one frame, it can be discarded before summation of the data. Whole-body imaging can lead to unusual appearances if the patient moves between bed scan positions with, for example, the upper part of an arm being visible in the higher scanning positions, but being absent or "amputated" lower down when moved out of the field of view scanning positions.

Problem with injections may interfere with image interpretation. A partly infiltrated injection not only may cause reconstruction artifacts across the trunk, but may result in a low-count study and inaccuracies in standardized uptake value (SUV) measurement. Local axillary lymph node uptake may occur following subcutaneous extravasation, and thus radiopharmaceuticals should be administered on the opposite side to the known or questioned pathologic lesion, if possible. Although rare, an inadvertent intra-arterial injection may be easily recognized.

PET Imaging With C-11 Methionine

A. Uptake mechanism

C-11 L- methionine represents the amino acid with which there is a sufficient clinical experience in PET imaging. Increased transport and utilization of amino acids are common in cancers. The use of L-methionine in cancer imaging is based on this observation and the increased activity of the transmethylation in some cancers. There is normally substantial uptake of C-11 methionine in the pancreas, salivary glands, liver, and kidneys. As a natural amino acid, there is some metabolism of L-methionine in the bloodstream. This tracer is mostly used in imaging of brain tumors, head and neck cancers, lymphoma, and lung cancers as well as several other clinical settings. Early clinical studies demonstrated the stereospecificity of tumor uptake. L-methionine uptake is much greater in brain tumors than the uptake of D-methionine when an intact brain–blood barrier was present [2].

B. Physiologic distribution of C-11 methionine

By far the greatest experience with C-11 methionine lies in brain tumor imaging. Uptake of ^{18}F-FDG into brain tumors is closely related to grade of malignancy. As there is high uptake of ^{18}F-FDG into the normal brain cortex and basal ganglia, it may be difficult to identify low- or intermediate-grade tumor with similar or less activity. The relatively high uptake of ^{18}F-FDG in normal structure may, however, allow better anatomic localization of those tumors that are visible or similarly may give a number of anatomic landmarks to aid image registration with magnetic resonance imaging (MRI) or computed tomography (CT). In contrast to ^{18}F-FDG, C-11 methionine typically shows low-grade uptake in the normal cortex and is better suited for detection of low- and intermediate-grade tumors. However, while tumor margins and extent may be more easily identified with C-11 methionine, the correlation between tumor grade and uptake appears less strong than that with ^{18}F-FDG.

One of the most difficult problems in the management of primary brain tumors is the assessment of tumor recurrence versus posttreatment scar and gliosis, which often remain problematic with anatomic imaging such as MRI and CT, and where functional imaging with PET has a role. Soon after radiation therapy, accumulation of ^{18}F-FDG may occur in macrophages surrounding necrotic areas in addition to any viable tumor cells. By contrast, methionine has low uptake by macrophages and other cellular components but accumulates in viable cancer cells. Uptake of C-11 methionine therefore correlates better with tumor extent when compared with surgical and biopsy findings. Unlike ^{18}F-FDG, there is no significantly increased uptake of C-11 methionine in stressed muscles.

Tumor imaging in the pelvis may be problematic because normal excreted activity in the urine may interfere with tumor identification. Because there is very little urinary C-11 methionine activity in the majority of patients, the use of this tracer has been evaluated in a number of urinary and gynecologic cancers. Besides the response of invasive bladder tumor to chemotherapy, ovarian and uterine cancers have been assessed with this radiopharmaceutical.

C. Physiologic variants

As with all imaging techniques, a thorough knowledge of normal distribution and anatomic, physiologic, and pathologic variants is required to avoid misinterpretation. As the clinical use of C-11 methionine PET develops, more and more potential pitfalls will be recognized. Here we summarize the status from our own and others' experience.

There are a number of structures in the head during brain tumor imaging that normally show accumulation of C-11 methionine. The lacrimal glands may show moderately intense uptake but may be easily recognized by virtue of the symmetric distribution and the anterior position below the frontal lobes. Normal bone marrow uptake within the sphenoid and clivus may cause confusion at the skull base, however. Pathologic variants that we have experienced include uptakes within a recent biopsy tract, into an incidental benign meningioma, and also within the pons to the surrounding area following radiotherapy.

In the neck, bone and bone marrow activity, which may appear quite focal at the medial tips of the clavicles, may cause false positive interpretations when investigating hyperparathyroidism or focal metastatic lymph node. The majority of patients show no thyroid C-11 methionine activity; however, a small percent show a low-grade activity that is lower than the activity seen in abnormal parathyroid glands. This may actually be helpful in identifying anatomic landmarks for the surgeon. Unfortunately, as with other nuclear medicine procedures for investigating hyperparathyroidism, the uptake within the thyroid may on occasion interfere with diagnosis. We have noted diffusely increased uptake in patients with coincidental Hashimoto's thyroiditis and thyrotoxicosis resulting from Grave's disease. Uptake may also be seen in benign thyroid nodules and thus correlative imaging may be required with this technique in specific cases.

High salivary gland activity is demonstrated by C-11 methionine PET. This is unlikely to cause confusion but asymmetric activity following unilateral radiotherapy or extensive surgery for head and neck cancers may be problematic.

In the abdomen, physiologic accumulation within the bowel may cause difficulties and limit the use of this tracer in the investigation of bowel cancer and pelvic tumors. High pancreatic uptake in the upper mid-abdomen is normally identified although this may obscure the uptake within pancreatic tumors. We have found that anatomic information obtained from a C-11 methionine scan complements an 18F-FDG scan where no significant pancreatic accumulation normally occurs.

Presence of urinary C-11 methonine activity is variable but occurs in the minority of patients. It may nevertheless lead to interpretative problems in the pelvis. In our experience, there is low-grade renal cortical activity which would not be expected to interfere with renal tumor evaluation.

References

1. Cook GJR, Fogelman I, Maisey MN. Normal physiological and benign pathological variants of F-18 deoxyglucose PET scanning: potential for error in interpretation. Semin Nucl Med. 1996;26:308–14.
2. O'Tuama LA, Phillips PC, Smith IR, et al. L-methionine uptake by human cerebral cortex. Maturation from infancy to old age. J Nucl Med. 1991;32:16–20.
3. Newberg A, Alvi A, Reivich M. Determination of regional cerebral function with FDG-PET imaging in neuropsychiatric disorders. Semin Nucl Med. 2002;32:13–34.
4. Tashiro M, Fujimoto T, Itoh M, et al. F-18 FDG PET imaging of muscle activity in runners. J Nucl Med. 1999;40:70–6.
5. Shreve PD, Anzai Y, Wahl R. Pitfalls in oncologic diagnosis with FDG PET imaging: physiologic and benign variants.
6. Loessner A, Alvi A, Lewandrowski KU, et al. Regional cerebral function determined by FDG-PET in healthy volunteers: normal patterns and changes with age. J Nucl Med. 1995;36:1141–9.
7. Hany TF, Gharehpapagh E, Kamel EM, et al. Brown adipose tissue: a factor to consider in symmetrical tracer uptake in the neck and upper chest region. Eur J Nucl Med. 2002;29:1393–8.
8. Yasuda S, Fuji H, Takahashi W, et al. Elevated F-18 FDG uptake in the posas muscle. Clin Nucl Med. 1998;23:716–7.
9. Kim S-K, Chung J-K, Kim B-T, et al. Relationship between gastrointestinal F-18 FDG accumulation and gastrointestinal symptoms in whole-body PET. Clin Pos Imaging. 1999;2:273–80.
10. Sugawara Y, Fisher SJ, Zasadny KR, et al. Preclinical and clinical studies of bone marrow uptake of F-18 FDG with or without granulocyte colony stimulating factor during chemotherapy. J Clin Oncol. 1998;16:173–80.

Artifacts in FDG PET and PET/CT

9

Masashi Kawaguchi, Ukihide Tateishi, Tomio Inoue, and E. Edmund Kim

As the number of clinical positron emission tomography (PET) units is increasing, interpretation of PET images requires knowledge of the possible pitfalls that may occur because of artifacts and mimic pathology. In addition, the advent of combined PET/computed tomography (CT) scanners in clinical imaging practice has brought its own specific pitfalls and artifacts. These artifacts may be caused by various factors such as injection, attenuation material, image reconstruction, contamination, patient movements, and pathologic variants. Knowledge of the normal distribution of fluorodeoxyglucose (FDG) and its pathologic variation is essential before interpreting PET scans as well as an awareness of potential false positive and negative cases that can occur. With attention to detail in the preparation of patients, together with appropriate imaging protocols and experience in interpretation, many pitfalls can be avoided.

M. Kawaguchi • U. Tateishi, M.D., Ph.D. (✉)
T. Inoue, M.D., Ph.D.
Department of Radiology, Yokohama City University Graduate School of Medicine, Yokohama 236-0004, Japan
e-mail: utateish@yokohama-cu.ac.jp; tomioi@yokohama-cu.ac.jp

E.E. Kim, M.D., M.S.
Departments of Nuclear Medicine and Diagnostic Radiology, The University of Texas MD Anderson Cancer Center and Medical School, Houston, TX 77030, USA

Graduate School of Convergence Science and Technology, Seoul National University, Seoul, South Korea
e-mail: ekim@mdanderson.org

Normal Whole-Body FDG Distribution

On whole-body PET performed between 1 and 2 h following intravenous administration of FDG, the brain, heart, and urinary tract are the most prominent sites of tracer accumulation (Fig. 9.1).

In the brain, there is high uptake in the cortex and basal ganglia irrespective of different substrates as glucose is the predominate substrate for brain metabolism. The liver and spleen are associated with slightly higher FDG activity than blood pool levels and are reliably identified in the abdomen, as are the kidneys. Some lymphoid tissue is normally quite active, including the tissues of Waldeyer's ring where the tonsils can show moderate uptake, and that is usually symmetrical. Salivary glands also show low to moderate symmetrical uptake. Thymic activity is commonly seen in children and can also be seen in adolescents and young adults after chemotherapy as a result of thymic rebound phenomenon [1]. Cardiac activity is variable and depends to some extent on substrate availability such as fatty acids and glucose. Glandular tissue of the breast is associated with low-level uptake in younger woman. Bone marrow is normally associated with modest FDG uptake, roughly equivalent to liver. The bowel is seen to varying degrees, as is the stomach because of widely variable levels of

E.E. Kim et al. (eds.), *Clinical PET and PET/CT: Principles and Applications*,
DOI 10.1007/978-1-4419-0802-5_9, © Springer Science+Business Media New York 2013

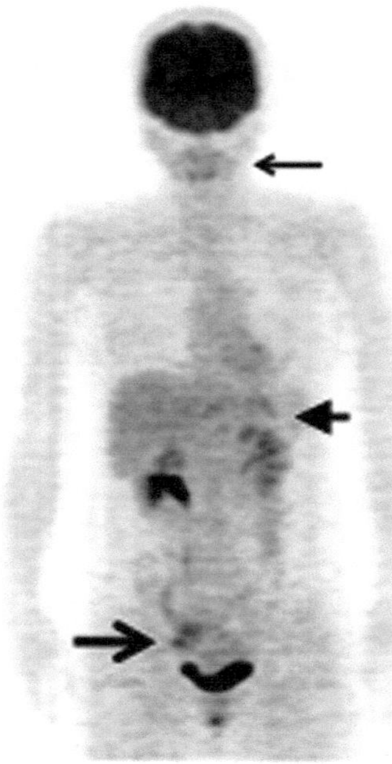

Fig. 9.1 48-y-old, female. Normal distribution of FDG 1 h following intravenous tracer administration. Attenuation-corrected anterior maximum intensity projection (MIP) image. Intense tracer activity in the brain and bladder. In the neck, palatine tonsil lymphoid tissue tracer activity (*small arrow*) is seen. Inferior to the heart is low-level gastric tracer activity (*arrowhead*) and the outlines of the liver, spleen, and kidneys are discernable. In premenopausal women cyclical right ovarian uptake of FDG is seen in pelvis (*large arrow*)

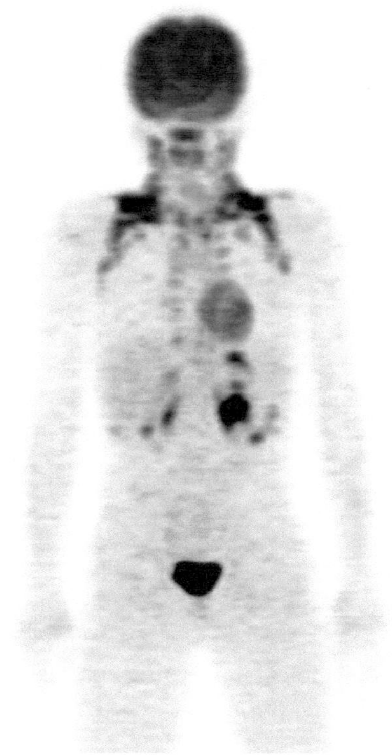

Fig. 9.2 Brown adipose tissue (BAT) FDG uptake. Anterior MIP image of 9-y-old boy. Intense FDG activity is present symmetrically at the base of neck, upper mediastinum, supraclavicular regions, axillae, paravertebral locations at the thoracic spine

FDG uptake in the alimentary tract. Marrow is commonly identified in the vertebral bodies, pelvis, hips, proximal long bones, and the sternum. The level of FDG uptake in children is higher in bone marrows than in adults. Uptake of FDG into active, non-rested muscle is a potential cause of misinterpretation of FDG PET scans although with combined PET/CT, this is less likely. Activities such as talking can lead to muscle uptake in the neck and larynx. Asymmetric uptake can be seen in laryngeal muscles in patients with vocal code palsies [2]. In premenopausal women, FDG uptake of cyclical ovarian and uterine has been described [3]. Activity of uterine cavity is seen at mid cycle and during menses and ovarian activity can be seen at mid cycle.

Brown adipose tissue (BAT) expresses a unique mitochondrial uncoupling protein that permits direct heat generation from fatty acid oxidation in response to cold exposure, ingestion of food, or increased sympathetic activity. This process requires an increased supply of adenosine triphosphate (ATP), which in turn is provided by an increase in glycolytic metabolism. It is recognized that intense increased FDG activity can localize to adipose tissue in the neck, supraclavicular regions, axillae, paravertebral locations at the thoracic spine, mediastinum, and occasionally subdiaphragmatic and perinephric fat (Fig. 9.2). This phenomenon is seen more often in young patients, females, and slender patients [4].

Artifacts in FDG PET and PET/CT

Injection-related artifacts may interfere with image interpretation (Fig. 9.3). A partly infiltrated injection causes a reconstruction artifact across the trunk. It also results in inaccuracy of the standard uptake value (SUV). If the injection leak on FDG PET images is demonstrated, the SUV derived from these images should be carefully evaluated. Following the subcutaneous extravasations of FDG solution, the tracer may flow into the lymphatic channel and may be trapped in local lymph nodes [5]. It mimics an abnormal FDG uptake in the lymph node metastases. The tracer should be administered on the opposite site to the known lesion. Increased levels of insulin in the peri-injection period cause extracardiac uptake in diabetic patients or patients who did not fast [6].

On PET/CT scanners, the emission data can be corrected for photon attenuation using the CT scan to generate an attenuation map. Doing so confers the following advantages: there is less statistical noise from the CT compared with germanium 68 (^{68}Ge) transmission data on standalone PET scanners; the scanning time for CT is much shorter then for radionuclide imaging, thus reducing overall scanning time by 15–20 min; and the need for PET transmission hardware and the cost of replacing germanium source rods are eliminated [7].

There is a potential risk of overestimating the true FDG activity with CT-based attenuation correction. When the CT images are used to perform attenuation correction of the PET projection data, dense objects can cause apparent hot spot artifacts on the PET, as well as beam hardening artifact on CT images. Metallic prosthetic implants and high-density medical devices such as dental fillings, hip prosthetics, surgical clips, metallic stents, drainage tubes, or chemotherapy ports cause high CT numbers and generate streaking artifacts on CT images because of their high photon absorption [8,9]. This increase in CT numbers results in high PET attenuation coefficients, which lead to an overestimation of the PET activity in that lesion and thereby to false-positive PET imaging (Figs. 9.4, 9.5, 9.6, and 9.7).

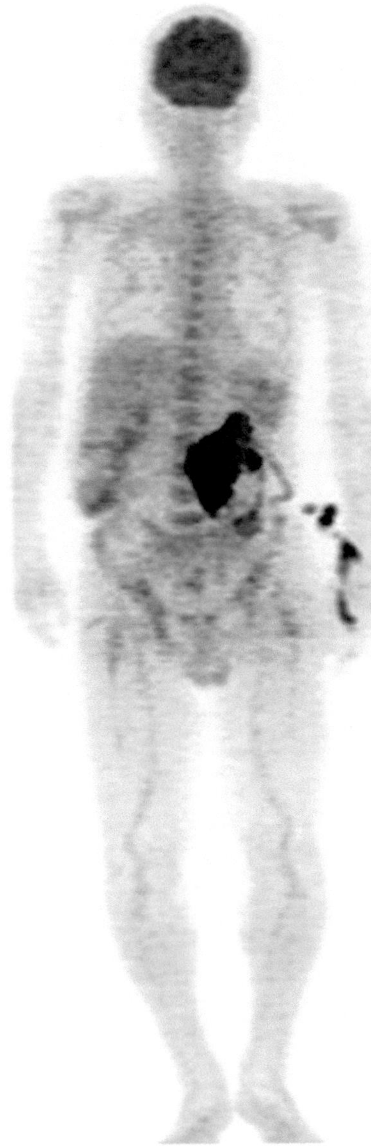

Fig. 9.3 Anterior MIP image of a patient with retroperitoneal tumor (*small arrow*). Note increased uptake in nephrostomy tube (*large arrow*). Subcutaneous extravasation and superficial contamination of FDG solution are seen in left forearm (*arrowhead*)

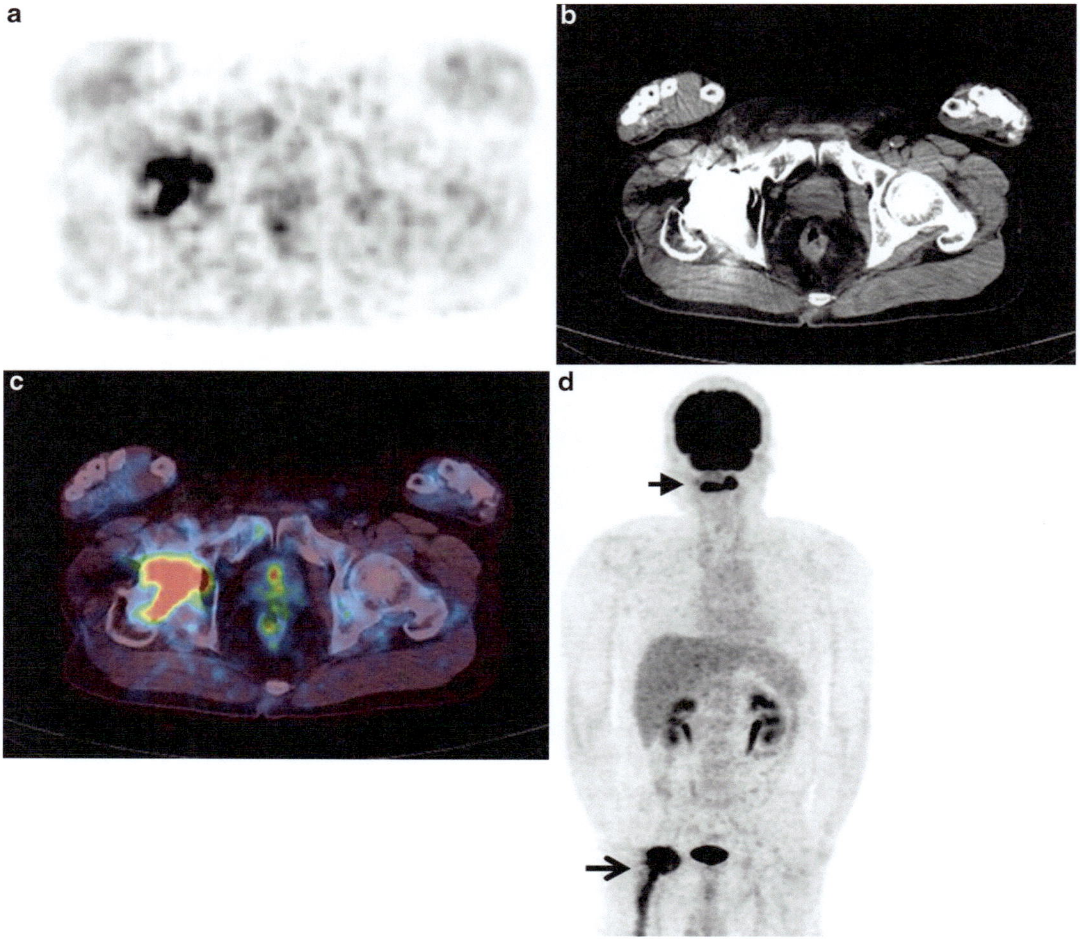

Fig. 9.4 Artifacts because of metallic dental fillings (*arrowhead*) and hip prosthetics (*arrows*). PET scan shows apparent increased activity in oral cavity and right hip joint

Intravenous or oral agents such as iodine and barium sulfate are administered to improve the quality of CT images by delineating vessels and soft tissues [10]. High contrast concentration results in high CT numbers and streaking artifacts on CT images. Therefore, contrast media also can cause an overestimation of tracer uptake and produce false-positive PET results similar to metallic implants (Fig. 9.8).

Such artifacts can be recognized by review of the non-attenuation-corrected filtered back projection PET images (Fig. 9.9). It is important to verify attenuation-corrected images against non-attenuation corrected images to avoid false-positive results. Regarding the image reconstruction, attenuation correction is essentially needed to obtain the quantitative image data such as the SUV.

Present statistical image reconstruction algorithms can yield focal apparent increased activity from movement artifacts or generalized noise. Transaxial attenuation-corrected images generated using ordered-subset expectation maximization reconstruction method with three interactions and eight subsets show multiple tiny apparent foci of increased FDG activity in the liver of a large patient. It is advisable to have non-attenua-

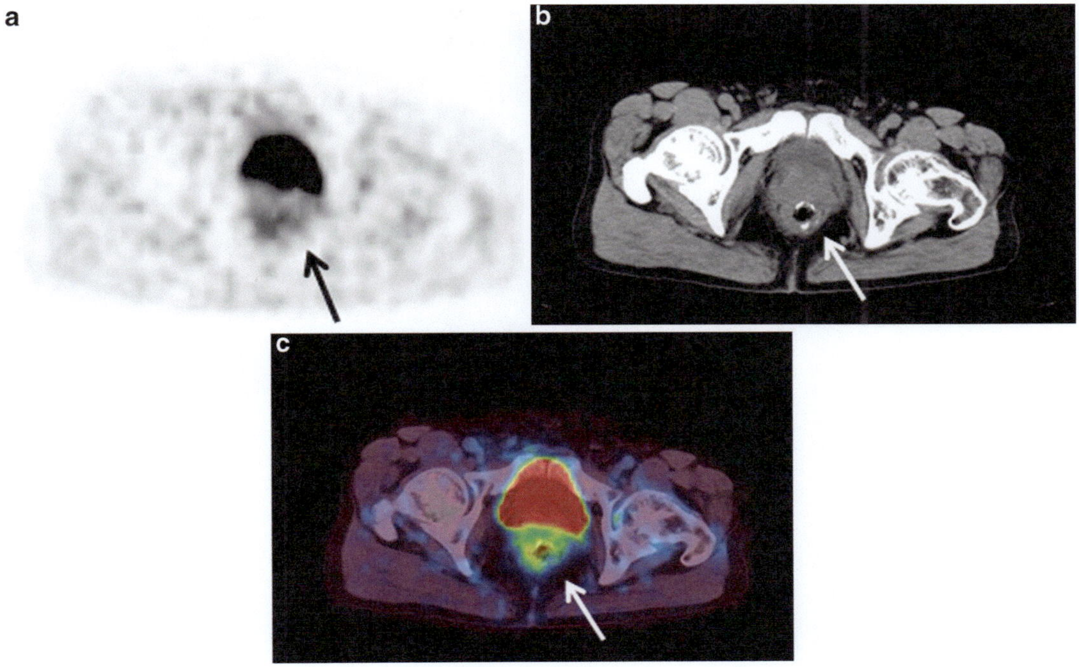

Fig. 9.5 55-y-old man who underwent resection for rectal cancer. Transaxial PET image through pelvis reveals focus of increased tracer uptake in rectum (*arrow*), suggestive of local recurrence. Corresponding CT scan shows surgical clip in place (*white arrow*)

tion-corrected filtered back projection images for confirmation of such suspect abnormalities.

Urinary contamination is sometimes observed on FDG PET images. Because urinary contamination is usually superficial activity on the skin or clothes, it is easily recognized as artifact.

Patient movements degrade the image quality of FDG PET. Whole-body FDG PET imaging can lead to an unusual appearance if the patient moves between the bed scan positions, with the upper part of an arm, for example, being visible in the higher scanning positions but absent or "amputated" lower down when moved out of the field of view for lower scanning positions (Fig. 9.10).

Respiratory motion during scanning causes artifact in PET/CT imaging. The artifact is caused by the discrepancy between the chest position on the CT image and the chest position on the PET image. Each bed position of the PET scan may take 2–5 min to acquire during free breathing and resulting in images representing an average position of respiratory cycle. This may lead to misregistration of lung nodules by 15 mm [11]. Difference between the PET and CT acquisitions may be maximal at the level of the diaphragm which may lead to artifacts, the most common being an apparent area of reduced activity at the diaphragmatic surface when the CT data are used for attenuation correction. Additionally, this can lead to apparent mispositioning of liver metastases into the lung base (Figs. 9.11 and 9.12).

Motion artifacts lead to two major effects: First, it affects the accuracy of quantification, producing a reduction of the measured SUV. Second, the apparent lesion volume is overestimated. Respiratory gating by applying a multiple-frame capture technique, with which PET data are

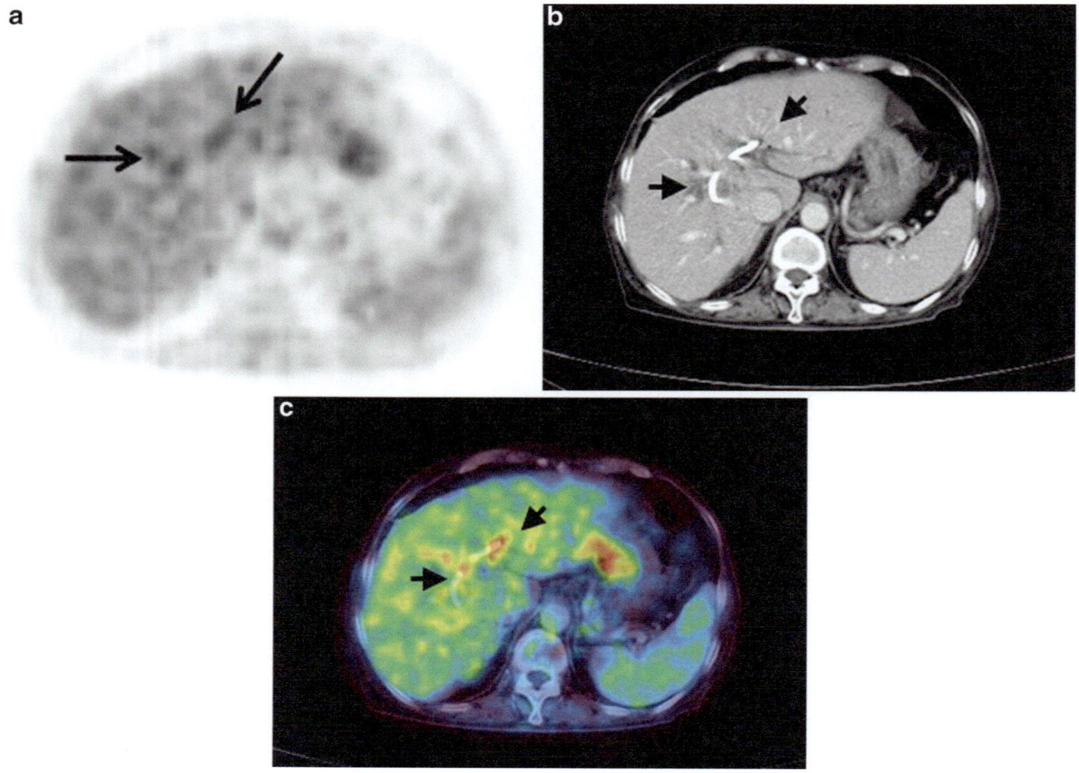

Fig. 9.6 73-y-old woman with extrahepatic bile duct cancer. Transaxial PET image reveals focus of increased tracer uptake in liver (*arrows*), suggestive of tumor invasion. Corresponding CT scan shows bile duct tube in place (*arrowheads*)

acquired in synchronization with the respiratory motion, compensates for these effects.

A number of benign diseases may cause significant uptake of FDG that may simulate malignant lesion. In the chest, active tuberculosis, sarcoidosis, and histoplasmosis have been reported as showing increased FDG uptake (Fig. 9.13) [12]. These disorders may lead to FDG uptake (SUV) in the borderline or low-malignant range. Inflammation in any tissue may cause increased FDG uptake. Common sites of inflammatory activity are surgical or radiotherapeutic areas (Fig. 9.14), and the activities may last for several weeks after therapy.

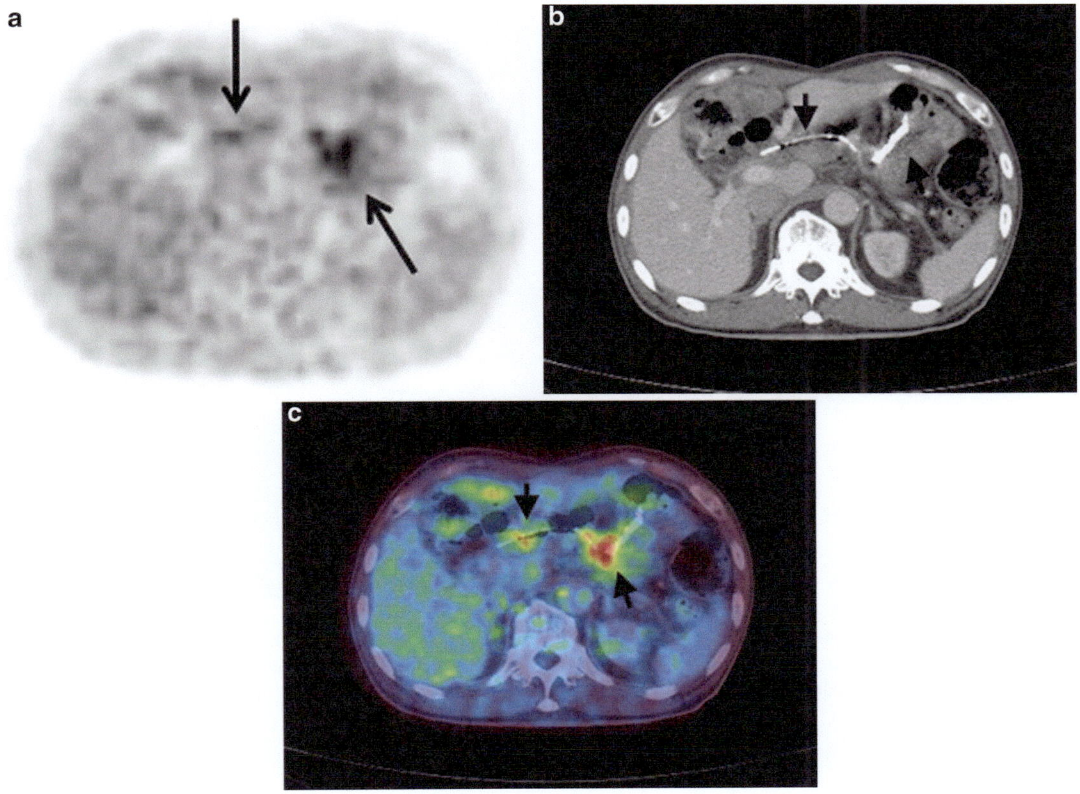

Fig. 9.7 76-y-old man after gastorectomy and pancreatoduodenectomy for gastric cancer and pancreatic cancer. Transaxial PET image reveals focus of increased tracer uptake in residual stomach and pancreas (*arrows*), suggestive of recurrence. Corresponding CT scan shows surgical clip in the stomach and pancreatic duct tube (*white arrow*)

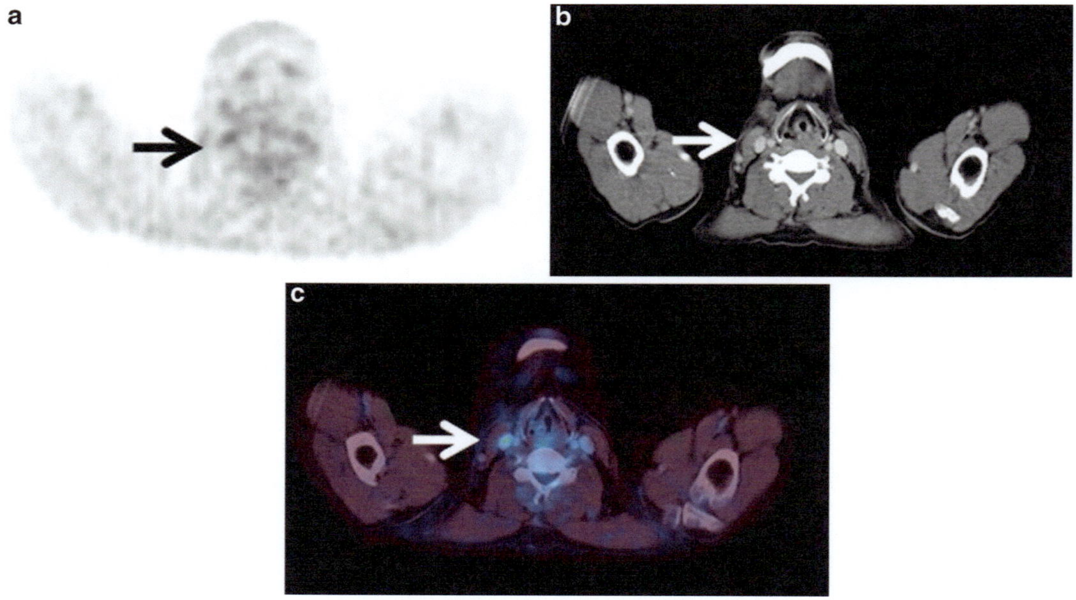

Fig. 9.8 Focal nodal uptake is seen in the right neck on FDG PET (*arrow*). It apparently seems to be lymph node metastasis although CT scan shows intravenous contrast medium in right common carotid artery and internal jugular vein (*white arrow*) at the site

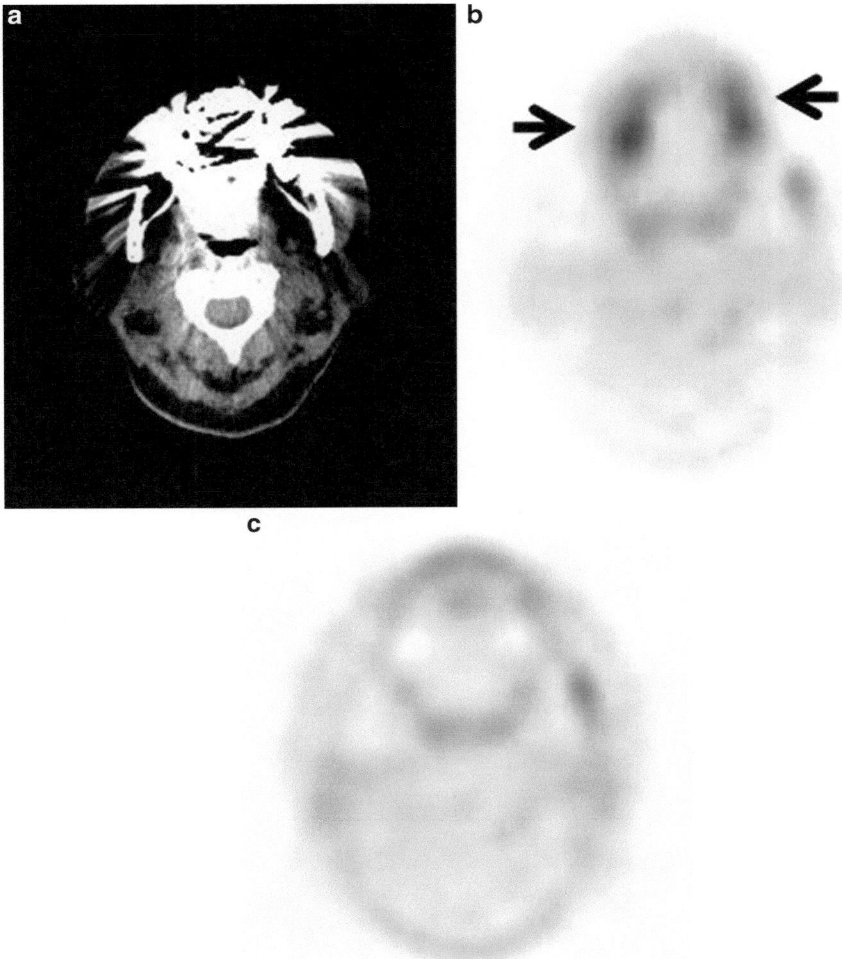

Fig. 9.9 High-density metallic implants generate streaking artifacts and high CT numbers on CT image. High CT numbers will then to be mapped to high PET attenuation coefficients, leading to overestimation of activity concentration (*arrows*). PET images without attenuation correction help to rule out metal induced artifacts

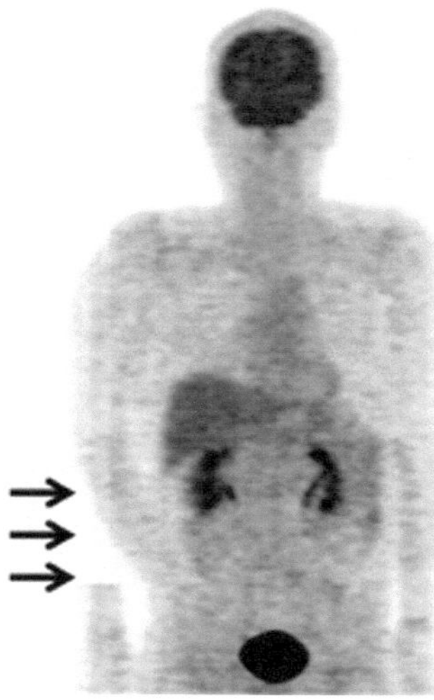

Fig. 9.10 FDG PET MIP image shows an unusual appearance with discontinuous activity in the right forearm (*arrows*) as a result of patient's movements between bed scan positions

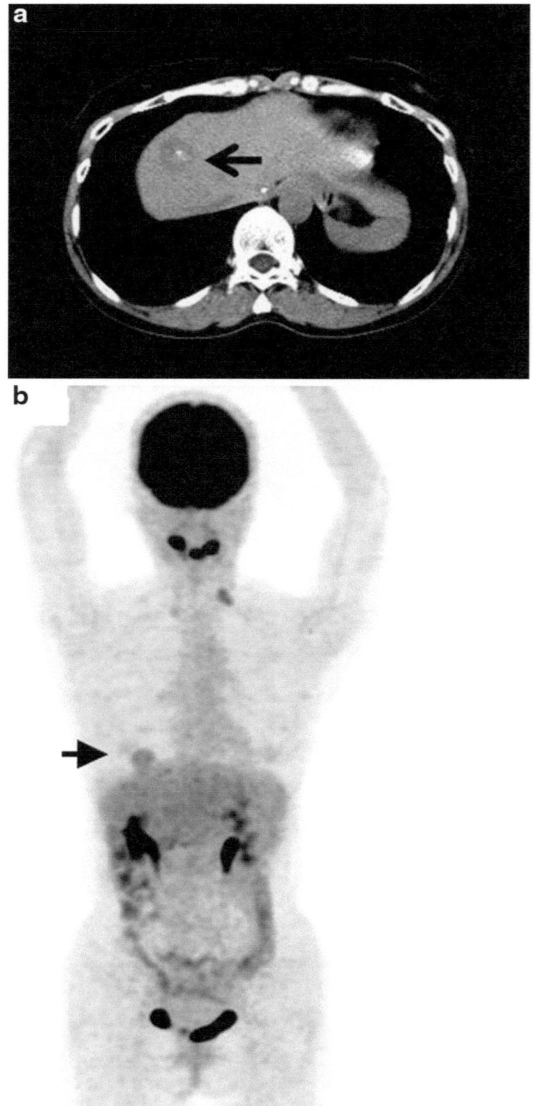

Fig. 9.11 55-y-old woman with liver metastasis of colon cancer. Lesion at dome of liver (*arrow*) is mislocalized to right lung base (*arrowhead*) because of respiratory mismatch on PET images with CT attenuation correction

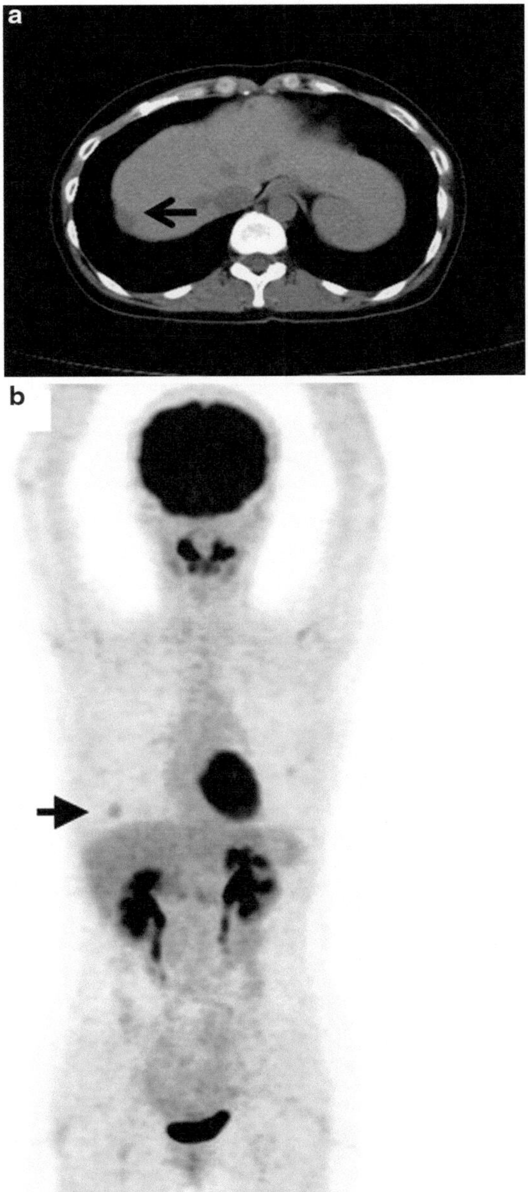

Fig. 9.12 46-y-old woman with peritoneal dissemination of ovary cancer. Lesion at dome of liver (*arrow*) is mislocalized to right lung (*arrowhead*) because of respiratory motion

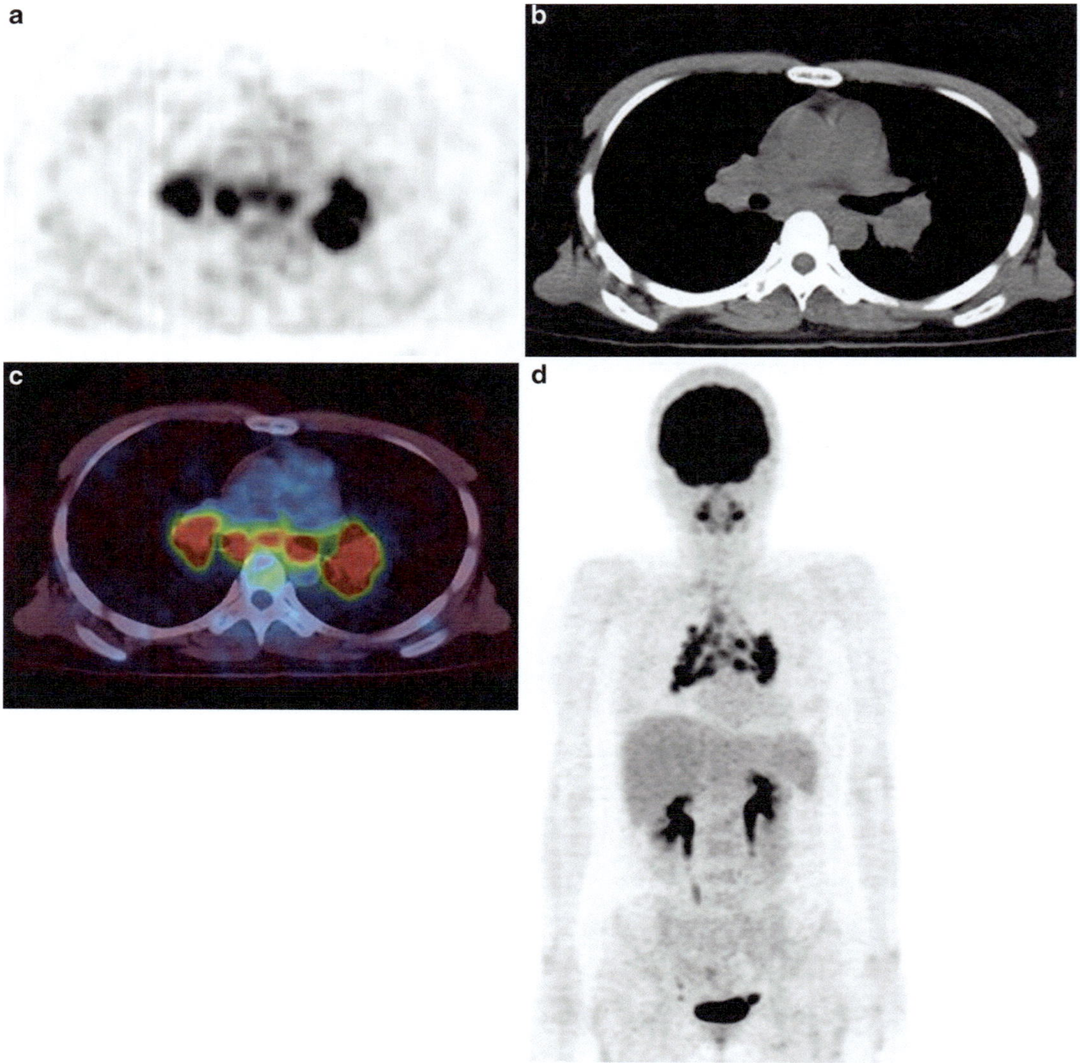

Fig. 9.13 Patterns of FDG PET in sarcoidosis. Increased FDG uptake involving enlarged lymph nodes in the bilateral mediastinum and pulmonary hila

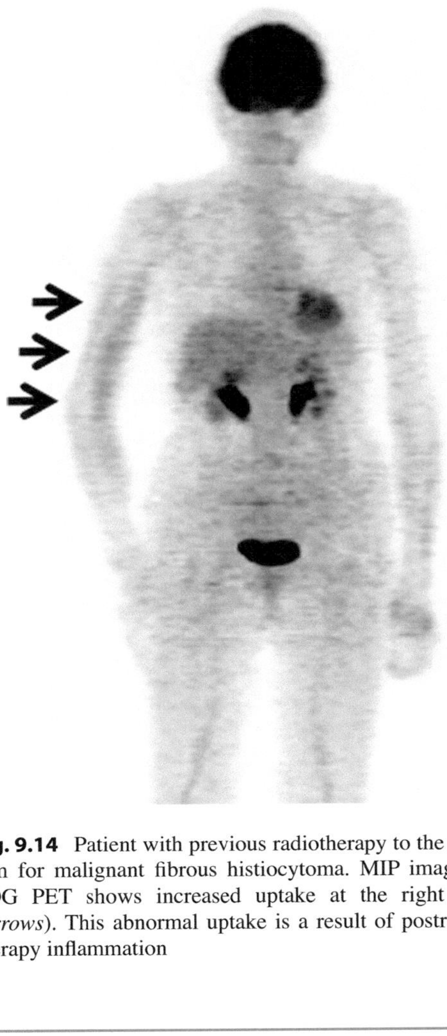

Fig. 9.14 Patient with previous radiotherapy to the right arm for malignant fibrous histiocytoma. MIP image of FDG PET shows increased uptake at the right arm (*arrows*). This abnormal uptake is a result of postradiotherapy inflammation

References

1. Kawano T, Suzuki A, Ishida A, Takahashi N, Lee J, Tayama Y, et al. The clinical relevance of thymic fluorodeoxyglucose uptake in pediatric patients after chemotherapy. Eur J Nucl Med Mol Imaging. 2004;31:831–6.
2. Kamel EM, Goerres GW, Burger C, von Schulthess GK, Stenert HC. Recurrent laryngeal nerve palsy in patients with lung cancer: detection with PET-CT image fusion: report of six cases. Radiology. 2002;224:153–6.
3. Lerman H, Mtese U, Grisaru D, Fishman A, Lievshitz G, Even-Sapir E. Normal and abnormal ^{18}F-FDG endometrial and ovarian uptake in pre- and postmenopausal patients: assessment by PET/CT. J Nucl Med. 2004;45:266–71.
4. Yeung HWD, Grewal RK, Gonen M, et al. Patterns of ^{18}F-FDG uptake in adipose tissue and muscle: a potential source of false-positives for PET. J Nucl Med. 2003;44:1789–96.
5. Alibazoglu H, Megremis D, Ali A, et al. Injection artifact on FDG-PET imaging. Clin Nucl Med. 1998;23:264–5.
6. Minn H, Nuutila P, Lindholm P, et al. In vivo effects of insulin on tumor and skeletal muscle glucose metabolism in patients with lymphoma. Cancer. 1994;73:1490–8.
7. Nakamoto Y, Osman M, Cohade C, et al. PETCT: comparison of quantitative tracer uptake between germanium and CT transmission attenuation-corrected scans. J Nucl Med. 2002;43(9):1137–43.
8. Goerres GW, Hany TF, Kamel E, et al. Head and neck imaging with PET and PET/CT: artefacts from dental metallic implants. Eur J Nucl Med. 2002;29:369–70.
9. Kamel EM, Burger C, Buck A, von Schulthess GK, Goerres GW. Impact of metallic dental implants on CT-based attenuation correction in a combined PET/CT scanner. Eur Radiol. 2003;13:724–8.
10. Antoch G, Freudenberg LS, Egelhof T, et al. Focal tracer uptake: a potential artifact in contrast-enhanced dual-modality PET/CT scans. J Nucl Med. 2002;43:1339–42.
11. Goerres GW, Kamel E, Seifert B, Burger C, Buck A, Hany TF, et al. Accuracy of image coresistration of pulmonary lesions in patients with non-small cell lung cancer using an integrated PET/CT system. J Nucl Med. 2002;43:1469–75.
12. Cook GJR, Fogelman I, Maisey MN. Normal physiological and benign pathological variants of F-18 deoxyglucose PET: potential for error in interpretation. Semin Nucl Med. 1996;26:308–24.

Radiation Dosimetry in ^{18}F-FDG PET/CT

10

Eunkyung (Angela) Park

The number of 18F-fluorodeoxyglucose (FDG) positron emission tomography (PET) and PET/computed tomography (CT) examinations that are performed is rapidly increasing. A total of 308,663 FDG PET and PET/CT examinations were performed in Korea in 2009 compared with 66 examinations conducted in 1994, when the first PET was installed [1]. In the US, probably more than 1.5 million PET and PET/CT patient studies were performed per year in recent years.

FDG PET and PET/CT examinations are now an integral part of daily oncology practice. Whole-body FDG PET or PET/CT is known to be useful during every stage of care in oncology patients, including diagnosis, staging workup, treatment response evaluation, restaging, follow-up for recurrence surveillance, and predicting prognosis [2, 3]. FDG PET and PET/CT examinations are also being used with benefit in patients with various neurologic and cardiovascular diseases.

Given the increasing number of FDG PET and PET/CT examinations, radiation safety has become an important issue. Many patients undergo multiple PET/CT examinations along with other radiologic examinations throughout the treatment and follow-up periods. The major concerns of FDG PET and PET/CT examinations are radiation-related long-term side effects, such as hematooncologic diseases and heritable effects.

Those concerns have led to as the following questions: What is the amount of radiation exposure per FDG PET or PET/CT examination? What are the potential hazards of radiation exposure associated with FDG PET or PET/CT examinations? From a radiation-effect perspective, is it acceptable to use FDG PET or PET/CT annually as a tool for cancer screening in healthy individuals? What kind of special attention must be paid to pediatric patients and pregnant women? What do the current risk estimates indicate? What can be done to minimize radiation dose and potential hazards while maintaining optimal image quality?

We will attempt to answer these questions by determining the following: (1) the basic radiation dosimetry of FDG PET and PET/CT in oncology patients; (2) the relationship between radiation dose and potential hazards; (3) the use of FDG PET or PET/CT as a cancer screening tool in healthy populations; and (4) special considerations for pediatric patients and pregnant women.

Basic Quantities of Radiation Dosimetry

Gamma rays from PET and x-rays from CT are forms of ionizing radiation. The basic radiation quantities for ionizing radiation are exposure

E. Park, M.D., Ph.D. (✉)
Yale PET Center, Department of Diagnostic Radiology,
Yale University School of Medicine,
New Haven, CT, USA
e-mail: angela.park@yale.edu

E.E. Kim et al. (eds.), *Clinical PET and PET/CT: Principles and Applications*,
DOI 10.1007/978-1-4419-0802-5_10, © Springer Science+Business Media New York 2013

dose, absorbed dose, equivalent dose, and effective dose [4]. Roentgen (R) is used to express the quantity of radiation exposure, which is defined in terms of the amount of ionization produced in air. R is an old unit and the International System of Units (SI) derived unit of radiation exposure is coulombs per kilogram (C/kg). One R equals 2.58×10^{-4} C/kg. The old unit for absorbed dose is rad and 1 R of exposure gives an absorbed dose of approximately 1 rad in water or human soft tissue. The SI unit of the absorbed dose is the gray (Gy), where 1 Gy equals 100 rad. Absorbed dose is used to evaluate the acute effect (deterministic effect) of radiation, while equivalent and effective doses are used to evaluate the late effects (stochastic effects).

When human soft tissue is exposed to radiation, the biologic effect is different according to the type of radiation (alpha particles, beta particles, neutrons, ultraviolet, gamma rays, and x-rays), which is why equivalent dose is needed to be calculated to evaluate the stochastic effect of radiation. The quality factor (Q) links radiation absorption and its biologic effect (absorbed dose and equivalent dose). Q takes into account the relative biologic effectiveness (RBE) of the type of radiation being used and is therefore an approximation. Equivalent dose is defined as the product of the absorbed dose (rad) and Q; the units are roentgen equivalent man (rem). The SI unit is the sievert (Sv) and 1 Sv equals 100 rem. Because Q is 1 for photons and electrons, the dose equivalent is numerically equal to the absorbed dose for both PET and CT.

This is not the final step for assessing radiation quantity. Generally, radiation dose to the body is not uniform. To evaluate the whole body dose, the radiation dose is needed, which reflects the different relative risk of each tissue or organ. The concept of effective dose has been derived to take this nonuniformity of each soft tissue or organ in the human body into account, and to evaluate the stochastic effect of radiation to the human body as a whole [4]. Tissue weighting factors to calculate effective dose are published in International Commission on Radiological Protection (ICRP) publication 60 [5]. The unit for effective dose is the rem or Sv, which is the same as the equivalent dose.

Effective Dose from FDG PET/CT

The effective doses from PET/CT imaging depend on the radiopharmaceutical, the activity administered, the patient weight, and the CT protocol used. For example, effective doses are higher in obese patients receiving a large amount of activity of a radiopharmaceutical with a long effective half-life. The estimated effective dose of ^{18}F-FDG is approximately 2.1×10^{-2} to 2.9×10^{-2} mSv/MBq [6, 7], but the measured actual effective doses vary. The bladder wall receives the highest dose, and differences in voiding amounts and voiding intervals largely explain the variations of dosimetry encountered.

For PET/CT imaging, the effective dose for the accompanying CT scan depends on the CT protocol used. CT protocols can be designed to produce diagnostic quality images, localization images, or attenuation correction data without imaging [8]. Brix et al. [9] reported that the effective dose for one FDG PET/CT examination ranged from 8.5 to 26.4 mSv, according to the CT protocol used.

Excess Lifetime Risks from FDG PET/CT

Brix et al. [10] calculated the excess lifetime risks for cancer incidence and mortality based on the risk model devised by the Biological Effects of Ionizing Radiation (BEIR) VII committee in 2006 [11] and disease and life table data for a German population. The excess lifetime risks for cancer incidence and mortality from FDG PET was quite small, but tended to be higher in women than in men of the same age. The excess lifetime risks for cancer incidence and mortality from FDG PET were also higher when patients were exposed to radiation at a younger age, especially before 30 years of age [10]. Huang et al. [12] examined several CT protocols by varying tube current and kV, and concluded that whole-body PET/CT scanning increases cancer incidence by 0.231–0.514% in 20-year-old US women and by 0.163–0.323% in 20-year-old US men based on lifetime attributable risk calculations. However, the true risk may be lower than these estimations. BEIR VII presumed that a small cancer risk does exist and is proportional to radiation dose, even <100 mSv, based on the linear no-threshold model [11]. Many researchers have been critical of overestimated radiation risks based on extrapolation of data from much higher level of radiation exposures, such as atomic bombs in Hiroshima and Nagasaki, which limits the estimation of risks at the low level of exposure encountered in medical examinations [4]. Published data indicate that an excess number of malignancies can be found only at doses exceeding approximately 200 mSv at a statistical significance level of 95% [5]. The Health Physics Society recommends against quantitative risk assessment of radiogenic health effects below an individual dose of 50 mGy in 1 year [13]. Furthermore, internal radiation exposure is alleged to induce less hazards than the same amount of external radiation exposure. Making an accurate estimation of radiation risk from low-level ionizing radiation is still a difficult problem to solve.

Reducing the Effective Dose by the 3D PET Acquisition Mode and Iterative Reconstruction Method

The acquisition of PET images in the three-dimensional (3D) mode provides a means of reducing the dose contribution from PET. The 3D PET acquisition mode does not have septae, therefore more counts are detected than in the two-dimensional (2D) mode, which has septae. 3D is more sensitive than 2D by a factor of 4–5, which enables a lower amount of ^{18}F-FDG to be injected with a shorter acquisition time [14]. This is especially advantageous for small pediatric patients and thin adult patients. Time reduction using 3D mode can also be beneficial to reduce the motion artifact and the amount of anesthesia, and to prevent possible nerve injury from a long-standing arm-held position [14]. The injection dose and/or scan time can also be reduced using an iterative reconstruction algorithm, which requires less overall count than the filtered back projection method [14].

From PET to PET/CT

As a result of the difficulty associated with the precise anatomic localization of hyper- or hypometabolic lesions on PET images, nuclear medicine physicians correlate PET and conventional CT or MR images by making one-by-one visual comparisons or using image fusion programs. Currently, hardware fusion PET/CT imaging is the general trend. Hardware fusion PET/CT not only increases diagnostic accuracy, but also significantly decreases the time required for attenuation correction as compared with standard PET imaging using a Ge-68 rod source [15]. Regarding radiation dosimetry, hardware fusion PET/CT increases the effective dose to patients because photon flux from the CT scanner is at least 10^4 higher than that from the Ge-68 rod source [16].

Reducing the Effective Dose by Modified CT Protocols

The radiation exposure from PET/CT imaging varies among radiotracers, however, the greater part of the total radiation exposure from the PET/CT examination is generally originating from the CT portion. Various PET radiotracers, including ^{18}F-FDG, account for a much lesser part of the radiation doses. Therefore, the CT protocols used significantly control the effective doses from FDG PET/CT examinations. Some specific examples follow. When a diagnostic-quality CT (a "standard" kVp of 140, 190 mA, and a pitch of 1.25) was used for a FDG PET/CT examination, CT delivered an effective dose of 22 mSv and PET delivered an effective dose of 11 mSV [17–21]. When a quantitatively accurate, but nondiagnostic CT scan (120 kVp, 60 mAs, and a pitch of 1.5) was used, the CT delivered an effective dose of 6 mSv, giving a total effective dose of 17 mSv [17–21]. Wu et al. [15] tried a 10 mA tube current (140 kVp and a pitch of 6) and reported a measured mean effective dose of 0.72 mSv, which was approximately 1/26th of the CT protocol based on an 80 mA tube current. They suggested a revised PET/CT protocol to minimize the radiation dose, while maximizing the diagnostic information with the sequence of the topogram, an ultra-low-dose CT pre-scan, PET acquisition, and additional CT scans [15].

PET image quality and diagnostic accuracy do not appear to be jeopardized by a low tube current. Hany et al. [22] decreased the CT tube current from 120 to 10 mA, but found no obvious decrease in the diagnostic accuracy of PET/CT examination. Kamel et al. [23] also reported that the tube current (120, 80, 40, and 10 mA) had no significant effect on the FDG standard uptake values (SUVs) or measured lesion sizes. They concluded that CT scans using tube currents as low as 10 mA yielded adequate attenuation correction for PET, which were consistent with the results of Wu et al. [15, 23]. It has been reported that although CT noise is highly dependent on acquisition parameters, the contribution of CT noise to PET noise is minimal. In fact, CT noise only caused a 2% variation in PET noise, which is acceptable for clinical purposes [21]. In addition, the lower sensitivity of low-dose localization CT scans with end tidal expiration for the diagnosis of pulmonary nodules is not because of the reduced dose, but rather because of the lack of full inspiration [24].

PET/CT With Contrast Enhancement

Additional CT scans with contrast enhancement are performed in some hospitals to obtain more detailed diagnostic information when performing FDG PET/CT. The scans significantly increase the total radiation dose; however, this may not always be true in the context of the total dose administered during the long course of treatment as a whole. Contrast-enhanced PET/CT can make definitive diagnoses alone without additional standard CT information in many cases, and PET/CT has nearly replaced CT in some steps of managing cancers where superior sensitivity/specificity has been proved [25, 26]. Thus, the total radiation exposure to a patient during the course of treatment can be reduced by omitting overlapping standard CT examinations, and thus it can bring both convenience and economic benefit for patients.

FDG PET/CT for Cancer Screening in an Asymptomatic Healthy Population

Radiation exposure from FDG PET/CT examinations in oncology patients is justified in almost all cases because the clinical benefit is definitely higher than the potential risk, as described in other chapters of this book. Then, what about the use of FDG PET/CT in an asymptomatic healthy population as a cancer screening method? In particular, would annual FDG PET/CT examinations be beneficial in terms of early cancer detection and a better prognosis, given the radiation risk?

Cancer is a leading cause of death worldwide, accounting for 13% of all deaths [27]. In 2009, an estimated 1,479,350 people in the US were newly diagnosed with cancer, and about 562,340 died of cancer [28]. The number one cause of death in Korea has been cancer since 2000 [29]. People are becoming increasingly concerned with health, and are ready to spend money to maintain health and to prevent oncologic, cardiovascular, and cerebrovascular diseases and other life-threatening diseases. According to the National Institutes of Health, the estimated overall cost of cancer in 2008 was $228.1 billion [28].

Ever since FDG PET/CT became available for clinical use, it has been widely adopted for cancer screening in adults, especially in Korea, Japan, and Taiwan, without any reported complications [30–32]. In Korea, FDG PET/CT has been available at the Health Promotion Centers as an elective examination for cancer screening tests since 1998, and today it is a popular choice, along with CT and MRI [33].

The number of FDG PET/CT examinations conducted for cancer screening in the normal population in Asian countries is increasing mainly because of the promotion and lowering the cost of the examination among hospitals with the wide availability of PET/CT and cyclotrons. However, regulatory restrictions in many other countries prohibit the use of ionizing radiation without a legitimate indication [34].

Malignant lesions are found in approximately 1–2% of patients who undergo FDG PET/CT for cancer screening [27, 35, 36]. FDG PET/CT is advantageous because it can detect a variety of malignancies and examine the whole body in one session in a comparatively short time period as a noninvasive method [35, 37]. However, FDG PET/CT also has disadvantages such as relatively high radiation exposure, high cost, and low sensitivity for some cancers such as urologic malignancies, low-cell density cancers, low-FDG avid tumors, and small-sized lesions [38, 39]. Despite the low cost effectiveness and the lack of definitive evidence regarding the usefulness of FDG PET/CT as a cancer screening tool [40], the reality is that FDG PET/CT is already in use for that purpose. At present, the judicious use of FDG PET/CT is suggested as a cancer screening aid combined with other selected modalities such as gastroscopy, abdominal sonography, pelvic MRI, and CA-125 level measurement in the older age group with a high cancer risk [27, 36, 40, 41]. Whether or not cancer screening with FDG PET/CT will contribute to the early initiation of treatment and the reduction of mortality remains to be seen.

Special Consideration: Pediatric Patients

As is typically done in other general nuclear medicine examinations, the ^{18}F-FDG injection dosage in children is basically scaled by body weight or body surface area (BSA), with a 70 kg and a 1.73 m^2 adult as a standard, respectively. Organ dose, effective dose, and image quality are also important factors in determining pediatric ^{18}F-FDG injection dosage. Organ and effective doses are not necessarily proportional to body weight or BSA because the geometry of the organs may change dramatically from birth to adulthood [42, 43]. Differences in organ size, shape, density, position, and chemical composition significantly influence the geometric and anatomic relationships [42, 43]. A tabulated organ dose of ^{18}F-FDG per unit activity administered is available for different age groups in ICRP publication 80 [44]. Each hospital makes its own policy to deal with these complex parameters, and the dosing scheme varies substantially among hospitals [45].

There is a minimal dose needed to acquire adequate images which are sometimes larger than the dose simply calculated by body weight or BSA, especially in infants and small children. The European Association of Nuclear Medicine (EANM) [46] set 26 MBq for 2D-acquisition and 14 MBq for 3D-acquisition as minimum recommended injection doses and the North American consensus guidelines [47] set 37 MBq as the minimum recommended injection dose. The recommended pediatric dosage of ^{18}F-FDG and other commonly used radiotracers can also be found in these guidelines.

Children are said to have a higher risk of getting radiation-induced cancer than adults because the rapidly dividing cells are more sensitive to radiation exposure and the longer life expectancy gives a chance for potential cancer to be realized [14]. However, there are a number of research results that suggest a position contrary to this. After reviewing the studies of low-level radiation exposure with large sample sizes and long follow-up, Ernst et al. [48] argued that no available data could confirm the hypothesis that children are more radiosensitive than adults. Charron [49] also asserted that there is no direct evidence that low-level radiation increases the incidence of cancer, even in children.

Special Consideration: Pregnancy and Breastfeeding

Whether it is by accident or out of necessity, FDG PET/CT examinations are performed during pregnancy. Of course, it is desirable to avoid unnecessary radiation exposure during pregnancy, but FDG PET/CT examinations are not an absolute contraindication, as are most other nuclear medicine and radiologic examinations. FDG does cross the placenta and gives direct and indirect radiation to the embryo or fetus, but data on fetal dosimetry is limited. Zanotti-Fregonara et al. [50] calculated the radiation dose received by an 8-week embryo from a mother who was injected with 320 MBq of ^{18}F-FDG. The resulting FDG dose to the embryo was 10.6 mGy (3.3×10^{-2} mGy/MBq) and they found that the positron (β+) dose comprised a higher portion than indirect radiation by photon emission from the maternal tissue, such as the uterus and bladder, by 55% and 45%, respectively [50]. This amount of fetal whole body dose is higher than the doses from the common general nuclear medicine examinations using Tc-99 m, I-123, and I-131 [51]; however, it remains well within the current consensus of safe levels, even after adding the CT dose of 8.3 mGy. The probability that a child will have malformations does not increase below 50 mGy. The cancer risk increases about 0.1–0.6% up to 100 mGy, but there is a greater than 99% chance that the exposed fetus will not develop childhood cancer or leukemia [51]. Therefore, termination of pregnancy at fetal doses <100 mGy is not justified based upon radiation risk. The probability of bearing healthy children as a function of radiation dose is announced in ICRP publication 84 [51].

Breast feeding is allowed after FDG PET/CT examinations. FDG is excreted via breast milk, but less than 1% of the total activity given to the mother is secreted in breast milk. Radiation dose to a 3-month-old infant is at most 0.2 mSv. Meanwhile, close contact needs to be avoided because radiation activity is higher in breast tissue than in breast milk. Radiation exposure to a child is negligible when close contact is avoided for about 4 h [52].

References

1. The Korean Society of Nuclear Medicine. Nuclear medicine procedures statistics over 48 years: year 2009; 2009.
2. Choi J, Kim B. Whole body positron emission tomography/computed tomography. J Korean Med Assoc. 2006;49:1027–34.
3. Czernin J, Phelps ME. Positron emission tomography scanning: current and future applications. Annu Rev Med. 2002;53:89–112.
4. Cameron J. Radiation dosimetry. Environ Health Perspect. 1991;91:45–8.
5. ICRP. Recommendations of the international commission on radiological protection. ICRP Publication 60. Ann ICRP. 1991;21(1–3).
6. Mejia AA, Nakamura T, Itoh M, et al. Absorbed dose estimates in positron emission tomography studies based on the administration of ^{18}F-labeled radiopharmaceuticals. J Radiat Res (Tokyo). 1991; 32(3):243–61.
7. Deloar HM, Fujiwara T, Shidahara M, et al. Estimation of absorbed dose for 2-[F-18]fluoro-2-deoxy-D-glucose using whole-body positron emission tomography and magnetic resonance imaging. Eur J Nucl Med. 1998;25(6):565–74.
8. Gelfand MJ. Dosimetry of FDG PET/CT and other molecular imaging applications in pediatric patients. Pediatr Radiol. 2009;39(Suppl 1):S46–56.
9. Brix G, Lechel U, Glatting G, et al. Radiation exposure of patients undergoing whole-body dual-modality ^{18}F-FDG PET/CT examinations. J Nucl Med. 2005;46(4):608–13.
10. Brix G, Nekolla EA, Nosske D, Griebel J. Risks and safety aspects related to PET/MR examinations. Eur J Nucl Med Mol Imaging. 2009;36(Suppl 1):S131–8.
11. Committee to assess health risks from exposure to low levels of ionizing radiation, National Research Council. Health risks from exposure to low levels of ionizing radiation: BEIR VII phase 2. Washington, DC: The National Academy Press; 2006.
12. Huang B, Law MW, Khong PL. Whole-body PET/CT scanning: estimation of radiation dose and cancer risk. Radiology. 2009;251(1):166–74.
13. Mossman KL. The linear no-threshold debate: where do we go from here? Med Phys. 1998;25(3):279–84. discussion 300.
14. Fahey FH. Dosimetry of pediatric PET/CT. J Nucl Med. 2009;50(9):1483–91.
15. Wu TH, Chu TC, Huang YH, et al. A positron emission tomography/computed tomography (PET/CT) acquisition protocol for CT radiation dose optimization. Nucl Med Commun. 2005;26(4):323–30.
16. Beyer T, Townsend DW, Brun T, et al. A combined PET/CT scanner for clinical oncology. J Nucl Med. 2000;41(8):1369–79.
17. Brix G, Beyer T. PET/CT: dose-escalated image fusion? Nuklearmedizin. 2005;44(Suppl 1):S51–7.
18. Fahey FH, Palmer MR, Strauss KJ, Zimmerman RE, Badawi RD, Treves ST. Dosimetry and adequacy of CT-based attenuation correction for pediatric PET: phantom study. Radiology. 2007;243(1):96–104.
19. Groves AM, Owen KE, Courtney HM, et al. 16-detector multislice CT: dosimetry estimation by TLD measurement compared with Monte Carlo simulation. Br J Radiol. 2004;77(920):662–5.
20. Huda W, Vance A. Patient radiation doses from adult and pediatric CT. AJR Am J Roentgenol. 2007; 188(2):540–6.
21. Zanzonico P, Dauer L, St Germain J. Operational radiation safety for PET-CT, SPECT-CT, and cyclotron facilities. Health Phys. 2008;95(5):554–70.

22. Hany TF, Steinert HC, Goerres GW, Buck A, von Schulthess GK. PET diagnostic accuracy: improvement with in-line PET-CT system: initial results. Radiology. 2002;225(2):575–81.
23. Kamel E, Hany TF, Burger C, et al. CT vs ^{68}Ge attenuation correction in a combined PET/CT system: evaluation of the effect of lowering the CT tube current. Eur J Nucl Med Mol Imaging. 2002;29(3):346–50.
24. Gelfand MJ, Lemen LC. PET/CT and SPECT/CT dosimetry in children: the challenge to the pediatric imager. Semin Nucl Med. 2007;37(5):391–8.
25. Rohren EM, Turkington TG, Coleman RE. Clinical applications of PET in oncology. Radiology. 2004;231(2):305–32.
26. Wechalekar K, Sharma B, Cook G. PET/CT in oncology–a major advance. Clin Radiol. 2005;60(11): 1143–55.
27. Lee JW, Kang KW, Paeng JC, et al. Cancer screening using ^{18}F-FDG PET/CT in Korean asymptomatic volunteers: a preliminary report. Ann Nucl Med. 2009;23(7):685–91.
28. American Cancer Society. Cancer facts and figures 2009. Atlanta: American Cancer Society; 2009.
29. Korea National Statistical Office. Causes of death statistics in 2008. In: Statistics Korea, editor. Annual report on the cause of death statistics, 14 Sept 2009.
30. Yasunaga H. Who wants cancer screening with PET? A contingent valuation surgery in Japan. Eur J Radiol. 2007;70:190–4.
31. Kojima S, Zhou B, Teramukai S, et al. Cancer screening of healthy volunteers using whole-body ^{18}F-FDG-PET scans: the Nishidai clinic study. Eur J Cancer. 2007;43(12):1842–8.
32. Chen YK, Ding HJ, Su CT, et al. Application of PET and PET/CT imaging for cancer screening. Anticancer Res. 2004;24(6):4103–8.
33. Chung J, Cho H, Shim J, et al. Detection of cancer with PET and PET/CT in asymptomatic volunteers. Nucl Med Mol Imaging. 2009;43(6):526–34.
34. Weckesser M, Schober O. Is whole-body FDG-PET valuable for health screening? Against. Eur J Nucl Med Mol Imaging. 2005;32(3):342–3.
35. Yasuda S, Ide M, Fujii H, et al. Application of positron emission tomography imaging to cancer screening. Br J Cancer. 2000;83(12):1607–11.
36. Minamimoto R, Senda M, Terauchi T, et al. Analysis of various malignant neoplasms detected by FDG-PET cancer screening program: based on a Japanese nationwide survey. Ann Nucl Med. 2011; 25(1):45–54.
37. Yasuda S, Shohtsu A. Cancer screening with whole-body ^{18}F-fluorodeoxyglucose positron-emission tomography. Lancet. 1997;350(9094):1819.
38. Robbins E. Radiation risks from imaging studies in children with cancer. Pediatr Blood Cancer. 2008;51(4):453–7.
39. Ide M, Suzuki Y. Is whole-body FDG-PET valuable for health screening? For. Eur J Nucl Med Mol Imaging. 2005;32(3):339–41.
40. Schoder H, Gonen M. Screening for cancer with PET and PET/CT: potential and limitations. J Nucl Med. 2007;48(Suppl 1):4S–18.
41. Nishizawa S, Kojima S, Teramukai S, et al. Prospective evaluation of whole-body cancer screening with multiple modalities including [18F]fluorodeoxyglucose positron emission tomography in a healthy population: a preliminary report. J Clin Oncol. 2009;27(11):1767–73.
42. Zhu X. Dosage of radiopharmaceuticals and internal dosimetry. In: Charron M, editor. Practical pediatric PET imaging. New York: Springer; 2006. p. 37–46.
43. Cristy M, Eckerman KF. Specific absorbed fractions of energy at various ages from internal photon sources. I. Methods. Oak Ridge National Laboratory Rep. ORNL/TM-8381/V1; 1987.
44. ICRP. Radiation dose to patients from radiopharmaceuticals (Addendum to ICRP Publication 53). ICRP Publication 80. Ann ICRP. 1998;28(3).
45. Treves ST, Davis RT, Fahey FH. Administered radiopharmaceutical doses in children: a survey of 13 pediatric hospitals in North America. J Nucl Med. 2008;49(6):1024–7.
46. Lassmann M, Biassoni L, Monsieurs M, Franzius C. The new EANM paediatric dosage card: additional notes with respect to F-18. Eur J Nucl Med Mol Imaging. 2008;35(9):1666–8.
47. Pediatric Nuclear Medicine Workgroup. North American consensus guidelines for administered radiopharmaceutical activities in children and adolescents 2010.
48. Ernst M, Freed ME, Zametkin AJ. Health hazards of radiation exposure in the context of brain imaging research: special consideration for children. J Nucl Med. 1998;39(4):689–98.
49. Charron M. The biologic effects of low-level radiation. In: Charron M, editor. Practical pediatric PET imaging. New York: Springer; 2006. p. 30–6.
50. Zanotti-Fregonara P, Champion C, Trebossen R, Maroy R, Devaux JY, Hindie E. Estimation of the beta+dose to the embryo resulting from 18F-FDG administration during early pregnancy. J Nucl Med. 2008;49(4):679–82.
51. ICRP. Pregnancy and medical radiation. ICRP Publication 84. Ann ICRP. 2000;30(1).
52. Leide-Svegborn S. Radiation exposure of patients and personnel from a PET/CT procedure with ^{18}F-FDG. Radiat Prot Dosimetry. 2010;139(1–3):208–13.

Current Status of PET in the World

11

Seok-Ki Kim, Keon W. Kang, and Myung-Chul Lee

The concept of fluorodeoxyglucose positron emission tomography (FDG PET) was conceived in the early 1970s by a number of researchers. In August 1976, the first brain and whole-body images were acquired successfully using the initial type of PET scanner optimized for in vivo imaging with positron-emitting radionuclides in humans [1]. This demonstrated the feasibility of the methodology, but it was still far from clinical study.

During most of the 1980s, FDG PET imaging was used to determine alterations in the brain function associated with a multitude of neuropsychiatric disorders. In the late 1980s, imaging of the entire body became a reality on the basis of refinement of the PET scanner. Under these circumstances, FDG PET was expected to play a major role in treating malignant disorders in the near future.

By the late 1990s, it became apparent that FDG PET imaging was substantially superior to conventional techniques in diagnosing, staging, treatment response monitoring, and detecting recurrence in a variety of cancer types. Although FDG PET was proved to be clinically useful in malignant disorders, there were few PET centers worldwide, which were focused predominantly on the research aspects of PET. Smaller institutions, which were interested in clinical usage of FDG PET, could not consider installing a PET system because of budget limitations.

By the 2000s, the introduction of PET/CT was a turning point, bringing great changes in the sociomedical status of FDG PET. FDG PET and PET/computed tomography (CT) have become popular clinical medical imaging tools, and recently have been accepted as the most important and innovative methods for cancer imaging. For instance, the striking increase of the number of FDG PET-related medical articles reflect the fact that FDG PET has had much attention brought to it by clinicians. Between 1995 and 1999, during the early stage of clinical usage, only 553 FDG PET-related articles were published, according to a PubMed search (National Center for Biotechnology Information, U.S. National Library of Medicine, and National Institutes of Health), whereas 1,374 and 2,981 articles were published between 2000–2004, and 2005–2009, respectively (Fig. 11.1).

S.-K. Kim, M.D. (✉)
Department of Nuclear Medicine,
National Cancer Center,
Gyeonggi-do 410-769, South Korea
e-mail: skim@ncc.re.kr

K.W. Kang, M.D., Ph.D.
Department of Nuclear Medicine, Seoul National University College of Medicine,
Seoul 110-744, South Korea
e-mail: kangkw@snu.ac.kr

M.-C. Lee, M.D., Ph.D.
Department of Nuclear Medicine, Gachon University School of Medicine,
1198 Guwol-dong, Namdong-Gu,
Incheon 405, South Korea
e-mail: mclee@gilhospital.com

E.E. Kim et al. (eds.), *Clinical PET and PET/CT: Principles and Applications*,
DOI 10.1007/978-1-4419-0802-5_11, © Springer Science+Business Media New York 2013

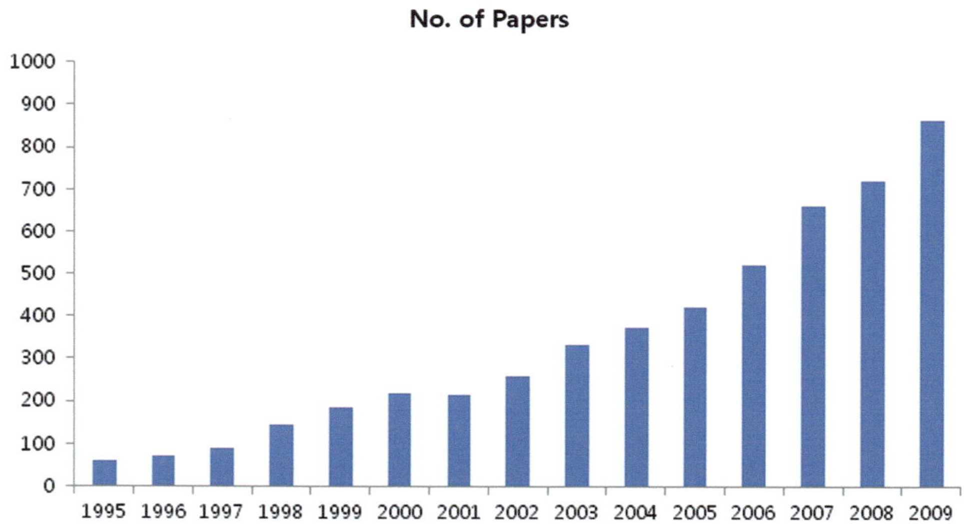

Fig. 11.1 Number of articles published annually in which the title contains fluorodeoxyglucose positron emission tomography (FDG PET)

Resolution of Technical Barrier to Popularization

Because the installation and management of a PET center is considerably more difficult than other medical imaging systems (e.g., magnetic resonance image [MRI] or CT), PET could not advance as quickly as MRI or CT in the beginning. Because positron-emitting radionuclide has a short half-life, cyclotron and radiosynthesis equipment need to be installed near the PET scanner. As a result of these shortcomings, PET systems were not easily assessable and not many clinicians had the opportunity to familiarize themselves with FDG PET. Therefore, only few obvious clinical roles and indications for FDG PET were originated. This resulted in less use of FDG PET, leading to a vicious cycle. The high installation cost and complexity of the system was still a barrier for further installation and administration.

In the 1990s, manufacturers began to build clinically relevant PET scanners for whole-body imaging, beyond the brain and the heart, which could acquire whole-body images within a 1-h time period. In parallel, small-sized relatively cost-effective cyclotrons were built, and automated radiopharmaceutical synthesis systems came to the market. FDG could be produced at an acceptable cost and companies began to make infrastructures for FDG distribution to several satellite PET sites within 3-h (or less) travel distances. Thus, from the late 1990s to the present, the initial technical barrier to PET spread was resolved and the PET scanner could become a clinical modality rather than only an investigational means.

Advent of PET/CT

Another important advancement has been attributed to the popularization of PET–the development of PET/CT. In most clinical settings, PET imaging is more beneficial when viewed with data from other imaging techniques, mainly CT and MRI, which have attained a high level of clinical relevance. For such clinical needs, PET was combined with CT into a single scanner (PET/CT), which further enhanced the utility of the methodology in daily practice. The integration of PET and CT images allows precise localization of the diseased sites for optimal management of patients with cancer and other disorders, which is essential for accurate planning of surgical and biopsy procedures. PET/CT imaging is becoming a standard of care in radiation oncology where utilizing conventional imaging techniques results in either over- or undertreating cancer patients.

PET/CT imaging is more clinically relevant than PET alone, and after its advent into the clinical world, has been replacing PET scans. It was presented at the European Association of Nuclear Medicine (EANM) Congress in 2005 that use of PET was heading toward a considerable decline, and was being rapidly overtaken by PET/CT throughout Europe. Sales figures for PET/CT scanners have surpassed those of "stand alone" PET systems, and it is predicted that greater than 90% of PET scanners would be substituted for PET/CT in the near future. At the same Congress meeting, von Schulthess highlighted the fact that the use of PET/CT was growing by 60%, whereas PET use was declining at a rate of 20%. In 2001, 91% of all PET scanners were stand-alone PET systems, whereas in 2004, 67% were PET/CT systems.

The other important aspect which must be mentioned is the higher throughput of PET/CT than stand-alone PET. PET/CT scanner uses fast CT for attenuation correction, as opposed to conventional time-consuming transmission scans. CT-based attenuation correction accomplished whole-body examination in less than 30 min. Although PET/CT carries a higher cost than stand-alone PET, PET/CT could be more cost effective than stand-alone PET because of its high throughput and clinical usefulness. PET/CT requires short scanning time, has high throughput, provides more clinical information including functional and anatomic aspects, and is more convenient to patients and the operator. These features are encouraging for the continued exploration of new clinical indications of PET.

Reimbursement and Insurance

After the 1990s, when FDG PET had been accepted as a clinical imaging modality, some developed countries had considered reimbursement by national or private insurance systems. Eventually, based on data that had been collected in the literature, Medicare became convinced of the technique's efficacy and granted reimbursement for this service by the late 1990s.

Although reimbursement for this service had been initiated in the US in the late 1990s, the reimbursement system was still in a transition state in the US and Europe until the early 2000s [2]. Public and private insurance systems are different among US and European countries. In the UK, both public and private insurance authorizes clinical PET to some extent. In Germany, private health insurance companies give authorization but public insurance does not. In Belgium, private health insurance companies do not exist but public insurance authorizes clinical PET.

Reimbursement seems to be one of the most important factors influencing the development of PET. Serious intervention or regulation by insurance systems could restrict the expensive modality, whereas reimbursement by public insurance systems may have a positive effect on the popularization of PET. Korea began reimbursement by public insurance systems in June of 2006. Between 2006 and 2007, there was a 45% increase in PET studies nationwide. The market share of PET in the imaging branch of nuclear medicine was 45% in 2006 (Table 11.1).

According to a survey conducted in 2006 by the World Federation of Nuclear Medicine and Biology (WFNMB), in 2005, 67% of developed countries in Europe initiated reimbursement for PET along with 31% of developing countries. At that time, Luxembourg, Belgium, The Netherlands, France, UK, Italy, Denmark, Finland, Czech Republic, Cyprus, Germany, Switzerland, Ireland, Israel, Japan, Spain, Indonesia, Poland, Taiwan, and Hungary had already initiated reimbursement. However, Mongolia, Pakistan, Vietnam, Singapore, United Arab Emirates, Slovenia, Bulgaria, Chile, Paraguay, Peru, Philippines, Romania, Serbia and Montenegro, South Africa, Thailand, Argentina, and Algeria had not. The reimbursement fee for PET varies considerably throughout Europe. For example, in Great Britain, reimbursement is €222; Belgium, €825; France, €1,050; Switzerland, €1,230; and Czech Republic, €2,050 [2]. In Korea, reimbursement is about 710,000 KRW (764 US dollar).

Table 11.1 Market share of PET in nuclear medicine departments in Korea

Year	1997	2001	2004	2005	2006
Image	239	481	742	815	941
Radioimmuno-assay	782	1,075	1,391	1,581	1,843
Treatment	22	26	31	36	41
PET	19	75	122	574	754
Total	1,062	1,657	2,286	3,006	3,579
					100 million won (KRW)

Table 11.2 Number of facilities/sites in various countries where PET has been installed

Country	1992	1996	2000	2005
US	60	82	176	1,080[a]
Japan	23	24	35	120
Germany	15	16	22	66
Belgium	6	6	8	11
England	8	8	6	11
Australia	2	2	5	7
Korea	0	2	5	52
China				60
Taiwan			8	20
Other	36	35	37	150
Total	150	175	302	1,577

Numbers were calculated or summed based on a ~ 2006 WFNMB survey, 2005 EANM Conference symposium, and 2003 German survey [8]

[a]Number based on a 2004 survey

The spectrum of reimbursement indications was different among countries. A relatively broad spectrum of indications was accepted in Europe (Belgium, The Netherlands, France, Great Britain, Italy, Finland, Switzerland, and Spain) and the US. In 2006, Korea also adopted broad indications. Reimbursement spectrums vary by the economic needs, cost-effectiveness of societies, and the recommendations of health professional groups.

Although reimbursement systems began in major leading countries, cost-effectiveness analysis of FDG PET had not yet been carried out. Until then, some researchers had reported that ovarian cancer, recurrent laryngeal cancer, locally advanced head and neck cancer, recurrent nasopharyngeal cancer, and suspected lung cancer are cost-effective indications for FDG PET [3–7]. It seemed that the more cost-effective data would accumulate, more indications would be revealed.

Popularization of PET

Until the early 2000s we had witnessed a rise in the number of PET/CT installations. Most of the 1,000 PET/CT units worldwide were operational in the US, and notably less in Europe. Only 17 PET/CT installations existed in Germany. There are about 300 stand-alone PET scanners installed in Europe at the present time, most of them operating in clinical practice [8].

According to the survey by the WFNMB, the number of PET installation sites increased dramatically after 2000 (Table 11.2). The installation sites increased between 1996 and 2000 in the US, and other countries followed between 2000 and 2005. More are expected to be installed in 2010. The market share of PET in nuclear medicine increased (Table 11.1) and is probably be the leading most portion of market share of nuclear medicine at the present time.

For example, in Korea, the number of PET applications did not increase during the 1990s, but the trend changed and began to increase exponentially since 2001 (Fig. 11.2). Profound distribution of PET or PET/CT scanners, on-site medical cyclotrons, and supporting delivery infrastructure of radiopharmaceuticals made the increase possible in Korea. Between 1994 and 2002, there were only seven PET centers in Korea and they distributed only around the area of the capital (Fig. 11.3). In 2008, the number of PET sites and PET scanners reached 78 sites with 127 scanners, and 113 of the 127 scanners were PET/CT. The PET sites were distributed regionally nationwide. There was a burst in the number of PET applications around 2006 as a result of reimbursement by public insurance systems. PET became an available technology for most Korean patients, geographically and financially.

The total number of scans per million head of population varied considerably from one country to another. The total number of scans per scanner or utilization rate also varied considerably from one European country to another. According to the EANM Congress of 2005, the Czech Republic performed about 3,400 scans per scanner, whereas Belgium performed 870 scans [8].

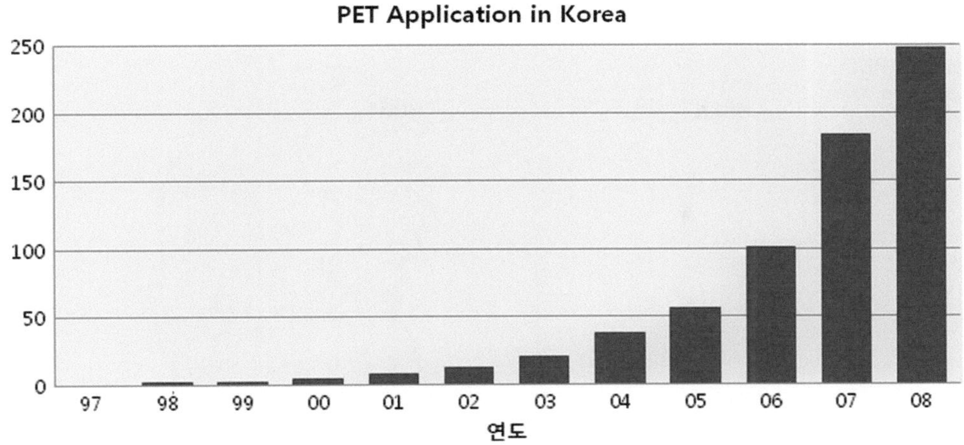

Fig. 11.2 Number of PET applications performed annually in Korea from 1997 to 2008

Infrastructures that deeply influence the popularity of PET, such as the delivery system, distribution of medical cyclotron, medical insurance coverage, medical care system, and economic status, are very different among countries. Although developed and developing countries have infrastructures and substantial PET sites, less developing countries do not. Moreover, the number of PET or PET/CT per capita is different between developed countries and developing countries. In Benelux, Austria, Switzerland, and Italy the number of PET studies per million inhabitants is more than 1,000; whereas in France, Iberia, and Scandinavia this number varies between 500 and 1,000; in Germany and the UK, it is less than 500 scans (Table 11.3).

Prospects and Collaboration

As mentioned previously, the popularization of PET is not geographically homogenous. However, despite the rising number of PET installations, PET imaging accounts for only a small part of the total expense of diagnostic imaging. Developing countries and less developed countries do not have substantial infrastructure, and PET technology is not yet clinically relevant. Until 2006, a considerable number of countries had substantial numbers of PET and infrastructure to influence the national medical care system. A commercial transportation and distribution system for FDG has been already been initiated in almost every country in Europe and Asia-Oceania, whereas in Japan, a typical developed country, neither transportation of FDG nor full reimbursement of clinical PET has been started or has been delayed. The coverage by insurance and regulatory approval systems varies among nations. Obviously, the applicability and recognition of PET as an imaging modality in diagnostic oncology (and neurology) is affected by the recommendations of professional groups regarding the different levels of oncologic scanning. Based on these facts, it would be much easier for less-developed countries to facilitate PET centers by obtaining help and experience from the leading countries by international collaboration.

To overcome this unequal level of popularization, a new PET application and radiotracer, which cannot be replaced by other modality, should be developed, and PET should be more popularly used. A new array of promising new positron-emitting radiotracers, other than FDG, as well as new imaging instruments would make the future of PET brighter than its current success. FDG is only one of many radiopharmaceuticals, and others are now in production or under active investigation. These new radiotracers have characteristic roles and the indications of PET will be wider. Current PET scanners are rapidly evolving as well, with new crystal materials,

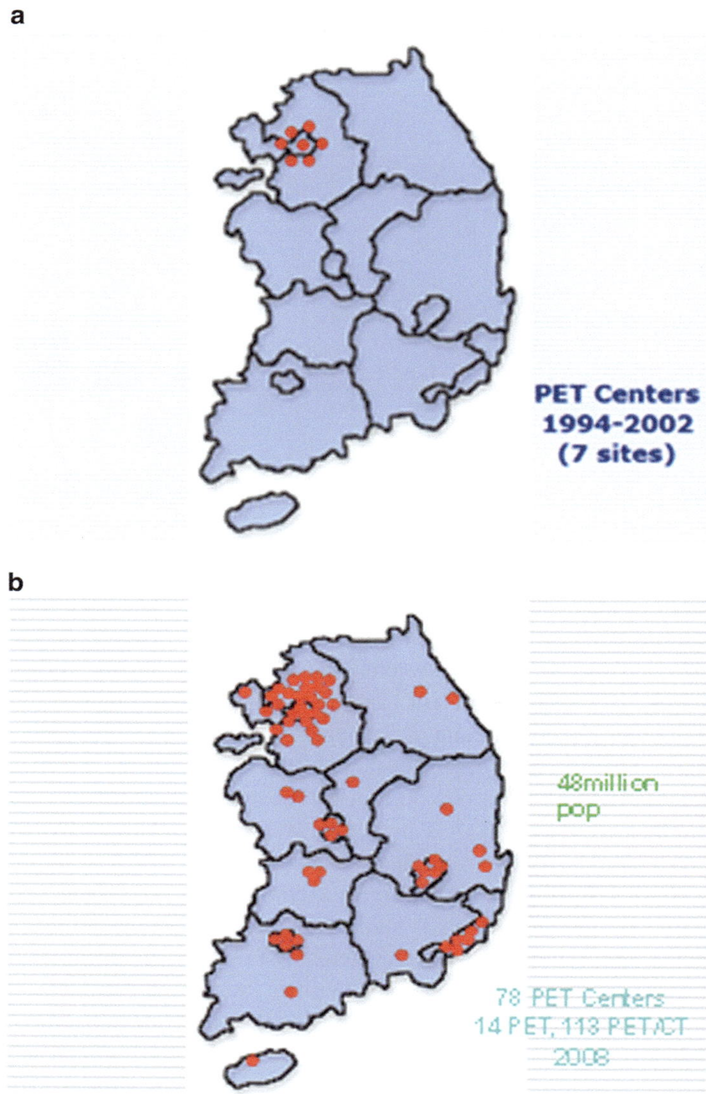

Fig. 11.3 Chronologic changes of regional distribution of PET scanners and medical cyclotrons in Korea

PET/CT combination systems, and other technical innovations that are already in use. Technology, such as PET and MRI combinations as well as new tabletop medical cyclotrons, will strengthen the usefulness of PET.

The lack of a unified international or domestic system and excessive requirements for regulatory approval of radiopharmaceuticals are serious obstacles that need to be addressed prior to reimbursement. Currently, ^{18}F-FDG manufacturers need to comply with more rigorous regulatory standards similar to those required for unlabelled drugs. Complying with such standards requires additional upfront costs for personnel, office space, and equipment. In addition, regulatory agencies have been increasingly moving toward a more stringent regulatory environment for manipulation and transport of radiopharmaceuticals [9].

Conclusion

The field of PET is relatively the newest, and will progress with many advantageous conditions. PET/CT was emerging as an investigational technology for four decades prior to maturing as

Table 11.3 FDG PET studies per million population

2006 WFNMB survey (2002)	
Country	No. per million
Argentina	35
Chile	34
Korea	487
Philippines	9
Singapore	35
Finland	371
German survey (2003) [8]	
Country	No. per million
Benelux	1,200
Austria	1,100
Switzerland	1,100
Italy	1,100
France	800
Iberia	800
Scandinavia	500
Germany	500
UK	300
Number of PET studies for the US, Korea, and Japan (2005)[a]	
Country	No. per million
US	3,571
Korea	1,166
Japan	202

[a]Personal survey performed in 2005

a clinical medical imaging modality, especially for oncology. In the future, promising new tracers and new instruments will continue to drive the sustainable success of PET technology. International collaboration and the sharing of experience will be helpful for promoting clinical PET worldwide and abolishing regional unequal diffusion.

References

1. Phelps ME, Hoffman EJ, Mullani NA, Ter-Pogossian MM. Application of annihilation coincidence detection to transaxial reconstruction tomography. J Nucl Med. 1975;16(3):210–24.
2. Tashiro M, Kubota K, Ito M, Fujimoto T, Yamaguchi K, Sasaki H, Moser E. Clinical PET activities in European and Asia-Oceanian countries. Kaku Igaku. 2001;38(3):255–67.
3. Mansuet M, Grimaldi A, Mangili G, Picchio M, Giovacchini G, Vigano R, Messa C, Fazio F. Positron emission tomography/computed tomography introduction in the clinical management of patients with suspected recurrence of ovarian cancer: a cost-effectiveness analysis. Eur J Cancer Care. 2009;18:612–9.
4. van Hooren ACG, Brouwer J, de Bree R, Hoekstra OS, Leemans CR, Uyl-de Groot CA. The cost-effectiveness of 18FDG-PET in selecting patients with suspicion of recurrent laryngeal carcinoma after radiotherapy for direct laryngoscopy. Eur Arch Otorhinolaryngol. 2009;266:1441–8.
5. Sher DJ, Tishler RB, Annino D, Punglia RS. Cost-effectiveness of CT and PET-CT for determining the need for adjuvant neck dissection in locally advanced head and neck cancer. Ann Oncol. 15 Oct 2009; 21(5):1072–7
6. Yen RF, Yen MF, Hong RL, Tzen KY, Chien CR, Chen TH. The cost-utility analysis of 18-fluoro-2-deoxyglucose positron emission tomography in the diagnosis of recurrent nasopharyngeal carcinoma. Acad Radiol. 2009;16(1):54–60.
7. Mansueto M, Grimaldi A, Torbica A, Pepe G, Giovacchini G, Messa C, Fazio F. Cost-effectiveness analysis in the clinical management of patients with known or suspected lung cancer: [18F]fluorodeoxyglucose PET and CT comparison. Q J Nucl Med Mol Imag. 2007;51(3):224–34. Epub 1 Jun 2007.
8. Dietlein M, Schicha H. Reimbursement of the PET in oncology in Europe; a questionnaire based survey. Nuklearmedizin. 2003;42:80–5.
9. Krug B, Van Zanten A, Pirson AS, Crott R, Vander Borght T. Activity-based costing evaluation of [18F]-fludeoxyglucose production. Eur J Nucl Med Mol Imaging. 2008;35(1):80–8.

Part II

Clinical Applications

Epilepsy

12

Dong Soo Lee, So Won Oh, and Myung-Chul Lee

Positron emission tomography (PET) has a key role in the management of patients with focal epilepsy as a well-established, functional imaging modality. Especially among various PET agents to evaluate brain function, ^{18}F-fluorodeoxy-glucose (FDG) has been widely used because it reflects neuronal activity and allows quantification of cerebral glucose metabolism using tracer kinetic modeling. In the management of patients with medically intractable epilepsy, FDG PET became a routine process to localize epileptogenic foci, particularly in cases of patients presenting with normal anatomic structures on magnetic resonance imaging (MRI). Recently, this pivotal role of FDG PET in presurgical evaluation had been challenged by high-quality MRI [1].

Despite this trend, the role of PET as a functional imaging modality in the management of patients with epilepsy seems secure in terms of both demonstrating the epileptogenic zones and better understanding of the neurobiology of epilepsy. FDG PET could provide useful information to localize the epileptogenic focus even in patients with medically intractable focal epilepsy who have unremarkable MRI scans [1]. To investigate neurochemistry, which is considered crucial in epileptogenesis and spread of epileptic activities, several PET tracers have been introduced and actively explored its feasibility in clinical practice [2]. Moreover, the introduction of an epoch-making experimental tool, a dedicated small animal PET scanner and animal model for epilepsy, has accelerated investigations to unveil secrets of epilepsy.

FDG PET

Surgical interventions would be an accepted treatment option to effectively alleviate seizures in approximately 20–30% of the patients with focal epilepsy who became resistant to antiepileptic drugs [3, 4]. Although the success rates of surgical interventions in patients with temporal lobe epilepsies reach almost 85% [5–8], those rates decrease 50% to 60% in patients with cortical origin epilepsies [9, 10]. In this regard, careful selection of eligible patients and precise localization of the epileptogenic zones are imperative to achieve

D.S. Lee, M.D., Ph.D. (✉)
Department of Nuclear Medicine, WCU Department of Molecular Medicine and Biopharmaceutical Sciences, Seoul National University College of Medicine, Seoul National University, Seoul 110-744, South Korea
e-mail: dsl@snu.ac.kr

S.W. Oh, M.D.
Department of Nuclear Medicine, Seoul Metropolitan Government-Seoul National University, Boramae Medical Center, Seoul 156-707, South Korea
e-mail: mdosw@snu.ac.kr

M.-C. Lee, M.D., Ph.D.
Department of Nuclear Medicine, Gachon University School of Medicine, 1198 Guwol-dong, Namdong-Gu, Incheon 405, South Korea
e-mail: mclee@gilhospital.com

E.E. Kim et al. (eds.), *Clinical PET and PET/CT: Principles and Applications*,
DOI 10.1007/978-1-4419-0802-5_12,

Table 12.1 Correct localization of MRI, 18F-FDG PET, and ictal SPECT

	Pathology (%)	Surgical outcome (%)
MRI	72	77
^{18}F-FDG PET	85	86
Ictal SPECT	73	78

(Modified from reference 12.15)

a seizure-free outcome and minimize side effects related with unsuccessful surgery, and thus meticulous presurgical evaluations including scalp electroencephalography (EEG) and various imaging studies are required.

FDG PET, as a noninvasive evaluation tool, has been reported to have high sensitivities with 60–90% in lateralizing temporal lobe epilepsy (TLE) [11]. On interictal FDG PET, the epileptogenic focus is usually seen as a hypometabolic area, which is considered to be seizure-related changes in the brain. The pathophysiologic basis of the hypometabolism remains elusive, but it has been suggested that the hypometabolism in the hippocampus may reflect the hippocampal neuronal loss, a histopathologic hallmark of medial temporal sclerosis [12].

In regard to the diagnostic performance of various imaging methods to localize the epileptogenic foci, sensitivities were varied between medial temporal lobe epilepsy and neocortical epilepsies [13]. The diagnostic performance for extratemporal neocortical epilepsy is not particularly high. Recently, the introduction of nuclear imaging analysis methods such as statistical parametric mapping (SPM) helped the localization of the epileptogenic foci with improved sensitivities [13]. In a previous study using SPM, we investigated the diagnostic performance of FDG PET in pediatric patients with TLE, and the introduction of SPM was found to be helpful for the localization of the epileptogenic zones [14].

The sensitivity of FDG PET was compared in a head-to-head fashion with MRI or ictal single-photon emission computed tomography (SPECT) using ^{99m}Tc-hexamethylpropyleneamine oxime (HMPAO) or ethylene cysteinate dimer [15] (Table 12.1). Among 118 patients who were operated on for medial temporal and neocortical epilepsies and were followed up for more than one year, the sensitivity of FDG PET was 85%.

Diagnostic Performance of FDG PET in Medial Temporal Lobe Epilepsy

Medial temporal lobe epilepsy is well known for its pathologic diagnostic criteria of hippocampal sclerosis and/or atrophy. These hippocampal changes are easily found by the recent generation MRI machines. Both the quantitative and the qualitative MRI interpretation give similar diagnostic effectiveness for TLE with the MRI machines. In cases of hipppocampal changes clearly identified on MRI, FDG PET reveals equally well the epileptogenic zones in medial temporal lobe epilepsy (Fig. 12.1a).

The advanced equipment and acquisition methods such as 3-T MRI have increased the sensitivity of localization of epileptogenic zones. However, despite these advancements, MRI reveals no significant anatomic structures in the 20–25% of the patients with medically intractable epilepsy [16]. For those patients, FDG PET could provide useful data for lateralizing the lesion as well as the desirable location for an invasive scalp EEG recording. The use of FDG PET is reported to be cost effective, especially in patients with unremarkable MRI scans [11].

In brief, FDG PET is helpful mainly for three types of medial TLE. The first type is represented by patients with ambiguous sclerosis (Fig. 12.1b). In a few patients with medial TLE, hippocampal sclerosis is not prominent even on MRI with the most recent techniques. The 3-T MRI with fluid-attenuated inversion recovery (FLAIR) and multiple channel coils could identify relevant abnormalities only in 20% of patients with previously unremarkable MRI scans [1]. The second type is of bilateral sclerosis and/or atrophy (Fig. 12.1c). Quite a few confusing cases have been filed among 600 fully investigated epilepsy patients at our institution. The third type is represented by those patients with inherently normal MRI findings (Fig. 12.1d). FDG PET and ictal SPECT were found to be similarly effective at localizing epileptogenic zones in nonlesional (MRI-negative) medial temporal lobe epilepsy [17].

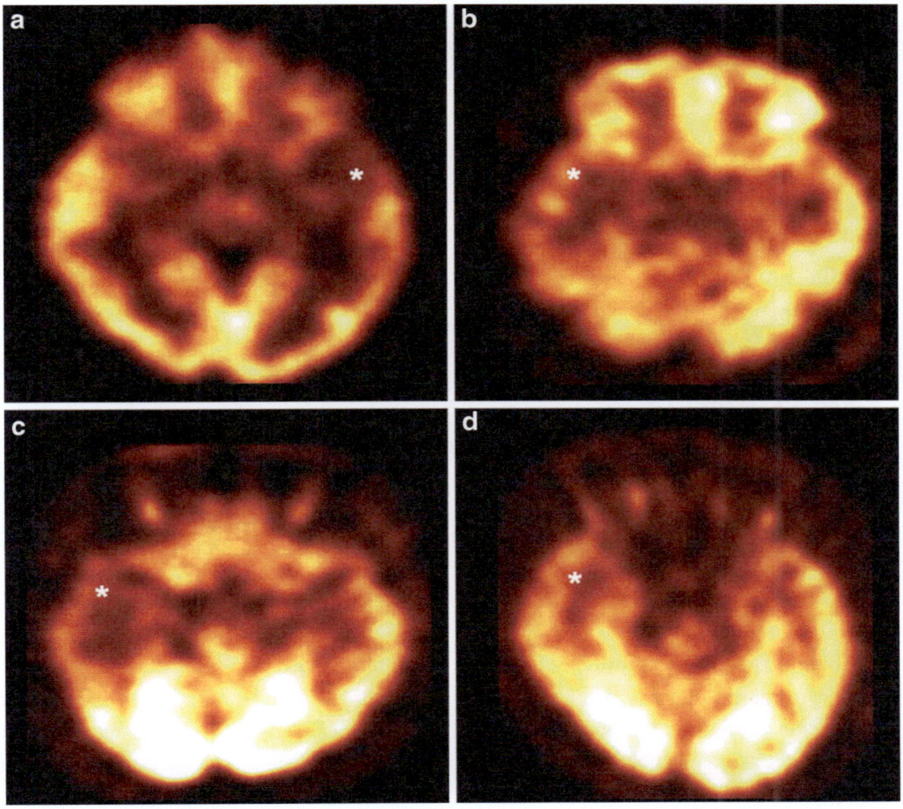

Fig. 12.1 Selected axial FDG PET images of lower brain for medial temporal lobe epilepsy. (**a**) A typical matching case with hippocampal atrophy and hypometabolism with decreased uptake of ^{18}F-FDG (*) in the left temporal lobe. (**b**) A case with ambiguous ictal EEG but with definite hypometabolism with decreased activity (*) in the right temporal lobe. (**c**) An example of bilateral hippocampal atrophy on MRI but unilateral hypometabolism (*) in the right temporal lobe. (**d**) A nonlesional cryptogenic case on MRI but with mild hypometabolism (*) in the right temporal lobe. All four patients underwent surgery with outcomes of Engel class 1

Diagnostic Performance of FDG PET in Neocortical Epilepsy

About one third to one half of medically intractable patients have neocortical epilepsy [18–20]. Neocortical epilepsy consists of lateral temporal, frontal, occipital, and parietal lobe epilepsy, in decreasing order of prevalence [19]. Neocortical epilepsy poses two types of problems in localization of epileptogenic zones. The first is that if MRI shows multiple candidate foci of the epileptogenic zones, it cannot be verified which is the culprit lesion for the seizure generation. The second is that if MRI does not show any structural lesion, that is to say, when the lesion is 'cryptogenic', it is difficult to determine where to apply subdural grids and strips to find the seizure focus during subdural EEG studies. In such cases, FDG PET is helpful in providing useful information on the virtual location of subdural electrodes to find the epileptogenic zone. FDG PET can at least lateralize cryptogenic lesions, although it cannot localize a lesion.

According to our previous study [21], positive predictive value of FDG PET in cryptogenic epilepsy is over 70%. Localization rates are different for various epileptogenic lobes. Lateral temporal lobe or frontal lobe epilepsies are relatively easy to diagnose among complex partial seizure patients. In frontal lobe epilepsy, the sensitivity of FDG PET was 36% in patients without structural lesions on MRI and 73% in patients with

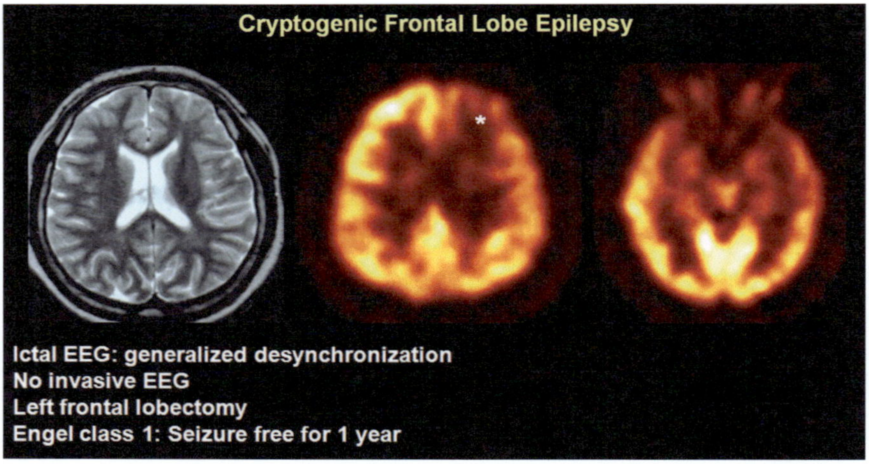

Fig. 12.2 A case with cryptogenic frontal lobe epilepsy. Selected axial T2-weighted, MR image of the brain was normal, and ictal EEG also was nonlocalizing. Selected axial FDG PET showed images of the head, definitive hypometabolism with decreased uptake of ^{18}F-FDG (*) in left frontal lobe. After successful frontal lobectomy, the patient became seizure-free

structural lesions in frontal lobe epilepsy [22]. In nonlesional cryptogenic cases, epileptogenic zones yield similar decreased metabolism to the lesions in explicit cases with subdural lesions (Fig. 12.2).

On the contrary, it is not easy to localize epileptogenic zones in occipital lobe epilepsy [23]. Areas showing the most severe hypometabolism are limited to the occipital lobes in some patients (Fig. 12.3), however, they are not limited in others. In those other cases, the areas of highest perfusion were also not limited to occipital lobes on ictal SPECT. The hypometabolism was localized even to the ipsilateral temporal lobes in a few patients (Fig. 12.4). Epileptogenic zones could have been misdiagnosed for temporal lobes in those patients. As for the occipital lobe epilepsy, the localization rate was found to be 47% by MRI and 60% by PET [23]. In such confusing cases of occipital lobe epilepsy, the examination of visual symptoms and visual field is mandatory [23].

Comparison of Interictal FDG PET with Interictal Perfusion SPECT

The diagnostic performance of interictal SPECT for localization of epileptogenic zones is somewhat disappointingly low as compared with that of interictal PET. The sensitivity of interictal perfusion SPECT was 44% on average by a meta-analysis [5], and 34% in our cohort study including both temporal and neocortical epilepsy cases. The sensitivities of interictal PET have been reported to be improved over those of interictal SPECT (73–97%) [24–26].

Considering the dogma of metabolism and perfusion coupling in the brain, it is important to figure out the significance of, or the reason for, this discrepancy in the sensitivities of the two functional imaging modalities representing metabolism and perfusion. The reason why interictal FDG PET is excellent but interictal SPECT is poor for the localization of epileptogenic zones could be explained as follows.

Among greater than 300 patients, we identified 14 patients with increased perfusion in the zones that was determined to be epileptogenic by surgical outcome or invasive studies [27]. Four of those were patients in whom interictal SPECT was performed on the second day after ictal episode. The other four patients, seemingly hyperperfused, were studied on the third to fifth day after ictus (Fig. 12.5a, b). This means that the interictal SPECT was in fact not performed at the interictal phase. Subclinical seizure activity just

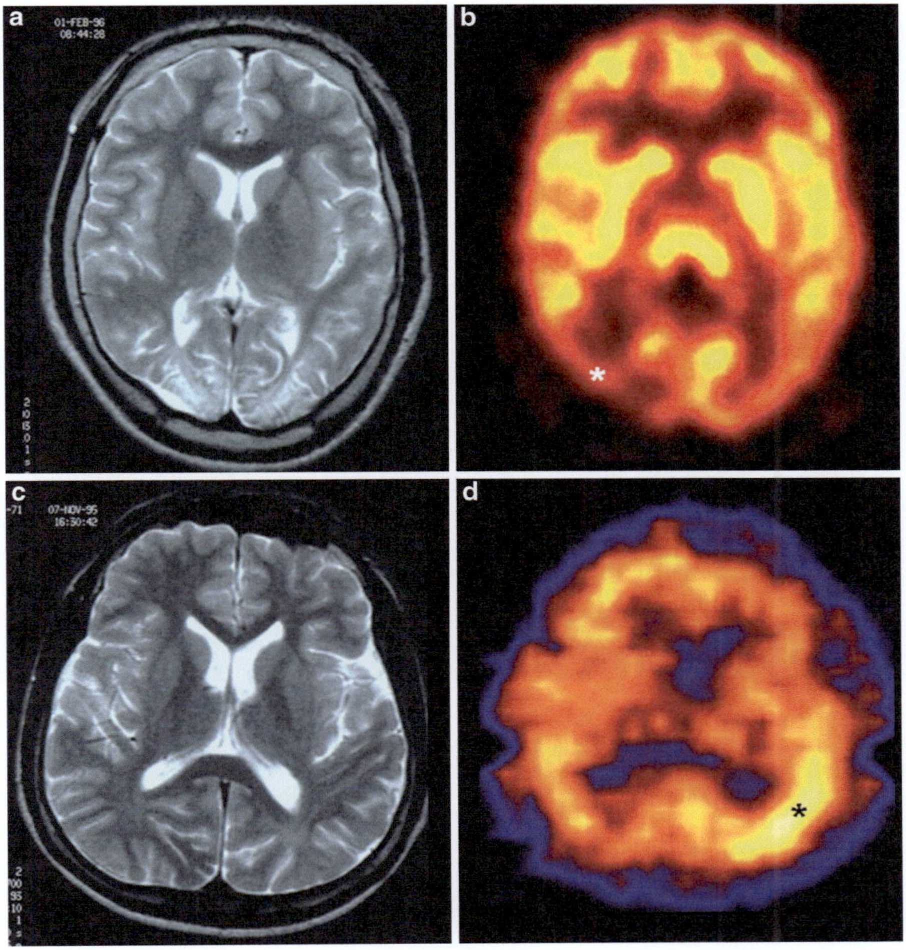

Fig. 12.3 Cases of occipital lobe epilepsy. Selected T2-weighted axial MR image of the brain (**a**) was normal, but metabolism with ^{18}F-FDG was decreased in the right occipital lobe epilepsy (*) on the axial image of the head (**b**). In another case, the MR image (**c**) was normal, but perfusion with ^{99m}Tc HMPAO was increased in the left occipital lobe (*) on ictal SPECT of the head (**d**). Both patients became seizure-free after neocortical resection

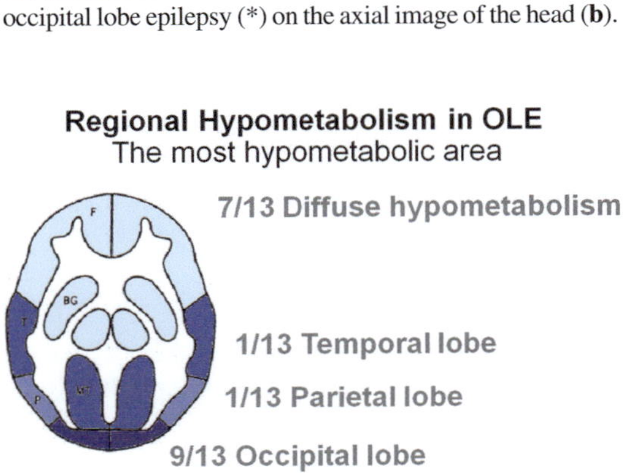

Fig. 12.4 Regional prevalence if interictal hypometabolism on ^{18}F-FDG PET in occipital lobe epilepsy. Occipital lobe is the most common site of hypometabolism

prior to or during interictal studies might have resulted in this increased perfusion at the epileptogenic zones.

On the other hand, 'delayed postictal perfusion abnormalities', even long after the previous ictus, could have resulted in the increased perfusion [28]. During the delayed postictal period at 6 h after ictal SPECT, we found remnant hyperperfusion in one half of patients (Fig. 12.5c–e). In one patient, severe hypoperfusion was found on delayed postictal SPECT, but showed recovery on interictal SPECT. Based on these findings, we suggest that even with EEG monitoring to

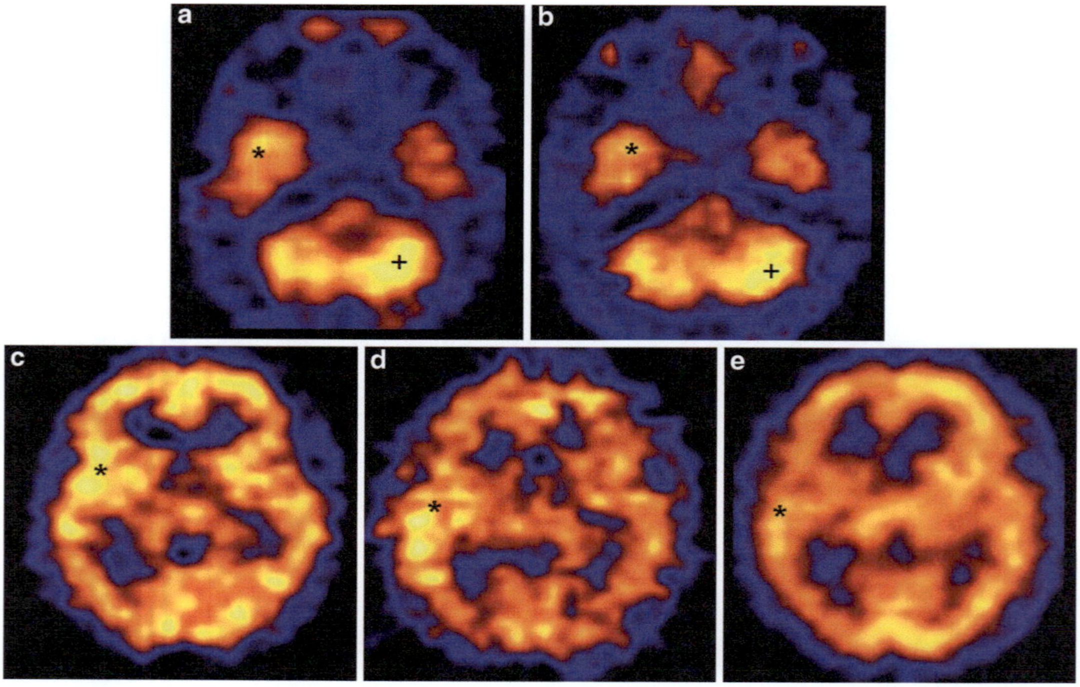

Fig. 12.5 Hyperperfusion on interictal SPECT using ^{99m}Tc HMPAO and delayed postictal hyperperfusion after ictus. In a patient with surgically confirmed right temporal lobe epilepsy, on the fourth day after ictal study (**a**), axial images of the head taken on interictal SPECT (**b**) showed similar increased perfusion in the right temporal lobe (*) and crossed cerebellar hyperperfusion (+). In the other patient with right temporal lobe epilepsy, perfusion was increased in the right temporal lobe (*) on ictal SPECT (**c**) and also on 6-h delayed SPECT (**d**). On interictal SPECT (**e**), perfusion was relatively decreased in this temporal lobe (*)

prove that there is no ictal discharge during interictal SPECT, it cannot be verified that the 'true' interictal SPECT has been obtained.

Voxel-Based Analysis of FDG PET

SPM is a voxel-based approach for determining the significantly different area from normal controls (Fig. 12.6). After spatially transforming and smoothing the individual PET data using the general linear model, the voxel count of the individual patient is compared with those of the normal controls. This analysis method is a very robust analytic tool to compare statistically abnormal cerebral perfusion with normal controls [22, 29, 30].

Interestingly, SPM analysis of ^{15}O-water PET, FDG PET, and ^{99m}Tc-HMPAO interictal SPECT revealed that in the same patients the areas of hypoperfusion were mostly concordant with but smaller than the areas of hypometabolism (Fig. 12.7) [31]. This apparent uncoupling of perfusion and metabolism in epileptogenic zones is another reason why interictal perfusion SPECT is inferior to interictal FDG PET in localizing epileptogenic zones.

On SPM analysis in frontal lobe epilepsy, using an uncorrected probability value of 0.005 as the threshold, the sensitivity of SPM analysis reached that of visual assessment. Sensitivity is decreasing as stricter thresholds are chosen to find abnormal area of decreased perfusion (Fig. 12.8).

Quantification Using Automatic Volume of Interest on Population-Based Atlas

This method is structured on population-based standard anatomy, which was developed by the Montreal Neurological Institute and named SPAM (Fig. 12.9). SPAM, an acronym for "statistical

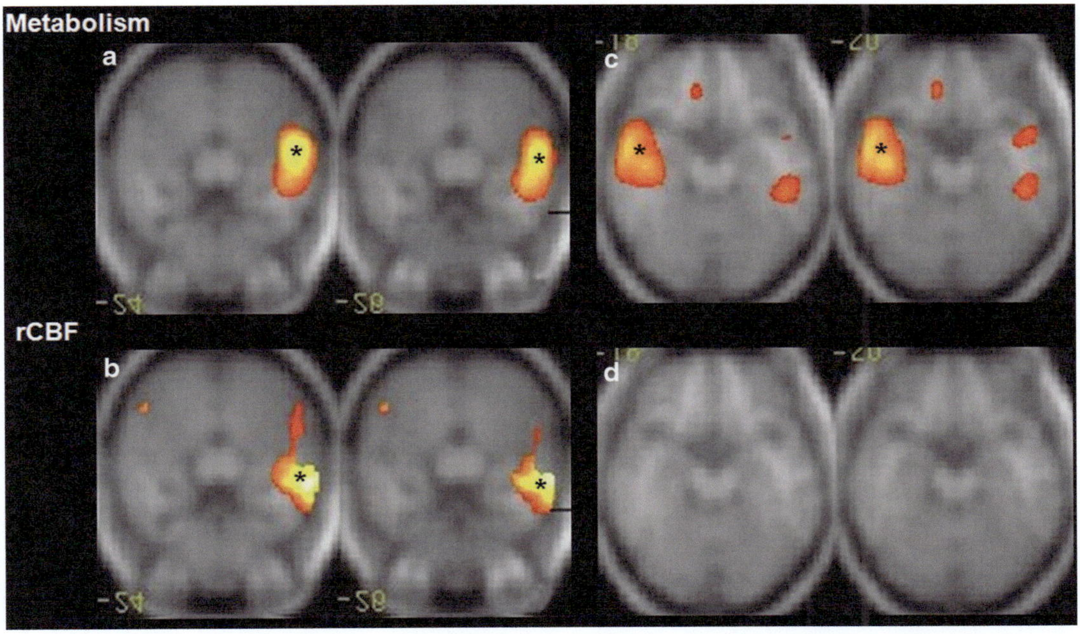

Fig. 12.6 SPM analysis results of ^{18}F-FDG PET and ^{15}O-water PET superimposed on MRI. Activities are the voxels that differ from the normal controls. In a coupled case, the left temporal lobe (*) was found to have hypometabolic voxels on axial FDG PET images (**a**) and hypoperfused voxels on water PET (**b**). In an uncoupled case, the right temporal lobe (*) was found to have hypometabolic voxels on FDG PET axial images (**c**), however, there was no area of hypoperfusion on water PET (**d**)

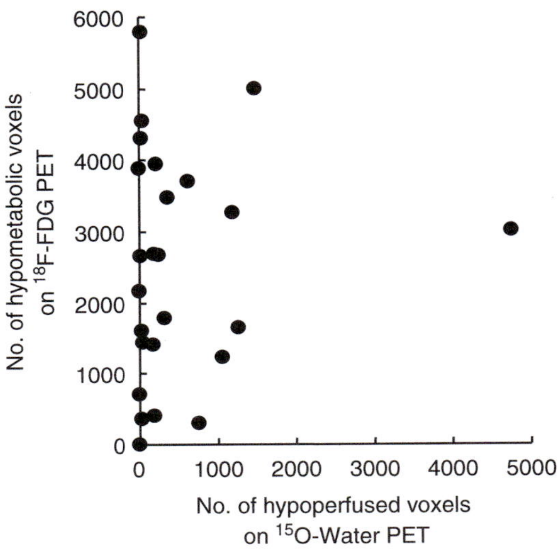

Fig. 12.7 Number of hypoperfused voxels and hypometabolic voxels on ^{15}O-water PET and ^{18}F-FDG PET in the epileptogenic temporal lobes. Each data point represents voxel number per epileptogenic whole temporal lobe per patient. Numbers of hypometabolic voxels tended to be much greater than those of hypoperfused voxels

probabilistic anatomic map," differs from SPM. SPM is a voxel-based approach, whereas SPAM is an area-based approach. SPAM is an objective and operator-independent method of volume of interest (VOI) drawing. We have a population-averaged anatomic definition of gyri and lobes in MRI template format. To construct SPAM, the Montreal group collected, parceled, and segmented normal MR images from 152 young subjects. Original PET images are transformed to an MRI template and the voxel counts are multiplied by the probabilities obtained from the SPAM template. For example, if the right hippocampus is chosen, the resulting image shows the probabilities of each voxel belonging to the right hippocampus. This method was first used to objectively quantify the asymmetric index, and these asymmetric indices could be used to localize epileptogenic zones on FDG PET [31].

The methods to use SPAM for evaluation of extent and severity of hypometabolism on FDG

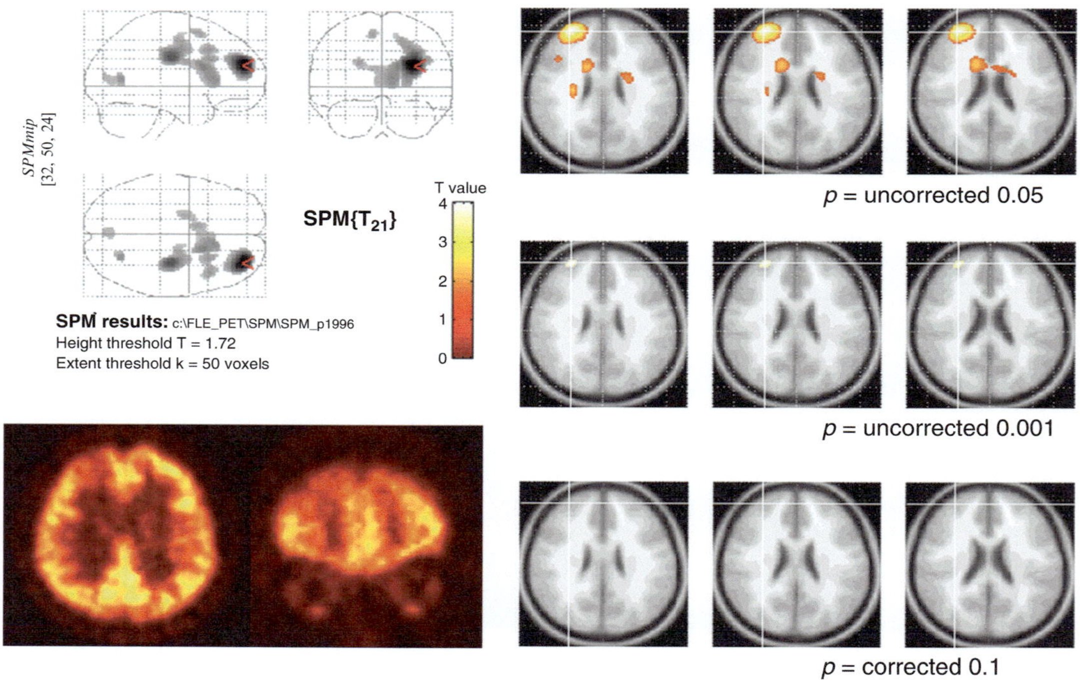

Fig. 12.8 Example of SPM analysis with varying threshold. According to cutoff value of voxel height, SPM analysis became less sensitive when stricter criterion was applied. Sensitivity decreases according to the decrease in probability value

Fig. 12.9 SPAM)as an objective VOI) in PET image processing. Frontal and parietal (*left*) as well as temporal and occipital (*right*) lobes were displayed on the MRI template. These SPAM masks can be used as a VOI on the MRI template

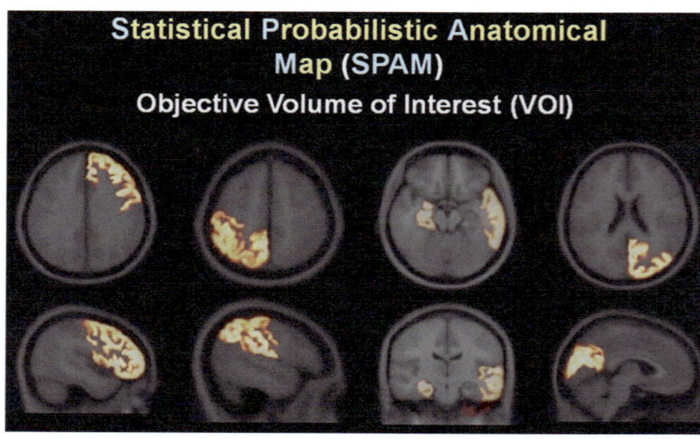

PET in the epileptogenic zones are depicted in Fig. 12.10. The relation of hypometabolism and surgical prognosis of medial temporal lobe epilepsy could be evaluated. By successful application of SPAM to six gyri of temporal lobes, this analysis revealed that focal severity and extent were not related to the surgical outcome in medial temporal lobe epilepsy [32].

Prognostic Values of FDG PET in Surgical Interventions

The prognostic values of FDG PET in presurgical evaluations have been investigated both in TLE and neocortical epilepsies. The focal hypometabolism on presurgical FDG PET are known to have a significant correlation with postoperative

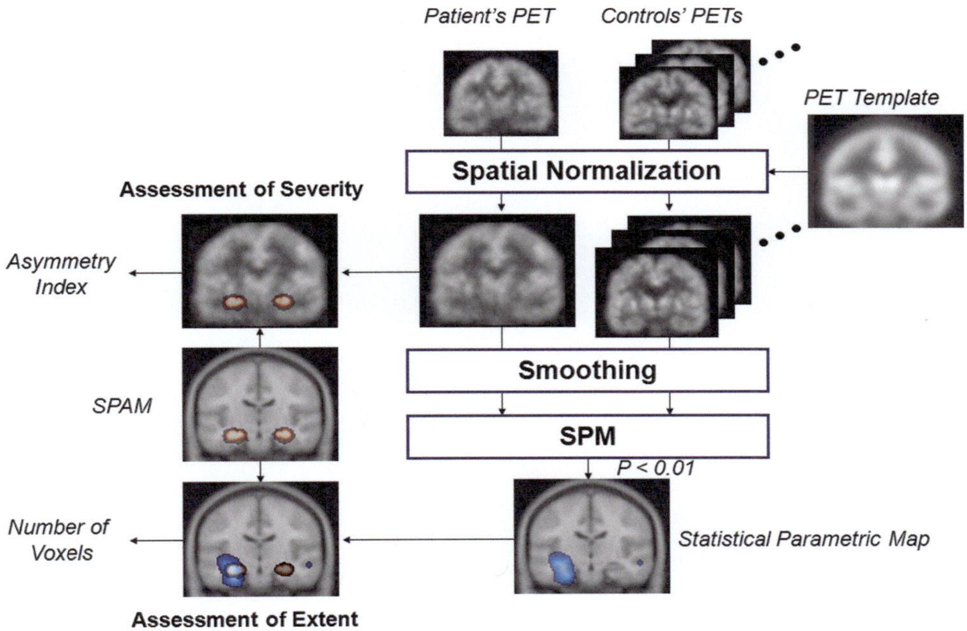

Fig. 12.10 Assessment of severity and extent of hypometabolism. Asymmetric indexes were calculated on six pairs of VOIs to represent the temporal lobe significant regional hypometabolism was estimated by comparing the PET images with those of controls by using SPM. The extent of hypometabolic area for each VOI was determined by counting the number of voxels with significantly decreased hypometabolism in each VOI segmented

seizure-free outcomes [33, 34]. By a meta-analysis dealing with predictive diagnostic values of FDG PET in TLE patients, unilateral temporal lobe hypometabolism could predict a good surgical outcome in 86% of patients, and in 80% of patients with normal MRI [35]. Although MRI itself is strongly predictive of surgical outcome in TLE [33], FDG PET seems to have a comparably high predictive value and even to achieve clinical benefit in the patients with suspected TLE and normal MRI. In addition, presurgical FDG PET is sure to be cost effective for localization of epileptogenic zones, especially if its use is restricted to the evaluation of patients in whom MRI and scalp EEG do not provide a definitive answer [11].

In neocortical epilepsies, surgical outcomes as well as localization rates of epileptogenic zones were lower than those of TLE. However, according to our previous study, the localizing values of FDG PET and interictal EEG were well correlated with a seizure-free outcome, and the positive predictive value of FDG PET was 63% in patients with cryptogenic neocortical epilepsy [36].

Beyond FDG PET in Epilepsy

In vivo neurochemistry, considered to be responsible for neuronal modulation, has had much attention in the past decades with the hope of revealing the pathophysiology of epilepsy. In particular, γ-aminobutyric acid (GABA), a major inhibitory neurotransmitter that plays a major role in regulating neuronal excitability throughout the central nervous system, is supposed to play the key role in epilepsy [37]. Besides the GABAergic system, other neurotransmitters such as serotoninergic, dopaminergic systems have also been suggested to have a significant pathophysiologic role in the epileptic brain. In this regard, PET agents for GABAergic, serotoninergic, dopaminergic systems, etc. have been actively investigated to evaluate the involvement of theses neurotransmitters in vivo.

PET with ^{11}C-flumazenil (FMZ), which binds to GABA$_A$ receptor, has been widely used to investigate the status of GABAergic system in TLE patients. On FMZ PET, epileptogenic zones

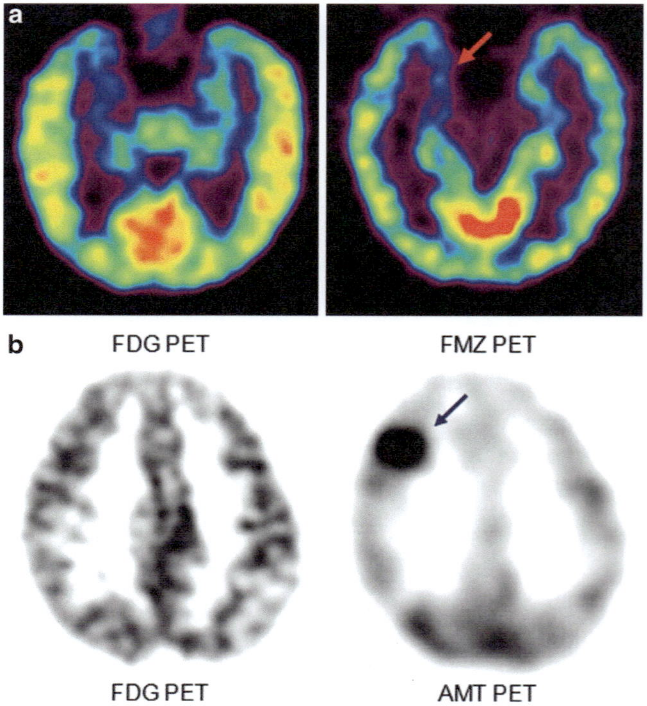

Fig. 12.11 PET scans using radiotracers other than FDG in patients with focal epilepcies. Epileptogenic focus in the right temporal lobe showed relatively decreased glucose metabolism and reduced FMZ uptake (**a**: Modified from Ref. [38]). Epileptogenic focus, proved to be cortical dysplasia later on histology, showed no abnormal glucose metabolism, but increased AMT uptake in the right frontal cortex (**b**: Modified from Ref. [45])

show decreased FMZ uptake as compared with the contralateral homotopic reference region and the remaining neocortex (Fig. 12.11a) [38]. However, careful interpretation is needed for the abnormalities on FMZ PET because decreased FMZ uptake could be seen not only in the epileptogenic zone but also in the remote area. Several hypostheses including a secondary epileptogenesis model, multifocal cortical dysplasia, and underlying pathology associated with increased susceptibility to seizures have been suggested to explain the presence of the multiple decreased FMZ sites remote from the epileptogenic zones [39]. Recently, a novel ^{18}F-labeled PET agent (^{18}F-flurorflumazenil) binding to GABA $_A$ receptor was reported and expected to facilitate the use of FMZ PET in clinical practice [40].

To evaluate the serotonergic system, PET agents for serotonin metabolism or serotonin receptor have been developed. ^{11}C-alpha-methyl tryptophan (AMT), an analog of tryptophan, reflects serotonin synthesis in vivo or induction of the kynurenine pathway [41, 42]. AMT PET has been suggested to be useful to localize epileptogenic zones in cortical malformations (Fig. 12.11b) [43–45]. Increased cortical AMT uptake was most sensitive in children with tuberous sclerosis [43]. For the evaluation of the serotonin receptor status, ^{18}F-MPPF, an antagonist of the 5HT$_{1A}$ receptor, has been investigated in patients with focal epilepsies. A recent study reported that MPPF PET could lateralize an epileptogenic lobe with a sensitivity of 90%, and proved its usefulness in the presurgical evaluation of TLE patients [46].

The pathophysiologic role of the dopaminergic system in the epileptic brain is not yet clearly understood. Recently, the striatal dopaminergic system became an important target for both basic and clinical research because it was reported to play a key role in modulation of seizure activity in animal studies [47]. To characterize the striatal dopaminergic system in vivo, ^{18}F-fallypride, a high-affinity dopamine D$_2$/D$_3$-receptor antagonist, has been actively used in animal studies as well as in the clinical setting. With the introduction of dedicated PET scanner for small animals, new PET agents for in vivo neurochemistry are expected to make advances in the understanding of the pathophysiology of epilepsy.

Conclusion

FDG PET is helpful in localizing epileptogenic zones, especially in patients with nonlesional epilepsy on MRI. Quantitative methods such as SPM and SPAM are believed to have the ability to enhance the objectivity of the analysis to find epileptogenic zones by revealing hypometabolic areas. In the near future, various PET agents other than FDG could be utilized to unveil the nature of the epilepsy.

References

1. Duncan J. The current status of neuroimaging for epilepsy. Curr Opin Neurol. 2009;22(2):179–84.
2. la Fougère C, Rominger A, Förster S, Geisler J, Bartenstein P. PET and SPECT in epilepsy: a critical review. Epilepsy Behav. 2009;15:50–5.
3. Kwan P, Brodie MJ. Early identification of refractory epilepsy. N Engl J Med. 2000;342(5):314–9.
4. Engel Jr J, Wiebe S, French J. The quality standards subcommittee of the American Academy of Neurology; American Epilepsy Society; American Association of Neurological Surgeons. Practice parameter: temporal lobe and localized neocortical resections for epilepsy: report of the quality standards subcommittee of the American Academy of Neurology, in association with the American Epilepsy Society and the American Association of Neurological Surgeons. Neurology. 2003;60(4):538–47.
5. Devous Sr MD, Thisted RA, Morgan GF, Leroy RF, Rowe CC. SPECT brain imaging in epilepsy: a meta-analysis. J Nucl Med. 1998;39(2):285–93.
6. Wiebe S, Blume WT, Girvin JP, et al. A randomized, controlled trial of surgery for temporal-lobe epilepsy. N Engl J Med. 2001;345:311–8.
7. Schramm J, Kral T, Grunwald T, et al. Surgical treatment for neocortical temporal lobe epilepsy: clinical and surgical aspects and seizure outcome. J Neurosurg. 2001;94:33–42.
8. Foldvary N, Nashold B, Mascha E, et al. Seizure outcome after temporal lobectomy for temporal lobe epilepsy: a Kaplan-Meier survival analysis. Neurology. 2000;54:630–4.
9. Engel Jr J. Surgery for seizures. N Engl J Med. 1996;334(10):647–52.
10. Duchowny M, Jayakar P, Resnick T, et al. Epilepsy surgery in the first three years of life. Epilepsia. 1998;39(7):737–43.
11. O'Brien TJ, Miles K, Ware R, Cook MJ, Binns DS, Hicks RJ. The cost-effective use of ^{18}F-FDG PET in the presurgical evaluation of medically refractory focal epilepsy. J Nucl Med. 2008;49(6):931–7.
12. O'Brien TJ, Jupp B. In-vivo imaging with small animal FDG-PET: a tool to unlock the secrets of epileptogenesis? Exp Neurol. 2009;220(1):1–4.
13. Spencer SS, Theodore WH, Berkovic SF. Clinical applications: MRI, SPECT, and PET. Magn Reson Imaging. 1995;13(8):1119–24.
14. Lee JJ, Kang WJ, Lee DS, et al. Diagnostic performance of ^{18}F-FDG PET and ictal ^{99m}Tc-HMPAO SPET in pediatric temporal lobe epilepsy: uantitative analysis by statistical parametric mapping, statistical probabilistic anatomical map, and subtraction ictal SPET. Seizure. 2005;14(3):213–20.
15. Won HJ, Chang KH, Cheon JE, et al. Comparison of MR imaging with PET and ictal SPECT in 118 patients with intractable epilepsy. AJNR Am J Neuroradiol. 1999;20(4):593–9.
16. Lehéricy S, Semah F, Hasboun D, et al. Temporal lobe epilepsy with varying severity: MRI study of 222 patients. Neuroradiology. 1997;39(11):788–96.
17. Son YJ, Chung CK, Lee SK, et al. Comparison of localizing values of various diagnostic tests in nonlesional medial temporal lobe epilepsy. Seizure. 1999;8:465–70.
18. Nam H, Lee SK, Chung CK, et al. Incidence and clinical profile of extra-medial-temporal epilepsy with hippocampal atrophy. J Korean Med Sci. 2001;16:95–102.
19. Kutsy RL. Focal extratemporal epilepsy: clinical features, EEG patterns, and surgical approach. J Neurol Sci. 1999;166:1–15.
20. Zentner J, Hufnagel A, Ostertun B, et al. Surgical treatment of extratemporal epilepsy: clinical, radiologic, and histopathologic findings in 60 patients. Epilepsia. 1996;37:1072–80.
21. Lee DS, Lee SK, Chung J-K, et al. Predictive values of F-18 FDG-PET and ictal SPECT to find epileptogenic zones in cryptogenic neocortical epilepsies (Abstract). J Nucl Med. 1997;38:272.
22. Kim YK, Lee DS, Lee SK, et al. F-18 FDG-PET in localization of frontal lobe epilepsy: comparison of visual and SPM analysis. J Nucl Med. 2002;43:1167–74.
23. Kim SK, Lee DS, Lee SK, et al. Diagnostic performance of [^{18}F]-FDG-PET and ictal [^{99m}Tc]-HMPAO SPECT in occipital lobe epilepsy. Epilepsia. 2001;42:1531–40.
24. Spanaki MV, Spencer SS, Corsi M, et al. Sensitivity and specificity of quantitative difference SPECT analysis in seizure localization. J Nucl Med. 1999;40(5):730–6.
25. Weil S, Noachtar S, Arnold S, Yousry TA, Winkler PA, Tatsch K. Ictal ECD-SPECT differentiates

between temporal and extratemporal epilepsy: confirmation by excellent postoperative seizure control. Nucl Med Commun. 2001;22(2):233–7.
26. Zaknun JJ, Bal C, Maes A, et al. Comparative analysis of MR imaging, ictal SPECT and EEG in temporal lobe epilepsy: a prospective IAEA multi-center study. Eur J Nucl Med Mol Imaging. 2008;35(1):107–15.
27. Lee DS, Kim SK, Lee SK, et al. Frequencies and implications of discordant findings of interictal SPECT and ictal SPECT in patients with intractable epilepsy (Abstract). Eur J Nucl Med. 1997;24:983.
28. Lee DS, Lee SK, Kim SK, et al. Late postictal residual perfusion abnormality in epileptogenic zone found on 6-hour postictal SPECT. Neurology. 2000;55:835–41.
29. Signorini M, Paulesu E, Friston K, et al. Rapid assessment of regional cerebral metabolic abnormalities in single subjects with quantitative and nonquantitative F-18 FDG-PET: a clinical validation of statistical parametric mapping. Neuroimage. 1999;9:63–80.
30. Van Bogaert P, Massager N, Tugendhaft P, et al. Statistical parametric mapping of regional glucose metabolism in mesial temporal lobe epilepsy. Neuroimage. 2000;12:129–38.
31. Kang KW, Lee DS, Cho JH, et al. Quantification of F-18 FDG-PET images in temporal lobe epilepsy patients using probabilistic brain atlas. Neuroimage. 2001;14:1–6.
32. Lee SK, Lee DS, Yeo JS, et al. FDG-PET images quantified by probabilistic atlas of brain and surgical prognosis of temporal lobe epilepsy. Epilepsia. 2002;43:1032–8.
33. Vinton AB, Carne R, Hicks RJ, et al. The extent of resection of FDG-PET hypometabolism relates to outcome of temporal lobectomy. Brain. 2007;130: 548–60.
34. O'Brien TJ, Hicks RJ, Ware R, Binns DS, Murphy M, Cook MJ. The utility of a 3-dimensional, large-field-of-view, sodium iodide crystal-based PET scanner in the presurgical evaluation of partial epilepsy. J Nucl Med. 2001;42(8):1158–65.
35. Willmann O, Wennberg R, May T, Woermann FG, Pohlmann-Eden B. The contribution of ^{18}F-FDG PET in preoperative epilepsy surgery evaluation for patients with temporal lobe epilepsy a meta-analysis. Seizure. 2007;16(6):509–20.
36. Lee SK, Lee SY, Kim KK, Hong KS, Lee DS, Chung CK. Surgical outcome and prognostic factors of cryptogenic neocortical epilepsy. Ann Neurol. 2005;58(4): 525–32.
37. Treiman DM. GABAergic mechanisms in epilepsy. Epilepsia. 2001;42(Suppl 3):8–12.
38. Ryvlin P, Bouvard S, Le Bars D, et al. Clinical utility of flumazenil-PET versus [^{18}F]fluorodeoxyglucose-PET and MRI in refractory partial epilepsy: a prospective study in 100 patients. Brain. 1998;121:2067–81.
39. Juhász C, Asano E, Shah A, et al. Focal decreases of cortical $GABA_A$ recpetor binding remote from the primary seizure focus:what do they indicate? Epilepsia. 2009;50(2):240–50.
40. Chang YS, Jeong JM, Yoon YH, et al. Biological properties of 2′-[^{18}F]fluoroflumazenil for central benzodiazepine receptor imaging. Nucl Med Biol. 2005;32(3):263–8.
41. Diksic M, Nagahiro S, Sourkes TL, Yamamoto YL. A new method to measure brain serotonin synthesis in vivo. I. Theory and basic data for a biological model. J Cereb Blood Flow Metab. 1990;10(1):1–12.
42. Chugani DC, Muzik O. Alpha[C-11]methyl-L-tryptophan PET maps brain serotonin synthesis and kynurenine pathway metabolism. J Cereb Blood Flow Metab. 2000;20(1):2–9.
43. Chugani DC, Chugani HT, Muzik O, et al. Imaging epileptogenic tubers in children with tuberous sclerosis complex using alpha-[^{11}C]methyl-L-tryptophan positron emission tomography. Ann Neurol. 1998;44(6):858–66.
44. Fedi M, Reutens D, Okazawa H, et al. Localizing value of alpha-methyl-L-tryptophan PET in intractable epilepsy of neocortical origin. Neurology. 2001;57(9):1629–36.
45. Juhász C, Chugani DC, Muzik O, et al. Alpha-methyl-L-tryptophan PET detects epileptogenic cortex in children with intractable epilepsy. Neurology. 2003;60:960–8.
46. Didelot A, Ryvlin P, Lothe A, Merlet I, Hammers A, Mauguière F. PET imaging of brain $5\text{-}HT_{1A}$ receptors in the preoperative evaluation of temporal lobe epilepsy. Brain. 2008;131:2751–64.
47. Starr MS. The role of dopamine in epilepsy. Synapse. 1996;22(2):159–94.

Neurodegenerative Diseases

13

Sang Eun Kim, Jong Jin Lee, and Yoo Sung Song

Dementia

Dementia is a major public health challenge, not only for clinicians, but also for society as a whole. Prevalence rates of dementia are dependent on age, and continuously increase. Twenty-four million people are suspected of suffering from dementia worldwide, with about 4.6 million new patients every year. The number is estimated to double every 20 years, and is expected to reach up to 81 million cases by the year 2040. The prevalence is likely to rise more rapidly in developing countries [1]. In the US, there are about 3.4 million patients, and the overall prevalence in the US between the ages of 71–79 years is 5.0%, and 24.2% for the ages of 80–89 years [2]. Furthermore, dementia is related to increased mortality [3]. Thus, there is an increasing demand on the health care system and public resources to care for the people with dementia.

A wide variety of disorders have been identified as causes of dementia, including primary brain disease and disease of other organ systems that lead to secondary brain dysfunction. Between 10% and 20% of dementias may be reversible, some of which may be caused by etiologies such as medication, vitamin deficiencies, and endocrinologic problems [4]. Therefore, distinguishing patients with potentially reversible conditions from those with degenerative dementia is crucial [5]. Some irreversible types of dementia may have important interventions (e.g., vascular dementia), and accurate diagnosis is necessary in degenerative disorders to provide prognostic and genetic counseling. Neuroimaging plays a critical role in the diagnostic evaluation of the patient with dementia, such as vascular dementia, hydrocephalus, and neoplasms. Subdural hematomas and some infectious and degenerative processes can be identified with contemporary imaging technology.

Dementia causes not only a severe disability in normal life, but is a major cause of death in the elderly. A 5-year follow-up study demonstrated that demented people had a twice as higher mortality rate than nondemented people [6]. As the percentage of elderly people rises, and because the incidence of dementia increases with age, the economic, social, and health care consequences of dementing illnesses and Alzheimer's disease (AD) in particular, will increase with time. The cost of care for patients with dementia is on a steady increase. The worldwide cost for dementia care

S.E. Kim, M.D., Ph.D. (✉)
Department of Nuclear Medicine, Seoul National University Bundang Hospital, Seongnam 463-707, South Korea
e-mail: kse@snu.ac.kr

J.J. Lee, M.D., Ph.D.
Department of Nuclear Medicine, University of Ulsan College of Medicine, Asan Medical Center, Seoul 138-736, South Korea
e-mail: jjwalking@naver.com

Y.S. Song, M.D.
Department of Nuclear Medicine, Seoul National University Hospital, Seoul 110-744, South Korea
e-mail: yosung99@hanmail.net

E.E. Kim et al. (eds.), *Clinical PET and PET/CT: Principles and Applications*,
DOI 10.1007/978-1-4419-0802-5_13,

has been estimated to be $156 billion US in 2003, and $315 US in 2005 [7]. This chapter describes the application of functional neuroimaging in the evaluation of AD and other types of dementia.

Alzheimer's Disease

Alzheimer's disease is characterized by a progressive, global, and irreversible deterioration of cognitive function, which usually begins with memory problems, followed by deficits in language, mathematical and visuospatial skills, abstract thinking and planning, as well as personality and behavioral changes [8]. AD is the leading cause for dementia and has 9.7% prevalence in the US in patients 70 years or older. It increases up to 18.1% in people between the ages of 80 and 89 years and up to 29.7% in people over the age of 90 years [2]. Since the original case report of AD in 1907, clinicians have sought to find accurate antemortem tests to aid in the diagnosis of this disorder. A biopsy or postmortem examination of cerebral tissue is needed if confirmation of the presumptive clinical diagnosis is required, making clinicians rely on clinical diagnostic criteria. Currently, there is clinical ambiguity in diagnosing AD in its early stages and it is essentially a diagnosis of exclusion. Until now, however, no peripheral biochemical or genetic marker for AD has been found. Some cerebral spinal fluid (CSF) and serum markers have been studied for the diagnosis of AD, however, there is no specific marker for AD [9]. The patients, the family, and the physician are typically faced with a battery of negative test results and an ambiguous clinical impression that leads to periodic repetition of tests involving cost, inconvenience, potential morbidity to the patient, and lack of a definitive diagnosis. The ability to diagnose AD noninvasively and reliably with PET early in its course will have significant impact on these medical and economic realities.

Neuropathology

Pathologic hallmarks of AD are extracellular deposition of the amyloid β peptide in senile plaques and intracellular NFTs [10]. Amyloid precursor protein (APP), presenilin 1, presenilin 2, and apolipoprotein E genes are known to be linked with autosomal dominant or familial early onset AD [10]. Amyloid β peptide is derived from the APP and deposits in a hierarchical manner. The sequence of brain regions involved in AD are the neocortex, diencephalic nuclei, striatum, cholinergic nuclei of the basal forebrain, brainstem nuclei, and cerebellum [11].

NFTs are formed from paired helical filament composed of neurofilament and hyperphosphorylated tau protein [10]. Tau protein normally takes a role in the stabilization of neurons, involved in microtubule assembly [12]. Transportation and dynamics of microtubules are regulated by tau, a microtubule associated protein. Interaction is regulated by posttranslational modifications such as phosphorylation. Aggregation of hyperphosphorylated tau has been histologically proved in AD. NFTs are mostly found in the medium-sized pyramidal neurons of the hippocampus, the entorhinal cortex and of layers III and V of the isocortex, and also in the olfactory bulb at the early stage of disease [13]. NFTs show a characteristic distribution pattern according to the following stages: transentorhinal, limbic, and isocortical [14].

The AD brain also is characterized by neuronal cell loss and change in neuronal morphology, which is reflected by a decreased brain weight and by atrophy of the cortex. Although the pattern and degrees of atrophy vary considerably from individual to individual, it is most prominent in the frontal, anterior temporal parietal lobe. Neuronal loss is most notable in the hippocampus, frontal, parietal, and anterior temporal cortices; amygdale; and the olfactory system. Profound loss also occurs in the nucleus basalis, a large cholinergic system at the base of the forebrain. This cell loss also occurs in the locus ceruleus and is likely to account for reduction in brain level of norepinephrine noted in some patients with AD. As might be expected, neuronal loss is generally seen in areas that show plaque or tangle pathology. In the hippocampus, the most prominently affected zones are the CA1 region, the subiculum, and the entorhinal cortex. Other areas of the limbic system that are also affected include olfactory bulbs, olfactory cortices, amygdala, cingulate gyrus, and hypothalamus.

Many individuals (at least 20–30%) diagnosed antemortem with AD demonstrate cortical Lewy bodies at autopsy in addition to the neuropathologic findings of AD. AD with Lewy bodies has been associated with excess cognitive burden, extrapyramidal symptoms, and more frequent psychotic symptoms [15].

Neurochemistry

AD is associated with deficits in several neurotransmitter systems, both those that project to the neocortex and those that reside within the cortex. Among the neurotransmitters, acetylcholine has an important relationship with cognition and memory. Previous studies have led to a 'cholinergic hypothesis' of AD [16]. Cholinergic neuron loss is found in the basal forebrain and associated neocortical areas. The basal forebrain contains a well-characterized group of magnocellular cholinergic neurons extending from the medial septal region through the nucleus basalis of Meynert (Ch1–Ch4) which provide the majority of cholinergic innervation to the hippocampus and neocortex [17]. Cholinergic deficits are not the only transmitter deficit in AD. There are cortical losses of norepinephrine and serotonin that can be traced to cell loss in the locus ceruleus and raphe nuclei. In addition to deficits in systems that project to the cortex, there are abnormalities in pathways that are intrinsic to the cortex. A large number of peptide transmitters are found in cortical interneurons. Of these, losses of somatostatin, neuropeptide Y, corticotropin-releasing factor, and substance P have been described in AD.

Presumably, the deficits in these various transmitter systems in AD are all a reflection of the degeneration and death of neuronal populations. Another indication of neuronal degeneration in AD is the loss of synapses and presynaptic marker proteins in the neocortex and hippocampus. The loss is likely a result of both deafferentation of cortical and hippocampal neurons and of atrophy of the neurons themselves. Decline of the synaptic density in the neocortex and hippocampus is associated with brain function in AD, but it is still unclear whether these synaptic changes are related to NFTs or amyloid plaques [18].

Identification of the loss of cholinergic neurons in the basal forebrain and of cholinergic innervation of the cerebral cortex in AD was followed by investigations into the involvement of cholinergic receptors. In contrast to choline acetyltransferase (ChAT), no major or consistent changes in muscarinic acetylcholine receptors were observed in the cerebral cortex [19], although moderate reductions in the cortical M2 receptor subtype have been reported [20]. In contrast, reductions in nicotinic acetylcholine receptors (nAChRs) with high affinity for agonists ranging between 20% and 50% were consistently observed at autopsy in a number of neocortical areas and hippocampi of patients with AD [19]. A reduction in the density of the presynaptic vesicular acetylcholine transporter binding sites measured by [^{3}H]vesamicol was also seen in the AD cortical tissue, but the decrease in [^{3}H]vesamicol binding was less than in nAChRs [21]. The observation suggests that the vesamicol binding sites may be more preserved in the existing presynaptic terminals of AD cortical tissue, thereby expressing a compensatory capacity to maintain cholinergic activity. Also, the reduction in vesicular acetylcholine transporter radioligand binding was less than in ChAT activity in AD neocortex [22]. Thus, there is the possibility that these two presynaptic cholinergic markers may be differentially regulated or differentially lost in AD. There may be up-regulation of vesicular acetylcholine transporter expression to compensate for cholinergic terminal losses, or alternatively, ChAT expression may be reduced within otherwise intact presynaptic nerve terminals [23].

Prominent reductions in postmortem measures of presynaptic dopamine have been reported in AD with Lewy bodies [24, 25]. These reductions, however, are not as severe as seen in Parkinson disease (PD) [25].

Clinical Diagnosis

There is no definitive antemortem diagnostic test for AD, and brain biopsy may miss subsequently proven cases. Clinicians must therefore rely on clinical diagnostic criteria for senile or presenile dementia of the Alzheimer type, the two most common of which are those of the *Diagnostic and Statistical Manual of Mental Disorders*, Fourth Edition, Revised (American Psychiatric Association, 2000) and those of the National Institute of Neurological and Communicative Disorders and Stroke and the AD and Related Disorders Association Work Group.When compared against the "gold standard" of pathologic AD, their diagnostic accuracy in dementia of the Alzheimer type varies widely. The diagnostic accuracy ranges from 65% and 96%. However, the specificity of these diagnostic criteria against other types of dementias is only 23–88% [26].

Structural Imaging

In AD, structural imaging such as magnetic resonance imaging (MRI) and computed tomography (CT) show progressive cortical atrophy associated with increases in ventricular and cortical cerebrospinal fluid space. These imaging techniques are excellent in identifying the causes of dementia that have a structurally identifiable basis on the microscopic level. Such entities include multiple infarcts, subdural hematomas, brain tumors, and hydrocephalus. Medial temporal lobe atrophy is a highly evocative feature of AD [27]. Evaluation of the entorhinal cortex is more accurate in the diagnosis of early AD. However, hippocampal volume measurement is more practical because of the anatomic ambiguity of entorhinal cortex [28]. MRI-based hippocampal volume measurements reflect hippocampal neuronal loss [29].

Structural imaging techniques are of little use in differentiating AD from other degenerative dementias such as dementia with Lewy bodies (DLB), frontotemporal dementia (FTD), early Huntington's disease (HD), and progressive supranuclear palsy (PSP). However, CT and MRI have an important role for exclusion of structural lesions in patients with cognitive decline, particularly if the clinical presentation is in any way unusual [30, 31].

Functional Imaging

Positron emission tomography (PET) assesses and maps regional brain function. The signal measured in PET is derived from the decay of radioactive positron-emitting nuclides that are introduced into the body via intravenous injection or inhalation. Common nuclides including ^{15}O, ^{11}C, and ^{18}F are used to label compounds such as glucose and oxygen for the purpose of evaluating cerebral metabolism or measuring regional cerebral blood flow (rCBF). Radiolabeled receptor ligands have been developed and widely used for the assessment of neurotransmitter systems. The short half-life of some of these tracers facilitates repeat studies within a single scanning session while ensuring low radiation exposure to the subject. A circumferential detector placed around the head maps the distribution of the positron-emitting nuclide with a resolution of approximately 5 mm. Currently, high-resolution research tomography brain dedicated PET scanners are in development for both academic and commercial use. Also, the combination of MRI with PET has been researched for additional anatomic information [32].

Metabolic and Blood Flow Imaging

[^{18}F]2-Fluoro-2-deoxy-D-glucose (FDG) PET has the ability to provide objective, accurate, and noninvasive diagnostic information about patients with dementia of various causes. Glucose metabolism is coupled with glutamate-driven astrocytic glucose uptake, so that FDG PET may be related with excitatory glutamate neurotransmitter release, and neuronal activity [33].

FDG PET studies have shown a characteristic pattern of metabolic impairment of cortical association areas in AD (Fig. 13.1). Impairment of glucose metabolism seen in AD (usually 1–2 years after onset of the disease) typically involves the temporoparietal cortex, and often is bilateral. As the disease progresses, the areas of cortical involvement with hypometabolism expand. Later, decreased metabolism is found in the frontal cortex, but the primary visual cortex and primary sensorimotor cortices typically appear to

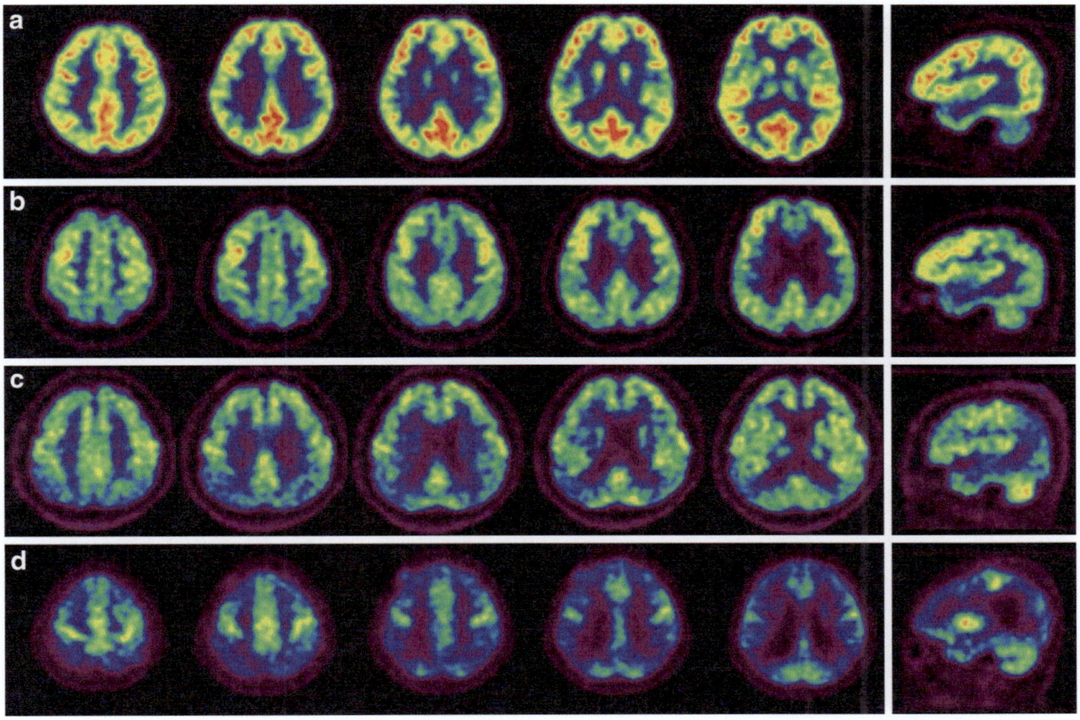

Fig. 13.1 ^{18}F-FDG PET images of normal control (**a**), and early-stage (**b**), midstage (**c**), advanced-stage (**d**) AD. AD shows a characteristic pattern of metabolic impairment in the bilateral temporoparietal association cortex, with relative sparing of primary sensorimotor and visual areas, basal ganglia, thalamus, and cerebellum. As disease progresses, temporoparietal hypometabolism is more prominent and frontal hypometabolism is also seen (**b**, **c**, **d**)

be relatively spared until the late stages of the disease, in accordance with pathologic data. The thalamus has been known to be relatively unaffected in FDG PET findings, which is inconsistent with the current understanding of AD pathology. MRI co-registered and voxel-based analysis revealed that glucose metabolism in the hypothalamus is reduced [33]. Cerebellar metabolism is relatively preserved in mild to moderate AD, and a significant reduction in cerebellar glucose metabolism has been reported in severe AD with no evident cerebellar atrophy [34]. In the early stages of the disease, the typical pattern may not yet be complete. In particular, frontal involvement may be missing and temporoparietal metabolism may only be unilaterally impaired. In spite of these limitations, it has been suggested that FDG PET may be used for early diagnosis of AD, which could be very valuable for therapeutic trials in the early stages of the disease.

PET may be helpful in predicting which patients are in the process of cognition decline. Patients in the stage of mild cognitive impairment show certain patterns on FDG PET findings. Even before the possible clinical diagnosis of probable AD, decrease of blood flow and glucose metabolism in the posterior cingulate and associative cortical activity has been reported [35–37]. The metabolic and flow reduction in these regions may be a result of functional deafferentation from the entorhinal cortex, which is among the first regions pathologically affected in AD [38]. Also, hypometabolism in these areas indicates that a patient is more likely to undergo cognitive decline faster than expected [39]. As the disease progresses, the medial temporal structures and parietotemporal association cortex show reductions in blood flow and FDG metabolism. Alterations in medial parietotemporal lobes and posterior cingulated gyrus also indicate fast

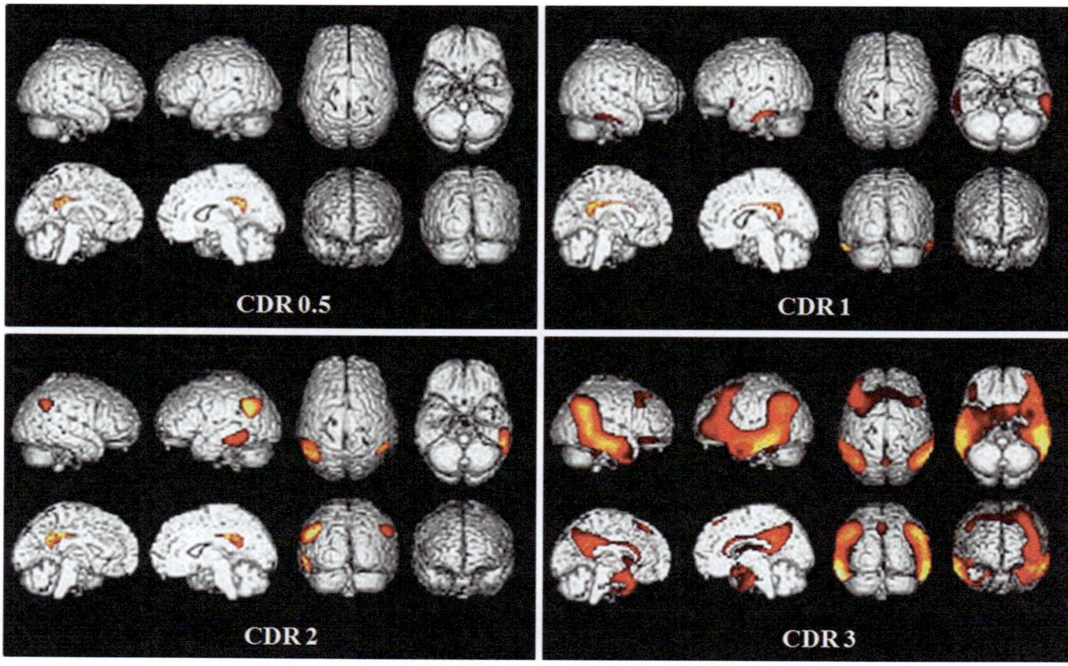

Fig. 13.2 SPM results of ^{18}F-FDG PET images of AD. Brain glucose hypometabolism correlates with clinical dementia rating

conversion to AD [40, 41]. Recent meta-analysis has shown that sensitivity of FDG PET for AD was 86% (95% CI: 76%, 93%), and specificity was 86% (95% CI: 72%, 93%) [42].

PET and single-photon emission computed tomography (SPECT) imaging of patients with AD demonstrates progressive reductions in resting-state brain glucose metabolism and blood flow in relation to dementia severity (Fig. 13.2), more so in association than in primary cortical regions. The metabolic and flow reductions correlate with high regional densities of NFTs and evidence for synaptic loss and dysfunction. During cognitive or psychophysic stimulation, however, blood flow and metabolism in the affected brain regions can increase to the same extent in mildly demented AD patients as in age-matched controls, despite reduced resting-state values. The extent of activation declines with dementia severity and is markedly reduced in severely demented patients. Thus, there appears to be an initial functionally responsive stage in AD in which direct brain analysis suggests is accompanied by reversible down-regulation because of reduced synaptic energy demand of enzymes mediating mitochondrial oxidative-phosphorylation. A later irreversible stage of AD is accompanied by marked synaptic loss, accumulation of intracellular NFTs, reduced general transcriptional capacity, and death of neurons.

Patients with early-stage AD present with memory decline and impairments of language and visuospatial functions [43]. However, some AD patients occasionally show frontal lobe dysfunctions in the early stage that are known to emerge only at the advanced stage. This subtype of AD is called frontal variant of AD. In such patients, hypometabolism in the frontal cortex, as well as temporoparietal regions, was seen on FDG PET scans. Visual variant of AD with prominent visual symptoms and metabolic impairment in occipital cortex has also been reported.

While structural imaging may show atrophy in the demented patient, this finding is nonspecific and overlaps with results seen in normal elderly subjects. Patients in whom the diagnosis of AD can be supported by PET may be given a chance for early treatment. Because it is known that metabolic decline precedes a patient's symptoms, early diagnosis may prevent or slower a patient's manifestations. Treatment with cholinesterase inhibitors delays cognitive decline and delays the need for hospitalization [44]. The effect of treatment may be assessed with FDG PET, and may be helpful in treating patients with early-stage dementia [45, 46]. FDG PET is expected to play an important role in early diagnosis and treatment.

SPECT measures of CBF can also be used to assess the functional effects of therapeutic drugs in AD. Regional CBF assessed by SPECT in AD patients improved after cholinesterase treatment after 4 months, thus reflecting the short-term effect of treatment [47]. Significant improvements of CBF were found in the left angular, right superior frontal gyrus; right occipital, left temporal lobe; and left orbital gyrus. Also, AD patients receiving cholinesterase treatment showed a different CBF change according to the progression of cognition loss. Patients who had a significant drop in Mini-Mental State Examination (MMSE) score despite treatment showed decreased levels of CBF in the frontal, temporal, and parietal superficial cortex in the right hemisphere and in frontal, medial temporal cortex in the left hemisphere compared with baseline pretreatment CBF. In contrast, patients who showed stable MMSE scores had no significant interval change of CBF before and after acetylcholinesterase treatment [48].

The magnitude of the health problem resulting from dementing illnesses is great in terms of medical practice, economics, and family hardship. The ability to diagnose AD early in its course, noninvasively and reliably with PET, will have significant impact on such medical and economic realities. In the US, the Centers for Medicare and Medicaid Services have approved FDG PET imaging as a routine examination tool for the early and differential diagnosis of AD [33].

Neurochemical Imaging

Behavioral studies provide evidence that acetylcholine participates in complex functions such as attention, memory, and cognition, and clinical and postmortem studies suggest its involvement in the cognitive deterioration seen in AD and in the memory loss associated with normal aging. Recent development in radiochemistry has made it possible to noninvasively evaluate the cholinergic system in the human brain using PET and SPECT. PET and SPECT studies have been performed to evaluate various elements involved with cholinergic neurotransmission in normal human aging and in dementia, including vesicular acetylcholine transporter, acetylcholinesterase, and muscarinic and nicotinic acetylcholine receptors.

Cholinergic neuronal integrity can be mapped using radiotracers for acetylcholinesterase and vesicular acetylcholine transporter and these biochemical markers have been shown to have a good correspondence with ChAT. Acetylcholinesterase, an enzyme that catalyzes the hydrolysis of acetylcholine to choline and acetic acid, is consistently reduced in the brain of AD patients. The activity of acetylcholinesterase can be measured by PET using labeled acetylcholine analogs that serve as substrates for acetylcholinesterase and hydrolyze to a hydrophilic product that is trapped in the cell. Another method is to use radioligands that bind to acetylcholinesterase.

[^{11}C]Physostigmine, [^{11}C]N-methyl-4-piperidyl acetate, and N-[^{11}C]-methylpiperidin-4-yl propionate (PMP) have been used in PET studies to measure acetylcholinesterase in the brains of healthy volunteers [49, 50]. PET studies of acetylcholinesterase activity using [^{11}C]PMP, a selective substrate for acetylcholinesterase, showed no changes in acetylcholinesterase with normal aging and a reduction of 30% in patients with mild to moderate AD. The smaller reductions reported by this PET study as compared with the postmortem studies (90–95%) most likely reflect the fact that postmortem studies are mostly of patients with very advanced disease. A progressive loss of cortical acetylcholinesterase activity has been observed in AD patients with cognitive decline. PET measurement of the acetylcholinesterase activity also allows assessment of the efficacy of the various acetylcholinesterase inhibitors that are used therapeutically and to determine the doses required to achieve optimal inhibition. They can also help identify patients in whom the concentration of acetylcholinesterase may be too low for acetylcholinesterase inhibitors to be effective.

Vesicular acetylcholine transporters are localized in the acetylcholine terminals and carry acetylcholine from the cytoplasm into the vesicles. (−)-5-[^{123}I]iodobenzovesamicol (IBVM), an analog of vesamicol that binds to the vesicular acetylcholine transporter, has been used to image the living human brain. A SPECT study showed that cortical binding of [^{123}I]IBVM in normal subjects declined only mildly with age (3.7% per decade), but was markedly reduced in AD patients in whom the reductions predicted dementia severity [50]. The binding levels also differed according to age of onset. With an onset age of less than 65 years, binding was reduced severely throughout the entire cerebral cortex and hippocampus (approximately 30%), but with an onset age of 65 years or older, binding reductions were restricted to temporal cortex and hippocampus. This most likely reflects the greater cholinergic loss in early- rather tha late-onset AD. Studies of the vesicular acetylcholine transporter are likely to be particularly useful for assessing neuroprotective treatments and may be of use in the detection of early disease.

From postmortem studies, it appears that nicotinic receptors are markedly reduced in the brain of AD patients, whereas muscarinic receptors are less affected. Several radiotracers have been developed for mapping muscarinic receptors. In accordance with postmortem findings, imaging studies have shown a reduction in muscarinic receptors due to aging; studies in AD subjects have shown reductions as well as no changes in receptor levels.

The neuronal nAChRs are involved in functional processes in brain including cognitive function and memory. A severe loss of nAChRs has been detected in the brains of patients with AD. There is a great interest in noninvasively imaging nAChRs for detection of receptor impairments even at a presymptomatic stage of AD as well for monitoring outcome of drug treatment. [^{11}C]nicotine has been used to study nicotinic receptors in both normal and AD brains with PET [51]. The labeling of the two enantiomers of nicotine, (S)(−) and (R)(+), which predominantly bind to the low- and high-affinity nicotinic sites, respectively, allowed the separate assessment of nicotinic receptor subtypes. Nicotine's binding to nicotinic receptors is quite selective and is predominantly seen at the $\alpha4\beta2$ nicotinic receptor subtype. A significant decrease in [^{11}C]nicotine binding was measured in the temporal cortex, frontal cortex, and hippocampus of AD patients. The changes in [^{11}C]nicotine binding were associated with cognitive function and interpreted as reflecting reductions in nicotinic receptors in AD. The studies also showed lower binding of the (R)(+) enantiomer of nicotine relative to the (S)(−) in the AD brain, which was interpreted as reflecting a predominant loss of high affinity for nicotinic receptors [52].

The binding of [^{11}C]nicotine is highly influenced by CBF and is limited by its rapid dissociation from the receptor and low specific-to-nonspecific binding ratio. This also has led to the search for new radiotracers with a higher affinity for nAChR. A ligand with a selectivity for the $\alpha4\beta2$ nAChRs would be particularly preferable because $\alpha4\beta2$ has been recognized as the predominant subtype that is deficient in AD [53]. Recently, several azetidine analogs have been labeled. The azetidine analogs, 2-[^{18}F]fluoro-3-(2(S)-azetidinylmethoxy)pyridine (2-[^{18}F]fluoro-A-85380), and 5-[^{125}I]iodo-A-85380 represent promising imaging agents for noninvasive, in vivo studies of $\alpha4\beta2$ nicotinic acetylcholine receptors because of their favorable kinetic properties, high specific-to-nonspecific binding ratio, low in vivo toxicity, and high selectivity for $\alpha4\beta2$ nAChRs. Several epibatidine analogs have also been developed. PET studies with analogs of epibatidine such as [^{18}F]norchlorofluoroepibatidine ([^{18}F]NFEP), [(±)]-exo-2-(2-[^{18}F]fluoro-5-pyridyl)-7-azabicyclo[2.2.1]heptane and N-methyl [^{18}F]NFEP ([^{18}F]N-methyl-NFEP) showed very high specific-to-nonspecific binding ratios in the nonhuman primate. However, it is still uncertain whether the epibatidine analogs can be applied in humans due to the risk of toxicity.

PET studies of nAChR can be useful for monitoring the outcome of drug treatment. Long-term treatment with tacrine (80 mg daily for 3 months) increased binding of [^{11}C]nicotine in the temporal cortex of AD patients, which was interpreted as reflecting a restoration of nicotinic receptors. These results are in agreement with preclinical data showing that cholinergic stimulation leads to up-regulation of nicotinic receptors. Tacrine also decreased the differences in the binding of the (R)(+) enantiomer of nicotine relative to (S)(−), suggesting a preferential effect on high-affinity sites [19]. The changes in synaptic acetylcholine concentration after interventions can be measured using a nAChR radioligand [^{18}F]NFEP, which is sensitive to competition with endogenous acetylcholine [54]. Because of the toxicity of [^{18}F]NFEP, these studies have been limited to nonhuman primates and have shown that the acetylcholinesterase inhibitor physostigmine (0.03 mg/kg intravenously) significantly increases synaptic acetylcholine concentration in the striatum, as is reflected by decreased binding of [^{18}F]NFEP in the striatum. The measure of extracellular acetylcholine is particularly promising for the evaluation of pharmacologic treatments because most drugs are targeted to enhance cholinergic function by increasing extracellular acetylcholine.

Amyloid Plaque Imaging

Confirmation of the clinical diagnosis of AD is based on the detection of amyloid plaques and NFTs in the brain. Unfortunately, until recently, such measures could only be performed postmortem. However, recent developments in radiotracers may now allow for the measurement of amyloid plaques and NFTs in the brain in vivo. [^{11}C]Pittsburgh Compound-B (PIB) and 2-(I-{6-[2-[^{18}F]fluoroethyl]-(methyl)-amino}-2-napthyl)ethylene)malononitrile ([^{18}F]FDDNP) is being used most widely [55, 56]. PIB is a neutral thioflavin that shows nanomolar affinity for neuritic amyloid plaques but low affinity to diffuse amyloid deposits and intracellular NFTs [57]. [^{11}C]PIB retention in the cerebral cortex in AD patients reflects the amyloid plaque retention (Fig. 13.3). AD patients show increased retention of tracer in association with cortical areas compared with controls [55]. It is also increased in the stage of early AD [57], supporting the fact that PIB retention in the brain is an earlier pathologic process than metabolic changes. There were no changes in [^{11}C]PIB uptake in a 2-year follow-up study, while glucose metabolism decreased with MMSE scores [58]. It can be suggested that the maximal amyloid deposit, in the associated cortical areas, is already reached in early-stage AD.

Interestingly, relatively low [^{11}C]PIB uptake by the hippocampus, amygdala, and parahippocampus compared with cortical association areas in AD was reported [57]. Low [^{11}C]PIB uptake by hippocampus is also reported in another study [59]. This is may be the result of relatively late deposition of amyloid in the hippocampus [14]. On the contrary, [^{11}C]PIB uptake in the middle frontal gyrus was prominent compared with the degree of glucose hypometabolism [59], which may be a result of earlier deposition of amyloid than NFTs in the frontal lobes.

PET studies with [^{18}F]FDDNP have shown good uptake in the human brain and greater accumulation and slower clearance of [^{18}F]FDDNP in AD patients than in control subjects. In AD patients, the accumulation was greater in the hippocampal region and was detected even in patients with mild AD [56]. The areas with high [^{18}F]FDDNP retention were the ones with low glucose metabolism. The binding of [^{18}F]FDDNP to amyloid plaques was confirmed in postmortem studies. The limitation of [^{18}F]FDDNP is the low specific signal, and is only 0.3-fold that of the reference tissue. Another limitation is its relatively high nonspecific binding as well as the potential contribution to the PET signal from tau protein [60].

Amyloid plaque imaging will be of use not only in the diagnosis of AD but also in the investigation of the temporal relationship between amyloid deposition, neuronal loss, and cognitive decline and assessment of the effects of drugs in disease progression. Also, this imaging technique may provide treatment for AD patients early in their disease, when response to treatment is usually better.

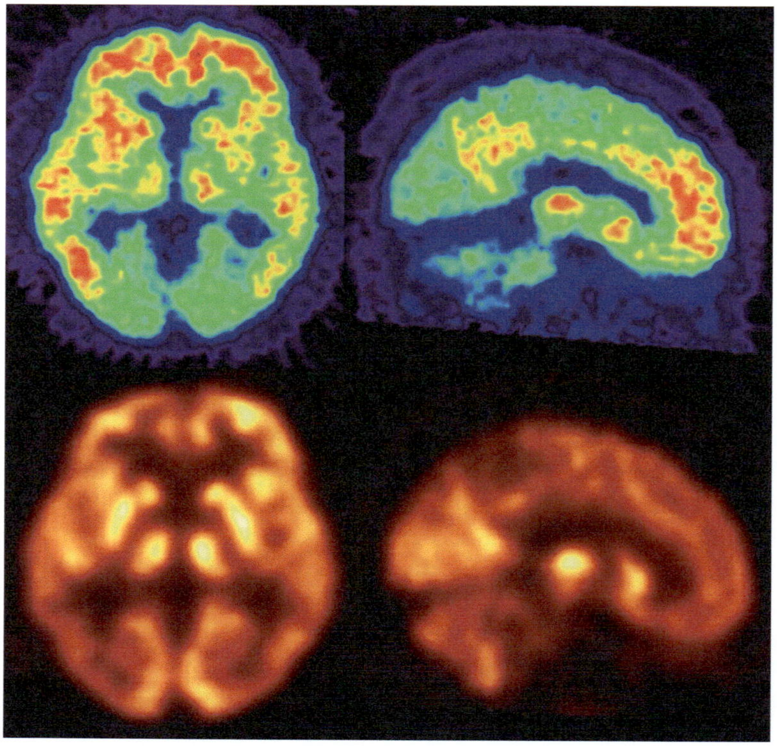

Fig. 13.3 [^{11}C]PIB PET (*upper row*) and ^{18}F-FDG PET images (*lower row*) of AD

Vascular Dementia

Vascular dementia is the second most common cause of dementia in the elderly, accounting for 15–30% of all cases [2]. There are various types of underlying damage to tissue and vessels in vascular dementia, including single or multiple infarcts that involve association and limbic cortices (multi-infarct dementia), small subcortical infarcts disrupting corticosubcortical circuits (lacunar type subcortical vascular dementia), and white matter lesions (Binswanger type subcortical vascular dementia). Vascular dementia develops when a threshold of total brain tissue destruction has been exceeded, or when critically located infarctions disrupt multiple cognitive functions (strategic infarct dementia). Damage to the medial frontal region (anterior cerebral artery territory infarction), the angular gyrus or the dorsolateral prefrontal region (middle cerebral artery territory infarction), the inferomedial temporooccipital region (posterior cerebral artery territory infarction), and the subcortical structure such as basal ganglia and thalamus can cause strategic infarct dementia.

PET studies in vascular dementia have shown global reductions in cerebral metabolism with additional focal and asymmetric areas of hypometabolism that are not limited to specific cortical or subcortical brain regions. This metabolic pattern differs from that in AD with hypometabolism affecting the association areas and relative sparing of subcortical structures. Metabolic impairment seen on PET is often more widespread than that shown on CT, MRI, or even neuropathologic techniques, suggesting that single lesions may have extensive and distant metabolic sequelae. These remote metabolic effects have been attributed to degeneration of fiber tracts with disconnection of distal structures and to microscopic infarcts not apparent on gross examination but manifested as hypometabolic regions.

Increasing severity of dementia correlates with global hypometabolism (i.e., the total volume of hypometabolic regions rather than the quantity of tissue destruction) and increasing involvement of the frontal cortex [61]. Also, SPECT in vascular dementia reveals diffusely diminished CBF with superimposed focal areas of more severe hypoperfusion. Vascular dementia could produce any pattern; however, the presence of one or more scattered perfusion defects, either unilateral or bilateral, with an asymmetric distribution is most suggestive of vascular dementia.

The clinical picture of vascular dementia varies, and the role of functional brain imaging of cerebral blood flow and metabolism would be expected to be different among subtypes of vascular dementia. In multi-infarct dementia (cortical infarcts), PET and SPECT are of value in detecting regions at risk, but the role would be supplementary in the evaluation of patients. Subcortical small infarcts that disrupt cortico-subcortical circuits result in cognitive dysfunction. Small infarcts involving the thalamus, caudate, and globus pallidus, which are central components of the corticosubcortical circuits, are classified into strategic lesions. Disruption of the frontal subcortical circuits leads to cognitive impairment with striking frontal lobe features, and disruption of the memory-related circuits leads to amnesia. In this type of vascular dementia, apart from detecting regions at risk, the role of PET and SPECT would be to prove functional deprivation of remote cortices. A frontal involvement is a functional brain imaging feature of subcortical strategic lesions leading to dementia [62]. In white matter lesions, documenting the presence of chronic ischemia and then illustrating a functional deprivation of cortices would be the most important roles of PET and SPECT. However, this needs to be determined in further studies.

Cerebrovascular disease and AD are common in the elderly and both frequently coexist. In addition to the features of dementia typical for AD and the accentuated atrophy in the parietal and medial temporal lobes demonstrated on MRI, temporoparietal and posterior cingulate abnormality indicates involvement of Alzheimer pathology. When frontal abnormality is lacking, effects of subcortical infarcts on cortical function would be negligible.

A longitudinal analysis of regional cerebral glucose metabolism in vascular dementia showed that the progression of dementia can be delayed by the adenosine uptake blocker propentofylline, and that neuropsychologic and metabolic changes are closely related [63].

Dementia with Lewy Bodies

Dementia with Lewy bodies is a common form of dementia, accounting for 10–15% of all dementia in old age [64]. The disorder shares clinical and pathologic features with both AD and PD. A consortium on DLB has revised a new criterion for the clinical and pathologic diagnosis of DLB [65]. Lewy bodies are neuronal inclusions composed of abnormally phosphorylated, neurofilament proteins aggregated with ubiquitin and α-synuclein. In DLB, significant Lewy body formation also occurs in paralimbic and neocortical structures, and extensive depletion of acetylcholine neurotransmission in neocortical areas occurs as a result of degeneration in the brainstem and basal forebrain cholinergic projection neurons. In PD, Lewy body accumulation is usually found in the substantia nigra and other brainstem nuclei such as the locus ceruleus and raphe. However, patients with PD typically have dementia symptoms 10 years or longer after the onset of motor symptoms, while DLB patients have dementia symptoms before or at the same time with motor symptoms [65].

Structural brain imaging in DLB reveals generalized atrophy, although 40% of patients show preservation of medial temporal lobe structures, unlike AD. There is no difference from AD in terms of degree of ventricular enlargement, frontal lobe atrophy, or presence of white matter changes on MRI [66].

FDG PET may be used for distinguishing AD from DLB in patients. In a study with autopsy-confirmed AD and DLB patients, metabolic

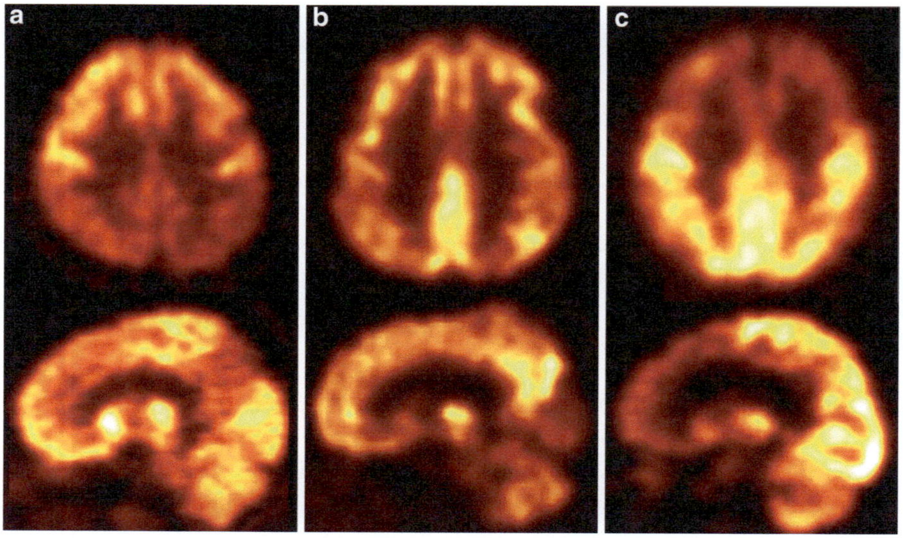

Fig. 13.4 ^{18}F-FDG PET images of AD (**a**), DLB (**b**), and frontotemporal dementia (**c**). FDG PET images of DLB show characteristic occipital hypometabolism (**b**). ^{18}F-FDG PET images of frontotemporal dementia show frontal hypometabolism (**c**)

reductions involving parietotemporal association, posterior cingulate, and frontal association cortices were found in both groups. However, metabolic reductions in the occipital cortex, particularly in the primary visual cortex, were found in only DLB patients [67]. Measuring the glucose metabolism in the occipital cortex may be an informative diagnostic aid to distinguish DLB from AD (Fig. 13.4).

There is a considerable degeneration of nigral neurons with depletion of striatal dopamine as well as cortical neuronal loss in DLB. In contrast, AD is not associated with significant changes in dopamine metabolism. Using SPECT, significant reduction in striatal uptake of a dopamine transporter (DAT) ligand [^{123}I]-2-carbomethoxy-3-(4-iodophenyl)-N-(3-fluoropropyl)nortropane was seen in DLB, but not in AD, indicating dopaminergic degeneration in DLB [68]. [^{18}F]FDOPA uptake is reduced in the caudate and putamen, which is not found in AD [69]. This may prove to be a useful diagnostic test for distinguishing DLB from AD in vivo. However, the reduced uptake of [^{18}F]FDOPA in DLB patients does not show a gradient pattern in the striatum such as in PD, which is discussed later.

Frontotemporal Dementia

FTD is a one of three major clinical syndromes of frontotemporal lobar degeneration, the other prototypical syndromes being nonfluent progressive aphasia and semantic dementia [70]. FTD is the most common form of primary degenerative dementia after AD that affects people in middle age, accounting for up to 20% of presenile dementia cases. The salient clinical characteristic is a profound alteration in character and social conduct such as social disinhibition, inappropriate behavior, and impulsiveness or with aphasia. Memory disturbance may be less prominent than in AD, or absent. Parkinsonian signs of akinesia and rigidity develop with disease progression and may be prominent in some portion of patients. A minority of patients with FTD develop neurologic signs of motor neuron disease. Postmortem pathologic examination reveals bilateral atrophy of the frontal and anterior temporal lobes and degeneration of the striatum. Only a minority of patients exhibit Pick-type histologic changes, hence, the term 'frontotemporal dementia' is preferred to 'Pick's disease' [71].

In a study of 45 patients with pathologically confirmed diagnosis, stereotactic surface projection analysis of FDG PET discriminated FTD from AD with a sensitivity of 73.2% and a specificity of 97.6% [72]. Hypometabolism was frequent in frontal, anterior cingulated, and anterior temporal regions in FTD, whereas, hypometabolism was frequent in temporoparietal and posterior cingulate regions in AD [72]. PET and SPECT studies have consistently shown anterior distribution of functional impairment in FTD (Fig. 13.4). Reductions in glucose metabolism and blood flow in the frontal and anterior temporal cortices with asymmetric patterns are seen frequency. In FTD, FDG PET showed hypometabolism in extensive cortical regions such as frontal and anterior temporal areas, cingulate gyri, uncus, and insula and subcortical areas, including basal ganglia and medial thalamic regions [73]. The hemispheric asymmetry of hypometabolism (more frequently lateralized to the left) was common in patients with FTD, which may help differentiate FTD from AD or other causes of dementia [73]. Also shown was reduction in the binding of the DAT ligand [^{11}C]WIN 35,428 in the striatum of FTD patients with relation to the severity of extrapyramidal symptoms of the patients [74].

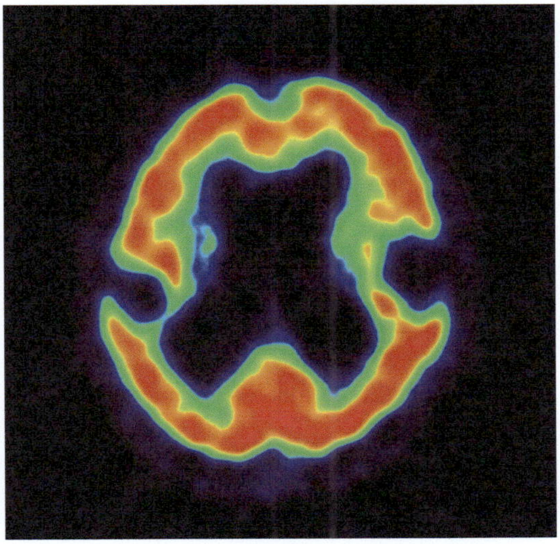

Fig. 13.5 ^{18}F-FDG PET images of normal pressure hydrocephalus

Normal Pressure Hydrocephalus

Normal pressure hydrocephalus (NPH) is an obstructive communicating hydrocephalus that classically produces the clinical triad of dementia, gait disturbance, and urinary incontinence. NPH is caused by obstruction of CSF absorption in the superior sagittal sinus. NPH may be idiopathic, may occur as a manifestation of the late decompensation of compensated congenital hydrocephalus, or may follow head trauma, subdural hematoma, subarachnoid hemorrhage, meningitis, or encephalitis.

Structural imaging reveals enlarged ventricles and is crucial to the identification and differential diagnosis of NPH. Ventricular enlargement in NPH is characterized by greater dilatation of the anterior horns (frontal and temporal) of the lateral ventricles than of the posterior horns. Usually, disproportionate enlargement of the ventricles and relatively modest sulcal dilatation, if any, are seen but atrophy of the cortical mantle occurs in the course of normal aging and the presence of some degree of peripheral atrophy does not exclude consideration of NPH.

SPECT reveals diffusely reduced CBF, and is more pronounced posteriorly than anteriorly. SPECT may aid in identifying patients who are likely to respond to shunting. It has been reported that patients with higher anterior than posterior blood flow were significantly less likely to improve following surgery than patients who had equal flow anteriorly and posteriorly, or greater posterior flow. PET reveals diffusely reduced glucose metabolism in hydrocephalus (Fig. 13.5). Restoration of normal metabolic rates after successful shunt surgery has been reported.

Infectious Dementias

Creutzfeldt-Jakob disease (subacute spongiform encephalopathy) is a prion infection of the brain that is rapidly progressive and usually fatal (within 1 year). Clinically, dementia, ataxia, myoclonus, and muscle rigidity are characteristic. Neuropathologic alterations include spongiform changes, nerve cell loss, and marked gliosis. SPECT and PET imaging has revealed diffuse and multifocal reductions in gray matter CBF and metabolism. These imaging techniques can be useful in selecting areas for diagnostic brain biopsy.

Acquired immunodeficiency syndrome (AIDS) dementia complex is a progressive dementing illness caused by infection from the human immunodeficiency virus (HIV). Between 70% and 90% of AIDS patients develop neuropsychologic impairment that is characterized by inattention, mental slowing, loss of spontaneity, reduced motor performance, and incoordination. At autopsy, mild to moderate cerebral atrophy is seen; neuropathology is found primarily in subcortical structures, particularly the basal ganglia and thalamus. CT and MRI studies revealed general atrophy, atrophy of the basal ganglia, and white matter lesions that appear to increase in severity with progression of HIV infection. SPECT showed multifocal cortical and subcortical areas of hypoperfusion. PET studies have demonstrated relative subcortical hypermetabolism in AIDS and early AIDS dementia complex, while more advanced AIDS dementia complex is associated with hypometabolism in cortical and subcortical gray matter and in the temporal lobe. In addition, PET and SPECT have been shown to be sensitive to reversal or improvement of abnormalities brought about by drug treatment, reflecting clinical improvement in neurologic and cognitive deficits.

Depressive Pseudodementia

A considerable portion of geriatric depression patients show a cognitive decline that is comparable in severity with primary degenerative dementia. However, this condition is differentiated from primary dementia by its reversibility. Reversible dementia syndrome of geriatric depression has been called depressive pseudodementia. A PET study showed decreased blood flow in the left anterior medial frontal lobe in depressive pseudodementia patients, while noncognitively impaired depressed patients showed decreased blood flow in the left anterior lateral prefrontal areas [75]. A SPECT study of elderly depressive pseudodementia patients revealed decreased blood flow in the temporoparietal region, a finding similar to that of AD and different from that of depression without cognitive impairment [76]. This functional imaging finding may have relevance to the report that elderly depressed patients with cognitive impairment that improves with treatment carry an increased chance of developing an irreversible dementia in the future when compared with age-matched patients with depression alone [77].

Movement Disorders

Functional neuroimaging can aid in the diagnosis of movement disorders associated with dementia. Imaging studies in PD, HD, PSP, Wilson's disease, and corticobasal degeneration (CBD) are described.

Parkinson Disease

PD is the second most common neurodegenerative disease in the United States [78]. The overall prevalence of PD is estimated to be 0.2%, but rises with increasing age, affecting as many as 0.5–1% of individuals 65–69 years and as many as 1–3% of individuals older than 80 years [79].

Clinical Diagnosis

Characteristic motor symptoms of PD are muscle rigidity, tremor, and bradykinesia. Diagnosis of PD is usually based on the clinical cardinal motor features, associated and exclusionary symptoms, and response to levodopa [80]. Clinical diagnostic accuracy made by a qualified neurologist was 65% at initial presentation and 76% after 12 years of follow-up in pathologically proved cases [81]. Differential diagnosis of parkinsonian syndromes includes idiopathic PD, symptomatic parkinsonism (drug-induced, toxic,inflammatory), pseudoparkinsonism (vascular, normal pressure hydrocephalus), atypical parkinsonism (multiple system atrophy, progressive supranuclear palsy, CBD, DLB), and monogenetically inherited forms of PD [82].

Neuropathology

The two main pathological hallmarks of PD are the loss of dopaminergic neurons in the substantia nigra and the presence of Lewy bodies. In addition to the selective cell loss of neuromelanin-containing neurons from the pars compacta of the substantia nigra, cell loss in the locus coeruleus, dorsal nuclei of the vagus, raphe nuclei, nucleus basalis of Meynert, and some other catecholaminergic brainstem structures including the ventrotegmental area, also exist [83].

Protein alpha-synuclein accumulates and binds to ubiquitin in the damaged cells. The alpha-synuclein-ubiquitin complex is not directed to the proteosome and forms cytoplasmic inclusions called Lewy bodies. These are mostly found in the dopaminergic neurons in the substantia nigra, as well as in the locus ceruleus, nucleus basalis, hypothalamus, cerebral cortex, cranial nerve motor nuclei, and central and peripheral components of the autonomic nervous system [84]. According to these findings, Braak et al. suggested pathology-based staging of PD [85]. Stage 1 is Lewy body in the medulla oblongata and olfactory structures, extending to the pons in stage 2. Stage 3 involves the substantia nigra and midbrain nuclei, with limbic areas in stage 4. Stages 5 and 6 involve the neocortex. However, the main concern in PD is the reduced dopaminergic neuron activity in the substantia nigra. It was reported that a constant proportion of nigral neurons (3–4%) contain Lewy bodies, irrespective of disease duration, which is consistent with the notion that, in contrast to NFTs, Lewy bodies are continuously forming and disappearing in the diseased substantia nigra [83].

Neurochemistry

Tyrosine is converted to DOPA by tyrosine hydroxylase, and DOPA is converted to dopamine by aromatic amino acid decarboxylase (AADC) in the presynaptic neuron. The synthesized dopamine is stored in the presynaptic vesicles, and is released to the synapse by certain signals. After neurotransmission, the dopamine in the synaptic area is reabsorbed into the presynaptic neuron by the DAT. Recent reviews show that these presynaptic dysfunctions may be caused by mutations in α-synuclein [86]. α-synuclein are thought to function in regulating presynaptic vesicles, and mutation in α-synuclein may result in a reduced number of vesicles. For these reasons, presynaptic and postsynaptic dopamine-related radiopharmaceuticals are used in clinical settings.

Neurochemical Imaging

FDG PET and cerebral blood perfusion images show no abnormality in PD. However, FDG PET was reported to be useful in differentiating parkinsonian type MSA from PD [87]. Presynaptic and postsynaptic dopamine agents are used in clinical settings. [^{18}F]FDOPA reflects the uptake of DOPA and conversion to dopamine in the nerve terminal. [^{18}F]FDOPA is converted to [^{18}F]fluorodopamine by DOPA decarboxylase. In patients with PD, [^{18}F]FDOPA uptake is decreased in the striatum, especially in the putamen [88]. The decreased uptake correlates with the degree of motor deficits of the patient [89]. [^{18}F]FDOPA is not affected by levodopa treatment, and can be used for follow-up of disease progression. However, in the early stage of PD, [^{18}F]FDOPA may increase in the striatum by a compensatory up-regulation [90–92].Striatal AADC activity is increased in the early stage to compensate for the decreased level of dopamine, but eventually becomes normal or decreased in the advanced stage. Compensatory increase in the early stage may also be seen in the prefrontal cortex, anterior cingulated area [93]. In addition, as serotonergic and noradrenergic neurons also display AADC activity, [^{18}F]FDOPA uptake may not wholly reflect dopaminergic AADC activity [94].

[^{11}C]DTBZ (dihydrotetrabenazine) is a vesicular monoamine transporter type 2 (VMAT2) antagonist. VMAT2 transports newly synthesized or re-uptaked dopamine to the vesicle. Loss of

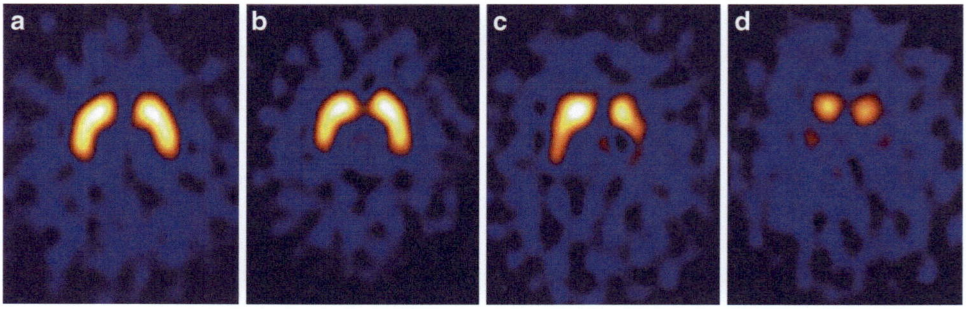

Fig. 13.6 [^{123}I]β-CIT images in normal control (**a**), essential tremor (**b**), and PD (**c**, **d**). DAT image shows rostrocaudal gradient in the early stage of PD (**c**). As disease progresses, DAT uptake of putamen disappears (**d**)

striatal dopamine correlates with decreased uptake of [^{11}C]DTBZ [95]. [^{11}C]DTBZ is also known not to be affected by levodopa therapy. VMAT2 is also contains serotonin and norepinephrine containing axons. However, over 95% of striatal VMAT2 binding sites are associated with dopaminergic terminals, and striatal VMAT2 binding site density is a linear function of mesencephalic nigrostriatal neuron number [96].

Dopamine transporters are located in the presynaptic dopamine neurons. DAT re-uptakes the dopamine in the synaptic area, and is down-regulated in PD. DAT is imaged by several radioligands such as [^{11}C]cocaine, [^{11}C]methylphenidate, [^{11}C] WIN 35,428, [^{18}F]FP-CIT (N-(3-fluoropropyl)-2β-carbomethoxy-3β-4-[^{123}I] iodophenylnortropane). SPECT agents such as [^{123}I] β-CIT (β-carbomethoxy-3-β-(4-iodophenyl)-tropane), [^{123}I]IPT (^{123}I-N-(3-iodopropen-2-yl)-2-carbomethoxy-3 β-(4-chlorophenyl) tropane), [^{99m}Tc]TRODAT are also in use. β-CIT (DOPASCAN) and FP-CIT (DaTSCAN) are commercially available in Europe. In a study using [^{123}I]β-CIT, DAT density loss showed good correlations with clinical PD symptoms such as akinesia, rigidity, axial symptoms and activities of daily living and correlated well with different stages of disease severity [97]. The sensitivity of [^{123}I]β-CIT in a quantitative manner for diagnosing PD was 92% and specificity was 100% [98]. In PD, DAT uptake shows a particular pattern called the "rostrocaudal gradient". Reduced uptake starts in the posterior putamen, advancing to the caudate nucleus. The decreased putamen to caudate nucleus ratio reflects the severity of disease. Reduced uptake usually begins in the unilateral striatum and involves the other side of the striatum as the disease progresses (Fig. 13.6).

D_2 receptor is the predominant dopamine receptor in the striatum. In PD, the D_2 receptor is upregulated before the initiation of levodopa treatment as a compensatory mechanism [99]. [^{11}C]raclopride, [^{18}F]fallypride are representative D_2 receptor PET imaging agents, and [^{123}I]-iodobenzamide (IBZM) is used for SPECT imaging. D_2 receptor imaging is used to differentiate other movement disorders that have postsynaptic neuron damage. The binding specificities of [^{11}C]raclopride and [^{123}I]IBZM for D_2 receptors are low, competing with levodopa or intrinsic dopamine, thus, it is not easy to perform in actual clinical settings because patients need to be taken off medication. Unlike raclopride, [^{18}F]fallypride has a high affinity for D2/D3 receptors, and can be used to image extrastriatal D2 receptors, which are important in etiology of diseases, substance abuse drug effects, therapeutic drug action, and others [100].

Multiple Systemic Atrophy

MSA is a neurodegenerative disease presenting with autonomic nervous system dysfunction, cerebellar ataxia,and parkinsonism. The disease progresses rapidly to death and there is no effective therapy. There are three subtypes of multiple system atrophy (MSA). Striatonigral degeneration (MSA-P) shows parkinsonism, olivopontocerebellar atrophy (MSA-C) shows cerebellar ataxia, and Shy-Drager syndrome (MSA-A) with predominant autonomic nervous system dysfunc-

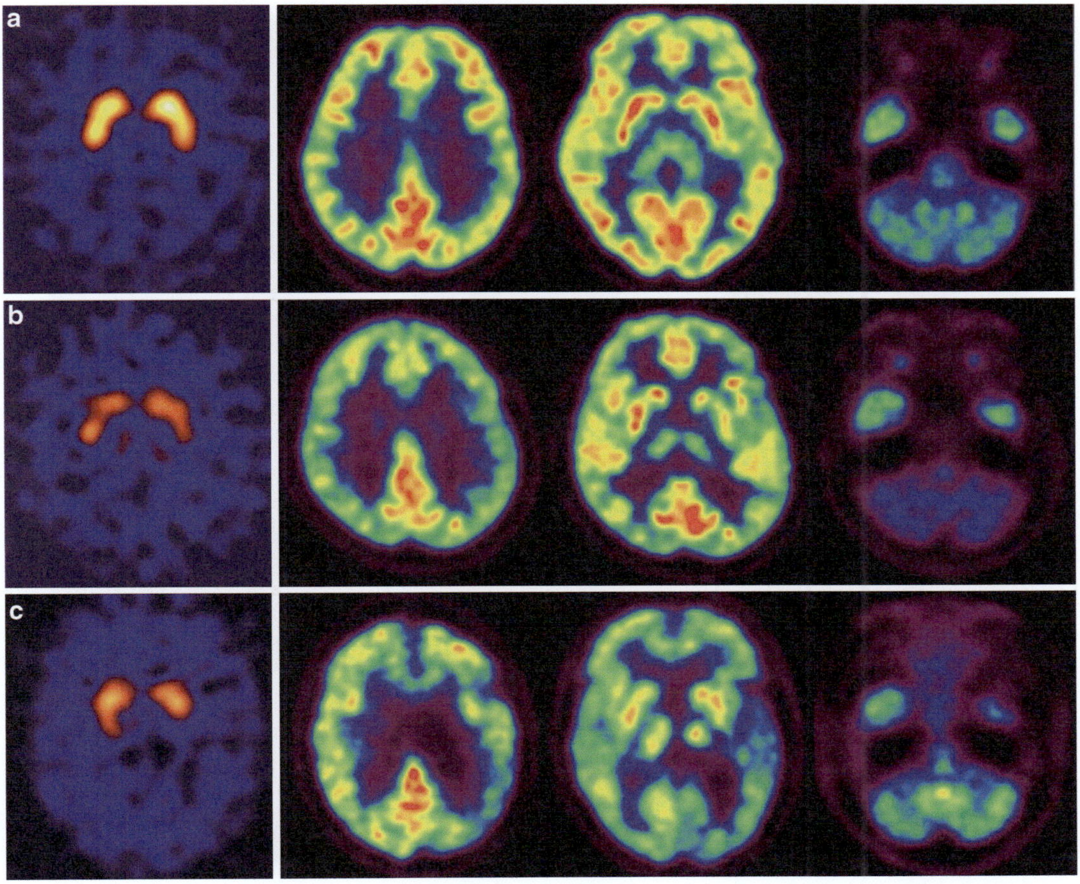

Fig. 13.7 [^{123}I]FP-CIT image (*left column*) and ^{18}F-FDG image of normal control (**a**), MSA (**b**), and corticobasal degeneration (**c**). In MSA, both DAT and FDG uptake decreases (**b**). In corticobasal degeneration, DAT and FDG uptake decreases asymmetrically in the striatum and temporoparietal cortices, which are contralateral to the affected limb (**c**)

tion. Postmortem neuropathology reports glial cytoplasmic inclusion bodies in striatonigral or olivonpontocerebellar systems [101]. Glial cytoplasmic inclusion bodies are prominent in areas with severe neuronal loss and correlate with the severity and duration of the disease [102]. MRI shows atrophy in the putamen, middle cerebellar peduncles, and pons. FDG PET shows hypometabolism in the cerebellum, brainstem, striatum, and frontal and motor regions in MSA. MSA-P shows hypometabolism in the bilateral putamen and MSA-C shows hypometabolism in the pons and cerebellum [103], in accordance with clinical features (Fig. 13.7). [^{18}F]FDOPA PET shows decreased uptake in the caudate nucleus and putamen. [^{11}C]raclopride PET also shows decreased uptake in the striatum. However, these dopamine PET images are not specific for MSA, and cannot discriminate from other parkinsonian syndromes [104, 105].

Progressive Supranuclear Palsy

Progressive supranuclear palsy, also designated Steele-Richardson-Olszewski syndrome, is clinically characterized by early postural instability and falls, supranuclear gaze palsy, parkinsonism, pseudobulbar palsy, and frontal lobe signs such as impairment of executive functions, forgetfulness, and slowing of thought processes. Pathologically, patients have neuronal loss, gliosis, intraneuronal neurofibrillary tangle formation, and granulovacuolar degeneration that are most marked in the midbrain.

CT reveals atrophy of the midbrain, with less severe volume loss of the pons, cerebellum, and cerebral hemispheres. FDG PET studies reveal a global decrease in cerebral glucose metabolism and blood flow but the decrease is more marked in the frontal cortex. Decreased activity in the striatum, thalamus, and midbrain is also seen. Frontal metabolism has been significantly correlated with disease duration, intellectual deterioration, and frontal neuropsychologic scores [106]. Reduced frontal metabolism could be the result of anatomic and/or functional impairment of the subcortical structures despite the well-recognized specific cortical pathology of PSP, predominating in the posterior frontal cortex. Striatal and thalamic hypometabolism is most likely a consequence of functional changes in the basal neural circuitry because these structures are usually relatively spared on the neuropathologic examination of PSP patients. On the contrary, midbrain hypometabolism could preferentially reflect the severe neuronal loss reported at that level. Midbrain hypometabolism is also reported as an early diagnostic sign for PSP, although the degree of midbrain hypometabolism has not been shown to correlate with clinical deterioration [107]. PET studies have demonstrated equally severe impairment of [^{18}F]fluorodopa uptake in the caudate, anterior putamen, and posterior putamen of patients with PSP, unlike PD patients who showed severe impairment in the posterior putamen with relative sparing of the anterior putamen and caudate [88]. Similar results were obtained from a PET study with DAT ligand [^{11}C]WIN 35,428 and [^{123}I]IPT [108, 109]. These findings suggest that there is more progressively extensive nigral involvement in PSP than in PD. Also, the severity of decrease in striatal [^{18}F]fluorodopa uptake in PSP patients paralleled the degree of reduction in frontal cerebral blood flow [110] and suggests that the impairment of cerebral function in PSP is to a large extent determined by brainstem pathology.

Corticobasal Degeneration

Corticobasal degeneration is an increasingly recognized neurodegenerative disease with both motor and cognitive dysfunction. The most characteristic initial motor symptoms are akinesia, rigidity, and apraxia. Dystonia and alien limb phenomena are frequently observed. There is often a parkinsonian picture with failure or lack of efficacy of dopaminergic medical therapy. Cognitive decline, prompting the diagnosis of dementia, may be the most common presentation of CBD that is misdiagnosed. Pathology is characterized by an asymmetric frontoparietal neuronal loss and gliosis with ballooned, achromatic cortical neurons, nigral degeneration, and variable subcortical involvement. Structural imaging reveals asymmetric atrophy in the frontoparietal cortex contralateral to the dominantly affected limb. Statistical parametric mapping analysis of FDG PET images comparing CBD with controls showed metabolic decrease in premotor, primary motor, supplementary motor, primary sensory, prefrontal, and inferior parietal cortices, and in the striatum and thalamus contralateral to the more affected limb [111–115] (Fig. 13.7). [^{18}F]fluorodopa uptake was also reduced in an asymmetric pattern, both the caudate nucleus and the putamen [111–114].

Huntington's Disease

HD is an autosomal, dominantly inherited, neurodegenerative disorder that is caused by a repeat of an unstable and abnormally expanded trinucleotide (CAG) in the *IT15* gene on chromosome 4. The three main clinical features of HD are movement disorder, progressive frontostriatal dementia, and psychiatric disturbance. HD results from the loss of specific sets of cholinergic and gamma-aminobutyric acid (GABA)-ergic neurons in the striatum.

CT and MRI reveal diminished volume of the caudate nuclei with loss of the convex bulge of the nucleus into the lateral aspects of the frontal horns of the lateral ventricles. The bicaudate index (width of both lateral ventricles divided by distance

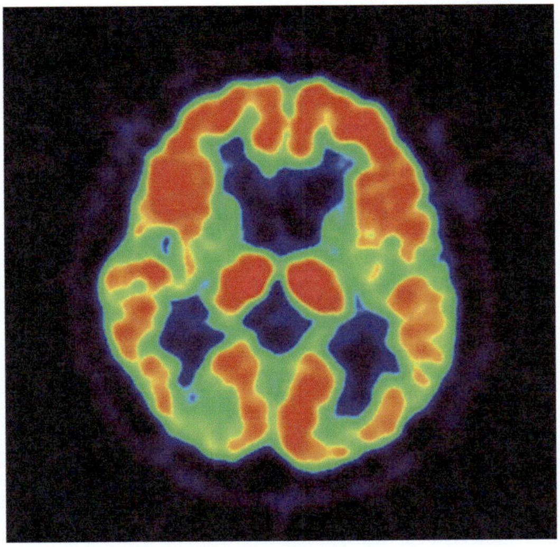

Fig. 13.8 ^{18}F-FDG PET images of HD. ^{18}F-FDG PET shows striatal hypometabolism

between the outer tables of the skull at the same level) distinguishes between HD and other disorders with cerebral atrophy. FDG PET studies show reduced striatal glucose metabolism (Fig. 13.8). Clinical scores of functional capacity, bradykinesia, rigidity, and dementia correlate with caudate hypometabolism, those of chorea and eye movement abnormalities correlate with putamen hypometabolism, and those of dystonia correlate with thalamic hypermetabolism. FDG PET measures of cortical metabolism are normal in preclinical disease, but patients later develop extensive hypometabolism in prefrontal and inferior parietal areas. Additionally, several studies have demonstrated that a percentage of relatives of patients with HD are at risk for the disease and have significantly reduced striatal glucose metabolism. Resting CBF, like glucose metabolism, is reduced in the striatum and cortex of patients with established HD.

The earliest histopathologic change seen in HD is the loss of medium spiny neurons from the striatum. These GABA-ergic projection neurons express dopamine receptors. Accordingly, severe loss of striatal D_1 and D_2 receptor binding in HD has been demonstrated postmortem and in vivo using PET and SPECT. Postmortem reductions in D_2 binding have also been found in the frontal cortex, and in vivo studies using PET have reported reduced D_1 binding in the frontal and temporal cortices in HD. PET has demonstrated that approximately 50% of at-risk asymptomatic adults and mutation carriers have reduced striatal D_1 and D_2 receptor binding. On the contrary, the striatal uptake of [^{18}F] DOPA is not impaired, which means that the nigrostriatal pathway in HD is preserved.

Wilson's Disease

Wilson's disease is an inherited defect in the copper-carrying serum protein ceruloplasmin, resulting in abnormal copper deposition in the basal ganglia, liver, and cornea. Neurologically, patients present with dysarthria, dystonia, rigidity, cebellar abnormalities, tremor, gait and postural disturbances, and mild dementia. FDG PET reveals globally diminished cerebral metabolism with relatively more marked changes in the lenticular nuclei. Severity of extrapyramidal symptoms was related to hypometabolism in the striatum. Even after improvement of extrapyramidal symptoms, hypometabolism in the striatum still remained [116]. [^{18}F]fluorodopa PET demonstrates diminished uptake in the striatum of symptomatic patients with Wilson's disease [117].

References

1. Ferri CP, Prince M, Brayne C, et al. Global prevalence of dementia: a Delphi consensus study. Lancet. 2005;366(9503):2112–7.
2. Plassman BL, Langa KM, Fisher GG, et al. Prevalence of dementia in the United States: the aging, demographics, and memory study. Neuroepidemiology. 2007;29(1–2):125–32.
3. Perkins AJ, Hui SL, Ogunniyi A, et al. Risk of mortality for dementia in a developing country: the Yoruba in Nigeria. Int J Geriatr Psychiatry. 2002;17(6):566–73.
4. Kabasakalian A, Finney GR. Reversible dementias. Int Rev Neurobiol. 2009;84:283–302.
5. Lowenthal DT, Paran E, Burgos L, Williams LS. General characteristics of treatable, reversible, and untreatable dementias. Am J Geriatr Cardiol. 2007;16(3):136–42.
6. Aguero-Torres H, Fratiglioni L, Guo Z, Viitanen M, Winblad B. Mortality from dementia in advanced age:

a 5-year follow-up study of incident dementia cases. J Clin Epidemiol. 1999;52(8):737–43.
7. Wimo A, Winblad B, Jonsson L. An estimate of the total worldwide societal costs of dementia in 2005. Alzheimers Dement. 2007;3(2):81–91.
8. Pietrini P, Alexander GE, Furey ML, Hampel H, Guazzelli M. The neurometabolic landscape of cognitive decline: in vivo studies with positron emission tomography in Alzheimer's disease. Int J Psychophysiol. 2000;37(1):87–98.
9. Teunissen CE, de Vente J, Steinbusch HW, De Bruijn C. Biochemical markers related to Alzheimer's dementia in serum and cerebrospinal fluid. Neurobiol Aging. 2002;23(4):485–508.
10. Parihar MS, Hemnani T. Alzheimer's disease pathogenesis and therapeutic interventions. J Clin Neurosci. 2004;11(5):456–67.
11. Thal DR, Rub U, Orantes M, Braak H. Phases of A beta-deposition in the human brain and its relevance for the development of AD. Neurology. 2002;58(12):1791–800.
12. Marx J. Alzheimer's disease. A new take on tau. Science. 2007;316(5830):1416–7.
13. Duyckaerts C, Delatour B, Potier MC. Classification and basic pathology of Alzheimer disease. Acta Neuropathol. 2009;118(1):5–36.
14. Braak H, Braak E. Neuropathological stageing of Alzheimer-related changes. Acta Neuropathol. 1991;82(4):239–59.
15. Heyman A, Fillenbaum GG, Gearing M, et al. Comparison of Lewy body variant of Alzheimer's disease with pure Alzheimer's disease: consortium to establish a registry for Alzheimer's disease, part XIX. Neurology. 1999;52(9):1839–44.
16. Terry Jr AV, Buccafusco JJ. The cholinergic hypothesis of age and Alzheimer's disease-related cognitive deficits: recent challenges and their implications for novel drug development. J Pharmacol Exp Ther. 2003;306(3):821–7.
17. Mesulam MM, Geula C. Nucleus basalis (Ch4) and cortical cholinergic innervation in the human brain: observations based on the distribution of acetylcholinesterase and choline acetyltransferase. J Comp Neurol. 1988;275(2):216–40.
18. Scheff SW, Price DA. Alzheimer's disease-related alterations in synaptic density: neocortex and hippocampus. J Alzheimers Dis. 2006;9(3 Suppl):101–15.
19. Nordberg A. Neuroreceptor changes in Alzheimer disease. Cerebrovasc Brain Metab Rev. 1992;4(4):303–28.
20. Flynn DD, Ferrari-DiLeo G, Levey AI, Mash DC. Differential alterations in muscarinic receptor subtypes in Alzheimer's disease: implications for cholinergic-based therapies. Life Sci. 1995;56(11–12): 869–76.
21. Ruberg M, Mayo W, Brice A, et al. Choline acetyltransferase activity and [3H]vesamicol binding in the temporal cortex of patients with Alzheimer's disease, Parkinson's disease, and rats with basal forebrain lesions. Neuroscience. 1990;35(2):327–33.
22. Efange SM, Garland EM, Staley JK, Khare AB, Mash DC. Vesicular acetylcholine transporter density and Alzheimer's disease. Neurobiol Aging. 1997;18(4): 407–13.
23. Frey KA, Minoshima S, Kuhl DE. Neurochemical imaging of Alzheimer's disease and other degenerative dementias. Q J Nucl Med. 1998;42(3):166–78.
24. Langlais PJ, Thal L, Hansen L, Galasko D, Alford M, Masliah E. Neurotransmitters in basal ganglia and cortex of Alzheimer's disease with and without Lewy bodies. Neurology. 1993;43(10):1927–34.
25. Perry EK, Marshall E, Perry RH, et al. Cholinergic and dopaminergic activities in senile dementia of Lewy body type. Alzheimer Dis Assoc Disord. 1990;4(2):87–95.
26. Dubois B, Feldman HH, Jacova C, et al. Research criteria for the diagnosis of Alzheimer's disease: revising the NINCDS-ADRDA criteria. Lancet Neurol. 2007;6(8):734–46.
27. Lehericy S, Marjanska M, Mesrob L, Sarazin M, Kinkingnehun S. Magnetic resonance imaging of Alzheimer's disease. Eur Radiol. 2007;17(2):347–62.
28. Anderson VC, Litvack ZN, Kaye JA. Magnetic resonance approaches to brain aging and Alzheimer disease-associated neuropathology. Top Magn Reson Imag. 2005;16(6):439–52.
29. Bobinski M, de Leon MJ, Wegiel J, et al. The histological validation of post mortem magnetic resonance imaging-determined hippocampal volume in Alzheimer's disease. Neuroscience. 2000;95(3):721–5.
30. Scheltens P, Fox N, Barkhof F, De Carli C. Structural magnetic resonance imaging in the practical assessment of dementia: beyond exclusion. Lancet Neurol. 2002;1(1):13–21.
31. Frisoni GB. Structural imaging in the clinical diagnosis of Alzheimer's disease: problems and tools. J Neurol Neurosurg Psychiatry. 2001;70(6):711–8.
32. Judenhofer MS, Wehrl HF, Newport DF, et al. Simultaneous PET-MRI: a new approach for functional and morphological imaging. Nat Med. 2008;14(4):459–65.
33. Mosconi L. Brain glucose metabolism in the early and specific diagnosis of Alzheimer's disease. FDG-PET studies in MCI and AD. Eur J Nucl Med Mol Imaging. 2005;32(4):486–510.
34. Ishii K, Sasaki M, Kitagaki H, et al. Reduction of cerebellar glucose metabolism in advanced Alzheimer's disease. J Nucl Med. 1997;38(6):925–8.
35. Silverman DH, Small GW, Chang CY, et al. Positron emission tomography in evaluation of dementia: regional brain metabolism and long-term outcome. JAMA. 2001;286(17):2120–7.
36. Herholz K, Nordberg A, Salmon E, et al. Impairment of neocortical metabolism predicts progression in Alzheimer's disease. Dement Geriatr Cogn Disord. 1999;10(6):494–504.
37. Minoshima S, Giordani B, Berent S, Frey KA, Foster NL, Kuhl DE. Metabolic reduction in the posterior cingulate cortex in very early Alzheimer's disease. Ann Neurol. 1997;42(1):85–94.

38. Gomez-Isla T, Price JL, McKeel Jr DW, Morris JC, Growdon JH, Hyman BT. Profound loss of layer II entorhinal cortex neurons occurs in very mild Alzheimer's disease. J Neurosci. 1996;16(14):4491–500.
39. Silverman DH, Truong CT, Kim SK, et al. Prognostic value of regional cerebral metabolism in patients undergoing dementia evaluation: comparison to a quantifying parameter of subsequent cognitive performance and to prognostic assessment without PET. Mol Genet Metab. 2003;80(3):350–5.
40. Chetelat G, Desgranges B, de la Sayette V, Viader F, Eustache F, Baron JC. Mild cognitive impairment: can FDG-PET predict who is to rapidly convert to Alzheimer's disease? Neurology. 2003;60(8):1374–7.
41. Drzezga A, Lautenschlager N, Siebner H, et al. Cerebral metabolic changes accompanying conversion of mild cognitive impairment into Alzheimer's disease: a PET follow-up study. Eur J Nucl Med Mol Imaging. 2003;30(8):1104–13.
42. Patwardhan MB, McCrory DC, Matchar DB, Samsa GP, Rutschmann OT. Alzheimer disease: operating characteristics of PET – a meta-analysis. Radiology. 2004;231(1):73–80.
43. Johnson JK, Head E, Kim R, Starr A, Cotman CW. Clinical and pathological evidence for a frontal variant of Alzheimer disease. Arch Neurol. 1999;56(10):1233–9.
44. Rogers SL, Friedhoff LT. Long-term efficacy and safety of donepezil in the treatment of Alzheimer's disease: an interim analysis of the results of a US multicentre open label extension study. Eur Neuropsychopharmacol. 1998;8(1):67–75.
45. Alexander GE, Chen K, Pietrini P, Rapoport SI, Reiman EM. Longitudinal PET evaluation of cerebral metabolic decline in dementia: a potential outcome measure in Alzheimer's disease treatment studies. Am J Psychiatry. 2002;159(5):738–45.
46. Silverman DH. Brain ^{18}F-FDG PET in the diagnosis of neurodegenerative dementias: comparison with perfusion SPECT and with clinical evaluations lacking nuclear imaging. J Nucl Med. 2004;45(4):594–607.
47. Cho H, Kwon JH, Seo HJ, Kim JS. The short-term effect of acetylcholinesterase inhibitor on the regional cerebral blood flow of Alzheimer's disease. Arch Gerontol Geriatr. 2010;50(2):222–6.
48. Nobili F, Koulibaly M, Vitali P, et al. Brain perfusion follow-up in Alzheimer's patients during treatment with acetylcholinesterase inhibitors. J Nucl Med. 2002;43(8):983–90.
49. Iyo M, Namba H, Fukushi K, et al. Measurement of acetylcholinesterase by positron emission tomography in the brains of healthy controls and patients with Alzheimer's disease. Lancet. 1997;349(9068):1805–9.
50. Kuhl DE, Minoshima S, Fessler JA, et al. In vivo mapping of cholinergic terminals in normal aging, Alzheimer's disease, and Parkinson's disease. Ann Neurol. 1996;40(3):399–410.
51. Kadir A, Almkvist O, Wall A, Langstrom B, Nordberg A. PET imaging of cortical ^{11}C-nicotine binding correlates with the cognitive function of attention in Alzheimer's disease. Psychopharmacology (Berlin). 2006;188(4):509–20.
52. Nordberg A, Hartvig P, Lilja A, et al. Decreased uptake and binding of ^{11}C-nicotine in brain of Alzheimer patients as visualized by positron emission tomography. J Neural Transm Park Dis Dement Sect. 1990;2(3):215–24.
53. Warpman U, Nordberg A. Epibatidine and ABT 418 reveal selective losses of alpha 4 beta 2 nicotinic receptors in Alzheimer brains. Neuroreport. 1995;6(17):2419–23.
54. Ding YS, Logan J, Bermel R, et al. Dopamine receptor-mediated regulation of striatal cholinergic activity: positron emission tomography studies with norchloro[^{18}F]fluoroepibatidine. J Neurochem. 2000;74(4):1514–21.
55. Klunk WE, Engler H, Nordberg A, et al. Imaging brain amyloid in Alzheimer's disease with Pittsburgh Compound-B. Ann Neurol. 2004;55(3):306–19.
56. Small GW, Kepe V, Ercoli LM, et al. PET of brain amyloid and tau in mild cognitive impairment. N Engl J Med. 2006;355(25):2652–63.
57. Edison P, Archer HA, Hinz R, et al. Amyloid, hypometabolism, and cognition in Alzheimer disease: an [^{11}C]PIB and [^{18}F]FDG PET study. Neurology. 2007;68(7):501–8.
58. Engler H, Forsberg A, Almkvist O, et al. Two-year follow-up of amyloid deposition in patients with Alzheimer's disease. Brain. 2006;129(Pt 11):2856–66.
59. Li Y, Rinne JO, Mosconi L, et al. Regional analysis of FDG and PIB-PET images in normal aging, mild cognitive impairment, and Alzheimer's disease. Eur J Nucl Med Mol Imag. 2008;35(12):2169–81.
60. Henriksen G, Yousefi BH, Drzezga A, Wester HJ. Development and evaluation of compounds for imaging of beta-amyloid plaque by means of positron emission tomography. Eur J Nucl Med Mol Imag. 2008;35(Suppl 1):S75–81.
61. Bench CJ, Dolan RJ, Friston KJ, Frackowiak RS. Positron emission tomography in the study of brain metabolism in psychiatric and neuropsychiatric disorders. Br J Psychiatry Suppl. 1990;9:82–95.
62. Kwan LT, Reed BR, Eberling JL, et al. Effects of subcortical cerebral infarction on cortical glucose metabolism and cognitive function. Arch Neurol. 1999;56(7):809–14.
63. Mielke R, Kittner B, Ghaemi M, et al. Propentofylline improves regional cerebral glucose metabolism and neuropsychologic performance in vascular dementia. J Neurol Sci. 1996;141(1–2):59–64.
64. McKeith IG. Consensus guidelines for the clinical and pathologic diagnosis of dementia with Lewy bodies (DLB): report of the consortium on DLB international workshop. J Alzheimers Dis. 2006;9(3 Suppl):417–23.
65. McKeith IG, Dickson DW, Lowe J, et al. Diagnosis and management of dementia with Lewy bodies: third report of the DLB consortium. Neurology. 2005;65(12):1863–72.
66. Barber R, Scheltens P, Gholkar A, et al. White matter lesions on magnetic resonance imaging in dementia

with Lewy bodies, Alzheimer's disease, vascular dementia, and normal aging. J Neurol Neurosurg Psychiatry. 1999;67(1):66–72.
67. Minoshima S, Foster NL, Sima AA, Frey KA, Albin RL, Kuhl DE. Alzheimer's disease versus dementia with Lewy bodies: cerebral metabolic distinction with autopsy confirmation. Ann Neurol. 2001;50(3):358–65.
68. Walker Z, Costa DC, Ince P, McKeith IG, Katona CL. In-vivo demonstration of dopaminergic degeneration in dementia with Lewy bodies. Lancet. 1999;354(9179):646–7.
69. Hu XS, Okamura N, Arai H, et al. ^{18}F-fluorodopa PET study of striatal dopamine uptake in the diagnosis of dementia with Lewy bodies. Neurology. 2000;55(10):1575–7.
70. Neary D, Snowden J, Mann D. Frontotemporal dementia. Lancet Neurol. 2005;4(11):771–80.
71. Snowden JS, Neary D, Mann DM. Frontotemporal dementia. Br J Psychiatry. 2002;180:140–3.
72. Foster NL, Heidebrink JL, Clark CM, et al. FDG-PET improves accuracy in distinguishing frontotemporal dementia and Alzheimer's disease. Brain. 2007;130(Pt 10):2616–35.
73. Jeong Y, Cho SS, Park JM, et al. ^{18}F-FDG PET findings in frontotemporal dementia: an SPM analysis of 29 patients. J Nucl Med. 2005;46(2):233–9.
74. Rinne JO, Laine M, Kaasinen V, Norvasuo-Heila MK, Nagren K, Helenius H. Striatal dopamine transporter and extrapyramidal symptoms in frontotemporal dementia. Neurology. 2002;58(10):1489–93.
75. Dolan RJ, Bench CJ, Brown RG, Scott LC, Friston KJ, Frackowiak RS. Regional cerebral blood flow abnormalities in depressed patients with cognitive impairment. J Neurol Neurosurg Psychiatry. 1992;55(9):768–73.
76. Cho MJ, Lyoo IK, Lee DW, et al. Brain single photon emission computed tomography findings in depressive pseudodementia patients. J Affect Disord. 2002;69(1–3):159–66.
77. Alexopoulos GS, Meyers BS, Young RC, Mattis S, Kakuma T. The course of geriatric depression with "reversible dementia": a controlled study. Am J Psychiatry. 1993;150(11):1693–9.
78. Menza M, Marin H, Kaufman K, Mark M, Lauritano M. Citalopram treatment of depression in Parkinson's disease: the impact on anxiety, disability, and cognition. J Neuropsychiatry Clin Neurosci. 2004;16(3):315–9.
79. Shih MC, Amaro Jr E, Ferraz HB, et al. Neuroimaging of the dopamine transporter in Parkinsons disease: first study using [^{99m}Tc]-TRODAT-1 and SPECT in Brazil. Arq Neuropsiquiatr. 2006;64(3A):628–34.
80. Rao G, Fisch L, Srinivasan S, et al. Does this patient have Parkinson disease? JAMA. 2003;289(3):347–53.
81. Rajput AH, Rozdilsky B, Rajput A. Accuracy of clinical diagnosis in parkinsonism – a prospective study. Can J Neurol Sci. 1991;18(3):275–8.
82. Lachenmayer L. Differential diagnosis of parkinsonian syndromes: dynamics of time courses are essential. J Neurol. 2003;250(Suppl 1):I11–4.
83. Lees AJ, Hardy J, Revesz T. Parkinson's disease. Lancet. 2009;373(9680):2055–66.
84. Olanow CW, Tatton WG. Etiology and pathogenesis of Parkinson's disease. Annu Rev Neurosci. 1999;22:123–44.
85. Braak H, Ghebremedhin E, Rub U, Bratzke H, Del Tredici K. Stages in the development of Parkinson's disease-related pathology. Cell Tissue Res. 2004;318(1):121–34.
86. Lotharius J, Brundin P. Pathogenesis of Parkinson's disease: dopamine, vesicles and alpha-synuclein. Nat Rev Neurosci. 2002;3(12):932–42.
87. Kwon KY, Choi CG, Kim JS, Lee MC, Chung SJ. Diagnostic value of brain MRI and ^{18}F-FDG PET in the differentiation of Parkinsonian-type multiple system atrophy from Parkinson's disease. Eur J Neurol. 2008;15(10):1043–9.
88. Brooks DJ, Ibanez V, Sawle GV, et al. Differing patterns of striatal ^{18}F-dopa uptake in Parkinson's disease, multiple system atrophy, and progressive supranuclear palsy. Ann Neurol. 1990;28(4):547–55.
89. Antonini A, Vontobel P, Psylla M, et al. Complementary positron emission tomographic studies of the striatal dopaminergic system in Parkinson's disease. Arch Neurol. 1995;52(12):1183–90.
90. Ribeiro MJ, Vidailhet M, Loc'h C, et al. Dopaminergic function and dopamine transporter binding assessed with positron emission tomography in Parkinson disease. Arch Neurol. 2002;59(4):580–6.
91. Tedroff J, Ekesbo A, Rydin E, Langstrom B, Hagberg G. Regulation of dopaminergic activity in early Parkinson's disease. Ann Neurol. 1999;46(3):359–65.
92. Lee CS, Samii A, Sossi V, et al. In vivo positron emission tomographic evidence for compensatory changes in presynaptic dopaminergic nerve terminals in Parkinson's disease. Ann Neurol. 2000;47(4):493–503.
93. Rakshi JS, Uema T, Ito K, et al. Frontal, midbrain and striatal dopaminergic function in early and advanced Parkinson's disease A 3D [(18)F]dopa-PET study. Brain. 1999;122(Pt 9):1637–50.
94. Tison F, Normand E, Jaber M, Aubert I, Bloch B. Aromatic L-amino-acid decarboxylase (DOPA decarboxylase) gene expression in dopaminergic and serotoninergic cells of the rat brainstem. Neurosci Lett. 1991;127(2):203–6.
95. Frey KA, Koeppe RA, Kilbourn MR, et al. Presynaptic monoaminergic vesicles in Parkinson's disease and normal aging. Ann Neurol. 1996;40(6):873–84.
96. Bohnen NI, Albin RL, Koeppe RA, et al. Positron emission tomography of monoaminergic vesicular binding in aging and Parkinson disease. J Cereb Blood Flow Metab. 2006;26(9):1198–212.
97. Brucke T, Asenbaum S, Pirker W, et al. Measurement of the dopaminergic degeneration in Parkinson's disease with [123I] beta-CIT and SPECT. Correlation with clinical findings and comparison with multiple system atrophy and progressive supranuclear palsy. J Neural Transm Suppl. 1997;50:9–24.
98. Jennings DL, Seibyl JP, Oakes D, Eberly S, Murphy J, Marek K. (123I) beta-CIT and single-photon emission computed tomographic imaging vs clinical evaluation in Parkinsonian syndrome: unmasking an early diagnosis. Arch Neurol. 2004;61(8):1224–9.

99. Kim YJ, Ichise M, Ballinger JR, et al. Combination of dopamine transporter and D2 receptor SPECT in the diagnostic evaluation of PD, MSA, and PSP. Mov Disord. 2002;17(2):303–12.
100. Mukherjee J, Christian BT, Dunigan KA, et al. Brain imaging of 18F-fallypride in normal volunteers: blood analysis, distribution, test-retest studies, and preliminary assessment of sensitivity to aging effects on dopamine D-2/D-3 receptors. Synapse. 2002;46(3):170–88.
101. Gilman S, Wenning GK, Low PA, et al. Second consensus statement on the diagnosis of multiple system atrophy. Neurology. 2008;71(9):670–6.
102. Wenning GK, Stefanova N. Recent developments in multiple system atrophy. J Neurol. 2009; 256(11):1791–808.
103. Kwon KY, Choi CG, Kim JS, Lee MC, Chung SJ. Comparison of brain MRI and 18F-FDG PET in the differential diagnosis of multiple system atrophy from Parkinson's disease. Mov Disord. 2007;22(16):2352–8.
104. Gilman S. Functional imaging with positron emission tomography in multiple system atrophy. J Neural Transm. 2005;112(12):1647–55.
105. Antonini A, Leenders KL, Vontobel P, et al. Complementary PET studies of striatal neuronal function in the differential diagnosis between multiple system atrophy and Parkinson's disease. Brain. 1997;120(Pt 12):2187–95.
106. Blin J, Baron JC, Dubois B, et al. Positron emission tomography study in progressive supranuclear palsy. Brain hypometabolic pattern and clinicometabolic correlations. Arch Neurol. 1990;47(7):747–52.
107. Mishina M, Ishii K, Mitani K, et al. Midbrain hypometabolism as early diagnostic sign for progressive supranuclear palsy. Acta Neurol Scand. 2004;110(2):128–35.
108. Ilgin N, Zubieta J, Reich SG, Dannals RF, Ravert HT, Frost JJ. PET imaging of the dopamine transporter in progressive supranuclear palsy and Parkinson's disease. Neurology. 1999;52(6):1221–6.
109. Im JH, Chung SJ, Kim JS, Lee MC. Differential patterns of dopamine transporter loss in the basal ganglia of progressive supranuclear palsy and Parkinson's disease: analysis with [(123)I]IPT single photon emission computed tomography. J Neurol Sci. 2006;244(1–2):103–9.
110. Leenders KL, Frackowiak RS, Lees AJ. Steele-Richardson-Olszewski syndrome. Brain energy metabolism, blood flow and fluorodopa uptake measured by positron emission tomography. Brain. 1988;111(Pt 3):615–30.
111. Laureys S, Salmon E, Garraux G, et al. Fluorodopa uptake and glucose metabolism in early stages of corticobasal degeneration. J Neurol. 1999;246(12):1151–8.
112. Nagahama Y, Fukuyama H, Turjanski N, et al. Cerebral glucose metabolism in corticobasal degeneration: comparison with progressive supranuclear palsy and normal controls. Mov Disord. 1997;12(5):691–6.
113. Garraux G, Salmon E, Peigneux P, et al. Voxel-based distribution of metabolic impairment in corticobasal degeneration. Mov Disord. 2000;15(5):894–904.
114. Nagasawa H, Tanji H, Nomura H, et al. PET study of cerebral glucose metabolism and fluorodopa uptake in patients with corticobasal degeneration. J Neurol Sci. 1996;139(2):210–7.
115. Lutte I, Laterre C, Bodart JM, De Volder A. Contribution of PET studies in diagnosis of corticobasal degeneration. Eur Neurol. 2000;44(1):12–21.
116. Hermann W, Barthel H, Hesse S, et al. Comparison of clinical types of Wilson's disease and glucose metabolism in extrapyramidal motor brain regions. J Neurol. 2002;249(7):896–901.
117. Snow BJ, Bhatt M, Martin WR, Li D, Calne DB. The nigrostriatal dopaminergic pathway in Wilson's disease studied with positron emission tomography. J Neurol Neurosurg Psychiatry. 1991;54(1):12–7.

Cerebrovascular Disease and PET

14

Hidehiko Okazawa and Yu-Kyeong Kim

Cerebrovascular Disease and O-15 PET

Measurement of Hemodynamic Parameters Using O-15 PET

Positron emission tomography (PET) and O-15 tracers have been used for greater than 30 years to evaluate human cerebral hemodynamics in patients with cerebral vascular disease (CVD). Quantitative measurement of cerebral blood flow (CBF) and metabolism is important because critical impairment of cerebral circulation induces irreversible damage to the cerebral cortex, causing neuronal deficits or functional damage. The cerebral regions of impaired hemodynamics, "misery perfusion" are visualized by mismatch between oxygen metabolism and CBF [1, 2], which is usually delineated by the elevation of oxygen extraction fraction (OEF) in O-15 gas PET [2–6]. Because patients with misery perfusion show a significantly higher incidence rate of stroke or recurrent stroke [7–9], evaluation of hemodynamic status in CVD patients is very important to determine indication of neurosurgical treatment. To quantitatively evaluate cerebral hemodynamic status, methods for precise measurement were developed and its accuracy has also been improved with the progression of PET scanner resolution.

The historic development of PET measurement of cerebral hemodynamic parameters is shown in Table 14.1 [10–25]. The impaired hemodynamic status of misery perfusion was at first determined using a count-based semiquantitative method [1, 2]. Quantitative methods for cerebral circulation and oxygen metabolism were proposed in the early 1980s, and the two common methods based on a single compartment model are known as the steady-state method and the bolus inhalation method (so-called 'autoradiographic' or 'three-step' method) (Fig. 14.1a). A quantitative steady-state method with continuous inhalation of O-15 labeled gases such as $^{15}O_2$, $C^{15}O_2$ and $C^{15}O$ was proposed [15, 16]. Lammertsma et al. corrected the effect of cerebral blood volume (CBV) on OEF in the O-15 gas steady-state method [17]. OEF is usually overestimated when CBV correction is not applied. Although this method is simple and easier than the bolus tracer administration method, specific equipment must be installed to keep radioactive gas at a constant rate of concentration during PET scans, and patients cannot avoid high exposure to radioactive gas. The autoradiographic method developed for measurement of CBF using O-15 water was applied [18, 19] to

H. Okazawa, M.D., Ph.D. (✉)
Division of Biomedical Imaging, The Faculty of Medical Sciences, University of Fukui, Fukui 910-1193, Japan
e-mail: okazawa@u-fukui.ac.jp

Y.-K. Kim, M.D., Ph.D.
Department of Nuclear Medicine, Seoul National University, Bundang Hospital, Gyeonggi-Do 463-707, South Korea
e-mail: yk3181@snu.ac.kr

E.E. Kim et al. (eds.), *Clinical PET and PET/CT: Principles and Applications*,
DOI 10.1007/978-1-4419-0802-5_14, © Springer Science+Business Media New York 2013

Table 14.1 Measurements of CBF and oxygen metabolism using O-15 tracers

Authors	Tracers	Method	Parameters	Year	References
Ter-Pogossian et al., Raichle et al.	$H_2{}^{15}O$, $^{15}O_2$	Bolus (No. image)	CBF, $CMRO_2$	1969–1976	[10–13]
Jones et al.	$^{15}O_2$, $C^{15}O_2$	Steady-state	Qualitative	1976	[14]
Frackowiak et al., Lammertsma et al.	$^{15}O_2$, $C^{15}O_2$	Steady-state	CBF, OEF, $CMRO_2$	1980, 1981	[15, 16]
Lammertsma et al.	$^{15}O_2$, $C^{15}O$	Steady-state(OEF-CBV correction)	OEF, $CMRO_2$	1983	[17]
Herscovitch et al., Raichle et al.	$H_2{}^{15}O$	Bolus, (ARG)	CBF	1983	[18, 19]
Mintun et al.	$H_2{}^{15}O$, $^{15}O_2$, $C^{15}O$	Bolus, (3-step)	CBF, CBV, OEF, $CMRO_2$	1984	[20]
Lammertsma et al.	^{11}CO, ^{11}C-HSA	Equilibrium	CBV, Htc ratio	1984	[21]
Gambhir et al.	$H_2{}^{15}O$	Bolus, (2-CM)	CBF, V_d	1987	[22]
Lammertsma et al.	$C^{15}O_2$	Build-up	CBF	1989	[23]
Ohta et al.	$^{15}O_2$, $H_2{}^{15}O$	Bolus, (1-step, 2-CM)	$CMRO_2$, OEF, CBF, V_0	1992, 1996	[24, 25]

CBF cerebral blood flow, *$CMRO_2$* cerebral metabolic rate of oxygen, *OEF* oxygen extraction fraction, *CBV* cerebral blood volume, V_d distribution volume, *Htc ratio* cerebral-to-large vessel hematocrit ratio, V_0 arterial-to-capillary volume, *ARG* autoradiographic method, *CM* compartment model

the measurement of oxygen metabolism with bolus administration of O-15 tracers (three-step method) [20]. This method does not require the specific equipment to maintain a constant concentration rate of radioactive gas.

Because various quantitative methods for measurement of CBF using O-15 water PET were proposed, the method for quantitative measurement was improved, as well as several methods for image calculation and correction of parameters to improve the image quality and calculation time [25–35]. A two-compartment (one-tissue compartment) model analysis increased the accuracy of CBF values by separating the vascular component from the blood flow value as shown in the following equation (Fig. 14.1b) [24, 25]:

$$C_b(t) = K_1 \cdot C_a(t) \otimes e^{-k2t} + V_0 \cdot C_a(t).$$

where $C_b(t)$ and $C_a(t)$ are the concentrations of tracer in the brain and arteries, K_1 and k_2 are rate constants, V_0 is arterial-to-capillary blood volume, and ⊗ denotes operation of convolution. A single-compartment model analysis can be described with elimination of the second term in this equation [18, 19]. Rate constant of K_1 linearly correlates with blood flow, which can be corrected by extraction of the tracer ($K_1 = E \cdot F$; E = extraction, F = blood flow). If this method is applied to the bolus $^{15}O_2$ inhalation method, the cerebral metabolic rate of oxygen ($CMRO_2$) can be calculated without measuring CBF and CBV by the equation of $CMRO_2 = tO_2c \cdot K_1$, where tO_2c is total arterial O_2 content (one-step method) [24]. This method includes an assumption that the metabolized and recirculating radioactivity of O-15 water is negligible during the scanning time. The $CMRO_2$ values tend to be overestimated because of this assumption as well as the fact that venous radioactivity cannot be eliminated completely despite separation of V_0 [24, 36]. This simple method, however, can evaluate changes in oxygen metabolism during neural stimulation by repeated measurement of $CMRO_2$ in activation studies [37]. Recently, a report from 11 PET centers in Japan, in which several representative methods for O-15 PET were used, showed no significant differences in quantitative values of hemodynamic parameters among the methods [38]. In this study, overall mean ± SD (standard deviation) values in

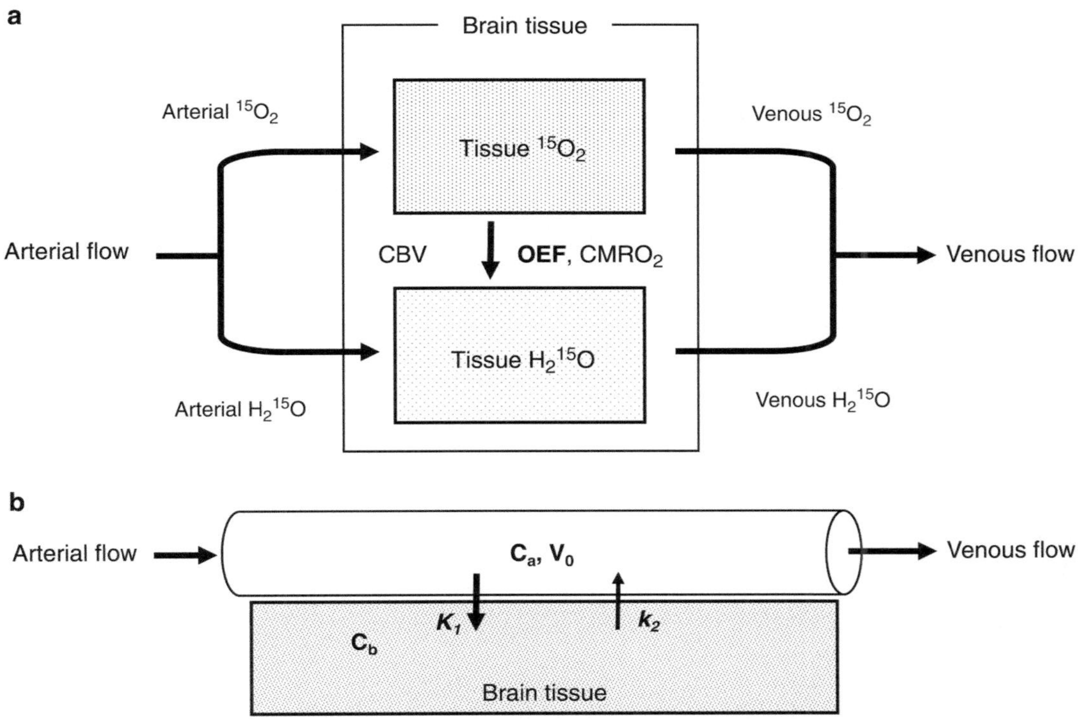

Fig. 14.1 Schematic of one-compartment (**a**) and two-compartment (one-tissue compartment) (**b**) models for calculation of CBF and oxygen metabolism. In model (**a**), CBF calculation using $H_2{}^{15}O$ or $C^{15}O_2$ can be explained by neglecting $^{15}O_2$ elements. C_a and C_b are the concentrations of arterial and brain tissue radioactivity, K_1 and k_2 are rate constants of tracers, and V_0 is the arterial-to-capillary blood volume

cerebral cortical regions for healthy human subjects were CBF = 44.4 ± 6.5 mL/100 g/min, CBV = 3.8 ± 0.7 mL/100 g, $CMRO_2$ = 3.3 ± 0.5 mL/100 g/min, and OEF = 0.44 ± 0.06.

Contrary to the development of precise quantification methods, one long-term prospective study reported that the diagnostic accuracy for misery perfusion was similar to, or rather, better with the count-based method compared with the quantitative evaluation [39, 40]. Recent reports on the application of count-based semi-quantitative methods have been controversial. A normalized method using cerebellar counts showed poor agreement with quantitative OEF elevation [41]. However, another study employing a simplified ipsilateral-to-contralateral asymmetry index (AI) comparison method using count-based ratio images showed good accordance with the AI of quantitative OEF in CVD patients [42, 43]. The advantage of these simplified methods is that the scanning protocol is simple and the procedure is noninvasive without arterial blood sampling. For precise evaluation of hemodynamic changes in the brain, quantitative methods with arterial blood sampling are required; however, in clinical studies, the simplified method is preferable for assessment of the hemodynamic status.

Chronic Cerebrovascular Disease

CBF autoregulation is the mechanism by which CBF is maintained during changes in systemic blood pressure. This physiologic function also can be applied to the relationship between changes in cerebral perfusion pressure (CPP) and CBF. CBF is maintained by autoregulatory vasoconstriction and vasodilatation of arterioles when CPP is changed; however, CBF decreases when

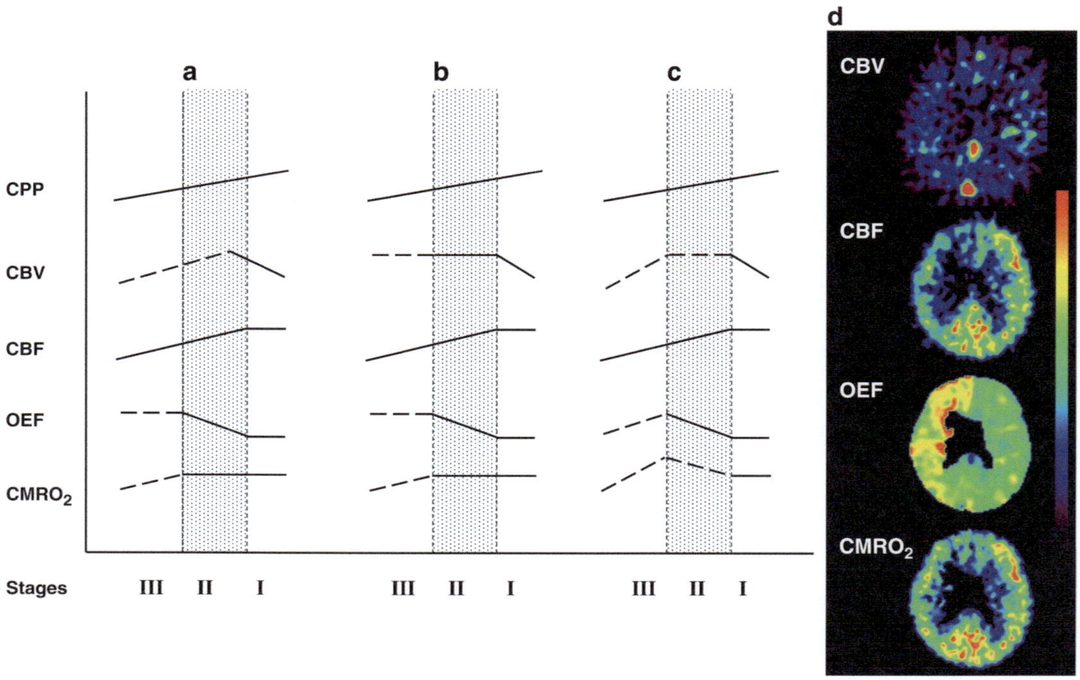

Fig. 14.2 Graph explaining changes in hemodynamic parameters induced by decreases in perfusion pressure (CPP). Powers et al. initially proposed the basic concept of hypothesis (**a**), and later revised the model with a minor change in CBV (**b**) [3–6, 40, 46]. Nemoto et al. modified this model based on their two-compartment analysis (**c**) [47]. *Dotted* area in the graph shows stage II impairment. Representative PET images for patients with misery perfusion (stage II) are presented in the right column (**d**). Misery perfusion shows a slight decrease in $CMRO_2$ at the region of CBF decrease and OEF elevation

CPP decreases below the lower limit of autoregulation (Fig. 14.2). Experiments on cerebrovascular autoregulation have shown an increase in the diameter of resistance arteries as a function of the decrease in systemic blood pressure [44, 45]. Although this vasodilatory change caused by a reduction in blood pressure is a well-known physiologic reaction in the acute phase, it is not clear whether the cerebral circulation in patients with chronic CVD shows similar vasodilatory compensation in the resistance arteries. To explain the cerebral hemodynamic changes in CVD patients, Powers et al. originally presumed that the dilatory change in resistance vessels continues even after the vasodilatation can no longer compensate for CBF autoregulation as described in animal experiments (Fig. 14.2a) [3, 5, 6]. They later modified this model with respect to hemodynamics in chronic CVD patients (Fig. 14.2b) [39, 46] and reported the importance of neurosurgical treatment for stage II ischemia. Recently, Nemoto et al. slightly corrected this hemodynamic assumption based on their analysis using a two-compartment model (Fig. 14.2c) [47]. However, most patients with misery perfusion usually show a slight decrease in $CMRO_2$ (Fig. 14.2d) as described by Powers et al. in their reports [3–5].

Several researchers and neurosurgeons reported that the extracranial-to-intracranial (EC/IC) bypass surgery is efficient for patients with misery perfusion caused by cerebral arterial occlusive lesions [3–6, 48]. However, the multicenter cohort study conducted in the mid-1980s for evaluation of prognosis of CVD patients contradicted the effectiveness of the EC/IC bypass surgery [49, 50]. The problem with the cohort study performed by the EC/IC bypass surgery group was that patient entry criteria were inappropriate. All patients with stenotic lesions in the internal carotid arteries were involved in the study, and there was no significant difference in outcome between the surgical treatment and simple medication groups. However, as many recent studies have suggested, if the patients do not show neurologic symptoms, stenoocclusive lesions do not necessarily cause hemodynamic impairment that may induce strokes in the brain [51–53]. Several long-term prospective studies have shown that patients without hemodynamic deficiency did not have a high incidence of subsequent infarction compared with those with misery perfusion. In their 5-year follow-up study ($n=40$), Yamauchi et al. (Kyoto University group) showed that the recurrence rate of stroke was significantly higher in patients with misery perfusion (57.1%) compared with those without OEF elevation (18.2%) [7, 8]. Grubb et al. (Washington University group) also showed a similar result with a larger patient sample ($n=81$) and 3-year follow-up period [9]. Their results suggest that a patient with stenoocclusive lesions in major cerebral arteries may not show neurologic deficits or hemodynamic impairment if the lesion advances slowly enough to generate sufficient collateral circulation.

This evidence shows the importance of evaluation of the cerebral circulation and oxygen metabolism; however, the degree of hemodynamic impairment can be evaluated by a reduction of cerebral vasoreactivity (CVR) after acetazolamide (ACZ) or CO_2 loading [54–56]. The vasodilatory effect of ACZ or CO_2 without changes in systemic blood pressure causes increases in CBF in normal circulation [54, 57, 58]. Recently, several long-term prospective studies were conducted using the quantitative measurement of baseline CBF and CVR to confirm the risk of developing cerebral infarction in hemodynamic impairment [59–67]. The studies were performed to contradict the prospective cohort study that denied the effectiveness and benefits of EC/IC bypass surgery for patients with cerebral arterial occlusion. The aim of the studies was to prove that symptomatic patients with CVD who have hemodynamic impairment should be treated by surgical or interventional methods to avoid recurrent strokes. The studies with alternative methods reported a benefit of measuring CVR to evaluate the hemodynamic condition and to predict the risk of subsequent strokes [59–64]. On the other hand, nonquantitative evaluation of CVR failed to predict any significant difference in recurrent stroke risk between normal and impaired CVR groups [65–67]. A recent study reported that diagnostic accuracy for detecting misery perfusion by using quantitative measurement of CBF and CVR after ACZ administration had a sensitivity of 56.3%, specificity of 88.2%, and accuracy of 78.0% [68].

Figures 14.3 and 14.4 show representative cases of stage I and stage II hemodynamic impairment. A patient with stage I showed a decrease in CVR without elevation of OEF (Fig. 14.3), while a patient with misery perfusion (stage II impairment) showed elevation of OEF as well as a decrease in CVR in the affected hemisphere.

Evaluation of Cerebral Glucose Metabolism Following Stroke

Stroke is caused by a variety of pathologic changes that produce a focal reduction of blood flow or multifocal regions of compromised perfusion. In most of these cases, the end result of reduced CBF and inadequate delivery of oxygen and glucose to the brain is cerebral infarction [69]. In stabilized infarction, [^{18}F]2-fluoro-2-deoxy-D-glucose (FDG) PET shows a focal area of hypometabolism in a location consistent with focal cerebral infarction [70]. However, the metabolic impairment in stroke patients is not limited to the area of infarction. PET and single-photon emission computed tomography studies have demonstrated remote effects in regional CBF and metabolism consequent to focal infarction [71]. From the early period after an acute brain lesion, diaschisis can develop because of reduced cerebral function resulting from the interruption of normal input to a region not directly involved in the stroke. Distinguishing between regional ischemia and depressed neurometabolic activity is

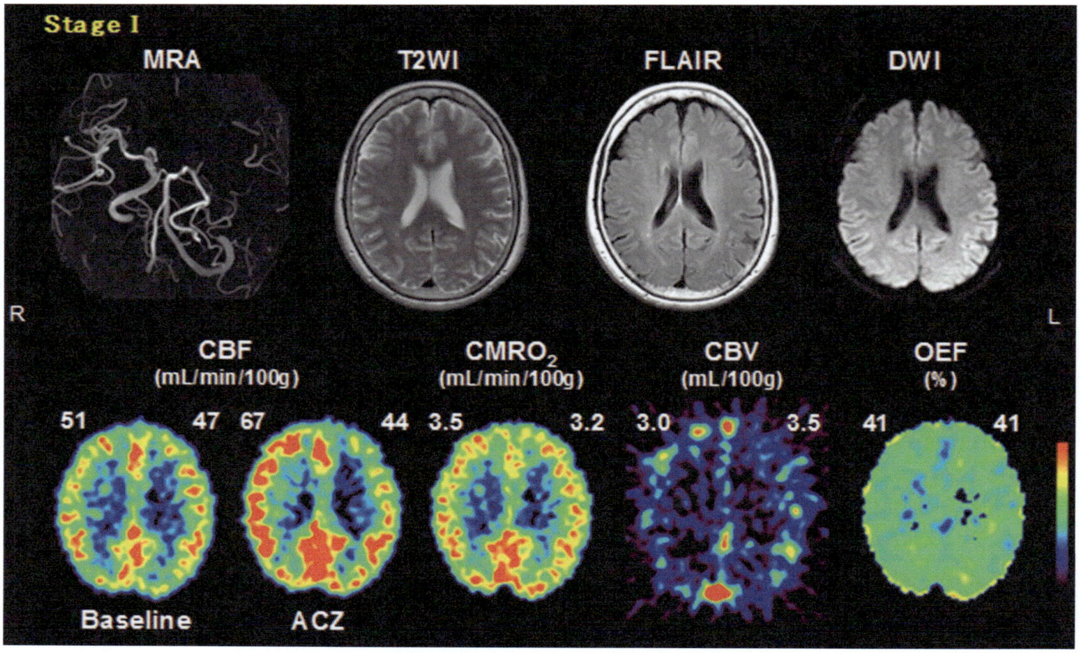

Fig. 14.3 A representative case of a stage I patient with stenosis in the left MCA. CBF and $CMRO_2$ did not show a significant decrease in the affected hemisphere, but CVR after ACZ administration showed the lack of vascular reactivity. Numbers are quantitative values for each hemisphere MRA: MR angiography

aided by the calculation of OEF with $CMRO_2$ and cerebral metabolism [48, 72, 73]. In the regions of diaschisis, the metabolic rate as measured by local glucose consumption was decreased, while OEF and $CMRO_2$ are preserved. Although there are reports of ischemic penumbra and luxury perfusion persisting after stroke [74, 75], normal oxygen extraction surrounding stroke suggests diaschisis [76].

It is likely that diaschisis is associated with functional impairment can determine the severity of the clinical images in the acute stage and its recovery [77]. Diaschisis can occur in the areas surrounding the "infarcted" lesion, in the outside of the lesion in the affected hemisphere as well as in the other hemisphere (e.g., "cross hemispheric" or "cross callosal" diaschisis). A regression of diaschisis is usually, although not invariably, found in the following months and may be related to the clinical recovery [78]. Immediately following stroke, extensive functional depression measured by glucose consumption and associated functional impairment can develop in the bilateral hemisphere [71, 79, 80]. In many reports, the improvement in function after left middle cerebral artery (MCA) stroke, e.g., progression from hand and leg weakness with aphasia to only hand weakness has been observed and seems linked to the anatomy adjacent to the cerebral infarction. Cortical diaschisis is particularly prominent with thalamic infarcts which often lead to pronounced thalamocortical diaschisis with corresponding cognitive deficits [81, 82]. In patients with cortical or subcortical infarction involved in the language area, regression of intrahemispheric and transhemispheric diaschisis may be associated with the recovery of a function that is subserved by an extensive network of interconnected regions in both hemispheres, at least in the first 6 months following stroke [78]. However, in cases of crossed (contralateral) cerebellar diaschisis (CCD) which can occur early after supratentorial ischemic lesions, particularly in the basal ganglia or frontal or parietal corticex, CCD can persist over a long period of time with eventual cerebellar atrophy, but usually lacks

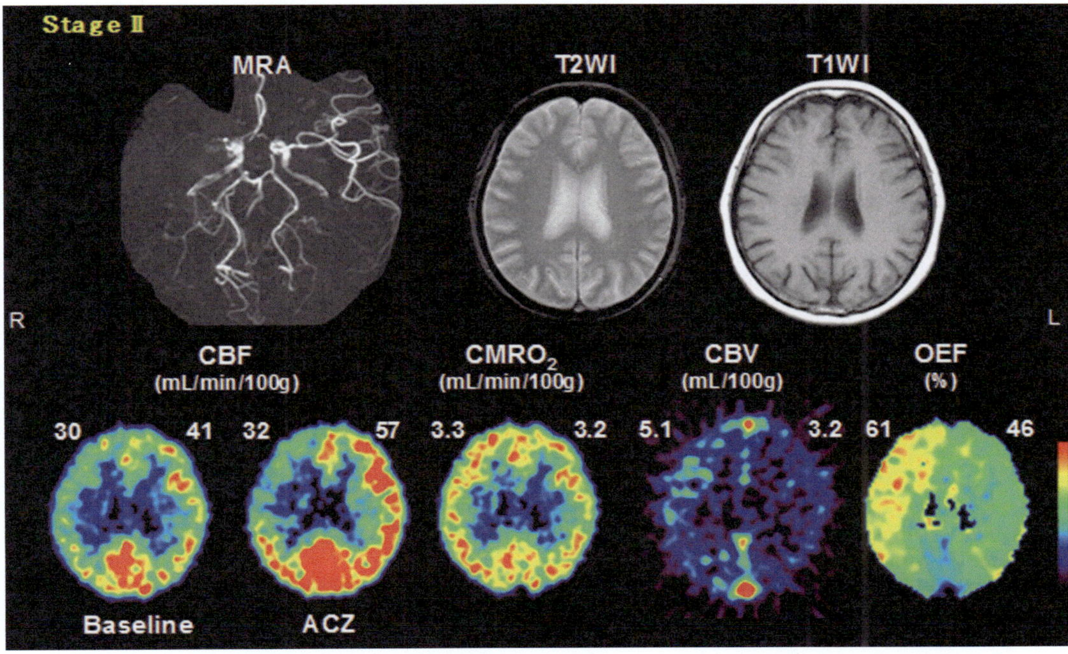

Fig. 14.4 A representative case of chronic CVD with misery perfusion (stage II) in the right cerebral hemisphere as a result of right MCA occlusion (see MRA). This patient did not show decrease in $CMRO_2$ in the impaired region (*right* frontal lobe). Numbers are quantitative values for each hemisphere

major correlates in neurologic functional impairment. The regional glucose metabolism in diaschisis in the early period following stroke may be associated with functional improvement during the recovery phase [83, 84]. Cerebral glucose metabolism in the left hemisphere outside the infarcted region, particularly temporoparietal metabolism, in the acute stage following stroke in the left hemisphere is thought to be the best predictor of recovery of auditory comprehension [85], and suggests an important role for intrahemispheric diaschisis in determining the severity of the clinical picture in the acute stage and its recovery [86].

Bilateral temporoparietal glucose metabolism shows a positive correlation with auditory comprehensive function in patients with aphasia following stroke.

Besides of the resolution of diaschisis, reorganization in the brain plays an important role in poststroke functional recovery. Changes in regional glucose metabolism in the contralateral hemisphere associated with poststroke reorganization have been detected by FDG PET [83]. The parallel change in glucose metabolism and high-energy phosphate metabolism associated with poststroke functional recovery is possibly explained by cerebral reorganization in the contralateral premotor cortex. The resulting cerebral reorganization may account for improved patient functional recovery from stroke. Similar findings can be observed in patients with aphasia following stroke. The changes in neuronal activities measured by glucose metabolism in the surrounding area of the "infarcted" region, in the contralateral mirror area and left Broca's area during activation were highly predictive of the recovery of auditory comprehension, indicating that the possibility to activate an extensive, bihemispheric neural network was crucial for recovery [84]. Hypermetabolism, measured by increased FDG uptake in the contralateral homologous area, indicates that there is increased energy being used, possibly because of increased neuronal plasticity.

References

1. Lenzi GL, Jones T, McKenzie CG, Moss S. Noninvasive regional study of chronic cerebrovascular disorders using the oxygen-15 inhalation technique. J Neurol Neurosurg Psychiatry. 1978;41:11–7.
2. Baron JC, Bousser MG, Rey A, Guillard A, Comar D, Castaigne P. Reversal of focal "misery-perfusion syndrome" by extra-intracranial arterial bypass in hemodynamic cerebral ischemia. A case study with ^{15}O positron emission tomography. Stroke. 1981; 12:454–9.
3. Powers WJ, Grubb Jr RL, Raichle ME. Physiological responses to focal cerebral ischemia in humans. Ann Neurol. 1984;16:546–52.
4. Powers WJ, Raichle ME. Positron emission tomography and its application to the study of cerebrovascular disease in man. Stroke. 1985;16:361–76.
5. Powers WJ, Press GA, Grubb Jr RL, Gado M, Raichle ME. The effect of hemodynamically significant carotid artery disease on the hemodynamic status of the cerebral circulation. Ann Intern Med. 1987; 106:27–34.
6. Powers WJ. Cerebral hemodynamics in ischemic cerebrovascular disease. Ann Neurol. 1991; 29:231–40.
7. Yamauchi H, Fukuyama H, Nagahama Y, Nabatame H, Nakamura K, Yamamoto Y, et al. Evidence of misery perfusion and risk for recurrent stroke in major cerebral arterial occlusive diseases from PET. J Neurol Neurosurg Psychiatry. 1996;61:18–25.
8. Yamauchi H, Fukuyama H, Nagahama Y, Nabatame H, Ueno M, Nishizawa S, et al. Significance of increased oxygen extraction fraction in five-year prognosis of major cerebral arterial occlusive diseases. J Nucl Med. 1999;40:1992–8.
9. Grubb Jr RL, Derdeyn CP, Fritsch SM, Carpenter DA, Yundt KD, Videen TO, et al. Importance of hemodynamic factors in the prognosis of symptomatic carotid occlusion. JAMA. 1998;280:1055–60.
10. Ter-Pogossian MM, Eichling JO, Davis DO, Welch MJ, Metzger JM. The determination of regional cerebral blood flow by means of water labeled with radioactive oxygen 15. Radiology. 1969;93:31–40.
11. Ter-Pogossian MM, Eichling JO, Davis DO, Welch MJ. The measure in vivo of regional cerebral oxygen utilization by means of oxyhemoglobin labeled with radioactive oxygen-15. J Clin Invest. 1970;49:381–91.
12. Raichle ME, Grubb Jr RL, Gado MH, Eichling JO, Ter-Pogossian MM. Correlation between regional cerebral blood flow and oxidative metabolism. In vivo studies in man. Arch Neurol. 1976;33:523–6.
13. Raichle ME, Grubb Jr RL, Eichling JO, Ter-Pogossian MM. Measurement of brain oxygen utilization with radioactive oxygen-15: experimental verification. J Appl Physiol. 1976;40:638–40.
14. Jones T, Chesler DA, Ter-Pogossian MM. The continuous inhalation of oxygen-15 for assessing regional oxygen extraction in the brain of man. Br J Radiol. 1976;49:339–43.
15. Frackowiak RS, Lenzi GL, Jones T, Heather JD. Quantitative measurement of regional cerebral blood flow and oxygen metabolism in man using ^{15}O and positron emission tomography: theory, procedure, and normal values. J Comput Assist Tomogr. 1980;4:727–36.
16. Lammertsma AA, Jones T, Frackowiak RS, Lenzi GL. A theoretical study of the steady-state model for measuring regional cerebral blood flow and oxygen utilisation using oxygen-15. J Comput Assist Tomogr. 1981;5:544–50.
17. Lammertsma AA, Wise RJ, Heather JD, Gibbs JM, Leenders KL, Frackowiak RS, et al. Correction for the presence of intravascular oxygen-15 in the steady-state technique for measuring regional oxygen extraction ratio in the brain: 2. Results in normal subjects and brain tumour and stroke patients. J Cereb Blood Flow Metab. 1983;3:425–31.
18. Herscovitch P, Markham J, Raichle ME. Brain blood flow measured with intravenous $H_2^{15}O$. I. Theory and error analysis. J Nucl Med. 1983;24:782–9.
19. Raichle ME, Martin WR, Herscovitch P, Mintun MA, Markham J. Brain blood flow measured with intravenous $H_2^{15}O$. II. Implementation and validation. J Nucl Med. 1983;24:790–8.
20. Mintun MA, Raichle ME, Martin WR, Herscovitch P. Brain oxygen utilization measured with O-15 radiotracers and positron emission tomography. J Nucl Med. 1984;25:177–87.
21. Lammertsma AA, Brooks DJ, Beaney RP, Turton DR, Kensett MJ, Heather JD, et al. In vivo measurement of regional cerebral haematocrit using positron emission tomography. J Cereb Blood Flow Metab. 1984; 4:317–22.
22. Gambhir SS, Huang SC, Hawkins RA, Phelps ME. A study of the single compartment tracer kinetic model for the measurement of local cerebral blood flow using ^{15}O-water and positron emission tomography. J Cereb Blood Flow Metab. 1987;7:13–20.
23. Lammertsma AA, Frackowiak RS, Hoffman JM, Huang SC, Weinberg IN, Dahlbom M, et al. The $C^{15}O_2$ build-up technique to measure regional cerebral blood flow and volume of distribution of water. J Cereb Blood Flow Metab. 1989;9:461–70.
24. Ohta S, Meyer E, Thompson CJ, Gjedde A. Oxygen consumption of the living human brain measured after a single inhalation of positron emitting oxygen. J Cereb Blood Flow Metab. 1992;12:179–92.
25. Ohta S, Meyer E, Fujita H, Reutens DC, Evans A, Gjedde A. Cerebral [^{15}O]water clearance in humans determined by PET: I. Theory and normal values. J Cereb Blood Flow Metab. 1996;16:765–80.
26. Herscovitch P, Raichle ME. Effect of tissue heterogeneity on the measurement of cerebral blood flow with the equilibrium $C^{15}O_2$ inhalation technique. J Cereb Blood Flow Metab. 1983;3:407–15.
27. Alpert NM, Eriksson L, Chang JY, Bergstrom M, Litton JE, Correia JA, et al. Strategy for the measure-

ment of regional cerebral blood flow using short-lived tracers and emission tomography. J Cereb Blood Flow Metab. 1984;4:28–34.

28. Carson RE, Huang SC, Green MV. Weighted integration method for local cerebral blood flow measurements with positron emission tomography. J Cereb Blood Flow Metab. 1986;6:245–58.
29. Huang SC, Feng DG, Phelps ME. Model dependency and estimation reliability in measurement of cerebral oxygen utilization rate with oxygen-15 and dynamic positron emission tomography. J Cereb Blood Flow Metab. 1986;6:105–19.
30. Koeppe RA, Holden JE, Ip WR. Performance comparison of parameter estimation techniques for the quantitation of local cerebral blood flow by dynamic positron computed tomography. J Cereb Blood Flow Metab. 1985;5:224–34.
31. Iida H, Kanno I, Miura S, Murakami M, Takahashi K, Uemura K. Error analysis of a quantitative cerebral blood flow measurement using $H_2{}^{15}O$ autoradiography and positron emission tomography, with respect to the dispersion of the input function. J Cereb Blood Flow Metab. 1986;6:536–45.
32. Iida H, Kanno I, Miura S, Murakami M, Takahashi K, Uemura K. A determination of the regional brain/blood partition coefficient of water using dynamic positron emission tomography. J Cereb Blood Flow Metab. 1989;9:874–85.
33. Cunningham VJ, Jones T. Spectral analysis of dynamic PET studies. J Cereb Blood Flow Metab. 1993;13:15–23.
34. Kimura Y, Hsu H, Toyama H, Senda M, Alpert NM. Improved signal-to-noise ratio in parametric images by cluster analysis. Neuroimage. 1999;9:554–61.
35. Shidahara M, Watabe H, Kim KM, Kudomi N, Ito H, Iida H. Optimal scan time of oxygen-15-labeled gas inhalation autoradiographic method for measurement of cerebral oxygen extraction fraction and cerebral oxygen metabolic rate. Ann Nucl Med. 2008; 22:667–75.
36. Okazawa H, Yamauchi H, Sugimoto K, Takahashi M, Toyoda H, Kishibe Y, et al. Quantitative comparison of the bolus and steady-state methods for measurement of cerebral perfusion and oxygen metabolism: PET study using ^{15}O-gas and water. J Cereb Blood Flow Metab. 2001;21:793–803.
37. Vafaee MS, Meyer E, Marrett S, Paus T, Evans AC, Gjedde A. Frequency-dependent changes in cerebral metabolic rate of oxygen during activation of human visual cortex. J Cereb Blood Flow Metab. 1999;19:272–7.
38. Ito H, Kanno I, Kato C, Sasaki T, Ishii K, Ouchi Y, et al. Database of normal human cerebral blood flow, cerebral blood volume, cerebral oxygen extraction fraction and cerebral metabolic rate of oxygen measured by positron emission tomography with ^{15}O-labelled carbon dioxide or water, carbon monoxide and oxygen: a multicentre study in Japan. Eur J Nucl Med Mol Imag. 2004;31:635–43.
39. Derdeyn CP, Videen TO, Simmons NR, Yundt KD, Fritsch SM, Grubb RL, et al. Count-based PET method for predicting ischemic stroke in patients with symptomatic carotid arterial occlusion. Radiology. 1999;212:499–506.
40. Derdeyn CP, Videen TO, Grubb Jr RL, Powers WJ. Comparison of PET oxygen extraction fraction methods for the prediction of stroke risk. J Nucl Med. 2001;42:1195–7.
41. Ibaraki M, Shimosegawa E, Miura S, Takahashi K, Ito H, Kanno I, et al. PET measurements of CBF, OEF, and $CMRO_2$ without arterial sampling in hyperacute ischemic stroke: method and error analysis. Ann Nucl Med. 2004;18:35–44.
42. Kobayashi M, Okazawa H, Tsuchida T, Kawai K, Fujibayashi Y, Yonekura Y. Diagnosis of misery perfusion using noninvasive O-15 gas PET. J Nucl Med. 2006;47:1581–6.
43. Kobayashi M, Kudo T, Tsujikawa T, Isozaki M, Arai Y, Fujibayashi Y, et al. Shorter examination method for the diagnosis of misery perfusion using count-based OEF elevation in ^{15}O-gas PET. J Nucl Med. 2008;49:242–6.
44. Grubb Jr RL, Phelps ME, Raichle ME, Ter-Pogassian MM. The effect of arterial blood pressure on the regional cerebral blood volume by x-ray fluorescence. Stroke. 1973;4:390–9.
45. MacKenzie ET, Farrar JK, Fitch W, Graham DI, Gregory PC, Harper AM. Effects of hemorrhagic hypotension on the cerebral circulation. I. Cerebral blood flow and pial arteriolar caliber. Stroke. 1979;10:711–8.
46. Derdeyn CP, Grubb Jr RL, Powers WJ. Cerebral hemodynamic impairment: methods of measurement and association with stroke risk. Neurology. 1999;53:251–9.
47. Nemoto EM, Yonas H, Kuwabara H, Pindzola RR, Sashin D, Meltzer CC, et al. Identification of hemodynamic compromise by cerebrovascular reserve and oxygen extraction fraction in occlusive vascular disease. J Cereb Blood Flow Metab. 2004;24:1081–9.
48. Baron JC, Bousser MG, Comar D, Soussaline F, Castaigne P. Noninvasive tomographic study of cerebral blood flow and oxygen metabolism in vivo. Potentials, limitations, and clinical applications in cerebral ischemic disorders. Eur Neurol. 1981;20:273–84.
49. The EC/IC bypass study group, Barnett HJM, Sackett DL, Taylor DW, Peerless SJ, Haynes RB, Gates PC, et al. Failure of extracranial-intracranial arterial bypass to reduce the risk of ischemic stroke. Results of an international randomized trial. The EC/IC bypass study group. N Engl J Med. 1985;313:1191–200.
50. The EC/IC bypass study group, Haynes RB, Taylor DW, Mukherjee J, Sackett DL, Cote R, Meguro K, et al. The international cooperative study of extracranial/intracranial arterial anastomosis (EC/IC bypass study): methodology and entry characteristics. The EC/IC bypass study group. Stroke. 1985;16:397–406.
51. Hennerici M, Hülsbömer HB, Rautenberg W, Hefter H. Spontaneous history of asymptomatic internal carotid occlusion. Stroke. 1986;17:718–22.

52. Hankey GJ, Warlow CP. Prognosis of symptomatic carotid occlusion: an overview. Cerebrovasc Dis. 1991;1:245–56.
53. Derdeyn CP, Yundt KD, Videen TO, Carpenter DA, Grubb Jr RL, Powers WJ. Increased oxygen extraction fraction is associated with prior ischemic events in patients with carotid occlusion. Stroke. 1998;29:754–8.
54. Vorstrup S. Tomographic cerebral blood flow measurements in patients with ischemic cerebrovascular disease and evaluation of the vasodilatory capacity by the acetazolamide test. Acta Neurol Scand. 1988;114(Suppl):1–48.
55. Yonas H, Smith HA, Durham SR, Pentheny SL, Johnson DW. Increased stroke risk predicted by compromised cerebral blood flow reactivity. J Neurosurg. 1993;79:483–9.
56. Yonas H, Pindzola RR. Physiological determination of cerebrovascular reserves and its use in clinical management. Cerebrovasc Brain Metab Rev. 1994;6:325–40.
57. Gotoh F, Meyer JS, Tomita M. Carbonic anhydrase inhibition and cerebral venous blood gases and ions in man. Demonstration of increased oxygen availability to ischemic brain. Arch Intern Med. 1966;117:39–46.
58. Okazawa H, Yamauchi H, Sugimoto K, Toyoda H, Kishibe Y, Takahashi M. Effects of acetazolamide on cerebral blood flow, blood volume and oxygen metabolism: a PET study with healthy volunteers. J Cereb Blood Flow Metab. 2001;21:1472–9.
59. Kuroda S, Kamiyama H, Abe H, Houkin K, Isobe M, Mitsumori K. Acetazolamide test in detecting reduced cerebral perfusion reserve and predicting long-term prognosis in patients with internal carotid artery occlusion. Neurosurgery. 1993;32:912–8.
60. Webster MW, Makaroun MS, Steed DL, Smith HA, Johnson DW, Yonas H. Compromised cerebral blood flow reactivity is a predictor of stroke in patients with symptomatic carotid artery occlusive disease. J Vasc Surg. 1995;21:338–44. discussion 344–345.
61. Kuroda S, Houkin K, Kamiyama H, Mitsumori K, Iwasaki Y, Abe H. Long-term prognosis of medically treated patients with internal carotid or middle cerebral artery occlusion: can acetazolamide test predict it? Stroke. 2001;32:2110–6.
62. Markus H, Cullinane M. Severely impaired cerebrovascular reactivity predicts stroke and TIA risk in patients with carotid artery stenosis and occlusion. Brain. 2001;124:457–67.
63. Ogasawara K, Ogawa A, Yoshimoto T. Cerebrovascular reactivity to acetazolamide and outcome in patients with symptomatic internal carotid or middle cerebral artery occlusion: a xenon-133 single-photon emission computed tomography study. Stroke. 2002;33:1857–62.
64. Ogasawara K, Ogawa A, Terasaki K, Shimizu H, Tominaga T, Yoshimoto T. Use of cerebrovascular reactivity in patients with symptomatic major cerebral artery occlusion to predict 5-year outcome: comparison of xenon-133 and iodine-123-IMP single-photon emission computed tomography. J Cereb Blood Flow Metab. 2002;22:1142–8.
65. Hasegawa Y, Yamaguchi T, Tsuchiya T, Minematsu K, Nishimura T. Sequential change of hemodynamic reserve in patients with major cerebral artery occlusion or severe stenosis. Neuroradiology. 1992;34:15–21.
66. Yokota C, Hasegawa Y, Minematsu K, Yamaguchi T. Effect of acetazolamide reactivity and long-term outcome in patients with major cerebral artery occlusive diseases. Stroke. 1998;29:640–4.
67. Yonas H, Pindzola RR, Meltzer CC, Sasser H. Qualitative versus quantitative assessment of cerebrovascular reserves. Neurosurgery. 1998;42:1005–10. discussion 1011–1012.
68. Okazawa H, Tsuchida T, Kobayashi M, Arai Y, Pagani M, Isozaki M, Yonekura Y. Can reductions in baseline CBF and vasoreactivity detect misery perfusion in chronic cerebrovascular disease? Eur J Nucl Med Mol Imag. 2007;34:121–9.
69. Mountz JM, Liu HG, Deutsch G. Neuroimaging in cerebrovascular disorders: measurement of cerebral physiology after stroke and assessment of stroke recovery. Semin Nucl Med. 2003;33:56–76.
70. Liu HG, Mountz JM. F-18 FDG brain positron emission tomography and Tl-201 early and delayed SPECT in distinguishing atypical cerebral tumor from cerebral infarction. Clin Nucl Med. 2003;28: 241–2.
71. Feeney DM, Baron JC. Diaschisis. Stroke. 1986;17:817–30.
72. Herold S, Brown MM, Frackowiak RS, Mansfield AO, Thomas DJ, Marshall J. Assessment of cerebral haemodynamic reserve: correlation between PET parameters and CO_2 reactivity measured by the intravenous 133 xenon injection technique. J Neurol Neurosurg Psychiatry. 1988;51:1045–50.
73. Ito H, Kanno I, Shimosegawa E, Tamura H, Okane K, Hatazawa J. Hemodynamic changes during neural deactivation in human brain: a positron emission tomography study of crossed cerebellar diaschisis. Ann Nucl Med. 2002;16:249–54.
74. Astrup J, Siesjo BK, Symon L. Thresholds in cerebral ischemia – the ischemic penumbra. Stroke. 1981;12:723–5.
75. Baron JC. Positron tomography in cerebral ischemia. A review. Neuroradiology. 1985;27:509–16.
76. Raynaud C, Rancurel G, Samson Y, Baron JC, Soucy JP, Kieffer E, et al. Pathophysiologic study of chronic infarcts with I-123 isopropyl iodo-amphetamine (IMP): the importance of periinfarct area. Stroke. 1987;18:21–9.
77. Seitz RJ, Azari NP, Knorr U, Binkofski F, Herzog H, Freund HJ. The role of diaschisis in stroke recovery. Stroke. 1999;30:1844–50.
78. Karbe H, Kessler J, Herholz K, Fink GR, Heiss WD. Long-term prognosis of poststroke aphasia studied with positron emission tomography. Arch Neurol. 1995;52:186–90.

79. Cappa SF, Perani D, Grassi F, Bressi S, Alberoni M, Franceschi M, et al. A PET follow-up study of recovery after stroke in acute aphasics. Brain Lang. 1997;56:55–67.
80. Carmichael ST, Tatsukawa K, Katsman D, Tsuyuguchi N, Kornblum HI. Evolution of diaschisis in a focal stroke model. Stroke. 2004;35:758–63.
81. Clarke S, Assal G, Bogousslavsky J, Regli F, Townsend DW, Leenders KL, et al. Pure amnesia after unilateral left polar thalamic infarct: topographic and sequential neuropsychological and metabolic (PET) correlations. J Neurol Neurosurg Psychiatry. 1994;57:27–34.
82. Stenset V, Grambaite R, Reinvang I, Hessen E, Cappelen T, Bjornerud A, et al. Diaschisis after thalamic stroke: a comparison of metabolic and structural changes in a patient with amnesic syndrome. Acta Neurol Scand Suppl. 2007;187:68–71.
83. Heiss WD, Emunds HG, Herholz K. Cerebral glucose metabolism as a predictor of rehabilitation after ischemic stroke. Stroke. 1993;24:1784–8.
84. Herholz K, Heiss WD. Functional imaging correlates of recovery after stroke in humans. J Cereb Blood Flow Metab. 2000;20:1619–31.
85. Karbe H, Szelies B, Herholz K, Heiss WD. Impairment of language is related to left parieto-temporal glucose metabolism in aphasic stroke patients. J Neurol. 1990;237:19–23.
86. Heiss WD, Thiel A, Kessler J, Herholz K. Disturbance and recovery of language function: correlates in PET activation studies. Neuroimage. 2003; 20(Suppl 1):S42–9.

Brain Tumors

15

Franklin C.L. Wong, Xiaoyi Duan, and E. Edmund Kim

Introduction

In 2009, about 61,414 new cases of primary brain tumors were expected to be diagnosed in the US, including 22,738 malignant brain tumors and 38,677 nonmalignant brain tumors [1]. Brain tumors are the most common solid tumors in children [2] and the second leading cause of cancer-related deaths in children under the age of 20 years [3]. In 2009, approximately 4,000 children younger than age 20 years were diagnosed with primary brain tumors, 2,875 of which were younger than 15 years [4].

F.C.L. Wong, M.D., Ph.D., J.D. (✉)
Departments of Nuclear Medicine and Neurooncology, The University of Texas MD Anderson Cancer Center, Houston, TX 77030, USA
e-mail: fwong@mdanderson.org

X. Duan, M.D.
Department of Nuclear Medicine, First Affiliated Hospital, Xi'an Jiaotong University, College of Medicine, Shaanxi 710061, China
e-mail: duanxt2009@hotmail.com

E.E. Kim, M.D., M.S.
Departments of Nuclear Medicine and Diagnostic Radiology, The University of Texas MD Anderson Cancer Center and Medical School, Houston, TX 77030, USA

Graduate School of Convergence Science and Technology, Seoul National University, Seoul, South Korea
e-mail: ekim@mdanderson.org

According to the 1993 World Health Organization (WHO) classification, primary brain tumors are classified according to their presumed cell of origin. Of all primary brain tumors, meningiomas are the most common, representing 33.4% of all primary brain tumors. Gliomas, which include all tumors arising from the glial cells or other supportive tissue of the brain, represent 33% of all brain tumors and 80% of all malignant brain tumors [1]. Astrocytomas and glioblastomas combined represent 77% of all gliomas [1]. Other brain tumors include pituitary tumors (12.2%), nerve sheath tumors (9%), lymphomas (2.5%), and oligodendrogliomas (2.1%) [1]. Medulloblastomas, embryonal, and primitive tumors represent 1% of all primary brain tumors [1]. The 2007 WHO Classification of Nervous System Tumors lists eight new entities including angiocentric glioma, atypical choroid plexus papilloma, extraventricular neurocytoma, papillary glioneuronal tumor, rosette-forming glioneuronal tumor of the fourth ventricle, papillary tumor of the pineal region, pituicytoma, and spindle cell oncocytoma of the adenohypophysis [5].

According to specific pathologic criteria, brain tumors are graded as low grade, or WHO grades I and II; high grade, or WHO grades III (anaplastic tumor) and IV (glioblastoma).

Metastatic brain tumors are the most common brain tumor with an annual incidence of more than four times that of primary brain tumors [1]. In all malignancy, 10–35% will develop brain metastases [6]. The most common metastatic brain tumor arises from primary lung tumors

E.E. Kim et al. (eds.), *Clinical PET and PET/CT: Principles and Applications*, DOI 10.1007/978-1-4419-0802-5_15, © Springer Science+Business Media New York 2013

(50–60%) and the second is breast cancer (15–20%) [7]. As more effective treatments are used for primary cancers and as larger numbers of people live longer, the number of metastatic brain tumors appears to be rising.

Radiologic Evaluation of Brain Tumors

MRI and CT

Magnetic resonance imaging (MRI) and computed tomography (CT) are still the most frequently used procedures for evaluation of primary or metastatic brain tumors. Benign brain tumors often show as hypodense mass lesions (darker than normal brain tissue) on CT. On MRI, they appear either hypo- (darker than brain tissue) or isointense (same intensity as brain tissue) on T1-weighted scans, and hyperintense (brighter than brain tissue) on T2-weighted scan. Contrast agent is often used in malignant primary and metastatic brain tumors because these tumors disrupt the normal blood-brain barrier, leading to an increase of its permeability. However, contrast enhancement is not useful to differentiate high- versus low-grade gliomas.

In most cases, contrast-enhanced MRI is more sensitive than CT, especially for detecting small tumors, tumor next to bone, brainstem tumors, low-grade tumors, and metastatic brain tumors. MRI can aid in determining the location, size, number, and probable type of brain tumors and may be used as the initial screening process when a patient has symptoms of brain tumor or the primary cancer has been diagnosed, however, CT is more effective at showing calcification and bony erosion.

Functional MRI

Functional MRI, also called real-time or fast MRI, acquires serial images in a fast sequence. This method may be useful prior to or during surgery to show the specific areas of the brain that control speech, movement, and memory. Functional MRI combined with imaging of cerebrospinal fluid (CSF) flow is called flow-sensitive MRI (FS MRI). FS MRI can show the flow of CSF through the ventricles and spinal cord and can therefore be used to plan the surgical removal of a skull base tumor, spinal cord tumor, or a tumor causing hydrocephalus.

Magnetic Resonance Angiography and Magnetic Resonance Spectroscopy

Magnetic resonance angiography (MRA) uses rapid MRI scans to follow the blood flow, thus help planning for the surgical removal of a tumor suspected of having a large blood supply or tumor growing into an area of the brain with an abundance of blood vessel. MRA can also be used to direct interventional effort to embolize or close-off large blood vessels that feed the brain tumor, making surgery easier.

As a noninvasive scanning technique, magnetic resonance spectroscopy evaluates ratios of minute amounts of tumor metabolites such as NAA/Cho [8], and can be used in characterizing low-grade gliomas, tumors with a large amount of surrounding edema, and in differentiating tumor recurrence from radiation necrosis. It may also be valuable in suggesting the degree of malignancy.

Single-Photon Emission Computed Tomography

Tools such as CT and MRI are excellent for brain tumor localization. However, they are unable to characterize the underlying histopathology. For example, it is difficult to define tumor grade or to differentiate tumor recurrence from necrosis or scar on CT or MRI [9]. With molecular specificity, single-photon emission computed tomography (SPECT) can provide additional information for the evaluation of brain tumor.

^{201}TI is a common tracer of cardiac SPECT. The cellular uptake of ^{201}TI depends on both blood flow and cellular extraction fraction which mainly occurs via the Na/K-ATPase active transport membrane pump in viable cells. In the late 1980s, a study reported that ^{201}TI uptake was able to distinguish low-grade from high-grade lesions with an accuracy of 89% [10]. ^{201}TI SPECT demonstrated a significantly better accuracy than contrast-enhanced CT in detecting residual tumor in brain tumor patients [11]. ^{99m}Tc-MIBI is another commonly used SPECT radiotracer for brain tumor imaging. It has better imaging properties than ^{201}TI. As illustrated in a pediatric tumor imaging report, ^{99m}Tc-MIBI showed greater uptake at the tumor site than did ^{201}Tl, and it defined the margins of the lesion more clearly, but may suffer interference from intense physiologic uptake by choroidal plexus [12].

PET and PET Radiotracer

The study of human brain tumor using PET began in the 1970s. Gross pathology such as perfusion abnormalities at the vascular level were reported with ^{15}O water PET [13]. Breakdown of blood barriers was reported by ^{68}Ga PET [14]. Differential vascular responses between vessels in tumor versus brain were reported under adenosine pharmacologic stimulation using ^{15}O water PET [15]. In the 1980s, reports indicated that increasing ^{18}F-fluorodeoxyglucose (FDG) uptake in gliomas correlated with tumor grades [16, 17].

FDG, which is used to evaluate glucose metabolism, remains the keystone of the PET radiotracer. ^{18}F-FDG identifies malignant lesions on the basis of glycolytic metabolism by the Warburg effect [18]. Normally, cerebral cortical and subcortical gray matter and the cerebellar cortex demonstrate physiologic high glucose metabolic activity. White matter with the centrum semiovale of the contralateral cerebral hemisphere has relative low glucose metabolism. Therefore, gray matter has higher ^{18}F-FDG uptake than white matter. Brain tumor may or may not have higher uptake than the surrounding normal, gray, or white matter. Extreme measures such as barbiturate coma have shown higher tumor-to-brain uptake ratios [19]. At times, because of the high FDG uptake in gray matter, the contrast of the signals from the tumor versus normal brain tissue decreases, leading to low sensitivity. With hybrid imaging such as PET/CT to clearly localize tumor, gray matter, and white matter, this problem can be partly overcome. Furthermore, comparison with prior studies and using standardized uptake value (SUV) or other quantitative parameters may help in assessing the contrast of the metabolic signals.

Other PET radiotracers have also been investigated, but none are used routinely in evaluating brain tumors. [C-11]-methionine is one of the most promising radiotracers as an alternative to ^{18}F-FDG because of its minimal background activity in the brain [20]. ^{11}C-labeled thymidine and ^{11}C-labeled choline have also been reported to show high tumor uptake [21, 22], but these radiotracers have been limited by a short physical half-life of 20 min for ^{11}C. Among the recent radiopharmaceutical developments for oncologic imaging, a thymidine analog, F-18 fluoro-3′-deoxy-3′-L-fluorothymidine (FLT), received much attention. It is trapped within the cell following its phosphorylation by thymidine kinase 1. ^{18}F-FLT has been applied in imaging human brain tumor and shows correlation with tumor proliferation [23–25].

In recent years, a new amino acid analog, F-18 fluoro dihydroxyphenylalanine (^{18}F-FDOPA), was introduced to evaluate brain tumor [26, 27]. The main advantage of ^{18}F-FDOPA was in low-grade brain tumors. A study published in 2009 evaluated ^{18}F-FDOPA, ^{18}F -FDG, and^{18}F-FLT in primary and recurrent low-grade gliomas using PET/CT. The conclusion was that the ^{18}F -FDOPA scan is superior to both ^{18}F-FDG and ^{18}F-FLT for the visualization of primary and recurrent low-grade gliomas [28].

In the literature, PET or PET/CT studies of human brain tumor have been reported with radiotracers of different molecular mechanisms including hypoxia, transporter for amino acids, enzymatic activities of glucose, and nucleosides and somatostatin receptor (Table 15.1).

Table 15.1 Radiotracers used in human brain tumor

Radiotracer	Imaging modality	Metabolism	Sensitivity %	Specificity %	Gold standard	References
^{18}F-FDG	PET/CT	Glucose	50	93	Pathology	[29]
^{18}F-FDOPA	PET/MRI	Amino acids	90	–	Pathology	[29]
^{18}F-FLT	PET	Nucleosides	79	63	Pathology	[30]
^{18}F-FMT	PET	Amino acids	74	82	Pathology	[31]
^{18}F-FMISO	PET	Hypoxia	47	–	Pathology	[32]
^{11}C-methionine	PET	Amino acids	90	92.3	Pathology	[33]
^{124}I-deoxyuridine	PET	Nucleosides	–	–	Pathology	[34]
^{68}Ga-DOTA-TOC	PET	Somatostatin	–	–	Pathology	[35]

^{18}F-FDG ^{18}F-fluorodeoxyglucose, *^{18}F-FDOPA*, *^{18}F-FLT* F-18 fluoro-3′-deoxy-3′-L-fluorothymidine, *^{18}F-FMT*, *^{18}F-FMISO*, *^{68}Ga-DOTA-TOC*

PET/CT Imaging in Brain Tumor

The combination of PET and CT allows obtaining both morphologic and metabolic images in a single imaging session, which reduces the incidence of false-positive findings and increases the confidence of the image to make an affirmative diagnosis. CT data are also used for attenuation correction of the coincident PET data. Compared with PET alone, PET/CT has shown dramatic improvement in diagnostic accuracy [36].

^{18}F-FDG is the most commonly used radiotracer in clinical PET/CT. In clinical processing, hyperglycemia may result in decreased cerebral FDG uptake and poor image quality. Therefore, for patients with diabetes mellitus, the blood glucose level is usually corrected to the normal range before imaging. A patient's mental status and mood may also affect the imaging result. Therefore, after ^{18}F-FDG is administered intravenously, the patient should rest in a quiet room with dim lights and minimal environmental stimulation during the uptake phase of 30–40 min before image acquisition. The patient's bowel and bladder control may require special attention. The patient may be fitted with a thermoplastic mask with an opening for the eyes, nose, and mouth to avoid motion. It is necessary to monitor patients closely for safety. The CT portion of the study is usually acquired immediately before or after the PET acquisition.

Clinical Application of 18F-FDG PET/CT in Brain Tumors

While historically brain tumor was the first human tumor extensively studied by ^{18}F-FDG PET, the routine clinical use of PET or PET/CT on brain tumors has been limited, partly by the higher background uptake and partly by limited reimbursement. Although ^{18}F-FDG PET is useful in the diagnosis and prognosis of hypermetabolic brain cancers, it is not used extensively for staging, rather, it is used more often in the differentiation of recurrent tumor from posttreatment necrosis, which contrast-enhanced MRI only performs with modest sensitivity and low specificity. The detection of cerebral metastasis is also limited because of the highly variable metabolic activities of metastatic tumors and high background brain activities. Nevertheless, ^{18}F-FDG PET is a good tool to monitor disease progression and treatment responses in brain tumors when the baseline study demonstrates hypermetabolism in suspected lesions.

Diagnosis, Staging, and Evaluating Prognosis

Currently, MRI remains the clinical "gold standard" for evaluating brain tumors. The images from PET/CT may offer valuable information for further evaluation. Earlier reports on the correlation of grades with ^{18}F-FDG showed that high-grade brain tumor demonstrated hypermetabolism with high FDG uptake, while low-grade brain tumors revealed low levels of glucose metabolism with less than, equal to, or slightly higher than that of white matter. Quantitative analysis, such as receiver operating characteristic (ROC) curves and SUV, can help to evaluate the PET/CT findings. Studies have shown when differentiating high-grade from low-grade brain tumor, ROC is a more effective quantitative index than SUV [37, 38]. ^{18}F-FDG PET can help to perform accurate biopsies of brain tissue and even allow a reduction in the number of samples acquired [39].

It is well established that ^{18}F-FDG uptake is a good indicator of prognosis and survival in patients with primary brain tumors [40]. For patients following surgery, persistent uptake of ^{18}F-FDG also has prognostic significance. Patients with high ^{18}F-FDG uptake have a significantly worse prognosis than those with low uptake lesions [41]. However, uptake of ^{18}F-FDG cannot be used as the sole independent predictor for evaluating prognosis of brain tumor because histologic grade is more important [42].

Differentiating Tumor Recurrence from Necrosis

Differentiating tumor recurrence from necrosis or scar is one of the most important utilities of ^{18}F-FDG PET/CT. Radiation necrosis is common in patients with brain tumor after radiotherapy, such as GliolSite irradiation with ^{125}I and gamma knife [43, 44]. Intense inflammatory response produces pathologic injury, resulting in disruption of the blood-brain barrier by vascular and astrocytic damage, thus producing radiation necrosis, edema, and cortical dysfunction. An earlier study showed that ^{18}F-FDG PET was clearly superior to CT and MRI in the distinction between tumor recurrence and radiation effects [45]. On ^{18}F-FDG images, the areas of necrosis reveal significantly reduced glucose metabolism while recurrent tumors show increased metabolism (Figs. 15.1 and 15.2) [46]. Areas where ^{18}F-FDG uptake is greater than adjacent normal brain are highly suspicious of recurrent tumors, with a sensitivity of 96% and specificity of 77% [47].

A recent study suggested using dual-phase imaging PET to evaluate radiation necrosis. In this procedure, ^{18}F-FDG excretion from necrotic tissue would be faster than that of brain tumor at delayed times [48]. Further study is needed to evaluate this approach.

Planning Treatment and Monitoring and Assessing Therapy Response

The result of PET/CT may have a direct impact on clinical treatment. For example, when a glioma is diagnosed by ^{18}F-FDG PET/CT, it may direct the subsequent treatment plans such as radiotherapy, chemotherapy, further surgery, or observation. PET/CT can also aid in achieving accurate dosimetry estimates, guiding interventional procedures, and delineating tumor volumes for radiation therapy [49, 50]. A study used MRI-defined volume and ^{18}F-FDG PET-defined volume at the same time to calculate the radiation dose of patients with glioblastomas. The finding was that volume defined by ^{18}F-FDG uptake showed a 0.5-cm larger margin than MRI, which resulted in a higher radiation dose for patients [51]. A combination of PET and CT would better define the radiotreated area than PET alone [52]. Currently, PET/CT-directed radiotherapy has entered the clinical market [53].

As a noninvasive method, ^{18}F-FDG PET/CT can be used in monitoring and assessing therapy response based on metabolic and volumetric changes of pre- and posttherapy. Reduction of glucose metabolism in lesions and/or shrinkage of tumor size can be considered a favorable response as early as 1 or 2 weeks after chemotherapy [54]. A recent study suggested that ^{18}F-FLT may be a better tracer for monitoring treatment response of brain tumor [55].

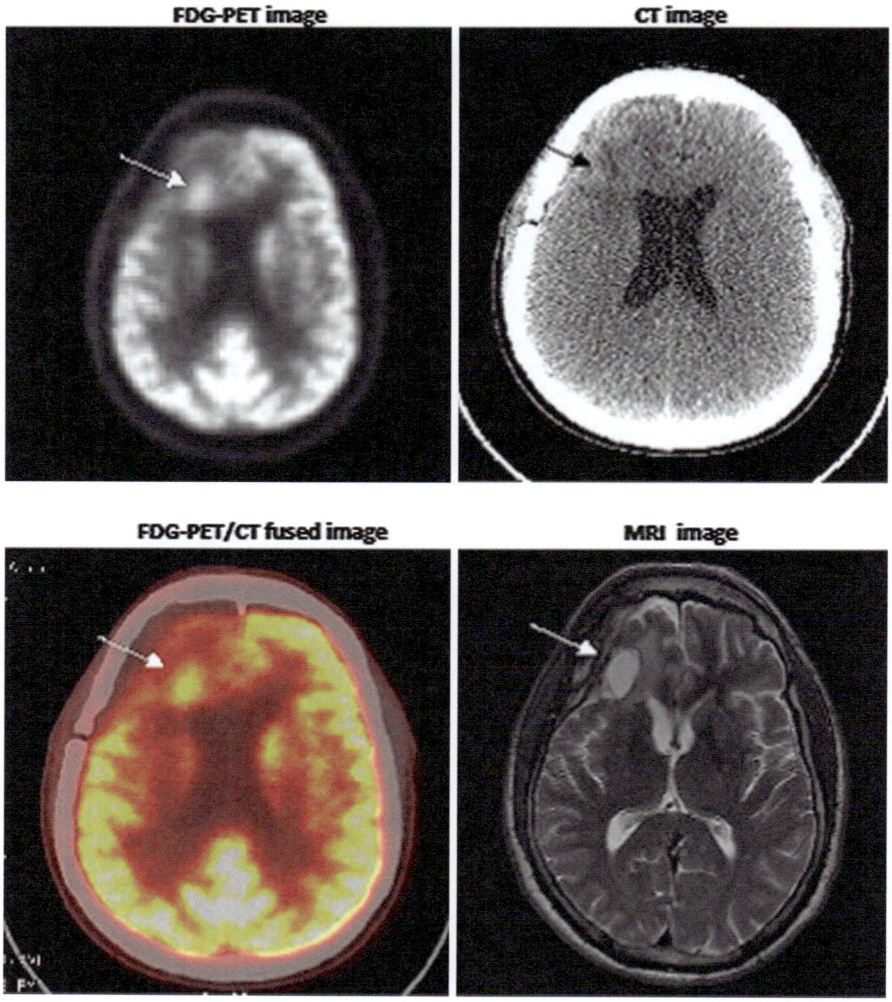

Fig. 15.1 ^{18}F-FDG PET/CT and MRI images of a 55-year-old male with right frontal glioblastoma multiforme. Recent MRI concerned for recurrent disease at the postsurgical site (*arrow*). FDG-PET images show focal increased hypermetabolism, similar to or just below normal cortical activity in the deep right frontal lobe (*arrow*), which corresponds to the enhancing lesion seen on MRI images. Noncontrast CT also show a small mass at this region (*arrow*). All these suggest recurrence at postsurgical site

Detecting Metastatic Brain Tumor

Clinically, metastatic brain tumor can be asymptomatic or it can present with headache, nausea or vomiting, or seizure [56]. Cerebral metastases occur in the supratentorial (80%), cerebellum (18%), and brainstem (2%) [57]. In ^{18}F-FDG images (Fig. 15.3), one or several foci of increased ^{18}F-FDG activity is highly suspicious of metastases. Using contrast-enhanced MRI as the gold standard, ^{18}F-FDG PET identified cerebral metastasis with a sensitivity of 75% and a specificity of 83% [58]. With PET/CT, sensitivity, specificity, and accuracy of ^{18}F-FDG in revealing metastatic brain tumor were 50%,

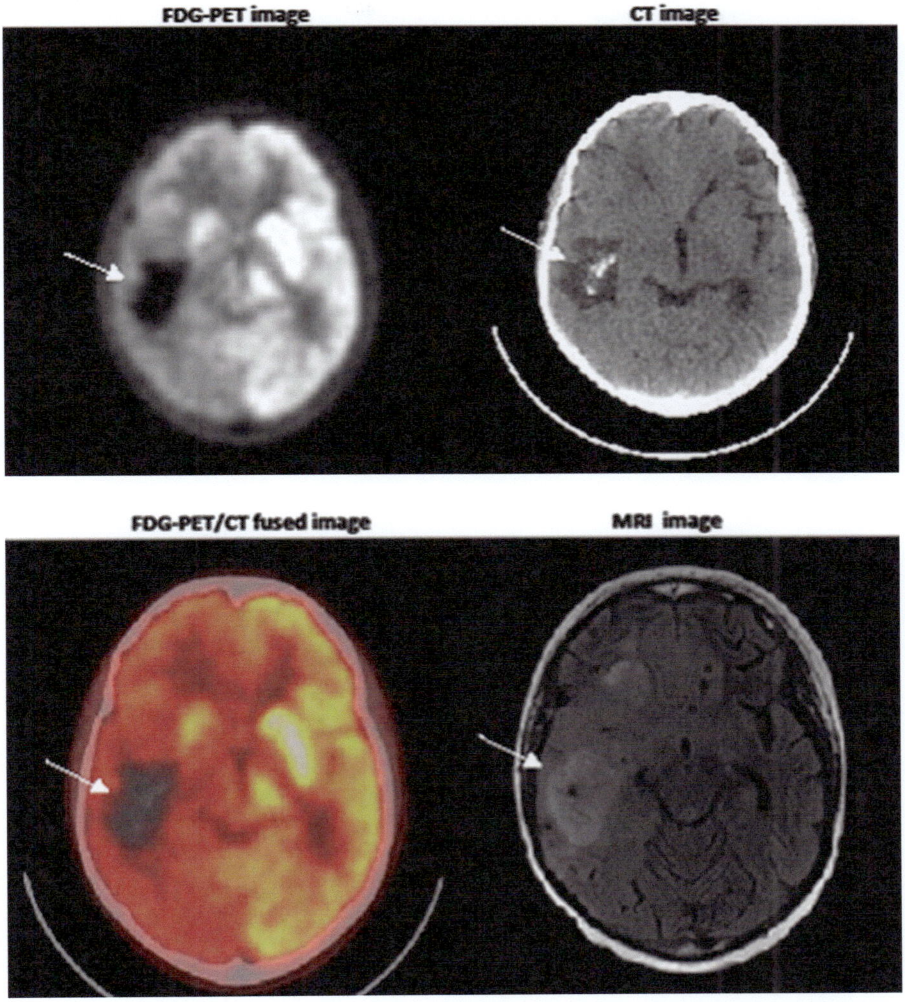

Fig. 15.2 ^{18}F-FDG PET/CT and MRI images of an 11-year-old female with metastatic glioblastoma gliomatous cerebri. FDG-PET image shows a decreased metabolic activity in the right cerebral cortex (*arrow*), suggesting necrotic masses secondary to radiation therapy . CT and MRI images show corresponding changes within this region (*arrow*)

93%, and 76%, respectively [29]. However, the lack of FDG hypermetabolism does not rule out metastasis.

At times, the primary site can be too small to be detected or to cause symptoms. In this situation, metastatic brain tumors may be found first, and the primary site may be discovered later. For patients with cerebral metastasis, whole-body ^{18}F-FDG PET scans were useful in finding the primary cancer in the body with a sensitivity of 79% [59], while the sensitivity of ^{18}F-FDG with PET/CT in search of the primary site increased to 93.3% [60]. On rare occasions, extracerebral metastases from primary gliomas have been identified.

Other Tumors of the Nervous System

Central nervous system (CNS) lymphomas most often occur in men. It has been found that 52% of cases were supratentorial, 34% were multiple,

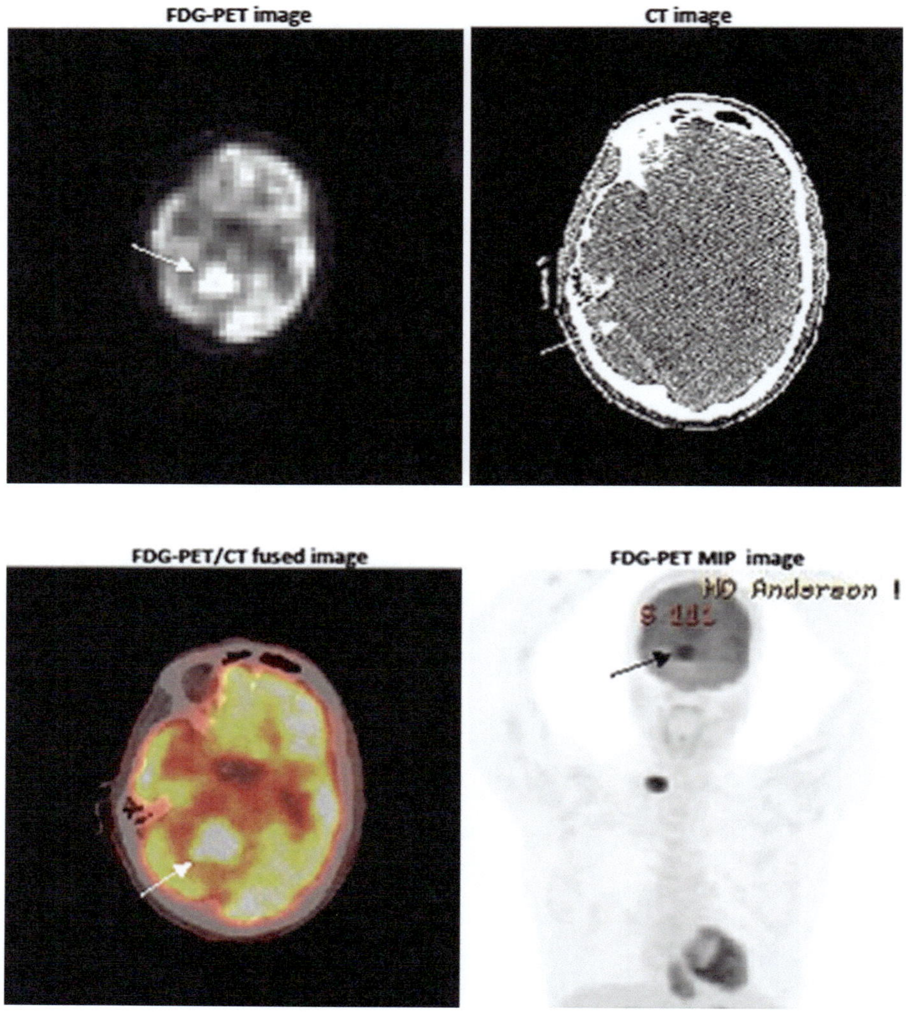

Fig. 15.3 ^{18}F-FDG PET/CT images of a patient with metastatic esophageal cancer. FDG-PET image demonstrates a focal hypermetabolism in right occipital lobe (*arrow*). On noncontrast CT images, edematous changes are seen within this region (*arrow*). Whole body image also shows the brain metastasis (*arrow*)

12% were cerebellar, 2% were in the brainstem, and less than 0.5% were spinal [61]. Only 1% of all non-Hodgkin's lymphomas are primary CNS lymphomas. Increased incidence of CNS lymphoma is correlated with the disappearance of intermediate-grade histology, suggesting a shift in the biology of the tumors [62]. The contrast-enhanced CT and MRI appearance of these lesions is sometimes distinctive. Multiple lesion and homogeneous enhancement of signal is suggestive of CNS lymphoma.

Meningiomas are readily diagnosed by contrast-enhanced MRI. However, recurrent meningiomas are more difficult to detect by MRI and they exhibit a variable degree of glucose hypermetabolism. A recent study of pre- and postsurgical FDG PET reported a sensitivity of 0.43 and a specificity of 0.95 in detecting recurrent meningiomas [63].

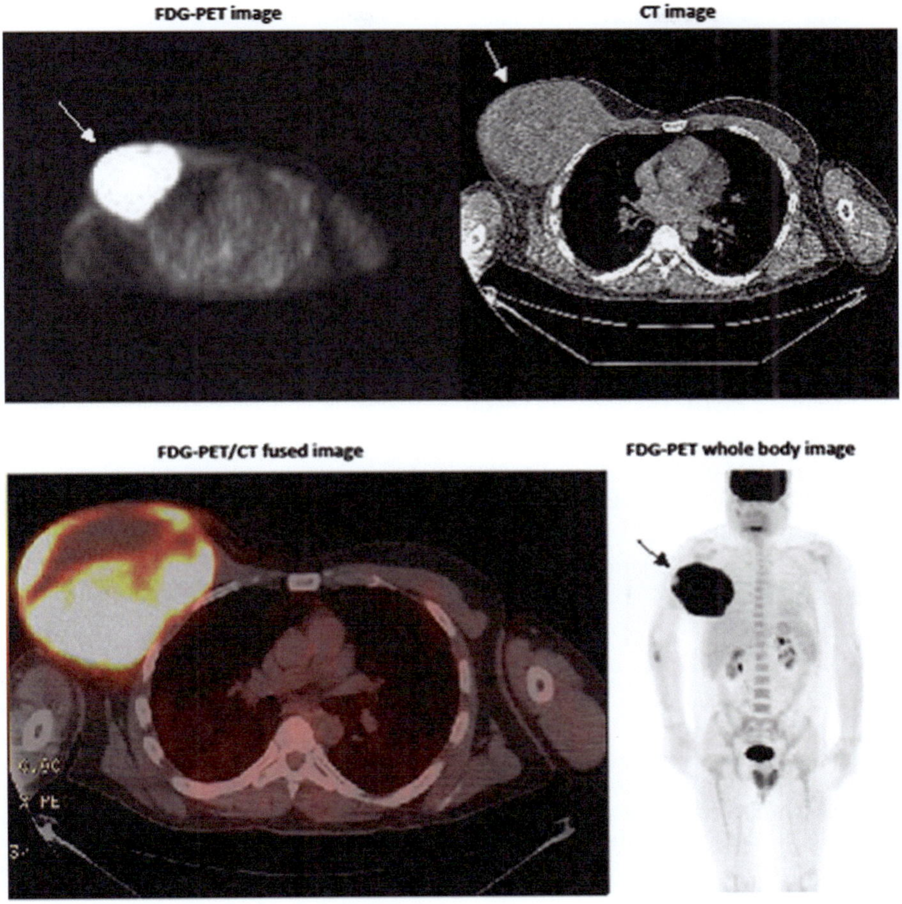

Fig. 15.4 A patient with diagnosed neurofibromatosis. FDG-PET/CT images note a large mass arising from the right pectoralis muscle measuring 17 × 13 × 13 cm with necrotic center and maximum SUV of 19.6 (*arrows*), which is consistent with the sarcomatoid changes in this patient with history of peripheral nerve sheath tumor. No other adenopathy is noted in whole-body images

Although in combination with CT, FDG PET is expected to further gain accuracy, it remains a diagnostic challenge of meningioma patients in routine clinical care. Nerve sheath tumors affect the CNS as acoustic neuroma or Schwannoma and the peripheral nervous system as neurofibromas (Fig. 15.4). Schwannomas may not be readily distinguished from malignant peripheral nerve cell tumors based on SUV from PET/CT. However, SUV is able to differentiate the latter from neurofibromas and determine the transformation of benign peripheral nerve sheath tumors to malignant tumors [64].

Conclusion

As a dominant clinical molecular imaging modality of cancer, PET/CT is rapidly growing and becoming more accepted in the study of brain tumor. In combination with precise anatomic information provided by contemporaneous CT, PET provides metabolic information for lesion localization and characterization. However, the use of PET/CT is currently limited by its complex equipment and high technologic requirement, which depends on the future development of hardware and software. Nonspecificity, false-negative and false-positive findings of ^{18}F-FDG affect clinical outcome. This limitation can be overcome by the development of other radiotracers including metabolism of lipids, amino acids and nucleosides, apoptosis, angiogenesis, and molecular retention schemes.

In addition to scientific and clinical concerns, cost effectiveness of PET/CT should also be considered as a major aspect of patient management. Currently in the US, PET/CT imaging is being widely used in oncologic diseases, including brain tumor. To make PET/CT a routinely useful clinical tool, efforts still need to be made to convince the public-at-large of its impact on the care of brain tumor. Furthermore, successful application of PET/CT in brain tumors also requires meticulous documentation and strict compliance with regulatory requirements.

References

1. CBTRUS (2009). CBTRUS statistical report: primary brain and central nervous system tumors diagnosed in the United States in 2004–2005. Source: central brain tumor registry of the United States, Hinsdale. Website: www.cbtrus.org.
2. Ries LAG, Melbert D, Krapcho M, Mariotto A, Miller BA, Feuer EJ, Clegg L, Horner MJ, Holader N, Eisner MP, Reichman M, Edwards BK, editors. SEER cancer statistics review, 1975–2004, National Cancer Institute. Bethesda, http://seer.cancer.gov/csr/1975_2004/, based on November 2006 SEER data submission, posted to the SEER web site, 2007.
3. Jemal A, Siegel R, Ward E, et al. Cancer statistics, 2009. CA: a cancer journal for clinicians. American Cancer Society. Published online May 2009.
4. Surveillance, Epidemiology, and End Results (SEER) Program (www.seer.cancer.gov) SEER*Stat Database: Incidence – SEER 17 Regs Limited-Use + Hurricane Katrina Impacted Louisiana Cases, Nov 2008 Sub (2000–2006) <Katrina/Rita Population Adjustment> – Linked To County Attributes – Total U.S., 1969–2006 Counties, National Cancer Institute, DCCPS, Surveillance Research Program, Cancer Statistics Branch, released April 2009, based on the November 2008 submission. Analyzed by CBTRUS July 13, 2009.
5. Louis DN, Ohgaki H, Wiestler OD, et al. The 2007 WHO classification of tumours of the central nervous system. Acta Neuropathol. 2007;114:97–109.
6. Norden AD, Wen PY, Kesari S. Brain metastases. Curr Opin Neurol. 2005;18:654–61.
7. Nathoo N, Toms SA, Barnett GH. Metastases to the brain: current management perspectives. Expert Rev Neurother. 2004;4(4):633–40.
8. Alger JR, Frank JA, Bizzi A. Metabolism of human gliomas: assessment with H-1 MR spectroscopy and F-18 fluorodeoxyglucose PET. Radiology. 1990; 177:633–41.
9. Ricci PE. Imaging of adult brain tumors. Neuroimaging Clin N Am. 1999;9:651–69.
10. Kim KT, Black KL, Marciano D, et al. Thallium-201 SPECT imaging of brain tumors: methods and results. J Nucl Med. 1990;31:965–9.
11. Datta NR, Pasricha R, Gambhir S, et al. Postoperative residual tumor imaged by contrast-enhanced CT and Tl-201 SPECT: can they predict progression-free survival in high grade glioma? Clin Oncol. 2004;16: 494–500.
12. O'Tuama LA, Packard AB, Treves ST. SPECT imaging of pediatric brain tumor with hexakis (methoxyisobutylisonitrile) technetium (I). J Nucl Med. 1990; 31:2040–1.
13. Ito M, Lammertsma AA, Wise RSJ, et al. Measurement of regional cerebral blood flow and oxygen utilization in patients with cerebral tumors: analytical techniques and preliminary results. Neuroradiology. 1982;23: 63–74.
14. Yamamoto YL, Thompson CJ, Meyer E, et al. Dynamic positron emission tomography for study of cerebral hemodynamics in a cross section of the head using positron-emitting ^{67}Ga-EDTA and ^{77}Kr. J Comput Assist Tomogr. 1977;1:43.
15. Baba T, Fukiu M, Takeshita I, et al. Selective enhancement of intratumoral blood flow in malignant gliomas using intra-arterial adenosine triphosphate. J Neurosurg. 1990;72(6):907–11.
16. Di Chiro G, De La Paz PL, Brooks RA, et al. Glucose utilization of cerebral gliomas measured by F-18 fluorodeoxyglucose and PET. Neurology. 1982;32: 1323–9.
17. Spence AM, Muzi M, Graham MM, et al. Glucose metabolism in human malignant gliomas measured quantitatively with PET, 1-[C-11]glucose and FDG: analysis of the FDG lumped constant. J Nucl Med. 1998;39(3):440–8.
18. Warburg O, Wind F, Negelein E. The metabolism of tumor in the body. J Gen Physiol. 1927;8:519–30.
19. Blacklock JB, Oldfield EH, Di Chiro G, et al. Effect of barbiturate coma on glucose utilization in normal brain versus gliomas. Positron emission tomography studies. J Neurosurg. 1987;67:71–5.
20. Inoue T, Kim EE, Wong FC, et al. Comparison of fluorine-18-fluorodeoxyglucose and carbon-11-methionine PET in detection of malignant tumors. J Nucl Med. 1996;37:1472–6.
21. Conti PS, Hilton J, Wong DF, et al. High performance liquid chromatography of carbon-11-labeled compounds. J Nucl Med. 1994;21(8):1045–51.
22. Heinisch M, Dirisamer A, Loidl W, et al. Positron emission tomography/ computed tomography with

F-18-fluorocholine for restaging of prostate cancer patients: meaningful at PSA<5 ng/ml? Mol Imaging Biol. 2006;8:43–8.
23. Jacobs AH, Thomas A, Kracht LW, Li H, Dittmar C, Garlip G, et al. ^{18}F-fluoro-L-thymidine and ^{11}C-methylmethionine as markers of increased transport and proliferation in brain tumors. J Nucl Med. 2005;46:1948–58.
24. Chen W, Cloughesy T, Kamdar N, et al. Imaging proliferation in brain tumors with ^{18}F-FLT PET: comparison with ^{18}F-FDG. J Nucl Med. 2005;46(6):945–52.
25. Backes H, Ullrich R, Neumaier B, et al. Noninvasive quantification of (18)F-FLT human brain PET for the assessment of tumour proliferation in patients with high-grade glioma. Eur J Nucl Med Mol Imag. 2009;12:1960–7.
26. Becherer A, Karanikas G, Szabo M, et al. Brain tumour imaging with PET: a comparison between [^{18}F]fluorodopa and [^{11}C]methionine. Eur J Nucl Med Mol Imag. 2003;30:1561–7.
27. Chen W, Silverman DH, Delaloye S, et al. ^{18}F-FDOPA PET imaging of brain tumors: comparison study with ^{18}F-FDG PET and evaluation of diagnostic accuracy. J Nucl Med. 2006;47:904–11.
28. Tripathi M, Sharma R, D'Souza M, et al. Comparative evaluation of F-18 FDOPA, F-18 FDG, and F-18 FLT-PET/CT for metabolic imaging of low gradr gliomas. Clin Nucl Med. 2009;34(12):878–83.
29. Ledezma CJ, Chen W, Sai V, et al. ^{18}F-FDOPA PET/MRI fusion in patients with primary/recurrent gliomas: initial experience. Eur J Radiol. 2009;71:242–8.
30. Choi SJ, Kim JS, Kim JH, et al. [^{18}F]3′-deoxy-3′-fluorothymidine PET for the diagnosis and grading of brain tumors. Eur J Nucl Med Mol Imag. 2005;32(6):653–9.
31. Inoue T, Koyama K, Oriuchi N, et al. Detection of malignant tumors: whole-body PET with fluorine 18 alpha-methyl tyrosine versus FDG – preliminary study. Radiology. 2001;220:54–62.
32. Cher LM, Murone C, Lawrentschuk N, et al. Correlation of hypoxic cell fraction and angiogenesis with glucose metabolic rate in gliomas using ^{18}F-fluoromisonidazole, ^{18}F-FDG PET, and immunohistochemical studies. J Nucl Med. 2006;47:410–8.
33. Ullrich RT, Kracht L, Brunn A, et al. Methyl-L-^{11}C-methionine PET as a diagnostic marker for malignant progression in patients with glioma. J Nucl Med. 2009;50:1962–8.
34. Blasberg RG, Roelcke U, Weinreich R, et al. Imaging brain tumor proliferative activity with [124I]iododeoxyuridine. Cancer Res. 2000;60:624–35.
35. Henze M, Dimitrakopoulou-Strauss A, Milker-Zabel S, et al. Characterization of 68 Ga-DOTA-D-Phe1-Tyr3-octreotide kinetics in patients with meningiomas. J Nucl Med. 2005;46:763–9.
36. Tsukamoto E, Ochi S. PET/CT today: system and its impact on cancer diagnosis. Ann Nucl Med. 2006; 20:255–67.
37. Meyer PT, Schreckenberger M, Spetzger U, et al. Comparison of visual and ROI-based brain tumor grading using ^{18}F-FDG PET: ROC analyses. Eur J Nucl Med. 2001;28:165–74.
38. Hustinx R, Smith RJ, Benard F, et al. Can the standardized uptake value characterize primary brain tumors on FDGPET? Eur J Nucl Med. 1999;26: 1501–9.
39. Pirotte B, Goldman S, Salzberg S, et al. Combined positron emission tomography and magnetic resonance imaging for the planning of stereotactic brain biopsies in children: experience in 9 cases. Pediatr Neurosurg. 2003;38:146–55.
40. Alavi JB, Alavi A, Chawluk J, et al. Positron emission tomography in patients with glioma. A predictor of prognosis. Cancer. 1988;62:1074–8.
41. Holzer T, Herholz K, Jeske J, et al. FDG-PET as a prognostic indicator in radiochemotherapy of glioblastoma. J Comput Assist Tomogr. 1993;17:681–7.
42. De Witte F, Lefranc F, Levivier M, et al. FDG-PET as a prognostic factor in high-grade astrocytoma. J Neurol Oncol. 2000;49:157–63.
43. Malkin MG. Interstitial irradiation of malignant gliomas. Rev Neurol. 1992;148:448–53.
44. Kobayashi T, Tanaka T, Kida Y. The early effects of gamma knife on 40 cases of acoustic neurinoma. Acta Neurochir Suppl. 1994;62:93–7.
45. Mogard J, Kihlström L, Ericson K. Recurrent tumor vs radiation effects after gamma knife radiosurgery of intracerebral metastases: diagnosis with PET-FDG. J Comput Assist Tomogr. 1994;18:177–81.
46. Glantz MJ, Hoffman JM, Coleman RE, et al. Identification of early recurrence of primary central nervous system tumors by [^{18}F]fluorodeoxyglucose positron emission tomography. Ann Neurol. 1991; 29:347–55.
47. Wang SX, Boethius J, Ericson K. FDG-PET on irradiated brain tumor: ten years' summary. Acta Radiol. 2006;47:85–90.
48. Spence AM, Muzi M, Mankoff DA, et al. ^{18}F-FDG PET of gliomas at delayed intervals: improved distinction between tumor and normal gray matter. J Nucl Med. 2004;45:1653–9.
49. Teh BS, Paulino AC, Lu HH, et al. Versatility of the Novalis system to deliver image-guided stereotactic body radiation therapy (SBRT) for various anatomical sites. Technol Cancer Res Treat. 2007;6(4):347–54.
50. Solberg TD, Agazaryan N, Goss BW, et al. A feasibility study of ^{18}F-fluorodeoxyglucose positron emission tomography targeting and simultaneous integrated boost for intensity-modulated radiosurgery and radiotherapy. J Neurosurg. 2004;101(Suppl 3):381–9.
51. Tralins KS, Douglas JG, Stelzer KJ, et al. Volumetric analysis of ^{18}F-FDG PET in glioblastoma multiforme: prognostic information and possible role in definition of target volumes in radiation dose escalation. J Nucl Med. 2002;43:1667–73.
52. Hwang AB, Bacharach SL, Yom SS, et al. Can positron emission tomography (PET) or PET/computed

tomography (CT) acquired in a nontreatment position be accurately registered to a head-and-neck radiotherapy planning CT? Int J Radiat Oncol Biol Phys. 2009;73:578–84.

53. Ciernik IF, Dizendorf E, Baumert BG, et al. Radiation treatment planning with an integrated positron emission and computer tomography (PET/CT): a feasibility study. Int J Radiat Oncol Biol Phys. 2003; 57:853–63.
54. Wieder HA, Brucher BL, Zimmermann F, et al. Time course of tumor metabolic activity during chemoradiotherapy of esophageal squamous cell carcinoma and response to treatment. J Clin Oncol. 2004;22:900–8.
55. Chen W, Delaloye S, Silverman DHS, et al. Predicting treatment response of malignant gliomas to bevacizumab and irinotecan by imaging proliferation with [^{18}F] fluorothymidine positron emission tomography: a pilot study. J Clin Oncol. 2007;25:4714–21.
56. Fadul C, Misulis KE, Wiley RG. Cerebellar metastases: diagnostic and management considerations. J Clin Oncol. 1987;5:1107–15.
57. Weisberg LA. Solitary cerebellar metastases: clinical and CT correlations. Arch Neurol. 1985;42:336–41.
58. Rohren E, Provenzale J, Barboriak D, et al. Screening for cerebral metastases with FDG-PET in patients undergoing whole-body staging of non-central nervous system malignancy. Radiology. 2003;226(1): 181–7.
59. Jeon H-J, Chung J-K, Kim Y-K, et al. Usefulness of whole-body F-18 FDG PET in patients with suspected metastatic brain tumors. J Nucl Med. 2003;43(11): 1432–7.
60. Nakagawa K, Aoyagi M, Inaji M, et al. The usefulness of whole body FDG-PET/CT in patients with brain metastasis. No Shinkei Geka. 2009;37:159–66.
61. Murray K, Kun L, Cox J. Primary malignant lymphoma of the central nervous system. Results of treatment of 11 cases and review of the literature. J Neurosurg. 1986;65:600–7.
62. Miller DC, Hochberg FH, Harris NL, et al. Pathology with clinical correlations of primary central nervous system non-Hodgkin's lymphoma. The Massachusetts General Hospital experience 1958–1989. Cancer. 1994;74:1383–97.
63. Lee JW, Kang KW, Park SH, et al. ^{18}F-FDG PET in the assessment of tumor grade and prediction of tumor recurrence in intracranial meningioma. Eur J Nucl Med Mol Imag. 2009;36:1574–82.
64. Benz MR, Czernin J, Dry SM, et al. Quantitative F-18 fluorodeoxyglucose PET accurately characterizes peripheral nerve sheath tumors as malignant or benign. Cancer. 2010;116:451–8.

Head and Neck Tumors

16

Franklin C.L. Wong, Xiaoyi Duan,
and E. Edmund Kim

Head and neck cancer is the sixth most common cancer worldwide and makes up 2–5% of cancers in the population. In 2009, the estimated number of new diagnosed head and neck cancers was 35,720 in the US, which includes 10,530 tongue cancers, 10,750 mouth cancers, 12,610 pharynx cancers, and 1,830 other oral cavity cancers [1]. Head and neck cancers are more common in men and account for 66–95% of all cases. Most patients with head and neck cancer are between the ages of 50 and 70 years and the number increases with age, especially after 50 years of age [2]. Head and neck cancers are strongly associated with certain environmental and lifestyle risk factors, including tobacco smoking, alcohol consumption, occupational exposure, and certain strains of viruses, such as the sexually transmitted human papillomavirus [3–5].

Most head and neck cancers occur in the tongue base or within the tonsillar fossa (75%). Head and neck squamous cell carcinomas (HNSCC) make up the vast majority of head and neck cancers (90%). It mostly occurs in males over the age of 40 years with a history of heavy alcohol use coupled with smoking.

Staging criteria for head and neck cancer based on the tumor node metastasis (TNM) system, which is outlined in Table 16.1.

There are more than 30,000 new cases of primary thyroid cancers in the US annually, and the incidence is increasing [6]. In 2009, there were 37,200 new cases of thyroid cancers in the US of which 27,200 were in women, accounting for 4% of all cancers occurring in women [1]. According to the histology or cell structure, thyroid cancers are classified into four types: Papillary cancer (70–80%), follicular (10%), medullary (5–10%), anaplastic (2–5%), metastases (3–5%). Papillary and follicular tumors, still named "differentiated thyroid cancer", are the most common types, with a more favorable prognosis than the medullary and undifferentiated types, but, if metastasis occurs, the prognosis is poor [7].

Staging of thyroid cancer depends on the type of cancer and the age of the patient. TNM staging for differentiated thyroid cancer and medullary thyroid cancer are outlined in Table 16.2.

F.C.L. Wong, M.D., Ph.D., J.D. (✉)
Departments of Nuclear Medicine and Neurooncology, The University of Texas MD Anderson Cancer Center, Houston, TX 77030, USA
e-mail: fwong@mdanderson.org

X. Duan, M.D.
Department of Nuclear Medicine, First Affiliated Hospital, Xian Jiaotong University, College of Medicine, Shaanxi 710061, China
e-mail: duanxt2009@hotmail.com

E.E. Kim, M.D., M.S.
Departments of Nuclear Medicine and Diagnostic Radiology, The University of Texas MD Anderson Cancer Center and Medical School, Houston, TX 77030, USA

Graduate School of Convergence Science and Technology, Seoul National University, Seoul, South Korea
e-mail: ekim@mdanderson.org

E.E. Kim et al. (eds.), *Clinical PET and PET/CT: Principles and Applications*,
DOI 10.1007/978-1-4419-0802-5_16, © Springer Science+Business Media New York 2013

Table 16.1 TNM staging for head and neck cancer

TX: Cannot be assessed
T0: No primary tumor
Tis: In situ
T1: <2 cm
T2: 2–4 cm
T3: >4 cm
T4: Invades adjacent structures (bone, deep muscle, sinus, skin)
NX: Cannot be assessed
N0: No evidence of regional lymph node metastasis
N1: Metastasis in a single ipsilateral lymph node (≤3 cm)
N2: a. Single ipsilateral lymph node (3–6 cm)
b. Multiple ipsilateral lymph nodes (<6 cm)
c. Bilateral or contralateral lymph nodes (<6 cm)
N3: Metastasis in a lymph node (>6 cm)
MX: Presence of distant metastasis cannot be assessed
M0: No evidence of distant metastasis
M1: Distant metastasis present

Table 16.2 Staging for thyroid cancers

Differentiated thyroid cancer
Less than 45 years of age
Stage I: Tumor of any size with regional node metastasis, no distant metastasis
Stage II: Tumor of any size with regional node metastasis, distant metastasis
45 years of age or older
Stage I: Tumor <2 cm, and remains localized to the thyroid
Stage II: Tumor 2–4 cm, and remains in the thyroid
Stage III: Tumor of any size with regional lymph node metastasis
Stage IV: Tumor of any size with distant metastasis
Medullary thyroid cancer
Stage 0: Cancerous cells have been found through a special screening but there is no tumor
Stage I: Tumor <2 cm, and remains in the thyroid
Stage II: Tumor 2–4 cm, and remains in the thyroid
Stage III: Tumor >4 cm, with regional tissues or lymph node metastasis
Stage IV: Distant metastasis

Imaging of Head and Neck Tumors

Computed Tomography and Magnetic Resonance Imaging

Currently, computed tomography (CT) and magnetic resonance imaging (MRI) with contrast enhancement are the standard imaging techniques for the evaluation of head, neck, and thyroid cancers, which can provide structural information at a high spatial resolution. MRI is superior to CT for laryngeal and hypopharyngeal tumor staging, with high sensitivity and specificity [8]. Soft tissue between the cricoids cartilage and the airway may represent subglottic carcinoma or extension. Thyroid adenomas may appear brighter than normal thyroid tissue on T1-weighted images, possibly related to hemorrhagic degeneration. Thyroid carcinomas show T1 and T2 prolongation. Parathyroid adenomas tend to have longer T2 relaxation times than thyroid adenomas. Tissue characterization of MRI, such as spin-echo sequences, is useful in distinguishing posttreatment fibrosis from recurrent cancer. Discrimination between adenomas and hyperplasia is not possible with MRI [9], because metastatic nodes show contrast enhancement in the rim. MRI has another advantage over CT in the differentiation of lymphadenopathy with various slice orientations and gradient echo techniques revealing vessels [10]. Magnetic resonance angiography allows excellent depiction of the carotid vessels, and is indicated in evaluating vascular displacement or compression by tumor growth and perfusion.

Magnetic Resonance Spectroscopy

Early experience with in vivo magnetic resonance spectroscopy (MRS) has shown its potential for obtaining biochemical information, thus enhancing the diagnostic sensitivity of MRI studies [11]. However, when applied in head and neck tumor, MRS is disappointing because MRS requires a homogeneous magnetic field, while susceptibility artifacts introduced by the paranasal sinuses, airway, and bone, and pulsation artifacts from the carotid artery, severely degrade data. Additionally, a large amount of fat within the neck produces a lipid peak that obscures the relatively small peaks of tumor markers, such as choline. Finally, MRS remains nonspecific. However, with the development of newer techniques, MRS may become practical for evaluating head and neck tumors [12].

Neck Ultrasound

Neck ultrasound (US) has been reported to be superior to palpation in the detection of lymph node metastases [13]. A study reported a sensitivity of 96.8% and a specificity of 93.3% for US in the diagnosis of head and neck cancers, and 91.7% and 91.7%, respectively, in the diagnosis of papillary thyroid cancers [14].

US-guided fine-needle aspiration biopsy (USGFNAB) of thyroid nodules is currently used by many clinicians, with accuracy of 98% in the diagnosis for primary thyroid cancers. The result from FNAB could affect clinical management in 85% of patients with thyroid nodules [15]. The false negative rate of FNAB for benign thyroid lesions is from 1% to 5% [16]. In addition to thyroid nodules, USGFNAB is also applied to neck masses, including cervical nodal metastases from thyroid and other head and neck cancers. Sufficient cells from lymph nodes as small as 3–4 mm can be obtained by USGFNAB [17].

The disadvantages of US include the following facts: First, procedures are time consuming and operator-dependent; Second, interpretation of US images is subjective, requiring experience and expertise with head and neck US and anatomy knowledge by individual acquiring the images; Third, regions, such as areas deep to bone or air-filled structures, are not well visualized by US; Fourth, it is limited to regional study, not a whole-body imaging technique.

Single-Photon Emission Computed Tomography

Functional imaging such as ^{99m}Tc-MIBI or ^{201}TI single-photon emission computed tomography (SPECT) has been reported as a useful modality in the staging of primary neck and head tumors, in the differentiation of metastatic from reactive lymph nodes, and is particularly useful for detection of occult head and neck tumors and for assessing recurrences. On the basis of whole-body scanning, SPECT is also helpful for screening of distant metastases [18, 19].

Fused SPECT/CT has emerged during the past decade, which correlates anatomic information from CT with functional information from SPECT. In recent years, SPECT/CT has been used for SN mapping, which is very important clinically if the tumor is located in body parts with ambiguous lymph node drainage. Fused SPECT/CT SN mapping is often performed before SN biopsy and could provide additional data that are of clinical relevance to SN biopsy in patients with trunk or head and neck melanoma and in patients with mucosal head and neck [20].

Some studies have reported on the role of ^{131}I SPECT/CT for investigation of differentiated thyroid cancers. This modality could accurately localize regional and distant metastases and, in the postsurgical patient, may identify residual thyroid tissues. This allows staging and risk stratification of patients prior to ^{131}I therapy [21]. With specific cancer types such as thyroid and parathyroid cancer, SPECT/CT is indeed a useful tool.

Positron Emission Tomography (PET) and PET/CT

The anatomic information from CT or MRI alone cannot completely reveal histopathologic and physiologic characteristics of tumors. Metabolism imaging such as PET might help to characterize the biologic behavior of both primary and metastatic diseases.

Head, neck, and thyroid tumors, either primary or metastatic tumors, have been studied with PET using ^{18}F-fluorodeoxyglucose (FDG) for viability, ^{11}C-methionine for amino acid transport [22], ^{18}F-fluorothymidine for cell proliferation [23], as well as ^{18}F-fluoromisonidazole for hypoxia [24]. The apparent advantages of these agents are their higher specificity and low background. To date, ^{18}F-FDG PET has become an accepted and widely used imaging modality for the evaluation of head and neck cancer [25–28]. However, because of the complex anatomy of the head and neck region, the clinical application of PET is limited by lack of anatomic detail.

Hybrid PET/CT is a promising imaging technique that permits almost synchronous image acquisition of anatomic and metabolic datasets. Compared with PET alone, PET/CT showed a higher accuracy for the detection of head and neck cancer (96% for PET/CT, 90% for PET alone) [29]. Another major advantage of PET/CT is the reduction of scanning time. Single PET examination alone still requires a transmission scan for attenuation correction. Combined CT and PET can obtain anatomic and functional images consecutively in one examination, and attenuation correction by incorporation of fast CT technology (2 min for a whole-body study), which is much faster than using a transmission scan. Therefore, the examination time of PET/CT is notably shortened [30].

Hybrid PET/CT is performed approximately 1 hour after the intravenous injection of ^{18}F-FDG, with acquisition of CT data immediately preceding acquisition of emission data. During the uptake period, patients are advised not to speak, as this may result in vocal cord uptake which could be misinterpreted as pathologic. Patients are also advised not to move or chew during the uptake period. In order for images to be easier illustrated, oral diazepam may be used before the injection of ^{18}F-FDG to help prevent unwanted uptake in neck muscles as a result of tension [31].

Clinically used radiopharmaceuticals include those involved in metabolism of glucose, nucleosides, amino acids, hypoxia, or transporters (Table 16.3).

Clinical Application of 18F-FDG PET/CT in Head and Neck Tumors

As MRI or CT can better evaluate local soft-tissue and bony anatomy, PET/CT is rarely used for initial T staging of primary tumors. Hybrid PET/CT may be helpful in delineation of extent of regional lymph node involvement, detection of distant metastases, identification of an unknown primary tumor, monitoring of the treatment response, long-term surveillance for recurrence and metastases, and planning radiotherapy.

Staging Primary Head and Neck Tumors

Accurate staging has a prognostic value and is important in selecting the appropriate treatment strategy. A recent multicenter prospective study showed that adding whole-body ^{18}F-FDG PET to the pretherapeutic conventional staging modality, such as US, CT, or MRI, can improve the TNM classification of HNSCC and it altered the management of 13.7% of 233 patients [39]. The result supports the implementation of ^{18}F-FDG PET in the routine imaging work-up of HNSCC. Compared with PET alone, PET/CT provides better localization of foci increased FDG uptake, thus reducing the number of equivocal PET [40]. A recent study reported that sensitivity of PET/CT was slightly higher than that of PET alone, while specificity of PET/CT was significantly higher than that of PET alone in patients with initial staging and follow-up of head and neck cancers (initial staging: 90.5% vs. 62.2%; follow-up: 97.2% vs. 74.4%) [41]. Results of PET/CT may alter the treatment plan in some patients with head and neck cancers [42]. For the detection of distant metastases, ^{18}F-FDG PET/CT had a sensitivity of 89%, a specificity of 97%, and an overall accuracy of 96%, while sensitivity and specificity were 61–97% and 21–100% for MRI or CT [43]. The initial staging and detecting metastases of head and neck tumors with ^{18}F-FDG PET/CT are demonstrated in Figs. 16.1 and 16.2.

It is clear that nodal size alone has not been a good discriminator in the assessment of possible malignant involvement. Small nodes can harbor a metastatic tumor and large nodes may simply reflect reactive change. ^{18}F-FDG PET/CT is helpful in the detection of nodal metastases as small as 10 mm. Its sensitivity, specificity, and accuracy were 84%, 91%, and 89% respectively [44]. While false-positives were notable in some patients with lymph nodes smaller than 3 mm [45]. In these cases, selective neck dissection or lymph node biopsy is more definitive.

Thyroid nodules are relatively common. The prevalence of incidental thyroid FDG uptake (including both focal and diffuse lesions) was

Table 16.3 Clinically used radiotracers for evaluation of head, neck, and thyroid tumors

Radiotracer	Imaging modality	Metabolism	Disease	Sensitivity %	Specificity %	Gold standard	References
^{18}F-FDG	PET/CT	Glucose	Head and neck tumor	89	95	Pathology	[41]
			Differentiated thyroid cancer	95	91	Pathology	[32]
^{18}F-FDOPA	PET/CT	Amino acids	Medullary thyroid cancer	81	–	Pathology	[33]
^{18}F-FLT	PET	Nucleosides	Head and neck tumor	95	–	Pathology	[34]
^{18}F-FMISO	PET	Hypoxia	Head and neck tumor	79	–	Pathology	[35]
^{18}F-FET	PET/CT	Amino acids	Head and neck tumor	64	100	Pathology	[36]
^{124}I NaI	PET/CT	Nucleosides	Differentiated thyroid cancer	90	–	Pathology	[37]
^{99m}Tc-MIBI	SPECT	Perfusion	Head and neck tumor	90	78	Pathology	[18]
^{131}I NaI	SPECT/CT	Nucleosides	Differentiated thyroid cancer	48	–	Pathology	[38]

^{18}F-FDG ^{18}F-fluorodeoxyglucose, *^{18}F-FDOPA* F-18 fluoro didroxyphenylalanine, *^{18}F-FLT* F-18 fluoro-3'-deoxy-L- fluorothymidine, *^{18}F-FMISO* F-18 fluoro-misonidazole, *^{18}F-FET* O-(2-[(18)F]-fluoroethyl)-L-tyrosine, *^{124}I NaI* I-124 sodium iodide, *^{99m}Tc-MIBI* Tc-99m sestamibi, *^{131}I NaI* I-131 sodium iodide

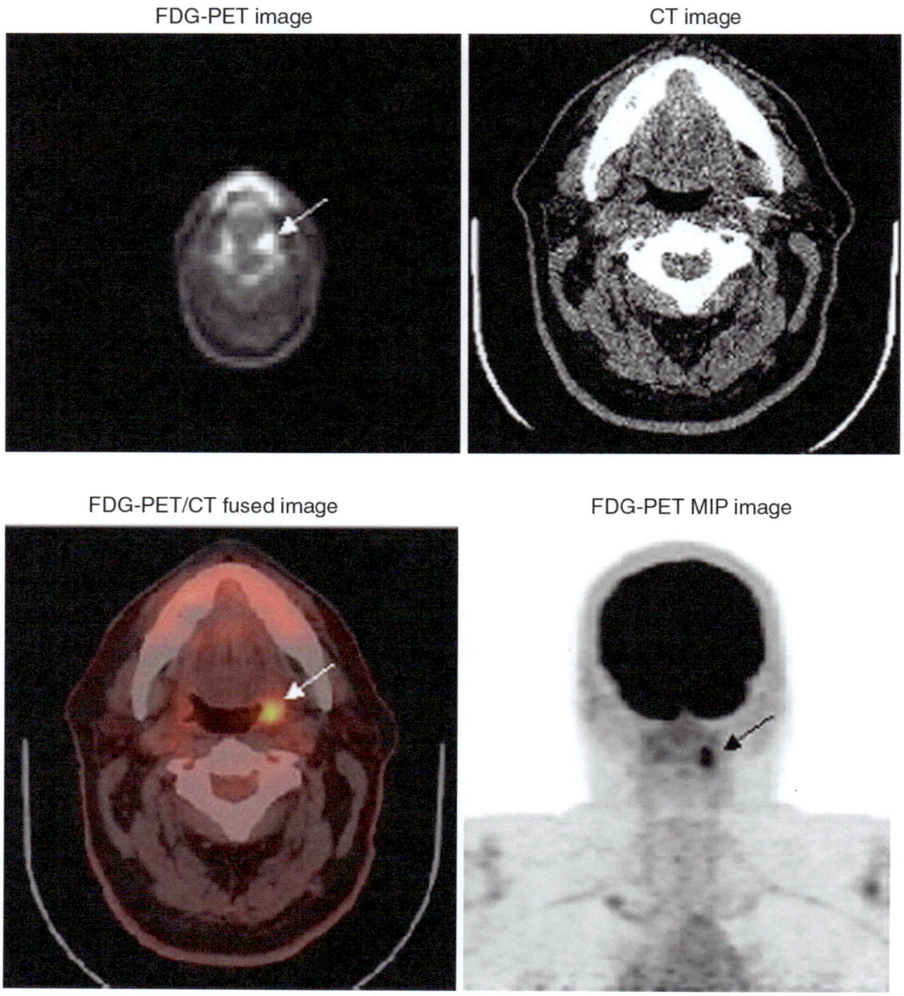

Fig. 16.1 A 62-year-old male with recently diagnosed left tonsillar carcinoma. FDG-PET images show a focal abnormal uptake at the left tonsil represents the patient's known primary tumor with maximum SUV of 5.1 (*arrow*). The corresponding lesion is noted on CT (*arrow*). Fused and MIP images show the lesion clearly (*arrows*). No evidence of active regional nodal or distant metastatic disease

3.8% on FDG PET/CT. Of focal lesions, the cancer risk is 63.6% on pathologic basis [46]. Diffuse thyroid FDG uptake is most probably benign and usually caused by thyroiditis [47].

In thyroid tumors, PET/CT is no better than US and CT for initial evaluation of cervical node [48]. Hybrid PET/CT may be used for detecting recurrent thyroid cancer and localizing neoplasm to facilitate biopsy of incidental findings. The correlation between standard uptake value (SUV) intensity and the risk for a malignant lesion is still controversial [49, 50]. In the case of focal FDG uptake, USGFNAB is likely to obtain a tissue diagnosis, with diagnostic accuracy of 98% [15]. For medullary tumor, PET/CT is superior to anatomic imaging in identifying the source of persistent measurable calcitonin in patients who have undergone total thyroidectomy [51, 52].

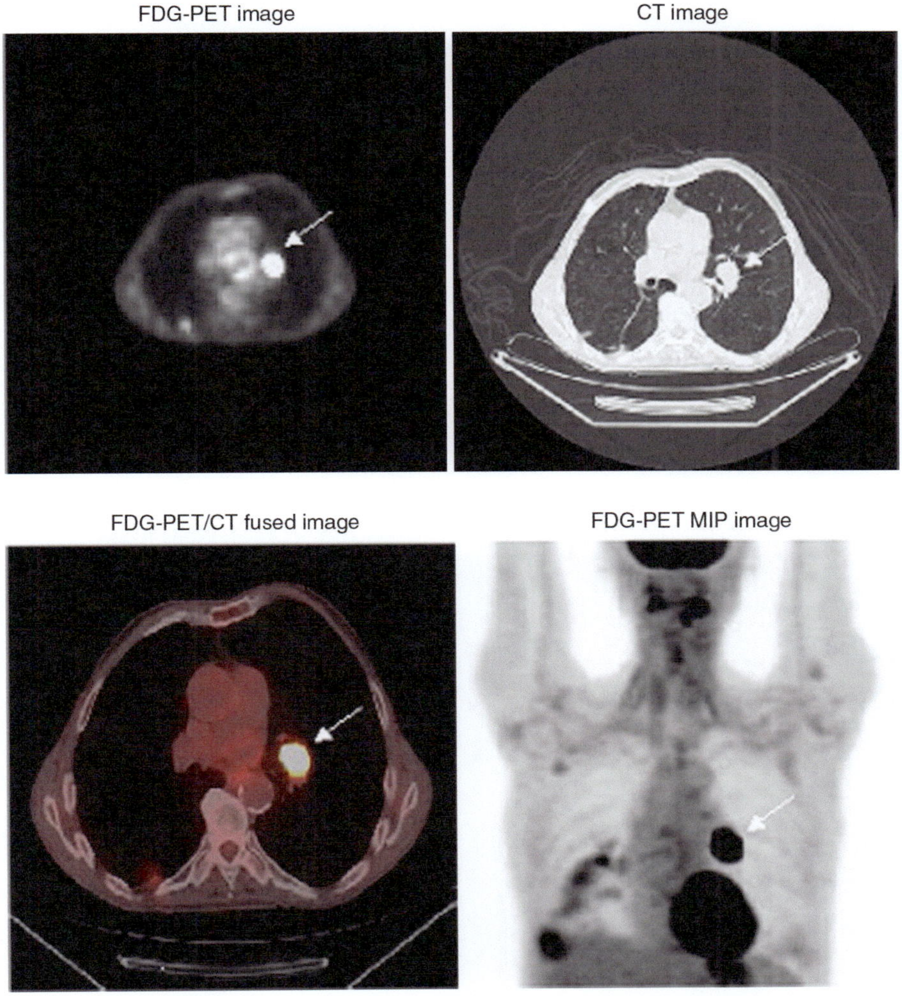

Fig. 16.2 A patient with squamous cell cancer in the tongue who has undergone chemoradiation. FDG-PET/CT images show an active area at left hilar with maximum SUV of 14.5, which may represents a head/neck metastatic lesion (*arrows*). Deep FNA confirms metastatic squamous carcinoma

Detecting Recurrent Tumors

After therapy, early detection of recurrence is critical to achieve an optimal outcome. After surgery or radiation therapy for head and neck tumors, the regional anatomy is distorted. Therefore, anatomic imaging such as CT and MRI has relatively poor specificity in the assessment of residual or recurrent disease [53, 54]. There is a relatively high sensitivity for ^{18}F-FDG PET/CT to detect recurrent disease at the primary tumor site (Fig. 16.3). It also finds regional lymph node metastases at earlier stage than conventional imaging [28, 55, 56]. Approximately 70% of patients with head and neck cancer with positive PET/CT findings were confirmed to have recurrent tumor by histopathology [57]. Abnormal physiologic uptake, metabolically active tissues such as brown adipose tissue and muscle contractions are the main reasons of false-positive results for PET/CT [58]. FNAB should be performed if PET/CT findings could not settle the issue.

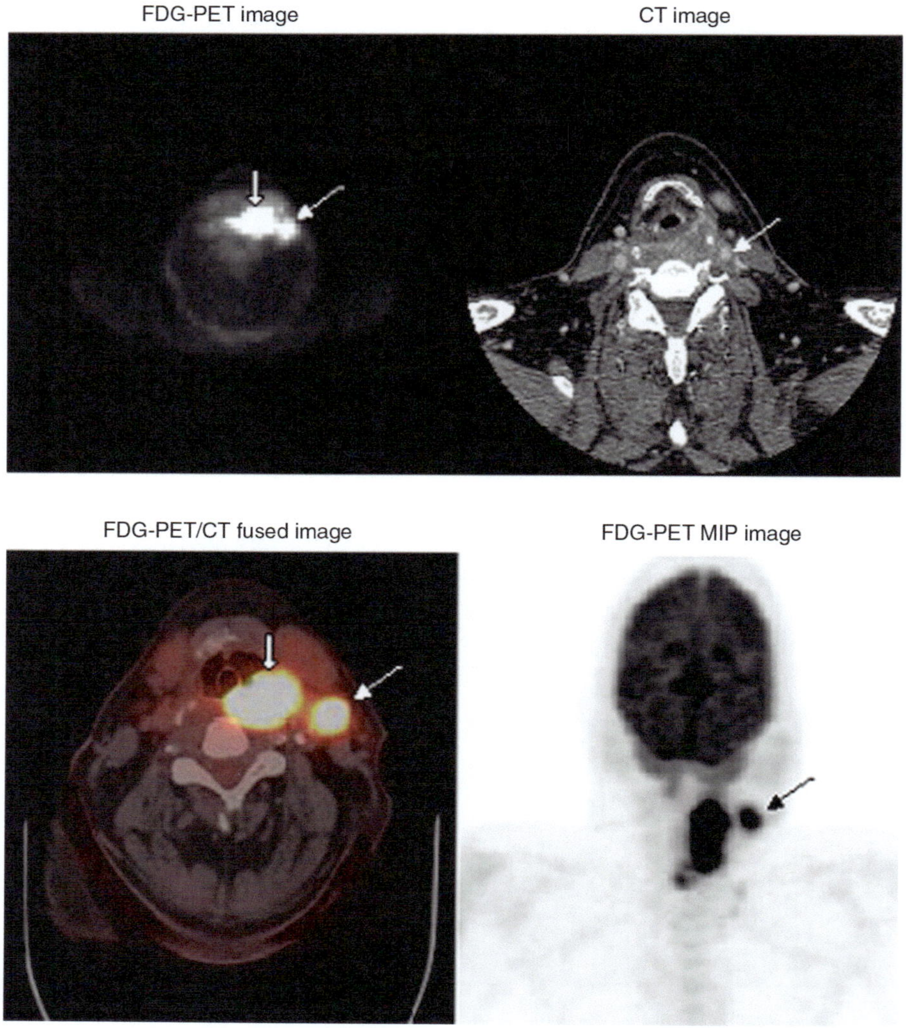

Fig. 16.3 A 54-year-old male with history of T1 squamous cell cancer in the left glottis and underwent laser resection in 09/2006. FDG-PET/CT images note a hypermetabolic lesion measuring 2.5×2 cm in the left oropharynx with SUV of 11, which is consistent with recurrence of tumor (*down arrows*). There is also hypermetabolic adenopathy in the left neck measuring 1.9×1.7 cm and SUV of 15.8 (*arrows*), which is confirmed to be metastatic squamous cell carcinoma by lymph node biopsy

Although well-differentiated papillary and follicular thyroid cancers are treatable, 20% of patients have a recurrence associated with an 8% death rate. Earlier detection and effective management of local recurrence can improve the prognosis for these patients. Whole-body ^{131}I scintigraphy (WBS) and serial thyroglobulin measurement are standard methods for detecting differentiated thyroid cancer recurrence. However, WBS is negative in 10–15% of patients with detectable serum Tg levels [59]. A meta-analysis reported the sensitivity and specificity of ^{18}F-FDG PET/CT in detection of recurrent or metastatic differentiated thyroid cancer were 93.5% and 83.9% respectively in patients with elevated serum thyroglobulin and negative ^{131}I scan [60], as demonstrated in Fig. 16.4. When used as a predictor for survival of thyroid cancer, ^{18}F-FDG

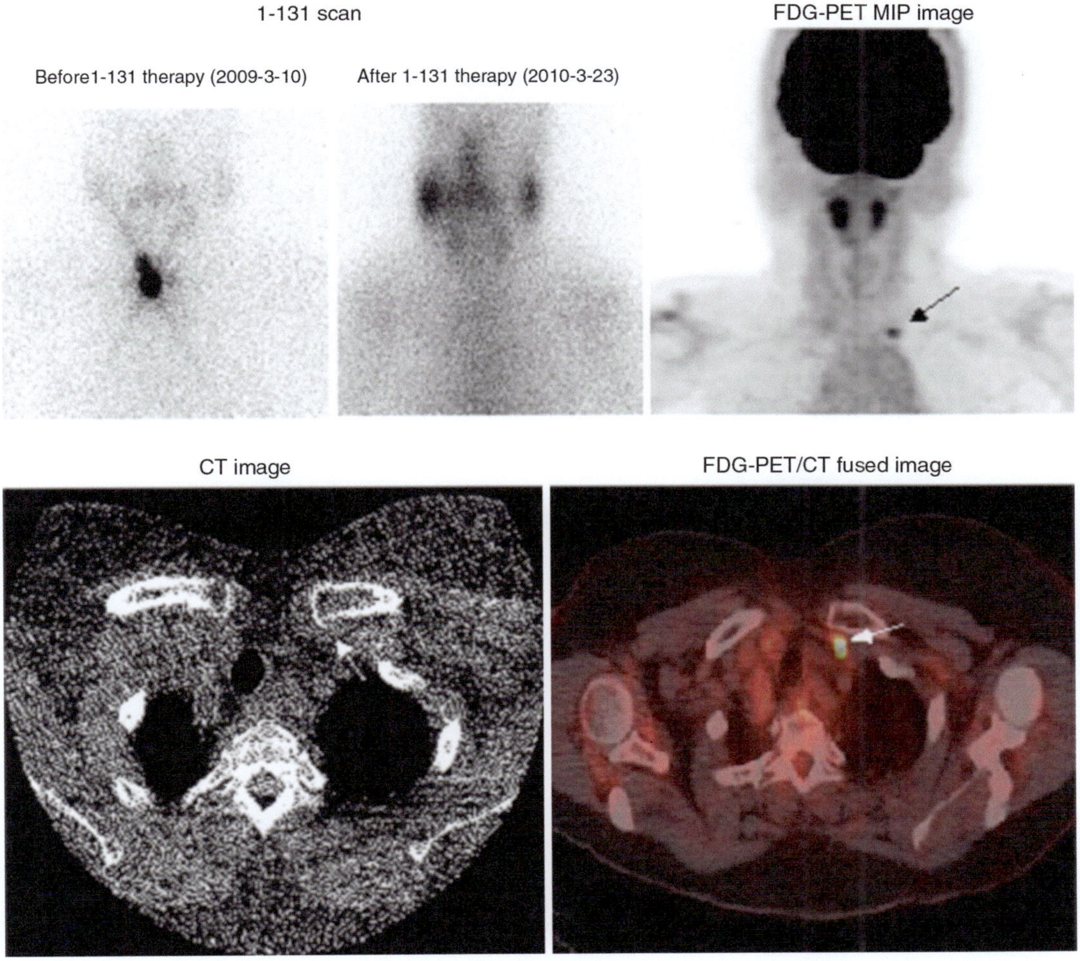

Fig. 16.4 A 64-year-old female with poorly differentiated thyroid cancer. Thyroidectomy was performed in 10/2008, followed by radioiodine ablation therapy. Of note, she has rising thyroglobulin level, with negative I-131 whole body scan. FDG-PET/CT images show focal hypermetabolism in the left supraclavicular region with SUV 6.3, which is consistent with recurrent thyroid cancer (*arrows*)

uptake of thyroid tumor correlated with elevated Tg and negative ^{131}I scan. High ^{18}F-FDG uptake may mean shorter survival [61].

Finding Unknown Primary Tumors

Approximately 2–9% of all HNSCCs present in the way how cervical malignant nodes have been detected but primary tumor site has failed to demonstrate [62]. Hybrid PET/CT is useful in these cases. A recent meta-analysis addressed 150 patients who had initial negative MRI findings, in which the primary tumors in 40 patients were detected by ^{18}F-FDG PET [63]. Another study reported patients with biopsy-proved metastatic disease from unknown head and neck primary tumor undergoing further evaluation with ^{18}F-FDG PET/CT. It showed that 57% of unknown primary tumors were detected by PET/CT [64]. The common sites for false-negative ^{18}F-FDG PET/CT scans are often the lingual and palatine tonsils because of their physiologic uptake. In such cases, asymmetric uptake may be an indicator of tumors. One precaution for salivary gland tumor is that the vast majority of FDG

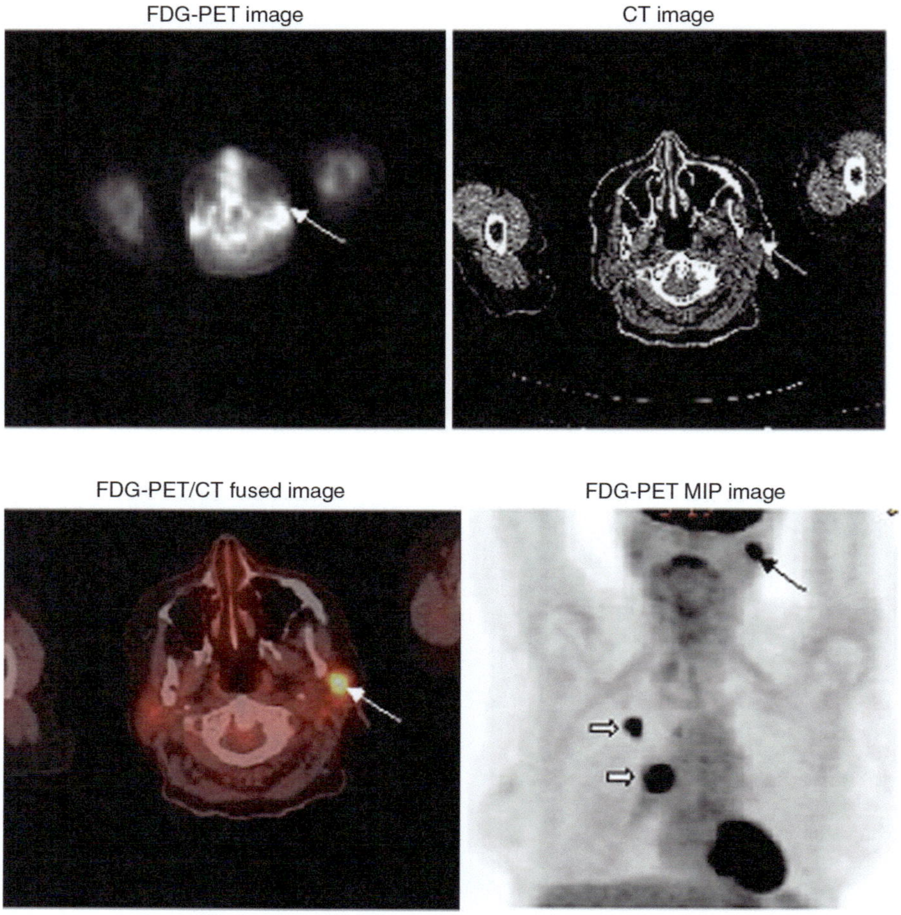

Fig. 16.5 A 73-year old female with diagnosed right non-small cell lung cancer and right hilar nodal metastases (*right arrows*). An incidental finding of pleomorphic adenoma with hypermetabolism is noted in the left parotid gland, likely representing benign lesion such as pleomorphic adenoma or Warthin's tumor (*arrows*)

hypermetabolic lesions in the salivary glands (especially the parotids) are benign tumors including pleomorphic adnoma (80%) or Warthin's tumor (<15%) (Fig. 16.5) [65].

Monitoring the Response to Therapy

Patients could benefit from periodic surveillance after treatment. For example, the early identification of nonresponders to a particular therapy would allow physicians to discontinue ineffective treatments and initiate alternative approaches. Theoretically, metabolic changes of tumor cells are earlier and better predictors of therapeutic effects than anatomic changes shown by CT or MRI [66]. Additionally, because often in cases there is residual fibrosis, edema, or tissue necrosis after surgery, chemotherapy, or radiation therapy, it is difficult for anatomic imaging to differentiate these conditions from tumor recurrence. Therefore, anatomic imaging is not sufficient for assessing response to therapy. Hybrid PET/CT could make up for this limitation and provide valuable information about the efficacy of radiation therapy or chemotherapy regimens (Fig. 16.6).

An early study has suggested that reduced FDG uptake after treatment appeared to coincide with a decline in the number of viable tumor cells

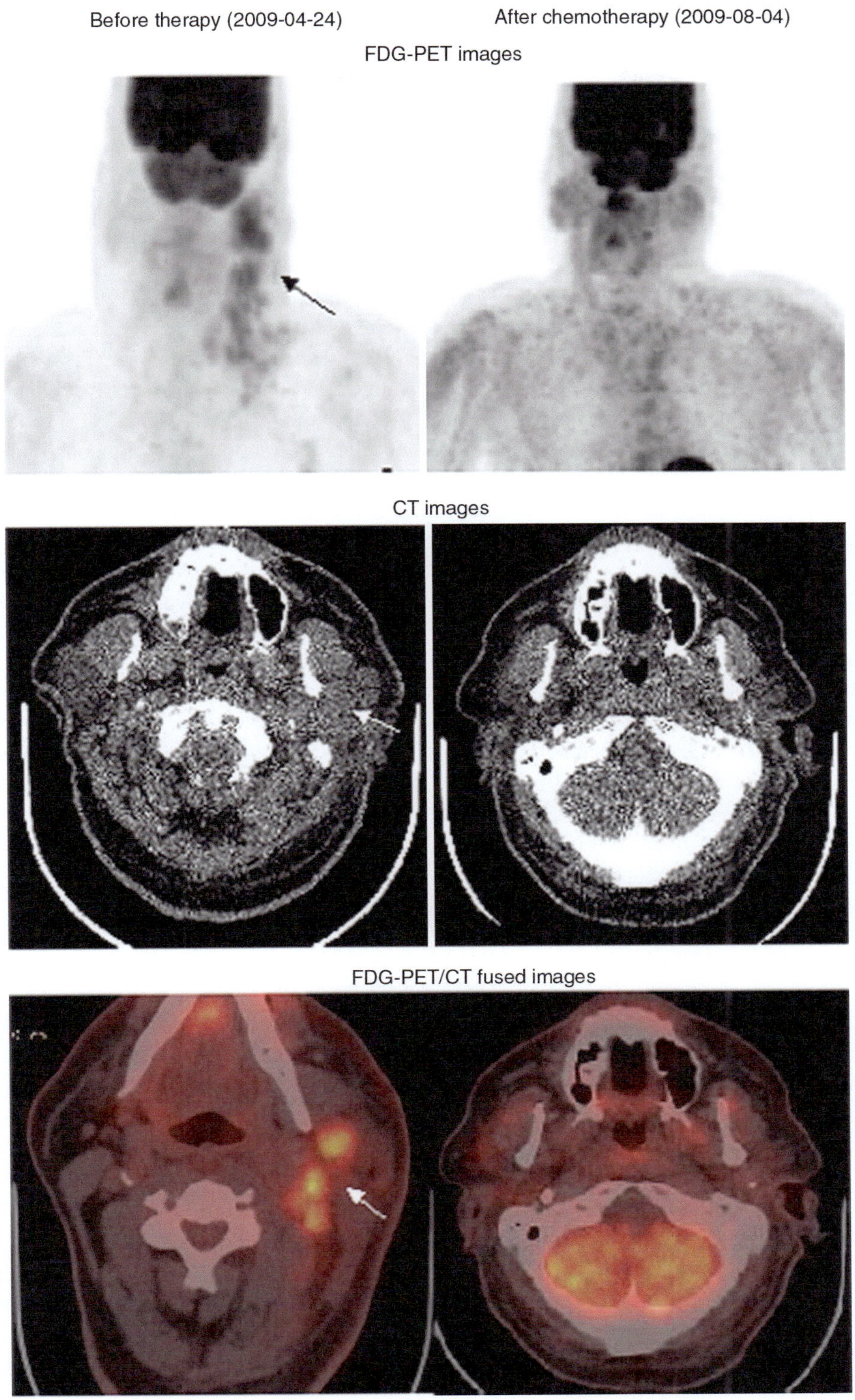

Fig. 16.6 A 69-year-old male with carcinoma of the left parotid. Before chemotherapy, FDG-PET/CT images show extensive nodular hypermetabolism involving left head and neck, extending from left temporalis muscle region to left axillary nodes (*arrows*). After chemotherapy, the primary left parotid tumor has decreased dramatically in intensity, and nodal hypermetabolism in the left neck and left axilla has resolved completely, which are consistent with an excellent response to treatment

[67]. A decline in ^{18}F-FDG uptake during chemotherapy was significantly associated with a clinical response and survival [28, 68]. SUV may be helpful in the evaluation of the response to therapy. A significant reduction in SUV after therapy would be a good response. Tissue inflammation in response to radiotherapy may lead to false-positive results. Normal variants of ^{18}F-FDG uptake in head and neck locations may also pose difficulty in interpreting images. So, there is no fixed quantitative scheme to use SUV to differentiate cancerous tissue from noncancerous tissue. Therefore, it is particularly important to have a baseline PET/CT scan to help differentiate incidental physiologic ^{18}F-FDG-avid foci from malignant foci on subsequent posttreatment scans.

The timing of PET/CT after therapy is very crucial for accurate assessment of treatment response. The metabolic activity of residual viable tumor might be decreased immediately after the completion of radiation therapy, and it may take several weeks to recover their metabolic activity. Additionally, inflammation caused by radiation may result in diffuse increased FDG uptake, which can impair the identification of residual tumor. A report noted an improvement in both sensitivity and specificity of ^{18}F-FDG PET when the scan was obtained at 8 weeks, as compared with 4–8 weeks, after the end of chemoradiotherapy. A false-positive or false-negative result on ^{18}F-FDG PET/CT did not occur later than 8 weeks after radiation therapy [69]. A recent study has the consensus opinion that PET/CT should be performed about 10–12 weeks after the end of therapy [70].

Planning Radiotherapy

Precise and accurate localization of radiotherapy targeted to the gross tumor volume (GTV) is critical for optimizing the radiation therapeutic ratio. With the development of molecular imaging, specific physiologic and molecular information about tumors can now be incorporated into radiation treatment planning. Hybrid PET/CT is a bridge between anatomic imaging and functional imaging, which can provide important information complementary to CT. Therefore, PET/CT appears to be ideally suited to radiotherapy planning in the era of conformal radiotherapy [71]. A recent study reported 42 patients with head and neck cancer of various stages and treated with ^{18}F-FDG PET/CT based intensity-modulated radiation therapy (IMRT). The 2-year overall survival and disease-free survival rates are 83% and 71%, respectively [72], which were notably higher than those in patients receiving standard fractionation (46.1% vs. 37.1%) or receiving accelerated fractionation with concomitant boost (50.9% vs. 39.3%) [73]. ^{18}F-fluoromisonidazole (^{18}F-FMISO) is a nitroimidazole PET tracer that is bound to cell constituents under hypoxic conditions. The feasibility of ^{18}F-FMISO PET/CT in detecting hypoxic subvolume for IMRT has been reported in select patients to achieve favorable outcome [74].

To date, the value of PET/CT for radiotherapy planning is still under investigation. Integrated PET/MRI may further improve the accuracy of GTV delineation, especially for oropharyngeal and oral cavity tumors, because of its higher spatial and temporal resolution.

There has been increasing concern about radiation exposure from PET/CT, especially from the CT portion. The total effective doses from CT and PET scanning ranged from 1.0 to 3.0 cGy [75]. The CT component contributed 54–81% of the total combined dose. However, in light of head and neck cancer, for a patient who is expected to receive 3,000–6,000 cGy to the treatment regions, the exposure from PET/CT should be less of a concern.

Conclusion

Hybrid PET/CT is an effective noninvasive clinical tool for the assessment of head, neck, and thyroid cancer. The primary benefits of this modality are detecting distant metastases, discovering unknown primary tumors, and monitoring response to therapy. This technique can also be used for long-term surveillance. However, the clinical application of PET/CT is currently limited because of its inadequate scanner resolution and nonspecificity of FDG. Ultimately, with the progression of hardware and software, and with the application of tumor-specific tracers, PET/CT may be more valuable in evaluation of head, head and thyroid tumors.

References

1. Jemal A, Siegel R, Ward E, et al. Cancer statistics, 2009. CA: a cancer journal for clinicians. American Cancer Society. Published online May 2009.
2. Ridge JA, Glisson BS, Lango MN, et al. Head and neck tumors. Cancer management: a multidisciplinary approach. 11 ed. 2008.
3. Maier H, Dietz A, Gewelke U, et al. Tobacco and alcohol and the risk of head and neck cancer. Clin Investig. 1992;70:320–7.
4. Cauvin JM, Guénel P, Luce D, et al. Occupational exposure and head and neck carcinoma. Clin Otolaryngol Allied Sci. 1990;15:439–45.
5. Gillespie MB, Smith J, Gibbs K, et al. Human papillomavirus and head and neck cancer: a growing concern. JSC Med Assoc. 2008;104:247–51.
6. Davies L, Welch HG. Increasing incidence of thyroid cancer in the United States, 1973–2002. JAMA. 2006;295:2164–7.
7. Hu MI, Vassilopoulou-Sellin R, Lustig R, et al. Head and neck tumors. Cancer management: a multidisciplinary approach. 11 ed. 2008.
8. Castelifns JA, Kaiser MC, Vakl J, et al. Magnetic resonance imaging of the laryngeal cancer. J Comput Assist Tomogr. 1987;11:134–40.
9. Glazer HS, Nimyer JH, Balfe DM. Neck neoplasms: MR imaging. Part II. Posttreatment evaluation. Radiology. 1986;160:349–54.
10. Vogl TJ, Steger W, Balzer J, et al. MRI of the neck, larynx and hypopharynx. In: Hasso AN, Stark DD, editors. Spine and body MRI. Boston: ARKS; 1991. p. 99–110.
11. Mafee MF, Barany M, Gotsis ED, et al. Potential use of in vivo proton spectroscopy for head and neck lesions. Radiol Clin North Am. 1989;27:243–54.
12. King AD, Yeung DKW, Ahuja AT, et al. In vivo proton MR spectroscopy of primary and nodal nasopharyngeal carcinoma. AJNR Am J Neuroradiol. 2004;25:484–90.
13. Prayer L, Winkelbauer H, Gritzmann N, Winkelbauer F, Helmer M, Pehamberger H. Sonography versus palpation in the detection of regional lymph-node metastases in patients with malignant melanoma. Eur J Cancer. 1990;26:827–30.
14. Hwang HS, Perez DA, Orloff LA. Comparison of positron emission tomography/computed tomography imaging and ultrasound in staging and surveillance of head and neck and thyroid cancer. Laryngoscope. 2009;119:1958–65.
15. Ogilvie JB, Piatigorsky EJ, Clark OH. Current status for fine needle aspiration for thyroid nodules. Adv Surg. 2006;40:223–38.
16. Gharib H, Goellner JR. Fine-needle aspiration biopsy of the thyroid: an appraisal. Ann Intern Med. 1993;118:282–9.
17. van den Brekel MW, Castelijns JA, Stel HV, et al. Occult metastatic neck disease: detection with US and US-guided fine-needle aspiration cytology. Radiology. 1991;180:457–61.
18. Leitha T, Glaser C, Pruckmayer M, et al. Technetium-99 m-MIBI in primary and recurrent head and neck tumors: contribution of bone SPECT image fusion. J Nucl Med. 1998;39:1166–71.
19. Valdés Olmos RA, Balm AJ, Hilgers FJ, et al. Thallium-201 SPECT in the diagnosis of head and neck cancer. J Nucl Med. 1997;38:873–9.
20. Even-Sapir E, Lerman H, Lievshitz G, et al. Lymphoscintigraphy for sentinel node mapping using a hybrid SPECT/CT system. J Nucl Med. 2003;44:1413–20.
21. Wong K, Zarzhevsky N, Cahill JM, Frey KA, Avram AM. The value of diagnostic 131-I SPECT-CT fusion imaging in the evaluation of differentiated thyroid carcinoma. AJR Am J Roentgenol. 2008;191:1785–94.
22. Leskinen-Kallio S, Lindholm P, Lapela M, Joensuu H, Nordman E. Imaging of head and neck tumors with positron emission tomography and [^{11}C]methionine. Int J Radiat Oncol Biol Phys. 1994;30:1195–9.
23. Shields AF, Grierson JR, Dohmen BM, et al. Imaging proliferation in vivo with [F-18]FLT and positron emission tomography. Nat Med. 1998;4:1334–6.
24. Koh WJ, Rasey JS, Evans ML, et al. Imaging of hypoxia in human tumors with [F-18]fluoromisonidazole. Int J Radiat Oncol Biol Phys. 1992;22:199–212.
25. Adams S, Baum R, Stuckensen T, et al. Prospective comparison of ^{18}F-FDG PET with conventional imaging modalities (CT, MRI, US) in lymph node staging of head and neck cancer. Eur J Nucl Med. 1998;25:1255–60.
26. Stokkel MP, ten Broek FW, Hordijk GJ, et al. Preoperative evaluation of patients with primary head and neck cancer using dual head 18 fluorodeoxyglucose positron emission tomography. Ann Surg. 2000;231 :229–34.
27. Wong RJ, Lin DT, Schoder H, et al. Diagnostic and prognostic value of [(18)F]fluorodeoxyglucose positron emission tomography for recurrent head and neck squamous cell carcinoma. J Clin Oncol. 2002;20: 4199–208.
28. Lowe VJ, Boyd JH, Dunphy FR, et al. Surveillance for recurrent head and neck cancer using positron emission tomography. J Clin Oncol. 2000;18:651–8.
29. Schöder H, Yeung HW, Gonen M, et al. Head and neck cancer: clinical usefulness and accuracy of PET/CT image fusion. Radiology. 2004;231:65–72.
30. Clarke JC. PET/CT "Cometh the hour, cometh the machine?". Clin Radiol. 2004;59:775–6.
31. Barrington SF, Maisey MN. Skeletal muscle uptake of fluorine-18-FDG: effect of oral diazepam. J Nucl Med. 1996;37:1127–9.

32. Palmedo H, Bucerius J, Joe A, et al. Integrated PET/CT in differentiated thyroid cancer: diagnostic accuracy and impact on patient management. J Nucl Med. 2006;47:616–24.
33. Beheshti M, Pöcher S, Vali R, et al. The value of ^{18}F-DOPA PET-CT in patients with medullary thyroid carcinoma: comparison with ^{18}F-FDG PET-CT. Eur Radiol. 2009;19:1425–34.
34. Linecker A, Kermer C, Sulzbacher I, et al. Uptake of (18)F-FLT and (18)F-FDG in primary head and neck cancer correlates with survival. Nuklearmedizin. 2008;47:80–5.
35. Rajendran JG, Schwartz DL, O'Sullivan J, et al. Tumor hypoxia imaging with [F-18] fluoromisonidazole positron emission tomography in head and neck cancer. Clin Cancer Res. 2006;12:5435–41.
36. Balogova S, Périé S, Kerrou K, et al. Prospective comparison of FDG and FET PET/CT in patients with head and neck squamous cell carcinoma. Mol Imaging Biol. 2008;10:364–73.
37. Capoccetti F, Criscuoli B, Rossi G, et al. The effectiveness of 124I PET/CT in patients with differentiated thyroid cancer. Q J Nucl Med Mol Imag. 2009;53:536–45.
38. Wong KK, Zarzhevsky N, Cahill JM, et al. Incremental value of diagnostic 131I SPECT/CT fusion imaging in the evaluation of differentiated thyroid carcinoma. AJR Am J Roentgenol. 2008;191:1785–94.
39. Lonneux M, Hamoir M, Reychler H, et al. Positron emission tomography with [^{18}F]fluorodeoxyglucose improves staging and patient management in patients with head and neck squamous cell carcinoma: a multicenter prospective study. J Clin Oncol 2010;28(7): 1190–95.
40. Schoder H, Yeung HW, Gonen M, et al. Head and neck cancer: clinical usefulness and accuracy of PET/CT image fusion. Radiology. 2004;231:65–72.
41. Ishikita T, Oriuchi N, Higuchi T, et al. Additional value of integrated PET/CT over PET alone in the initial staging and follow up of head and neck malignancy. Ann Nucl Med. 2010;24:77–82.
42. Gordin A, Golz A, Keidar Z, et al. The role of FDG-PET/CT imaging in head and neck malignant conditions: impact on diagnostic accuracy and patient care. Otolaryngol Head Neck Surg. 2007;137:130–7.
43. Ryan WR, Fee JR WE, Le QT, et al. Positron-emission tomography for surveillance of head and neck cancer. Laryngoscope. 2005;115:645–50.
44. Piao Y, Bold B, Tayier A, et al. Evaluation of ^{18}F-FDG PET/CT for diagnosing cervical nodal metastases in patients with oral cavity or oropharynx carcinoma. Oral Surg Oral Med Oral Pathol Oral Radiol Endod. 2009;108:933–8.
45. Schoder H, Carlson DL, Kraus DH, et al. ^{18}F-FDG PET/CT for detecting nodal metastases in patients with oral cancer staged N0 by clinical examination and CT/MRI. J Nucl Med. 2006;47:755–62.
46. Chen W, Parsons M, Torigian DA, et al. Evaluation of thyroid FDG uptake incidentally identified on FDG-PET/CT imaging. Nucl Med Commun. 2009;30:240–4.
47. Karantanis D, Bogsrud TV, Wiseman GA, et al. Clinical significance of diffusely increased ^{18}F-FDG uptake in the thyroid gland. J Nucl Med. 2007;48:896–901.
48. Jeong HS, Baek CH, Son YI, et al. Integrated ^{18}F-FDG PET/CT for the initial evaluation of cervical node level of patients with papillary thyroid carcinoma: comparison with ultrasound and contrast-enhanced CT. Clin Endocrinol (Oxford). 2006;65:402–7.
49. Kim TY, Kim WB, Ryu JS, et al. ^{18}F-fluorodeoxyglucose uptake in thyroid from positron emission tomogram (PET) for evaluation in cancer patients: high prevalence of malignancy in thyroid PET incidentaloma. Laryngoscope. 2005;115:1074–8.
50. Eloy JA, Brett EM, Fatterpekar GM, et al. The significance and management of incidental [^{18}F]fluorodeoxyglucose-positron-emission tomography uptake in the thyroid gland in patients with cancer. AJNR Am J Neuroradiol. 2009;30:1431–4.
51. Diehl M, Risse JH, Brandt-Mainz K, et al. Fluorine-18 fluorodeoxyglucose positron emission tomography in medullary thyroid cancer: results of a multicentre study. Eur J Nucl Med. 2001;28:1671–6.
52. Szakall Jr S, Esik O, Bajzik G, et al. ^{18}F-FDG PET detection of lymph node metastases in medullary thyroid carcinoma. J Nucl Med. 2002;43:66–71.
53. Kao CH, ChangLai SP, Chieng PU, Yen RF, Yen TC. Detection of recurrent or persistent nasopharyngeal carcinomas after radiotherapy with 18-fluoro-2-deoxyglucose positron emission tomography and comparison with computed tomography. J Clin Oncol. 1998;16:3550–5.
54. Anzai Y, Carroll WR, Quint DJ, et al. Recurrence of head and neck cancer after surgery or irradiation: prospective comparison of 2-deoxy-2-[F-18]fluoro-D-glucose PET and MR imaging diagnoses. Radiology. 1996;200:135–41.
55. Li P, Zhuang H, Mozley PD, et al. Evaluation of recurrent squamous cell carcinoma of the head and neck with FDG positron emission tomography. Clin Nucl Med. 2001;26:131–5.
56. Fukui MB, Blodgett TM, Meltzer CC, et al. PET/CT imaging in recurrent head and neck cancer. Semin Ultrasound CT MR. 2003;24:157–63.
57. Zimmer LA, Snyderman C, Fukui MB, et al. The use of combined PET/CT for localizing recurrent head and neck cancer: the Pittsburgh experience. Ear Nose Throat J. 2005;84:108–10.
58. Castellucci P, Zinzani P, Pourdehnad M, et al. ^{18}F-FDG PET in malignant lymphoma: significance of positive findings. Eur J Nucl Med Mol Imag. 2005;32:749–56.
59. Pacini F, Agate L, Elisei R, et al. Outcome of differentiated thyroid cancer with detectable serum Tg and negative diagnostic 131I whole body scan: comparison of patients treated with high 131I activities versus untreated patients. J Clin Endocrinol Metab. 2001;86:4092–7.
60. Dong MJ, Liu ZF, Zhao K, et al. Value of ^{18}F-FDG-PET/PET-CT in differentiated thyroid carcinoma with

radioiodine-negative whole-body scan: a meta-analysis. Nucl Med Commun. 2009;30:639–50.
61. Wang W, Larson SM, Fazzari M, et al. Prognostic value of [^{18}F]fluorodeoxyglucose positron emission tomographic scanning in patients with thyroid cancer. J Clin Endocrinol Metab. 2000;85:1107–13.
62. Jereczek-Fossa BA, Jassem J, Orecchia R. Cervical lymph node metastases of squamous cell carcinoma from an unknown primary. Cancer Treat Rev. 2004;30:153–64.
63. Menda Y, Graham MM. Update on ^{18}F-fluorodeoxyglucose/positron emission tomography and positron emission tomography/computed tomography imaging of squamous head and neck cancers. Semin Nucl Med. 2005;35:214–9.
64. Nanni C, Rubello D, Castellucci P, et al. Role of ^{18}F-FDG PET-CT imaging for the detection of an unknown primary tumour: preliminary results in 21 patients. Eur J Nucl Med Mol Imag. 2005;32:589–92.
65. Uchida Y, Minoshima S, Kawata T, et al. Diagnostic value of FDG PET and salivary gland scintigraphy for parotid tumors. Clin Nucl Med. 2005;30:170–6.
66. Findlay M, Young H, Cunningham D, et al. Noninvasive monitoring of tumor metabolism using fluorodeoxyglucose and positron emission tomography in colorectal cancer liver metastases: correlation with tumor response to fluorouracil. J Clin Oncol. 1996;14:700–8.
67. Abe Y, Matsuzawa T, Fujiwara T, et al. Assessment of radiotherapeutic effects on experimental tumors using ^{18}F-2-fluoro-2-deoxy-d-glucose. Eur J Nucl Med. 1986;12:325–8.
68. Brun E, Kjellén E, Tennvall J, et al. FDG PET studies during treatment: prediction of therapy outcome in head and neck squamous cell carcinoma. Head Neck. 2002;24:127–35.
69. Andrade RS, Heron DE, Degirmenci B, et al. Posttreatment assessment of response using FDG-PET/CT for patients treated with definitive radiation therapy for head and neck cancers. Int J Radiat Oncol Biol Phys. 2006;65:1315–22.
70. Ong SC, Schöder H, Lee NY, et al. Clinical utility of ^{18}F-FDG PET/CT in assessing the neck after concurrent chemoradiotherapy for locoregional advanced head and neck cancer. J Nucl Med. 2008;49:532–40.
71. Ciernik IF, Dizendorf E, Baumert BG, et al. Radiation treatment planning with an integrated positron emission and computer tomography (PET/CT): a feasibility study. Int J Radiat Oncol Biol Phys. 2003;57:853–63.
72. Vernon MR, Maheshwari M, Schultz CJ, et al. Clinical outcomes of patients receiving integrated PET/CT-guided radiotherapy for head and neck carcinoma. Int J Radiat Oncol Biol Phys. 2008;70:678–84.
73. Fu KK, Pajak TF, Trotti A, et al. A Radiation Therapy Oncology Group (RTOG) Phase III randomized study to compare hyperfractionation and two variants of accelerated fractionation to standard fractionation radiotherapy for head and neck squamous cell carcinomas: First report of RTOG 9003. Int J Radiat Oncol Biol Phys. 2000;48:7–16.
74. Lee NY, Mechalakos JG, Nehmeh S, et al. Fluorine-18-labeled fluoromisonidazole positron emission and computed tomography-guided intensity-modulated radiotherapy for head and neck cancer: a feasibility study. Int J Radiat Oncol Biol Phys. 2008;70:2–13.
75. Huang B, Law MW, Khong PL. Whole-body PET/CT scanning: estimation of radiation dose and cancer risk. Radiology. 2009;251:166–74.

Lung and Pleural Cancers

17

E. Edmund Kim and Franklin C.L. Wong

Lung cancer is the most frequently diagnosed cancer in the world, and the prevalence of lung cancer is increasing globally [1]. It is the leading cause of death from cancer, and the death occurs at a higher frequency in men than in women in most parts of the world [2]. There were 169,400 estimated new cases of lung cancer in 2002. Lung cancer claims approximately 150,900 lives each year in the US, and 20,000 more women died of lung cancer than breast cancer in 2002 [3]. The survival rate is poor, largely because lung cancer is usually diagnosed at an advanced stage. The overall 5-year survival of patients with lung cancer is approximately 14% and has remained unchanged over several decades despite aggressive treatment protocols [3]. Therefore, new diagnostic and treatment strategies are needed if an impact is to be made on the survival of patients with lung cancer. A cure may be achieved by surgery, which is feasible only in patients who present at an early stage. However, even in the early stage, approximately 75% of patients will die of recurrent disease [1, 4]. Lung cancer is rare before the age of 40 years, after which age-specific rates rise sharply. The ages with the greatest incidence are between 65 and 79 years [1].

There are several extrinsic risk factors for lung cancer. There is general agreement that lung cancer risks are increased by 60% from long-term environmental tobacco smoke exposure, making secondhand smoke a significant added risk factor. Other extrinsic factors include exposure to radon, asbestos, arsenic, and chromium compounds. Radon and asbestos share the distinction of having a synergistic relationship with cigarette smoking. There is increasing evidence that genetic factors can also contribute to lung cancer risk. However, research has not yet identified the gene locus or the mechanism [1, 4].

Malignant mesotheliomas are highly aggressive tumors that arise primarily from the surface serosal cells of the pleural, peritoneal, and pericardial cavities. Epidemiologic studies have established that exposure to asbestos fibers is the primary cause of mesothelioma.

Imaging plays a critical role in the initial detection and diagnosis of thoracic malignancies, as well as in pretreatment staging, which is important in identifying patients with localized disease who are likely to benefit from surgical resection [5]. Chest radiography, computed tomography (CT), and magnetic resonance imaging (MRI) are frequently used in patients with suspected lung

E.E. Kim, M.D., M.S. (✉)
Departments of Nuclear Medicine and Diagnostic Radiology, The University of Texas MD Anderson Cancer Center and Medical School, Houston, TX 77030, USA

Graduate School of Convergence Science and Technology, Seoul National University, Seoul, South Korea
e-mail: ekim@mdanderson.org

F.C.L. Wong, M.D., Ph.D., J.D.
Departments of Nuclear Medicine and Diagnostic Radiology, The University of Texas MD Anderson Cancer Center and Medical School, Houston, TX 77030, USA
e-mail: fwong@mdanderson.org

E.E. Kim et al. (eds.), *Clinical PET and PET/CT: Principles and Applications*,
DOI 10.1007/978-1-4419-0802-5_17,

cancer. These modalities provide anatomic and morphologic information, but they cannot accurately characterize lung, pleural, or lymph node abnormalities as benign or malignant. The diagnosis of lung cancer is usually obtained by sputum cytology, bronchoscopy, percutaneous needle biopsy, thoracoscopy, or open lung biopsy [6]. Because than 50% of radiographically indeterminate lesions resected at thoracosopy were benign [1], the accurate method of noninvasively characterizing these lesions could result in the avoidance of unnecessary and expensive procedures that are not always diagnostic. Several radionuclide imaging techniques using Tl 201 chloride, technetium (Tc)-99 m sestamibi, Tc-99 m P-829 (Neo-Tect), and ^{18}F-2-fluoro-2-deoxyglucose (FDG) have been proposed to evaluate solitary pulmonary nodules and stage lung cancer. The increased glucose metabolism results from increased expression of glucose transporter messenger RNA, enhanced levels of glucose transporter proteins, Glut-1 and -3, high levels of hexokinase II, and down-regulation of glucose-6-phosphatase enzyme [7]. The biochemical differences of FDG between normal and neoplastic tissue have resulted in its routine use for characterizing lesions that are indeterminate by conventional imaging modalities and to stage the tumors.

Pathology of Lung Cancer

Lung cancer arises from epithelial tissue in the lining of the bronchi, bronchioles, alveoli, and trachea. Approximately 90–95% of all primary lung cancers are bronchogenic carcinomas. Histologically, approximately 20% of them are small cell carcinomas, and the other 80% are grouped together as non-small cell lung cancers (NSCLCs), which are divided into adenocarcinoma (40%), squamous cell carcinoma (30%), and large cell undifferentiated carcinoma (10%). The classification of lung cancer by the World Health Organization has been accepted worldwide (Table 17.1) [8].

Small cell lung cancer has almost always spread systemically at the time of diagnosis, and chemotherapy is almost always used.

Table 17.1 World Health Organization classification of epithelial lung tumors

I. Preinvasive lesions
Carcinoma in situ and squamous dysplasia
Atypical adenomatous hyperplasia
II. Invasive malignant lesions
(A) Adenocarcinoma
1. Acinar
2. Papillary
3. Bronchoalveolar: nonmucinous (Clara cell) and mucinous (goblet cell) types
4. Mucus-secreting solid adenocarcinoma
5. Adenocarcinoma with mixed subtypes
(B) Squamous cell carcinoma
Variants: papillary, clear cell, small cell, basaloid
(C) Large cell carcinoma
Variants: neuroendocrine, basaloid, lymphoepithelioma
(D) Small cell carcinoma
(E) Adenosquamous carcinoma
(F) Others
1. Carcinoid tumors
2. Adenoid cystic carcinoma
3. Mucoepidermoid carcinoma
4. Spindle or giant carcinoma
5. Unclassified

Approximately 90% of small cell carcinomas are located centrally and tend to invade longitudinally along submucosal and intramural portions of the bronchial walls and in the supporting tissues and lymphatics [9]. They are often characterized by extensive and bulky mediastinal lymphadenopathy. Small cell and squamous cell carcinomas have a dose–response relationship to increasing tobacco exposure. Adenocarcinoma is increasing worldwide, despite the fact that it does not have a significant dose–response relationship with smoking. This increasing incidence of adenocarcinoma is more often seen in women in the US. Most adenocarcinomas are peripheral in origin and arise from alveolar surface epithelium or bronchial mucosal glands. They also can arise as peripheral scar tumors. Squamous cell carcinoma arises most frequently in the proximal segmental bronchi and is associated with squamous metaplasia. It tends to be slow growing and requires 3–4 years from its onset before clinical detection as an in situ carcinoma. It can be detected early by cytologic examination because its cells exfoliate. Squamous cell carcinomas are located centrally and are frequently associated with bronchial obstruction. A specific subtype of adenocarcinoma, known as bronchoalveolar carcinoma, presents in three different forms: a solitary peripheral nodule, multifocal disease, or a progressive pneumonic form spreading from lobe to lobe and affecting the bilateral lungs. Large cell tumors also tend to be peripheral, and many tumors previously characterized as large cell carcinomas are being classified as adenocarcinoma or squamous cell carcinoma with the improved histologic techniques. The prognosis of large cell undifferentiated carcinomas is similar to that of adenocarcinoma [8].

Adenocarcinomas from primary lung, breast, ovary, stomach, kidney, or prostate cancer frequently metastasize to the pleura and can be extremely difficult to differentiate from epithelial mesothelioma. Metastatic adenocarcinoma with extensive pleural involvement may grossly resemble mesothelioma and has been called pseudomesothelioma.

Diagnosis and Staging of Lung Cancer

Lung cancer growing within the lung parenchyma or the bronchial wall eventually invades the lymphatic channels and vascular structures, resulting in distant metastases. The lymphatic drainage follows the bronchoarterial branching pattern with lymph nodes situated at the origin of these branchings. Lower lobe lymphatics drain into the posterior mediastinum and ultimately to the subcarinal lymph nodes. Right upper lobe lymphatics drain into the superior mediastinum, whereas left upper lobe lymphatics run along the great vessels in the anterior mediastinum and along the main bronchus into the superior mediastinum. Metastatic lymphatic spread of lung cancer follows these lymphatic channels with tumor involving bronchopulmonary (N1), mediastinal (N2-3), and supraclavicular (N3) lymph nodes [10]. Lymphatic spread to the pleural surface can occur in peripheral tumors. Autopsy has revealed lung cancer metastases in every organ system, and the most frequent metastatic sites of NSCLC are bone, liver, adrenal glands, and brain [8]. In 1997, staging of lung cancer was revised by anatomic extent of the primary lung tumor (T), regional lymph nodes (N), and metastases (M) has been used worldwide in the management of lung cancer (Table 17.2). Tumor node metatsasis (TNM) staging (Table 17.3) includes clinical, surgical, and pathologic assessment. Clinical staging typically understages patients compared with the final staging obtained at surgery and pathology. The 5-year survival rate is highly correlated with the stage of lung cancer: 60–70% for stage I, 25–50% for stage II, 18–20% for stage IIIa, and 3–7% for stage IIIb or IV [8] (Table 17.3). The medical history and physical examination are very important in evaluating a patient with suspected lung cancer. Sputum cytology (three samples) will be positive in 80% of central tumors, but the yield is less than 20% for small peripheral tumors [8].

Imaging studies are essential in the evaluation of patients with suspected lung cancer. The detection and diagnosis of lung cancer usually begins with a chest radiograph. The appearance of lung cancer is variable and can range from a subtle finding to the dramatic, depending on location, stage at presentation, and associated findings. In many cases, the major radiographic abnormality is abnormal parenchymal opacification resulting from atelectasis or postobstructive pneumonitis, which may obscure the central tumor. Central tumors may be visible as an abnormal convexity or density in the hilar region. Often the first indication that a cancer exists is the finding of a solitary pulmonary nodule (SPN), measuring usually less than 3 cm in diameter. This is seen in up to 1 in 500 chest radiographs, with an estimated malignancy rate between 20% and 40% [11]. Lung cancer is most often located in the upper lobes, particularly the right upper lobe, and, not surprisingly, most missed cancers are in the right upper lobe. The right lower lobe is the next most common site. Size alone is insufficient for differentiation of benign and malignant lung tumors, although a lesion less than 3 cm is more likely to be malignant. Lamellation or central calcification in granulomas and a popcorn pattern in

Table 17.2 TNM classification of lung cancer

Primary tumor (T)	
Tx	Positive cancer cells but no lesion visualized
T0	No evidence of tumor
Tis	Carcinoma in situ
T1	<3 cm in greatest dimension
T2	<3 cm; invasion of main bronchus or visceral pleura; distal atelectasis
T3	Extension into chest wall, diaphragm; mediastinal pleura or pericardium; <2 cm from carina or total atelectasis
T4	Invasion of mediastinal organs; pleural effusion
Lymph node (N)	
Nx	Cannot be evaluated
N0	No involvement
N1	Ipsilateral bronchopulmonary or hilar
N2	Ipsilateral mediastinal, subcarinal, or supraclavicular
N3	Contralateral mediastinal, hilar, or supraclavicular
Distant metastasis (M)	
Mx	Cannot be evaluated
M0	None
M1	Present

Table 17.3 Current and proposed TNM staging and 5-year survival rate for lung cancer

Staging	T,N,M	5-year survival rate (%)
I,A	T1,N0,M0	65
I,B	T2,N0,M0	45
II,A	T1,N1,M0	46
II,B	T2,N1,M0	30
	T3,N0,M0	22
III,A	T3,N1,M0	20
	T1-3,N2,M0	18
III,B	T4,N0-2,M0	7
	T1-4,N3,M0	3
IV	T1-4,N0-3,M1	1

hamartomas are highly specific, but growing lung cancer may surround a calcified granuloma, and dystrophic calcifications can rarely be seen in primary or metastatic tumor. A minority of carcinoid also calcify. Lobulation of a nodule suggests uneven growth and supports malignancy. Spiculations are thought to represent a desmoplastic response to local tumor extension [12].

Cavitation is seen in a minority of lung cancers, mostly squamous cell carcinoma, but also occasionally in adenocarcinoma or large cell carcinoma. The cavity wall is usually thick (>5 mm) and may show a nodular internal margin. A maximum wall thickness of less than 4 mm is unlikely to be malignant except for rare cases [12]. Growth correlates with doubling time, which is a measure of volumetric growth, not diameter. Most tumors have a doubling time of between 30 and 490 days (mean value of 120 days). A 9-mm SPN with a doubling time of 100 days will measure 1.1 cm at 3 months and 1.4 cm at 6 months. The absence of growth over a 2-year period is the most reliable indicator of benignity [4, 12].

Cancers arising in the lung apex, known as superior sulcus or Pancoast tumors, are a distinct subgroup with constellation of symptoms.

Radiographic findings can be quite subtle and are frequently obscured by overlying musculoskeletal structures, brachiocephalic vessels, or pleural thickening. Findings suggestive of malignancy include an apical cap of greater than 5 min, asymmetry of apical caps, apical mass, or adjacent bone destruction [12]. Arm pain secondary to involved brachia plexus or Horner's syndrome (meiosis, ptosis, and anhydrosis) are classically associated with Pancoast tumors because of involvement of the stellate ganglion. Although the most common appearance of bronchoalveolar carcinoma is an SPN (43%), consolidation is the second most common pattern (30%) caused by tumor growth along the peripheral airways and alveoli. Air bronchograms and alveolograms are characteristic but not specific. Bronchorrhea (copious white mucoid or watery expectoration) is an unusual and late manifestation. The consolidative pattern has a poorer prognosis than the solitary nodular pattern [12, 13]. Hilar or mediastinal adenopathy is sometimes the sole manifestation of lung cancer. Small cell carcinoma tends to show a central adenopathy, but all cell types can have metastatic spread centrally.

Enlargement of the aortopulmonary window, right paratrachial thickening or soft tissue density, double density adjacent to the aortic knob, and abnormal convexity in the azygoesophageal recess are frequent findings of mediastinal metastasis of lung cancer [12]. Pleural involvement usually manifests as a pleural effusion, but a nonmalignant effusion can result from central lymphatic obstruction, pneumonia, congestive heart failure, or pulmonary embolus. Pancoast tumors are often associated with direct extension to ribs or vertebral bodies. Metastatic disease may show destruction or osteolytic lesions in the humerus, sternum, clavicle, or scapula. Lung cancer can also involve the heart by direct extension, or show an enlarging cardiac silhouette by malignant pericardial effusion. Elevation of the diaphragm can indicate phrenic nerve involvement, or be mimicked by a subpulmonic effusion. Hoarseness can be caused by tumor involvement of the recurrent laryngeal nerve in the aortopulmonary window [12].

It is well accepted that CT is the imaging modality of choice for the staging of lung cancer. Compared with MRI, CT is faster, less expensive, has better spatial resolution, offers superior evaluation of the lung parenchyma, and is more sensitive in detecting calcification. CT plays several vital roles in the evaluation of patients with known or suspected lung cancer. One role is to further characterize a suspicious abnormality seen on a chest radiograph. A second and indispensable role is that of pretreatment or preoperative staging. Additionally, CT provides a roadmap for other procedures such as bronchoscopy, mediastinoscopy, video-assisted thoracoscopy, and transthoracic needle biopsy. CT is more accurate in measuring nodular size and quantifying interval growth than chest radiography. It also can better detect and evaluate calcifications within a nodule. The wall thickness of a cavitary lesion can be measured more accurately with CT. A new technique for the assessment of SPN is based on differential nodular enhancement, as measured with thin-slice CT. Malignant nodules tend to enhance more significantly (20 Hounsfield unit increase) than benign nodules at 2-min postinjection of the contrast agent [14]. The CT angiogram sign of branching pulmonary vessels extending more than 3 cm in the midst of consolidated pulmonary parenchyma has been noted in the majority of bronchoalveolar carcinoma, but can also be seen in pneumonia, infarction, or lymphoma [15]. With CT, the primary tumor is evaluated for initial size and location as well as metastasis to pleura, chest wall, mediastinum, vertebral bodies, adrenal glands, or liver.

The best criterion for diagnosing chest wall invasion is bony destruction. Less reliable signs are pleural thickening, loss of the extrapleural fat plane, an obtuse angle between mass and chest wall, and more than 3 cm of contact between mass and chest wall. Chest wall invasion does not necessarily exclude resection, but there is increased morbidity and mortality with en bloc resection and chest wall reconstruction [16]. There are CT criteria that distinguish subtle mediastinal invasion from mere mediastinal contiguity. Tumor contact of less than 3 cm with the mediastinum, less than 90% of contact with the aorta, and the presence of mediastinal fat between the mass and mediastinal structures suggest technically feasible resectability of the lesion.

Lymph nodes are generally identified as nonenhancing soft-tissue densities surrounded by mediastinal fat. A node measuring more than 1 cm is usually considered abnormal, but enlarged nodes may represent benign reactive adenopathy. Nodes less than 1 cm in size also may contain microscopic metastases. Central low density can represent fat in a normal node or necrosis in a malignant node. With the advent of helical CT, particularly multidetector-row helical CT, the possibility of accurate mass screening of the at-risk population has been revisited for the prevention of, or delay of developing, lung cancer by means of earlier detection. Current estimates of the prevalence of detectable preclinical lung cancer in at-risk populations based on the ages of 50–55 years, history of smoking, or prior lung cancer range from 2% to 4% [17]. This prevalence results in a positive predictive value of 50% if the screening test is good, with 95% sensitivity and specificity [17]. The cost of lung cancer screening depends on the fee for CT scans, how many false-positive results occur, and how the at-risk population being screened is defined. Screening could cost more than $39 billion per year, but it may be cost effective because the cost associated with caring for late-stage lung cancer patients is very high [18]. Most academic radiology societies have suggested that CT screening for lung cancer be reserved for patients enrolled in clinical trials.

MRI may play a complementary role to CT in certain circumstances because of its superior tissue contrast, multiplanar imaging capability, and superb delineation of thoracic vessels. For example, for the evaluation of Pancoast tumors, direct coronal and sagittal MRI facilitates the assessment of invasion of the chest wall, brachial plexus, subclavian vessels, vertebral bodies, arid neural foramina. The superior contrast resolution of MRI suggests an advantage over CT in detecting subtle mediastinal invasion, but its poorer spatial resolution limits this advantage. The replacement of high-signal mediastinal fat by lower signal tumor on T2-weighted images suggests mediastinal invasion. MRI is also believed to be more accurate in establishing superior vena caval potency or obstruction resulting from thrombus, soft-tissue mass, or direct tumor invasion [19]. MRI may also demonstrate chest wall invasion better, and signs include loss of subpleural fat stripe and visualization of soft-tissue tumor extension into the chest wall. MRI can differentiate a low-signal benign pleural nodule from high-signal malignant nodules on T2-weighted images [19]. Several studies compared CT with MRI for detection of mediastinal nodal metastases and reported similar sensitivities and specificities of these modalities.

Fluorodeoxyglucose positron emission tomography (FDG PET) is now being used in the evaluation of patients with focal pulmonary opacities on chest radiographs and in the staging of lung cancer, and is replacing some of the invasive procedures previously used in the evaluation of lung cancer.

It has been advocated that radionuclide bone scans be used in clinical stage III disease before considering curative therapy. The role of bone scans in asymptomatic patients with early-stage disease is controversial.

Percutaneous fine-needle aspiration biopsy of pulmonary nodules is used to obtain tissue for identification of malignancy in pulmonary nodules and other abnormalities detected by CT. It is usually performed using CT guidance, and the positive yield is approximately 95%. A definite benign diagnosis is rarely made using this technique. An indeterminate biopsy must be further evaluated.

Bronchoscopy provides a greater than 90% diagnostic yield when a lesion is identified during the procedure. Peripheral lesions larger than 2 cm in diameter can be reached by brushes, needles, or forceps. It is also useful in staging because of the location of the cancer in the major airway as well as the ability to biopsy enlarged mediastinal lymph nodes.

The most accurate method of staging the superior mediastinal lymph nodes is mediastinoscopy. Anterior mediastinal lymph nodes are evaluated by the extended mediastinoscopic technique, anterior mediastinostomy, or video-assisted thoracoscopy, which also is used to excise peripheral nodules and evaluate pleural disease. Posterior mediastinal nodes can be biopsied by ultrasonograph-guided transesophageal endoscopy.

Thoracotomy is used for diagnosis and staging in less than 5% of patients being evaluated for lung cancer, and unexpected involvement of structures is frequently found, changing the stage of disease at thoracotomy.

FDG PET

FDG PET is one of the more recent advances in oncologic imaging and has generated renewed interest in diagnosis, staging, and response to treatment. It allows for the evaluation of the relative level of metabolic activity of a lesion compared with other tissues. It is based on the principle that there is increased utilization of glucose in malignant cells compared with most normal tissues due to the increased number of glucose transporters (I, III) in malignant cells [20]. There is also an increase in the glycolytic rate as a result of increased hexokinase (II) activity. When FDG is administered intravenously, it competes with glucose for transport into the cells. Once intracellular, it competes with glucose for phosphorylation by hexokinase to FDG-6-phosphate, which is not a substrate for glycolysis and is not further metabolized. Thus, it becomes trapped in the cancer cells, and the accumulated ^{18}F-FDG-6-phosphate allows for imaging. Malignant lesions demonstrating increased glucose metabolism appear as focal areas of abnormally increased activity.

Technique

FDG PET is performed on patients who have been fasting to minimize competitive inhibition of FDG uptake by serum glucose. Fasting for 4 h prior to the procedure is generally recommended, but 12-h fasting may decrease the myocardial activity to improve the detection of mediastinal metastases. A serum glucose level is routinely obtained at our institution before FDG injection. If the serum level is less than 200 mg/dL, then FDG is administered. If the serum glucose level is greater than 200 mg/dL, the study is delayed through insulin injection and FDG is not advised because it leads to increased activity in skeletal muscle, and thus FDG is less available in tumors. The blood sugar in diabetic patients should be well controlled by oral hypoglycemic agents or insulin before scheduling FDG PET.

The FDG dose is 145 μCi (5.4 MBq) to a maximum of 20 mCi (740 MBq) for dedicated PET. Smaller doses are required for camera-based PET. Attenuation-corrected whole-body scans provide more accurate detection of small lesions and lesions deep within the body. For a whole-body scan on a PET scanner with a 15-cm axial field of view, 10 bed positions are needed. Segmentation of transmission scans for 1–2 min per bed position reduces the scan time to approximately 100 min for whole-body PET. The nonattenuation-corrected whole-body scan at 8–10 bed positions usually last for 32–48 min of acquisition time. In a patient with lung cancer, a 4-min brain scan using the three-dimensional (3D) acquisition mode ideally begins 30 min after FDG injection. The 3D mode without septa provides approximately four-fold increased sensitivity for detection of annihilation radiation. There is certainly increased scatter radiation, and improved sensitivity yields better image quality. The scatter radiation in the body is greater than that in the head, and thus 3D acquisition is not currently used for body imaging. After the brain scan, nonattenuation-corrected scans are obtained in two-dimensional (2D) acquisition mode for 4 min per bed position from the level of the skull base through the midthighs, and then an attenuation-corrected chest scan at two bed positions is obtained in the 2D mode lasting 8 min for the emission scan and 10 min for the transmission scan at each bed position [21].

FDG PET scans are usually interpreted qualitatively. If the FDG uptake in the lesion is greater than that in the mediastinal blood pool, a malignancy is suggested. The semiquantitative parameter, which is an index of glucose metabolism called the standard uptake ratio or standard uptake value (SUV) normalizes the amount of FDG uptake in the lesion to the total injected dose and the patient's body weight after the lesion or region of interest (ROI) is outlined on the attenuation-corrected image and the mean activity is measured. The decay-corrected activities are then used to compute the SUV by the following formula:

$$SUV = \frac{MeanROIActivity(mCi\,/\,mL)}{InjectedDose(mCi)BodyWeight(g)}$$

The use of lean body weight and as well as correction for serum glucose has been suggested, and the time of acquisition also must be standardized because the SUV may change with time after FDG injection [22].

Solitary Pulmonary Nodules

Focal lung opacities including solitary nodules are usually identified on routine chest radiographs. They are found in approximately 130,000 patients every year in the US [22]. Studies to further characterize SPN are often performed with chest CT. If the SPN is stable in size for 2 years or longer, it is likely benign. By morphologic criteria, many lesions are indeterminate as to whether they are benign or malignant. Patients may require invasive biopsy, mediastinoscopy, thoracoscopy, or even thoracotomy to determine the nature of the lesion. More than half of radiographically indeterminate lesions that are thoracoscopically resected are found to be benign [6]. FDG PET has been shown to be an accurate, noninvasive tool for the assessment of pulmonary nodules.

A comprehensive meta-analysis by Gould et al. [23] of 40 eligible studies, including 1,474 focal pulmonary lesions of any size, found that the mean sensitivity and specificity for detecting malignancy were 96.0% and 73.5%, respectively. However, in this analysis, there was little data for nodules smaller than 1 cm in diameter. In a prospective, multicenter study of 89 patients who underwent evaluation of intermediate SPN, FDG PET had a sensitivity of 92% and a specificity of 90% using the SUV of 2.5 as the cutoff value [21]. Visual analysis of the images demonstrated a sensitivity of 98% and a specificity of 69%, and these results were not significantly different from the results using the SUV data. When the data were evaluated by separating the nodules into those 0.7 to smaller than 1.5 cm in diameter and compared with those greater than or equal to 1.5 cm in diameter, the sensitivity and specificity were not statistically significantly different.

Although there is much enthusiasm about the use of FDG PET in oncology, the technique has its limitations. False-positive results from FDG PET can occur with infectious or inflammatory processes. Abnormally increased FDG uptake with the SUV in the abnormal range can be seen with sarcoidosis, tuberculosis, histoplasmosis, cryptococcosis, aspergillosis, and other infections [21]. However, most chronic or indolent inflammatory processes and most acute infectious processes do not have significant FDG accumulation. False-negative FDG PET results have been seen with primary pulmonary carcinoid and bronchoalveolar cell cancer [21, 23]. Six of seven carcinoids had SUVs less than 2.5. The typical carcinoid is slow growing and demonstrates minimal mitotic activity, resulting in less FDG uptake than in NSCLC. Of seven bronchoalveolar lung carcinomas, four were negative using FDG PET because of less proliferative potential and longer mean doubling time than for other NSCLCs [21, 23]. False-negative PET findings are also a problem if the lesion is too small for the resolution of the instrument.

A relationship between prognosis and the amount of FDG uptake in nodules has been documented. Of the 118 patients with SUV less than 10, a median survival of 24.6 months was found, whereas 37 patients with SUV greater or equal to 10 had a statistically significant shorter median survival of 11.4 months. Multivariate analysis demonstrated that the results of a PET scan provided prognostic information independent of other clinical and imaging findings. Nodules with increased FDG uptake require a biopsy for diagnosis and PET aids in directing the biopsy. FDG PET precludes the need for invasive biopsy in patients with metabolically inactive lesions. The cost savings of FDG PET in the evaluation of SPN result in the prevention of unnecessary thoracotomies.

Staging of Lung Cancer

When a lung mass is found to be malignant, it is important to stage the extent of disease accurately. Appropriate clinical management depends on whether there is mediastinal involvement and/or distal disease. Several studies have shown that PET is more accurate than CT for the staging of NSCLC. A tabulated summary of FDG PET literature concentrating on lung cancer from 1993 to 2000 showed 83% sensitivity and 91% specificity for NSCLC staging, versus 64% and 74%, respectively, for CT [24]. The mediastinum is the most common site for metastases, and PET appears more accurate than CT in detecting metastatic mediastinal lymphadenopathy. In one retrospective study of 96 patients, 66 with histologically proved malignant tumors and 30 with benign masses, the sensitivity and specificity of PET for detecting malignancy was 97% and 89%, respectively. In that study, 111 lymph nodes were surgically sampled and the accuracy of FDG PET in predicting malignancy of nodes was 91% compared with 64% for CT. The sensitivity and specificity of FDG PET in detecting metastatic mediastinal lymph nodes was 98% and 94%, respectively [25].

In a prospective study by Pieterman et al. [26], a logistic regression analysis was used to evaluate the ability of PET and CT to identify malignant mediastinal lymph nodes and distant sites in 102 patients with resectable NSCLC. The sensitivity and specificity of PET for the detection of mediastinal metastases were 91% and 86%, respectively. Detection of unsuspected metastatic disease by PET may permit a reduction in the number of thoracotomies performed for nonresectable disease. For broad groupings of NSCLC stage, 10% of cases were downstaged and 33% upstaged after PET. Stating that incorporated PET provided a more accurate prognostic stratification than did staging with conventional means [27], PET may reduce the need for mediastinoscopy when the primary NSCLC SUV is less than 2.5 and the mediastinum is negative on PET [28]. The high negative predictive values of PET are benign, biopsy is not needed, and radiographic follow-up is recommended. Some reports have noted that up to 60% of patients with NSCLC develop adrenal metastases, and PET showed 100% sensitivity and 80% specificity for the diagnosis of adrenal metastasis in CT-detected adrenal lesions between 1 and 9 cm in size.

Detection of Residual or Recurrent Lung Cancer

After potentially curative therapy of NSCLC, abnormalities or symptoms suggesting recurrence can be difficult to characterize. Early detection is important because salvage therapies are available for localized recurrence. PET better assesses the status of disease and stratifies prognosis than does conventional staging, affects patient management, and should be incorporated into paradigms for suspected recurrence of NSCLC. Lesions with higher tumor-to-muscle ratios responded better to treatment than those with lower ratios. The decrease in FDG uptake after therapy correlated with a partial response to therapy. The relapse rate was higher in tumors with higher uptake ratios before and/or after therapy. The results of a pilot study of PET use in monitoring response to chemotherapy in 13 patients with primary lung cancer and mediastinal metastases are encouraging. Patz et al. [29] studied 43 patients on whom FDG PET was performed between 4 and 182 months after initial diagnosis and treatment of NSCLC. Thirty-five patients had recurrent or persistent cancer. The median SUV in the 35 patients who had recurrent or persistent cancer was 7.6 (range 1.9–18), whereas the median SUV in patients who had fibrosis after therapy was 1.6 (range 0.6–2.4). Using an SUV of greater than 2.5 to indicate malignancy, FDG PET had a sensitivity of 97% and a specificity of 100% for the detection of recurrent or persistent disease. In another study of 39 lesions in 38 patients using PET after therapy, a sensitivity of 100% and a specificity of 62% were found for the detection of recurrent or persistent lung cancer [30].

False-Positive and Negative FDG PET and PET/CT

FDG PET may yield false-positive findings in patients with florid inflammatory diseases such as tuberculosis, histoplasmosis, and aspergillosis. These infectious processes can be difficult to distinguish from an early stage of lung cancer in the absence of clinical information because they are also associated with the morphologic finding of nonspecific nodular lesions in the lungs. Most chronic inflammatory diseases are characterized by little or no increased FDG uptake.

Stressed muscular activity also leads to increased FDG uptake and is often found in the lower anterior neck. PET/CT was able to localize increased FDG uptake to the internal laryngeal muscles due to compensatory activation of the ipsilateral laryngeal muscle [31]. The same applies to the anatomic localization of brown fat which can be easily identified as a physiologic source.

The limited spatial resolution and acquisition times of FDG PET may lead to false-negative findings, especially in the detection of nodal micrometastases. PET/CT cannot completely replace mediastinoscopy for the staging of nodal involvement. Only 38% of lymph node metastases smaller than 1 cm in size could be identified with PET/CT [32]. Pulmonary carcinoids and bronchoalveolar carcinomas are a potential source of false-negative findings because of the relatively low metabolic activity and proliferation rates.

Small cell lung cancer is an aggressive tumor that grows rapidly and usually has metastasized by the time it is diagnosed. Given the frequent presence of overt metastases, it is customarily investigated by thoracic and abdominal CT, brain MRI, and nuclear bone scan. FDG PET was found to have a sensitivity of 98% and specificity of 92% in the detection of distant metastases, compared with 83% and 79%, respectively, for CT [33].

Lung Metastases

Metastases account for the highest percentage of malignant lung nodules. The lung is the most frequent site for hematogenous metastasis from extrapulmonary cancers such as nasopharynx, thyroid, breast, prostate, kidney, uterus, ovary cancers, as well as bone and soft-tissue sarcomas.

CT is the imaging modality of choice for diagnosing lung metastases with a sensitivity of 94% for 6–10 mm-sized metastases but 100% for metastases larger than 1 cm in size [34]. FDG PET is of limited accuracy for metastases smaller than 1 cm as well as for low metabolic tumors such as carcinoids. It has a sensitivity of 95–100% and a specificity of 90–96% for the detection of lung metastases from colon or breast cancer [35].

Pleural Mesothelioma

Malignant pleural mesothelioma is the most common pleural cancer and accounts for less than 2% of all thoracic tumors. It typically spreads within the pleural cavity, and hemorrhagic effusion is almost invariably present. Initial nodal metastasis is usually to lymph nodes that drain the parietal pleura, and distant metastases are rare. There are epithelial, mesenchymal, and mixed types, with the epithelial type being the most common.

CT shows a complete encasement of the lung or multiple sites of nodular pleural thickening, and the tumor usually demonstrates intense and inhomogeneous contrast enhancement. The tumor will also show increased FDG uptake. A sensitivity of 91% and a specificity of 100% were achieved, with the epithelial type revealing lower FDG uptake than the other types [36].

PET/CT was more accurate than PET and CT separately in establishing an indication for extrapulmonary pneumonectomy [37]. PET/CT also provides useful information for evaluating lymph node status. However, it is difficult to differentiate mesothelioma from pleural metastases using PET/CT, therefore, the diagnosis should be confirmed by biopsy.

Conclusion

PET is an exciting diagnostic tool that can quantify the metabolic activity of a tumor or node, and may reveal additional sites of disease not suspected on CT, thereby increasing the accuracy of the staging process. Familiarity with the various manifestations of lung cancer on chest radiography may help suggest the initial diagnosis. Once a suspicious abnormality is detected, CT is necessary to help confirm diagnosis by identifying CT findings that would most likely suggest cancer, and to stage the disease. The role of MRI is generally limited to specific problem-solving areas or when CT findings are equivocal or indeterminate.

References

1. Smith RA, Glynn TJ. Epidemiology of lung cancer. Radiol Clin North Am. 2000;38:453–70.
2. Magrath I, Litvak J. Cancer in developing countries: opportunity and challenge. J Natl Cancer Inst. 1993;85:862–73.
3. Jemal A, Thomas A, Murray T, Thun M. Cancer statistics, 2002. CA Cancer J Clin. 2002;52:23–47.
4. Bepler G. Lung cancer epidemiology and genetics. J Thorac Imaging. 1999;14:228–34.
5. Quint LE, Francis IR. Radiologic staging of lung cancer. J Thorac Imaging. 1999;14:235–46.
6. Mack MJ, Hazelrigg JR, Lartdreneau RJ, Acuft TE. Thoracoscopy for the diagnosis of the indeterminate solitary pulmonary nodule. Ann Thorac Surg. 1993;56:825–32.
7. Smith TAD. FDG uptake, tumor characteristics, and response to therapy: a review. Nucl Med Commun. 1998;19:97–105.
8. Ginsberg RS, Vokes EE, Rosenzweig K. Non-small cell cancer of the lung. In: DeVita VT, Hellman S, Rosenberg SA, editors. Cancer principles and practice of oncology. 6th ed. Philadelphia: Lippincott-Raven; 2002. p. 925–82.
9. Sone S, Sakai F, Takashima S, et al. Factors affecting the radiologic appearance of peripheral bronchogenic carcinomas. J Thorac Imaging. 1997;12:159–72.
10. Mountain C, Libshitz HI, Hermes KE. Lung cancer: a handbook for staging and imaging. Houston: University of Texas M.D. Anderson Cancer Center; 1992.
11. Yankelevitz DF, Henschke CI. Small solitary pulmonary nodules. Radiol Clin North Am. 2000;38:471–8.
12. Romney BM, Austin JH. Plain film evaluation of carcinoma of the lung. Semin Roetgenol. 1990;25:45–63.
13. Bouchard EW, Falken S, Molina PL. Lung cancer: a radiologic overview. Appl Radiol. 2007;7–19.
14. Swensen SJ, Morin RL, Schueller B, et al. Solitary pulmonary nodule: CT evaluation of enhancement with iodinated contrast material: a preliminary report. Radiology. 1992;182:343–7.
15. Schuster MR, Scanlan KA. "CT angiogram sign" establishing the differential diagnosis. Radiology. 1991;178:90–5.
16. Park BJ, Louie D, Altorki N. Staging and the surgical management of lung cancer. Radiol Clin North Am. 2000;38:545–58.
17. Obuchowski NA, Graham RJ, Baker ME, Powell KA. Ten criteria for effective screening: their application to multislice CT screening for pulmonary and colorectal cancers. AJR Am J Roentgeno. 2001;176:1357–62.
18. Henschke CI, Yartkelevitz DF. Screening for lung cancer. J Thorac Imaging. 2000;15:21–7.
19. Hatabu H, Syock KW, Sher S, et al. Magnetic resonance imaging of the thorax. Radiol Clin North Am. 2000;38:593–616.
20. Flier JS, Mueckler MM, Usher P, et al. Elevated levels of glucose transport and transporter messenger RNA are induced by ras or src oncogenes. Science. 1987;235:1492–5.
21. Coleman RE. PET in lung cancer. J Nucl Med. 1999;40:814–20.
22. Lowe VJ, DeLong DM, Hoffman JM, Coleman RE. Optimum scanning protocol for FDG-PET evaluation of pulmonary malignancy. J Nucl Med. 1995;36:883–7.
23. Gould MK, Maclean CC, Kuschner WG, et al. Accuracy of positron emission tomography for diagnosis of pulmonary nodules and mass lesions: a meta analysis. JAMA. 2001;285:914–24.
24. Gambhir SS, Czernim J, Schwimmer J, et al. A tabulated summary of the FDG-PET literature. J Nucl Med. 2001;42(Suppl):1S–92.
25. Graeber GM, Gupta NC, Murray GF. Positron emission tomographic imaging with fluorodeoxyglucose is efficacious in evaluating malignant pulmonary disease. J Thorac Cardiovasc Surg. 1999;117:719–27.
26. Pieterman RM, VanPutten JWG, Meuzelaar JJ, et al. Preoperative staging of non-small cell lung cancer with positron emission tomography. N Engl J Med. 2000;343:254–61.
27. Hicks RJ, Kalff V, MacManus MP, et al. ^{18}F-FDG-PET provides high-impact and powerful prognostic stratification in staging newly diagnosed non-small cell lung cancer. J Nucl Med. 2001;42:1596–604.
28. Kernstine KH, McLaughlin KA, Menda Y, et al. Can FDG-PET reduce the need for mediastinoscopy in potentially resectable nonsmall cell lung cancer? Ann Thorac Surg. 2002;73:394–402.
29. Patz Jr EF, Lowe VJ, Hoffman JM, et al. Persistent or recurrent bronchogenic carcinoma: detection with PET and 2-[F-18]-2-deoxy-D-glucose. Radiology. 1994;191:379–82.
30. Inoue T, Kim EE, Komaki R, et al. Detecting recurrent or residual lung cancer with FDG-PET. J Nucl Med. 1995;36:788–93.
31. Kamel EM, Goerres GW, Burger C, von Schulthess GK, Steinert HC. Recurrent laryngeal nerve palsy in patients with lung cancer: detection with PET-CT image fusion- report of six cases. Radiology. 2002;224(1):153–6.

32. Kim B-T, Lee KS, Shim SS, et al. Stage T1 non-small cell lung cancer: preoperative mediastinal nodal staging with integrated FDG PET/CT- a prospective study. Radiology. 2006;24(2):501–9.
33. Brink C, Schumacher T, Mix M, et al. Impact of F-18 FDG-PET on the primary staging of small-cell lung cancer. Eur J Nucl Med Mol Imaging. 2004;31(12):1614–20.
34. Diederich S, Semik M, Lentschig MG, et al. Helical CT of pulmonary nodules in patients with extrathoracic malignancy: CT-surgical correlation. AJR Am J Roentgeno. 1999;172(2):353–60.
35. Schirmeister H, Kuhn T, Guhlmann A, et al. F-18 FDG PET in the preoperative staging of breast cancer: comparison with the standard staging procedures. Eur J Nucl Med Mol Imaging. 2001;28(3):351–8.
36. Benard F, Sterman D, Smith RJ, Kaiser LR, Albelda SM, Alavi A. Prognostic value of FDG PET imaging in malignant pleural mesothelioma. J Nucl Med. 1999;40(8):1241–5.
37. Steinert HC, Santos DMM, Burger C, Stahel R. Therapy response evaluation in malignant pleural mesothelioma with integrated PET-CT imaging. Lung Cancer. 2005;49(Suppl 1):S33–5.

18 Breast Cancer

E. Edmund Kim and Masashi Yukihiro

In 2003, breast cancer was the most frequently diagnosed cancer (212,600 new cases), and the second leading cause of cancer death (40,200 deaths) in American women [1]. In women ages 40–55 years, breast cancer is the leading cause of mortality [1]. There has been a slight decline in breast cancer mortality overall [1], that can be attributed both to the success of early detection and to advanced treatment, particularly systemic therapy. Caucasian women in the US have a 13.1% lifetime incidence of developing breast cancer, whereas African-American women have a 9.6% lifetime incidence [1]. However, the lifetime risk of dying from breast cancer is 3.4% for both African-American and Caucasian women in the U.S. While the incidence of invasive breast cancer has leveled off, the number of ductal carcinomas in situ (DCIS) has been on the rise, probably a result of the increasing use of screening mammography.

The most common modality for detecting breast cancer is mammography, which has a high sensitivity rate but has a low positive predictive value [2]. It is difficult to distinguish the difference between malignant and benign breast tumors using sonography [3]. The sensitivity of magnetic resonance imaging (MRI) is almost 90%, but the specificity is 70% [3]. A reliable noninvasive imaging technique is needed to differentiate benign from malignant breast tumors. Nuclear medicine methods, including positron emission tomography (PET), have been developed for evaluating biochemical and physiologic characteristics of tumors, and they have added unique functional information to the anatomic abnormalities provided by conventional imaging.

Technetium (Tc)-99 m hexakis-isobutyl isonitrile (MIBI) is the most popular contrast agent for scintimammography, but Tl 201 chloride and Tc-99 m ethylene-bis [bis (2-ethoxyethyl)] phosphine (tetrofosmin) are also used with single-photon emission computed tomography (SPECT) [4]. ^{18}F-fluorodeoxyglucose (FDG) and ^{11}C-methionine have also been widely used as tumor-seeking agents with PET. Few comparative studies have described the uptake of radiopharmaceuticals as a method of detecting breast cancer. Among SPECT agents, tumor uptake of tetrofosmin was higher than that of MIBI and Tl in mice implanted with MCF-7 breast cancer cells [4]. The order of tumor uptake, from greatest to least, was L-^{18}F-α-methyltyrosine = ^{11}C-methionine > ^{18}F-FDG = tetrofosmin > MIBI = Tl. Tl 201 chloride showed the highest tumor-to-blood ratio (12.8). Tumor-to-muscle ratio, from highest to lowest, was ^{18}F-methyltyrosine = ^{11}C-methionine > ^{18}F-FDG > MIBI > tetrofosmine = Tl [4]. Various

E.E. Kim, M.D., M.S. (✉)
Departments of Nuclear Medicine and Diagnostic Radiology, The University of Texas MD Anderson Cancer Center and Medical School, Houston, TX 77030, USA

Graduate School of Convergence Science and Technology, Seoul National University, Seoul, South Korea
e-mail: ekim@mdanderson.org

M. Yukihiro, M.D., Ph.D.
Department of Radiology, School of Medicine, Gunma University, Ihara Shizouka 421-3306, Japan

E.E. Kim et al. (eds.), *Clinical PET and PET/CT: Principles and Applications*,
DOI 10.1007/978-1-4419-0802-5_18, © Springer Science+Business Media New York 2013

radiopharmaceuticals for breast cancer detection have been used for scintimammography and PET.

Although breast cancer is frequently characterized by increased FDG uptake, it displays considerable variation, with many variables affecting the cellular level as well as the microenvironment of tumor masses. Nontumoral tissue such as necrotic and fibrotic tissue may reduce tracer uptake, whereas the presence of inflammatory cells may result in increased FDG accumulation. Similar to glucose, FDG is a substrate for the first enzyme of glycolysis, hexokinase, and is phosphorylated intracellularly to FDG-6-phosphate. However, because FDG lacks a hydroxyl group in the second position, FDG-6-phosphate is not a substrate for either the second enzyme of glycolysis, glucose-6-phosphate isomerase, or for other intracellular metabolic pathways. FDG-6-phosphate is a charged molecule and does not diffuse out of the cell. Because glucose-6-phosphatase activity is minimal in cancer cells and most normal tissues, the reverse transformation of FDG is relatively slow. Therefore, FDG-6-phosphate remains trapped within the cell, and the cellular level of ^{18}F activity is related to the rate of glucose uptake and use by the cell. The expression of different types of glucose transporters and hexokinases has been suggested to determine the level of FDG uptake in cancer tissue. PET has attracted considerable attention because of its ability to study a variety of biologic and functional characteristics of breast cancer, such as blood flow, glucose metabolism, and receptor status. Study of tumor blood flow and oxygen utilization does not appear to be clinically relevant.

Staging refers to the grouping of patients according to the extent of their disease, and it is useful in determining the choice of treatment for individual patients, estimating their prognosis, and comparing the results of different treatment programs. Clinical staging includes physical examination, imaging, and pathologic examination of the breast or other tissues to establish the diagnosis of breast carcinoma. The extent of tissue examined pathologically for clinical staging is less than that required for pathologic staging. Appropriate surgical findings are elements of clinical staging, including the size of the primary tumor and chest wall invasion, and the presence or absence of local or distant metastasis. Pathologic staging includes all data used for clinical staging, surgical exploration, and resection as well as pathologic examination (Table 18.1).

PET Techniques

Patients must fast for at least 4–6 h prior to receiving an intravenous injection of 370–555 MBq of (10–15 mCi) ^{18}F-FDG over 2 min so that the serum insulin concentration will be at the basal level and the blood glucose level will be within the normal range (<130 mg/dL). An intravenous cannula is placed in the arm contralateral to the breast tumor, and blood samples are drawn. Patients are positioned supine or prone with a foam rubber support after comfortable positioning on the scanner table with both arms at their sides. A 25-min transmission study for attenuation correction is performed either before the study or after the completion of the emission study injection, using a connection for emission counts during transmission.

Dynamic imaging of metabolism is performed for 60 min after the start of ^{18}F-FDG infusion. The standard clinical protocol is started 60 min after tracer injection, and images are acquired over 6–8 bed positions and displayed in axial, coronal, and sagittal planes. Transmission scans are obtained with Ge 68 and rod sources, and images are reconstructed using algebraic algorithms. Attenuation correction is required for quantitative or semiquantitative assessment of tracer uptake. Blood flow imaging is performed using 962–1,998 MBq of ^{15}O-water. Dynamic ^{15}O-water images are collected for 7.75 min after injection, and peak total coincidence counting rates do not exceed 700 kilocycles per second (kcps). Background counts from the ^{15}O water study are less than or equal to 4 kcps at the start of the ^{18}F-FDG studies with a typical ^{18}F-FDG peak counting rate of 80 kcps. Also, 1,500–2,000 mL of 0.45% or 0.9% saline over 1.5–2 h and 20 mg furosemide given over 20 min are helpful in facilitating clearance of the activity from the renal collecting system and ureter.

Table 18.1 Staging of breast cancer

Primary tumor (T)	
T0	No evidence of tumor
Tis	Carcinoma in situ
T1mic	Microinvasion < 1 mm
T1	≤2 cm (0.1 < 1a < 0.5, 0.5 < b < 1, 1 < 1c < 2)
T2	2–5 cm
T3	>5 cm
T4	Extension to chest wall (4a), skin (4b), both (4c), or inflammatory carcinoma (4d)
Regional lymph node (N)	
N0	No node metastasis
N1	Movable ipsilateral axillary node
N2	1a: 1–3 axillary; 1b: internal mammary, fixed ipsilateral axillary nodes
N3	2a: 4–9 axillary; 2b: internal mammary, ipsilateral internal mammary nodes, >10
Distant metastasis (M)	
Mx	Cannot be assessed
M0	No distant metastasis
M1	Metastasis including ipsilateral supraclavicular node
Stage 0	Tis, N0, M0
Stage I	T1, N0, M0
Stage IIA	T0 or T1, N1, M0; T2, N0, M0
Stage IIB	T2, N1, M0; T3, N0, M0
Stage IIIA	T0 or T1, or T2, N2, M0; T3, N1 or N2, M0

A Foley catheter in the bladder is also useful to ensure adequate clearance of bladder activity.

Breast Cancer Diagnosis and Staging Using PET

PET of the breast offers physiologic information and therefore can act as an adjunct to conventional imaging, which provides morphologic information. PET can identify larger breast tumors with high accuracy and has also shown encouraging results in detecting regional lymph node metastases [5]. However, PET is currently restricted in detecting small breast tumors by its limited sensitivity. Partial-volume effects play an important role, but an increase in metabolic activity with tumor growth may also occur. There was no significant relationship between FDG accumulation and tumor size, but a significant difference in FDG uptake was found to be dependent on the microscopic growth pattern of breast cancer [5]. Nodular tumors with clearly visible tumor borders had a higher FDG uptake than did breast carcinomas with diffuse infiltration of surrounding tissue [standard uptake value (SUV) 4.1 ± 2.3 vs. 0.8 ± 0.2] [5]. Invasive lobular carcinomas had significantly lower FDG uptake (SUV 3.8) compared with invasive ductal carcinomas (SUV 5.6) [6]. Invasive lobular carcinoma is generally more difficult to diagnose than invasive ductal carcinoma by imaging procedures including mammography, sonography, and MRI [7].

Tissue heterogeneity is an important factor contributing to the total FDG uptake in tumors. The relative composition of malignant tumors ranges from a few transformed cells to greater than 90% of malignant cells. Because of the limited spatial resolution of PET scanners, the signal derived from tumors represents an average FDG uptake in all tumor components. Components with low metabolic activity, namely, cells containing mucine, connective tissue, and necrosis, may reduce the total FDG uptake in tumors, resulting in false-negative PET findings [8]. A weak relationship was found between FDG uptake and the percentage of tumor cells [5]. It has been suggested that the number of tumor cells may gain substantial importance only if the percentage of tumor cells is low (<30%); above this level, the PET signal from tumors reflects primarily the metabolic activity rather than the number of malignant cells. Breast carcinomas consisting of only scattered malignant cells are difficult to identify on PET images [5]. Inflammatory cells may significantly contribute to FDG uptake in tumors. Newly formed granulation tissue around the tumor as well as macrophages in the margins of necrosis showed an increased FDG uptake; however, no relationship was found between the presence of inflammatory cells and the intensity of FDG uptake [5]. A weak inverse relationship was found between FDG uptake and the density of microvessels [5]. Under anaerobic conditions, most malignant tumors metabolize glucose primarily to lactate, which results in higher utilization rates for glucose molecules. Hypoxia is present in tumor tissue beyond 100–200 μm of functional blood supply and is commonly found in solid tumors. A significant increase in FDG accumulation was found under moderately hypoxic conditions [9]. Studies with ^{15}O-water in human squamous cell carcinoma of the head and neck revealed no correlation between tumor perfusion and FDG uptake [10].

Recent clinical data indicate that tumor hypoxia negatively affects the therapeutic outcome of both radiotherapy and chemotherapy in various cancers. There was a more than twofold increase in ^{3}H-FDG uptake in MCF7 breast cancer cells under hypoxic conditions, partly due to an increase in glucose transporter activity by reduction of the thiol group in the glucose transport protein [11]. Modulation of hexokinase activity was probably not involved.

Radiodense breasts are found in women undergoing hormone replacement therapy and in those who have had breast augmentation or breast-conserving therapy for breast cancer. Mammographic evaluation of the postbiopsy or postsurgical breast is very difficult because of scar formation or the high density of implants. In such situations, FDG PET seems to be particularly useful and may obviate biopsy. FDG PET can image tumors in the augmented breast without implant displacement and without obvious degradation of image quality by the implant [12]. The potential role of FDG PET in breast imaging would be for the detection of multicentric or multifocal lesions and thus demonstrate the true extent of breast cancer. The finding of multifocal cancer may alter the therapy from lumpectomy to mastectomy. Another potential role of FDG PET in detecting occult primary breast cancer in a patient with known metastasis to axillary lymph node has been investigated.

One of the most important roles of FDG PET is the accurate staging of regional lymph node metastasis. Approximately 60% of patients with breast cancer have regional nodal metastasis at initial diagnosis. The axillary lymph nodes are involved in 40% of patients with breast cancer. The 10-year survival rate is significantly higher in patients with no involvement of nodes (65–80%) than in those with involvement of one to three nodes (38–63%) or more than three axillary nodes (13–27%) [13]. The axillary lymph node status is the single most important prognostic indicator in breast cancer patients. Using qualitative FDG PET in 51 patients, Avril et al. [14] reported an overall sensitivity of 79% and a specificity of 96% for detection of axillary nodal involvement. However, the sensitivity was only 33% without any change of specificity in patients with tumors smaller than 2 cm. In a prospective study of 124 patients, Utech et al. [15] demonstrated a weak correlation between the quantitative FDG uptake in the metastatic axillary nodes and the size and the S-phase fraction of the primary breast tumor in the 44 patients who had axillary nodal involvement. Guided by PET results, axillary dissection might be limited to patients with positive PET studies. However, PET is notable in detecting micrometastatic disease in lymph nodes. No imaging technique is routinely used to image internal mammary nodes, and sampling is not routinely performed.

FDG PET can not only detect the primary breast cancer and nodal metastases, but also bone and liver metastases. The overall sensitivity of FDG PET for the detection of all malignant lesions is reportedly greater than 85%, with a positive predictive value of 94% [16]. Many reports have suggested that PET is more sensitive than conventional staging imaging at detecting the true extent of disease and often reveals unsuspected metastases.

PET for Monitoring Therapy

PET offers the ability to quantitatively assess tumor metabolic activity, and thus may predict tumor behavior and therapeutic response. After therapy, the amount of tumor FDG uptake reflects the number of viable tumor cells present with the glucose metabolic rate of tumor cells [17]. It has been shown that an increase in FDG uptake in breast cancer over time is associated with tumor progression [18]. Semiquantitative and qualitative FDG PET of primary breast cancers showed a rapid and significant decrease in tumor glucose metabolism shortly after instituting chemohormonotherapy [19]. We have compared FDG PET with mammography and sonography in 16 patients with locally advanced breast carcinoma who received preoperative chemotherapy. FDG PET was superior to both mammography and sonography for the detection of primary breast cancer. There was a substantial decrease in tumor metabolism early in the course of effective chemotherapy [20]. Those reports suggest that based on tumor response at the biochemical level, PET could be used to guide changes in treatment regimen during the early course of therapy. Recent studies also reported that FDG PET can be used to improve prediction of the clinical outcome of previously treated breast cancer patients relative to what is achievable through conventional imaging alone. The positive and negative predictive values of PET were 93% and 84%, respectively. The prognostic accuracy of single whole-body PET was superior to that of multiple procedures with conventional imaging (90% vs. 75%) [21].

Receptor Imaging

Most breast cancers are hormone dependent, as shown by increases in the estrogen and progesterone receptors in the tumor. Estrogen receptor (ER)-positive breast cancers are less aggressive than ER-negative cancers, and are likely to respond to hormonal therapy. Quantitative and qualitative assays provide limited information about the functional status of the receptors and responsiveness to hormone therapy: only 55–60% of patients with ER-positive breast cancer respond to such treatment [22]. Therefore, a noninvasive method for the functional status of receptors would be of critical importance in identifying patients who will benefit from hormone therapy. Various steroidal and nonsteroidal estrogens labeled with ^{77}Br, ^{75}Br, ^{18}F, ^{123}I, and Tc-99 m have been synthesized. 16d-^{18}F-fluro-17B-estradiol (FES) has high specific activity and high affinity for ER-positive target tissues. FES PET has been shown to be highly sensitive (93%) for the detection of ER-positive metastatic foci in patients with breast cancer [23]. In addition, FES accumulation within metastatic lesions decreased after instituting tamoxifen therapy [24]. However, there was no significant relationship between FDG uptake and either ER status or FES uptake [25]. The overall rate of agreement between the results of in vitro ER assays and the results of FES PET was 88% [25]. Tumor heterogeneity and ER concordance between primary and metastatic breast cancers have been observed. The information about the intrinsic heterogeneity of receptor expression within individual lesions as well as the concordance or discordance between the primary and metastatic or recurrent lesions may be useful in selecting the mode of therapy, and the biologic availability of the receptors in vivo may more reliably predict hormone responsiveness than in vitro assay results. The discordance between primary and metastatic or recurrent lesions has been reported in 20–25% of breast cancer patients [25].

The clinical flare reaction is seen in 5–20% of patients with ER-positive metastatic breast cancer and generally occurs within 7–10 days after instituting antiestrogen therapy [26]. Clinically and radiographically, the flare reaction is not distinguishable from progression of disease, and is presumably due to temporary agonist effects of the antiestrogen agent on the tumor. It has been shown that tamoxifen and estrogen cause a similar increase in FDG uptakes in ER-rich organs early in the course of therapy [27]. Response to tamoxifen was correctly predicted by the presence of metabolic flare (increased FDG uptake) and the degree of ER blockade (decreased FES uptake) after tamoxifen therapy [28].

Future

Conventional FDG PET or PET/CT often fails to provide relevant information on small breast tumors because of the limited resolution of current scanners, resulting in less contrast between tumor and background. Positron emission mammography achieves a spatial resolution of 1.5 mm. It can be combined with conventional mammographic technology for the precise anatomic localization of positive findings. There are several other PET agents that image other metabolic mechanisms: F-18 fluoro-L-thymidine for tumor proliferation, F-18 annexin V for apoptosis, and matrix metalloproteinase for metastasis.

References

1. Jemal A, Thomas A, Murray T, et al. Cancer statistics. CA Cancer J Clin. 2002;52:23–47.
2. Kopans DB. The positive predictive value of mammography. AJR Am J Roentgenol. 1992;1158:521–6.
3. Stavros AT, Thickman D, Sisney GA, et al. Solid breast nodules: use of sonography to distinguish between benign and malignant lesions. Radiology. 1995;196:123–33.
4. Amano S, Inoue T, Tomiyoshi K, et al. In vivo comparison of PET and SPECT radiopharmaceuticals in detecting breast cancer. J Nucl Med. 1998;39:1424–7.
5. Avril N, Menzel M, Dose J, et al. Glucose metabolism of breast cancer assessed by F-18 FDG PET: histologic and immunohistochemical tissue analysis. J Nucl Med. 2001;42:9–16.
6. Crippa F, Seregini E, Agresti R, et al. Association between F-18 flurodeoxyglucose uptake and postoperative histopathology, hormone receptor status, thymidine labelling index and p53 in primary breast cancer; a preliminary observation. Eur J Nucl Med. 1998;25:1429–34.
7. Paramagul CP, Helvic MA, Adler DD. Invasive lobular carcinoma: sonographic appearance and role of sonography in improving diagnostic sensitivity. Radiology. 1995;195:231–4.
8. Brown RS, Leung JY, Fisher SJ, et al. Intratumoral distribution of tritiated fluorodeoxyglucose in breast carcinoma. Are inflammatory cells important? J Nucl Med. 1995;36:1854–61.
9. Clavo AC, Wahl RL. Effects of hypoxia on the uptake of tritiated thymidine, L-leucine, L-methionine and FDG in cultured cancer cells. J Nucl Med. 1996;37:502–6.
10. Haberkorn U, Strauss LG, Reisser C, et al. Glucose uptake, perfusion, and cell proliferation in head and neck tumors: relation of positron emission tomography to flow cytometry. J Nucl Med. 1991;32: 1548–55.
11. Burgman P, O'Donoghue JA, Humm JL, et al. Hypoxia-induced increase in FDG uptake in MCF7 cells. J Nucl Med. 2001;42:170–5.
12. Wahl RL, Helvie MA, Chang AE, et al. Detection of breast cancer in women after augmentation mammoplasty using F-18 fluorodeoxyglucose PET. J Nucl Med. 1994;35:872–5.
13. Flanagan FL, Dehdashti F, Siegel BA. PET in breast cancer. Semin Nucl Med. 1998;28:290–302.
14. Avril N, Dose J, Jäniicke F, et al. Assessment of axillary lymph node involvement in breast patients with positron emission tomography using radiolabeled 2-(fluorine-18)-fluoro-2-deoxy-D-glucose. J Natl Cancer Inst. 1996;88:1204–9.
15. Utech CI, Young CS, Winter PF. Prospective evaluation of F-18 FDG PET in breast cancer for staging of the axilla related to surgery and immunocytochemistry. Eur J Nucl Med. 1997;23:1588–93.
16. Hoh K, Hawkins RA, Glaspy JA, et al. Cancer detection with whole-body PET using F-18 FDG. J Comput Assist Tomogr. 1993;17:582–289.
17. Haberkorn U, Reinhardt M, Strauss LG, et al. Metabolic design of combination therapy: use of enhanced fluorodeoxyglucose uptake caused by chemotherapy. J Nucl Med. 1992;33:1981–7.
18. Minn H, Soini I. F-18 FDG scintigraphy in diagnosis and follow up of treatment in advanced breast cancer. Eur J Nucl Med. 1989;15:61–6.
19. Jansson T, Westlin JE, Ahlstrom H, et al. PET studies in patients with locally advanced and/or metastatic breast cancer: a method for early therapy evaluation? J Clin Oncol. 1995;13:1470–744.
20. Bassa P, Kim EE, Inoue T, et al. Evaluation of preoperative chemotherapy using PET with F-18 FDG in breast cancer. J Nucl Med. 1996;37:931–8.
21. Vranjesevic D, Filmont JE, Meta J, et al. Whole-body F-18 FDG PET and conventional imaging for predicting outcome in previously treated breast cancer patients. J Nucl Med. 2002;43:325–9.
22. Ravdin PM, Green S, Dorr TM, et al. Prognostic significance of progesterone receptor levels in

estrogen receptor positive patients with metastatic breast cancer treated with tamoxifen: results of a prospective Southwest Oncology Group study. J Clin Oncol. 1992;10:1284–91.

23. McGuire AH, Dehdashti F, Siegel BA, et al. Positron tomographic assessment of estrogen receptors in breast assays. J Nucl Med. 1995;36:1766–74.
24. Dehdashti F, Mortimer JE, Siegel BA, et al. Positron tomographic assessment of estrogen receptors in breast cancer. Comparison with FDG PET and in vitro receptor assays. J Nucl Med. 1995;36: 1766–74.
25. Butler JA, Trezona T, Vargas H, et al. Value of measuring hormone receptor levels of regional metastatic carcinoma of the breast. Arch Surg. 1989; 124:1131–6.
26. Welch MJ, Bonasera TA, Sherman EIC, et al. F-18 FDG and 162-(F-18) fluoroestradiol-17B (FES) uptake in estrogen-receptor (ER)-rich tissues following tamoxifen treatment: a preclinical study. J Nucl Med. 1995;36:39–44.
27. Wahl RL, Cody R, Fisher S. Uptake before and after estrogen receptor stimulation: feasibility studies for functional receptor imaging. J Nucl Med. 1991;32:1011–5.
28. Dehdashti F, Flanagan FL, Siegel BA. PET assessment of metabolic flare in advanced breast cancer. Radiology. 1997;205:220–5.

Coronary Artery Disease

19

Won Woo Lee, Dong Soo Lee, and Myung-Chul Lee

Introduction

Positron emission tomography (PET) is a promising tool for evaluating coronary artery disease (CAD). Assessments of the myocardial uptakes of PET tracers such as N-13 ammonia, O-15 water, and Rb-82 (Table 19.1) have proven to be useful for evaluating myocardial perfusion. Quantitative measurements of myocardial perfusion using PET have been performed successfully in basic and clinical research [1–3]. Because of its high accuracy at detecting jeopardized myocardial perfusion, PET is viewed with promise with respect to the noninvasive diagnosis of CAD [4]. Furthermore, the integration of function and anatomy as offered by state-of-the-art PET/CT demonstrates the potential clinical utility of PET/CT [5].

W.W. Lee, M.D. (✉)
Department of Nuclear Medicine, Seoul National University College of Medicine, Bundang Hospital, Gyeonggi-Do 463-707, South Korea
e-mail: wwlee@snu.ac.kr

D.S. Lee, M.D., Ph.D.
Department of Nuclear Medicine, Seoul National University College of Medicine, Seoul 110-744, South Korea

WCU Department of Molecular Medicine and Biopharmaceutical Sciences, Seoul National University, Seoul, South Korea
e-mail: dsl@snu.ac.kr

M.-C. Lee, M.D., Ph.D.
Department of Nuclear Medicine, Gachon University School of Medicine, 1198 Guwol-dong, Namdong-Gu, Incheon 405, South Korea
e-mail: mclee@gilhospital.com

Myocardial Perfusion PET

N-13 ammonia is a widely used PET tracer for the assessment of myocardial perfusion. The initial distribution of N-13 ammonia demonstrates the perfusion status of myocardium. Because N-13 has a short half-life of 10 min, N-13 ammonia PET can be performed under rest and stress conditions. The delayed uptake of N-13 ammonia was reported to demonstrate myocardial retention, and consequently a type of myocardial metabolism.

N-13 ammonia is present in plasma as a form of NH_4^+ or NH_3, and taken up in tissue in the form of N-13 glutamine through the glutamate-glutamine reaction. This process is demonstrated by a 2-compartment model (Fig. 19.1). In Figure 19.1, C_a and C_E represent unmetabolized free ammonia in the artery and tissue, respectively, and C_M represents metabolized N-13 compounds. V is the volume of distribution for free ammonia, and the constant of 0.8 is usually used.

When considering the spillover effect from the blood pool to the myocardial area, the total radioactivity demonstrated on PET images is:

$$C_{tiss}(t) = C_E(t) + C_M(t) + Sp \cdot C_a(t)$$

E.E. Kim et al. (eds.), *Clinical PET and PET/CT: Principles and Applications*,
DOI 10.1007/978-1-4419-0802-5_19,

Table 19.1 PET tracers used for myocardial perfusion measurements

	N-13 ammonia	O-15 water	Rb-82
First-pass extraction (maximum)	80–100%	100%	50–60%
Physical half-life	10 min	2 min	75 s
Positron energy (maximum)	1.19 MeV	1.72 MeV	3.35 MeV
Positron range in water (root mean square)	0.57 mm	1.02 mm	2.60 mm
Uptake mechanism	Passive diffusion, metabolism	Free diffusion	Na/K ATPase
Production	Cyclotron	Cyclotron	Sr-82/Rb-82 generator

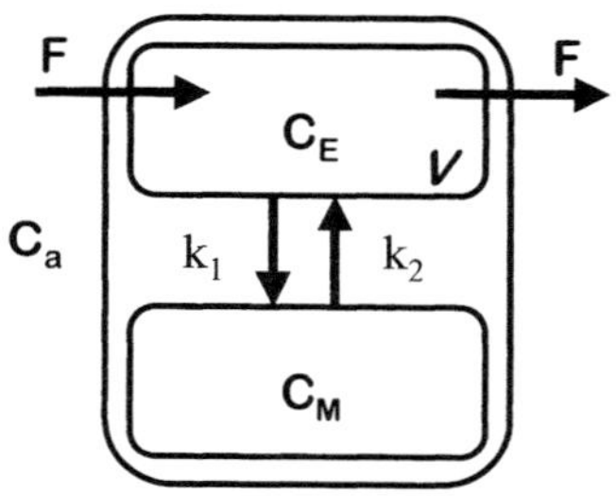

Fig. 19.1 Metabolism of ammonia in 2-compartment model Ca and CE represent unmetabolized free ammonia in the artery and tissue, respectively, and CM represents metabolized N-13 compounds. V is the volume of distribution for free ammonia

With the results of the differential equation for C_E and C_M, it is calculated with the assumption of $k_2=0$ as:

$$\frac{C_{tiss}(t)}{C_a(t)} = K\cdot\frac{\int_0^t C_a(\tau)d\tau}{C_a(t)} + \frac{F^2V}{(F+K_1)^2} + Sp$$

In this equation, K is a slope of a first order function and it can be acquired by the linear regression method. Subsequently, the regional myocardial blood flow can be calculated by the relationship between K and blood flow, FL:

$$K = F\cdot(1-0.607e^{125/F})$$

O-15 water PET can also be used as a tracer for perfusion as the water is taken up in the myocardium through free diffusion. Therefore, the single compartment model can be adopted for the assessment of myocardial perfusion. As in the protocol for stress-rest SPECT, stress and rest perfusion can be assessed. Perfusible tissue index (PTI) can be calculated from a single compartment model and constant of partial volume effect.

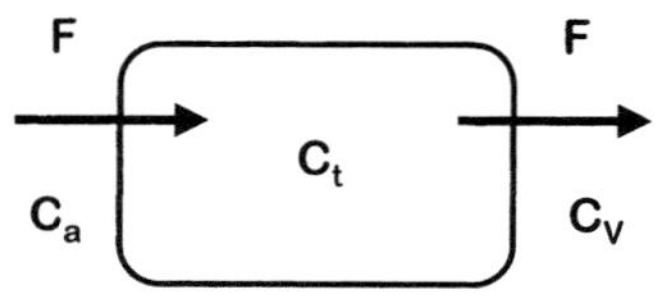

Fig. 19.2 Kety-Schmidt model for the calculation of perfusible tissue index (PTI). Water diffuses freely into tissue

PTI has been reported to demonstrate a myocardial viability and demonstrate heterogeneity of perfusion in another study.

As water diffuses freely into tissue, a Kety-Schmidt model can be used (Fig. 19.2). In this model, C_t is expressed as:

$$\frac{dC_t(t)}{dt} = F\cdot C_a(t) - F\cdot C_V(t)$$

This differential equation can be solved by assuming that tracer concentrations in tissues and veins are in an instantaneous equilibrium as:

$$C_t(t) = F\cdot C_a(t)\otimes e^{-\frac{Ft}{\lambda}} = F\cdot\int_0^t C_a(\tau)e^{-\frac{F}{\lambda}(t-\tau)}d\tau$$

where λ is the partition coefficient and usually set as 0.92. This equation can be written using correction parameters for partial volume effect (FMM) and spill-over as:

$$C_t(t) = FMM\cdot F\cdot C_a(t)\otimes e^{-\frac{F\cdot t}{\lambda}} + Sp\cdot C_a(t)$$

Rb-82 is also used as a perfusion tracer. Its short physical half-life of only 75 s made it possible to obtain repetitive studies such as stress-rest protocol in less than 30 min. Rb-82 is taken up by myocardial cells via Na/A ATPase. The first-pass extraction fraction of Rb-82 is approximately 50–60% at rest, but this reduces to 25–30% as blood flow increases in a nonlinear manner. The positron emitted by Rb-82 has a high kinetic energy [6] and a long range [7] before annihilation (Table 19.1). However, Rb-82 can be easily obtained by elution from a commercialized Sr-82/Rb-82 generator, and PET technical advances compensate for the physical shortcomings of Rb-82. Thus, Rb-82 became one of the most popular PET perfusion tracers, particularly in the US.

Diagnostic Accuracy of Myocardial Perfusion PET for the Detection of CAD

Myocardial perfusion PET has been widely used for the detection of CAD (Table 19.2). According to a summary result, the sensitivity, specificity, and accuracy of perfusion PET for the detection of CAD are found to be 92%, 85%, and 90%, respectively. This lower specificity is attributable to posttest referral bias. Two studies have evaluated the normalcy rates in patients with a low likelihood of CAD (<5%), and both found a normalcy rate of 100% (Table 19.2) [8, 9].

The diagnostic accuracy of perfusion PET has been reported to be superior to that of perfusion SPECT in head-to-head comparative studies [8–10]. Furthermore, the image quality of perfusion PET is usually better than that of perfusion SPECT because of its greater counting efficiency, robust attenuation correction, and higher spatial resolution [8]. However, further studies are required to clarify the cost effectiveness of perfusion PET over perfusion SPECT.

Integration of PET and CT for the Assessment of CAD

CT information obtained from current PET/CT scanners is primarily used for the attenuation correction of perfusion PET images. However, the simultaneous acquisition of perfusion PET and cardiac CT data may dramatically change the diagnosis of CAD in the near future because the presence of an obstructive coronary anatomy is effectively diagnosed by CT angiography (CTA) and atherosclerotic burden can be determined through coronary calcium scoring [7]. Furthermore, radiation overexposure resulting from the integration of cardiac PET/CT can be effectively minimized by using a stress-only perfusion protocol, prospective electrocardiography (ECG)-triggering, ECG-gated tube modulation, and other techniques [11].

Functionally relevant coronary stenosis or a subtending coronary artery responsible for perfusion abnormality can be readily demonstrated using the three-dimensional (3D) fusion images of integrated PET/CT (Fig. 19.3) [5]. Furthermore,

Table 19.2 Diagnostic accuracy of perfusion PET for the detection of CAD

Author	Year	Patient no.	PET perfusion tracer	Sensitivity	Specificity	PPV	NPV	Accuracy
Gould et al. [12]	1986	31	N-13 NH3/Rb-82	0.95	1.00	1.00	0.90	0.97
Tamaki et al. [13]	1988	51	N-13 NH3	0.98	1.00	1.00	0.75	0.98
Go et al. [10]	1990	202	Rb-82	0.93	0.78	0.93	0.80	0.90
Stewart et al. [14]	1991	81	Rb-82	0.85	0.86	0.94	0.67	0.85
Marwick et al. [15]	1992	74	Rb-82	0.90	1.00	1.00	0.36	0.91
Grover-McKay et al. [16]	1992	31	Rb-82	1.00	0.73	0.80	1.00	0.87
Bateman et al. [8]	2006	112	Rb-82	0.87	0.93 (normalcy rate 1.00)	0.95	0.81	0.89
Sampson et al. [9]	2007	102	Rb-82	0.93	0.83 (normalcy rate 1.00)	0.80	0.94	0.87
Total		684		0.92	0.85	0.93	0.81	0.90

PPV positive predictive value, *NPV* negative predictive value

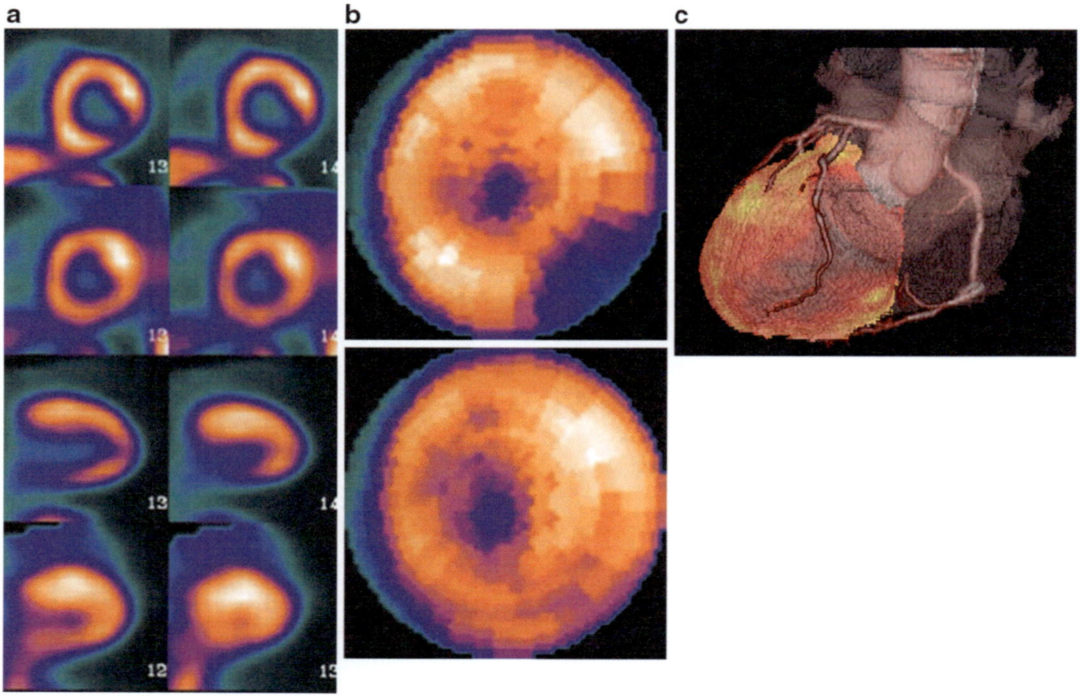

Fig. 19.3 Integrated PET/CT images demonstrating a subtending coronary artery responsible for a reversible perfusion defect. A reversible perfusion defect is observed at the inferolateral wall on tomographic images (**a**) and on the polar map (**b**) of adenosine stress-rest N-13 ammonia PET and 3D cardiac N-13 ammonia/CTA combined images (**c**) (Reprinted with permission of Nucl Med Mol Imaging)

coronary calcium scoring plays a crucial role in determining the intensity of medical therapy. Thus, a one-stop approach for the evaluation of CAD can be achieved using integrated PET/CT. However, it remains to be determined whether integrated PET/CT affects survival or clinical outcomes.

References

1. Ahn JY, Lee DS, Lee JS, et al. Quantification of regional myocardial blood flow using dynamic H2(15) O PET and factor analysis. J Nucl Med. 2001; 42(5):782–7.
2. Lee JS, Lee DS, Ahn JY, et al. Blind separation of cardiac components and extraction of input function from H(2)(15)O dynamic myocardial PET using independent component analysis. J Nucl Med. 2001;42(6):938–43.
3. Lee JS, Lee DS, Ahn JY, et al. Generation of parametric image of regional myocardial blood flow using H(2)(15)O dynamic PET and a linear least-squares method. J Nucl Med. 2005;46(10):1687–95.
4. Demer LL, Gould KL, Goldstein RA, et al. Assessment of coronary artery disease severity by positron emission tomography. Comparison with quantitative arteriography in 193 patients. Circulation. 1989;79(4):825–35.
5. Cho IH, Kong EJ. Myocardial perfusion PET. Nucl Med Mol Imaging. 2009;43(3):207–14.
6. Lee DS, Kang WJ, Lee WW, Paeng JC. Cardiovascular and other circulatory system. In: Chung JK, Lee MC, editors. Nuclear medicine. Seoul: Korea Medical Book Publisher; 2008. p. 349–394.
7. Di Carli MF, Dorbala S, Meserve J, El Fakhri G, Sitek A, Moore SC. Clinical myocardial perfusion PET/CT. J Nucl Med. 2007;48(5):783–93.
8. Bateman TM, Heller GV, McGhie AI, et al. Diagnostic accuracy of rest/stress ECG-gated Rb-82 myocardial perfusion PET: comparison with ECG-gated Tc-99 m sestamibi SPECT. J Nucl Cardiol. 2006;13(1):24–33.
9. Sampson UK, Dorbala S, Limaye A, Kwong R, Di Carli MF. Diagnostic accuracy of rubidium-82 myocardial perfusion imaging with hybrid positron emission tomography/computed tomography in the detection of coronary artery disease. J Am Coll Cardiol. 2007;49(10):1052–8.
10. Go RT, Marwick TH, MacIntyre WJ, et al. A prospective comparison of rubidium-82 PET and thallium-201 SPECT myocardial perfusion imaging utilizing a

single dipyridamole stress in the diagnosis of coronary artery disease. J Nucl Med. 1990;31(12):1899–905.
11. Husmann L, Herzog BA, Gaemperli O, et al. Diagnostic accuracy of computed tomography coronary angiography and evaluation of stress-only single-photon emission computed tomography/computed tomography hybrid imaging: comparison of prospective electrocardiogram-triggering vs. retrospective gating. Eur Heart J. 2009;30(5):600–7.
12. Gould KL, Goldstein RA, Mullani NA, et al. Noninvasive assessment of coronary stenoses by myocardial perfusion imaging during pharmacologic coronary vasodilation VIII Clinical feasibility of positron cardiac imaging without a cyclotron using generator-produced rubidium-82. J Am Coll Cardiol. 1986;7(4):775–89.
13. Tamaki N, Yonekura Y, Senda M, et al. Value and limitation of stress thallium-201 single photon emission computed tomography: comparison with nitrogen-13 ammonia positron tomography. J Nucl Med. 1988;29(7):1181–8.
14. Stewart RE, Schwaiger M, Molina E, et al. Comparison of rubidium-82 positron emission tomography and thallium-201 SPECT imaging for detection of coronary artery disease. Am J Cardiol. 1991;67(16):1303–10.
15. Marwick TH, Nemec JJ, Stewart WJ, Salcedo EE. Diagnosis of coronary artery disease using exercise echocardiography and positron emission tomography: comparison and analysis of discrepant results. J Am Soc Echocardiogr. 1992;5(3):231–8.
16. Grover-McKay M, Ratib O, Schwaiger M, et al. Detection of coronary artery disease with positron emission tomography and rubidium 82. Am Heart J. 1992;123(3):646–52.

Myocardial Viability

20

Won Jun Kang

Introduction

Ischemic heart disease is the most common cause of heart failure. For the treatment of heart failure, medical treatment, heart transplantation, and revascularization can be a therapeutic method [1]. Because of the ease of the procedure and good therapeutic performance, revascularization has been widely used in ischemic heart disease [2]. However, revascularization has a substantial degree of risk associated with the procedure, especially in patients with severe heart failure, and heart function is recovered only in some of the patients who undergo revascularization [3].

Myocardium with decreased contractility that can be recovered after revascularization, such as stent or coronary artery bypass grafting, is called viable myocardium although myocardial scar is not recovered even after successful revascularization. In view of the histology, viable myocardium is composed of viable myocytes, while myocardial scar is composed of extensive fibrosis [4]. Differentiation of viable myocardium and scarred myocardium is of great importance because selecting appropriate patients for revascularization can reduce the possible risks that might be caused by an unnecessary procedure.

The mechanism of viable myocardium is explained by 'hibernation' that has contractility dysfunction caused by long-standing chronic ischemia and 'stunning', which has contractility dysfunction after an ischemic episode [5, 6]. Hibernation and stunning are not separate processes, but can be present in the same patient [7]. Hibernation is thought to be a natural protecting mechanism by which ventricular work and energy consumption can be reduced. A repetitive ischemic episode can cause myocardial dysfunction even after restoration of resting blood flow, which is called 'repetitive stunning' [8]. Stunned myocardium with preserved resting blood flow is thought to be converted into hibernation with decreased resting blood flow after the passing of a certain period of time (Table 20.1).

The prevalence of viable myocardium is of value in selecting patients with viable myocardium, which can be influenced by the characteristics of enrolled patients, and the method to evaluate viable myocardium. A meta-analysis involving four different studies reported that approximately 50% of enrolled patients had viable myocardium [9].

W.J. Kang, M.D., Ph.D. (✉)
Division of Nuclear Medicine, Department of Nuclear Medicine, Yonsei University, Severance Hospital, 134 Shinchon-dong, Seodaemun-gu, Seoul 120-752, South Korea
e-mail: mdkwj@yuhs.ac

E.E. Kim et al. (eds.), *Clinical PET and PET/CT: Principles and Applications*,
DOI 10.1007/978-1-4419-0802-5_20, © Springer Science+Business Media New York 2013

Table 20.1 Myocardial perfusion SPECT findings according to perfusion status

	Definition	SPECT findings
Ischemic myocardium	Myocardium with insufficient oxygen supply by coronary stenosis	Defect on stress image
Infarction	Myocardial necrosis by coronary obstruction	Defect on stress and rest images
Hibernation	Myocardium with contractile dysfunction by chronically decreased perfusion abnormality	Rest perfusion defect; Improved perfusion on delayed thallium image or reinjection image
Stunning	Myocardium with persistent contractile dysfunction despite restoration of perfusion after ischemic injury	Normal SPECT (left ventricular dysfunction)

Gold Standard for Viable Myocardium

As the gold standard to determine presence of viable myocardium, improvement of regional left ventricular wall contractility, improvement of left ejection fraction, symptomatic improvement, improvement of exercise capacity, improvement of left ventricular remodeling, prevention of sudden cardiac death, and long-term prognosis were suggested. The most widely used endpoint for viable myocardium studies is assessment of regional left ventricular functional improvement following revascularization. In terms of clinical application, patient-based global function, such as ejection fraction, is most important. However, many studies measured segmental wall motion improvement after revascularization. A meta-analysis studying 15,045 segments from 3,003 patients showed a sensitivity of 84% and a specificity of 69% by using segmental wall motion improvement as the gold standard [10]. Generally, nuclear imaging has had reports of higher sensitivity than other imaging modalities, while dobutamine stress echocardiography showed higher specificity.

To expect an increase in the ejection fraction, a substantial amount of viable myocardium is needed in the patient base. Studies reported that over 25–30% of overall myocardium would be needed to show improvement in ejection fraction [11].

However, Samady et al. reported that the survival rate was improved even in patients without ejection fraction improvement. In addition to ejection fraction improvement, improvements in myocardial remodeling, prevention of arrhythmia, and prevention of sudden cardiac death should also be considered as parameters for viability studies [12]. A viability study using fluorodeoxyglucose (FDG) positron emission tomography (PET) showed predictive value in the improvement of exercise capacity and heart failure symptoms following revascularization [13].

Assessment of Viability with Myocardial SPECT

A persistent or fixed perfusion defect on myocardial single-photon emission computed tomography (SPECT) is likely to have scar tissue. However, about 20% of persistent perfusion defects can be caused by hibernating myocardium rather than scar. In hibernating myocardium, cardiac myocytes have preserved cell membrane potential and preserved metabolism status to support cellular survival despite decreased perfusion. Hibernating myocardium with decreased perfusion and contractile dysfunction is viable myocardium that can restore contractile function by means of revascularization.

For the evaluation of viable myocardium, thallium-201 myocardial SPECT is most widely used. The procedure of thallium absorption to myocardium is an energy-dependent process and requires preserved cell membrane integrity. Therefore, myocardium with thallium uptake represents viable myocardium. The degree of thallium uptake depends on tissue survival, and thallium myocardial perfusion SPECT can be

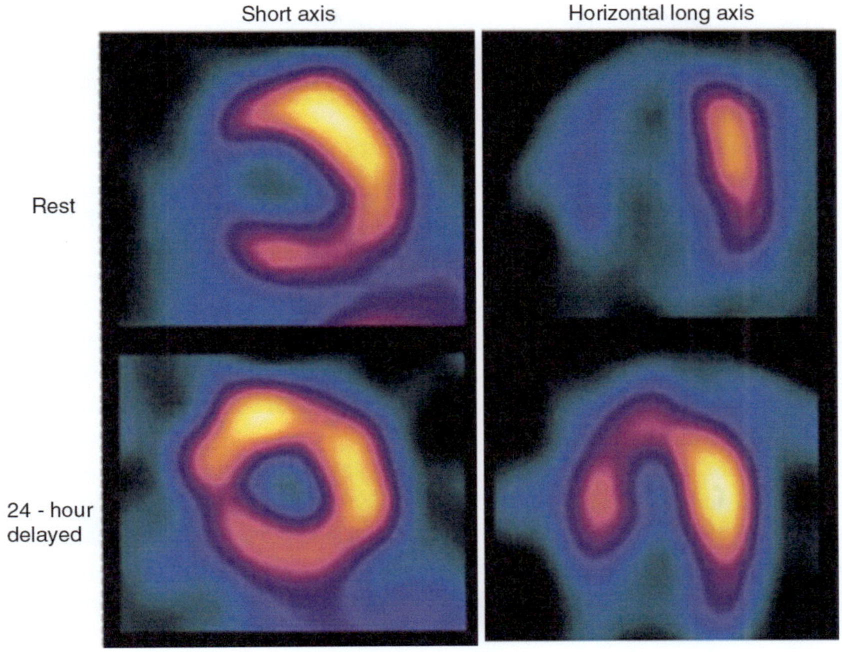

Fig. 20.1 Thallium-201 rest (*top*) and 24-h delayed (*bottom*) images. Severe perfusion decrease was noted on rest image, but perfusion was almost restored on 24-h delayed image. According to findings, significant amount of viable myocardium was expected on septum

used for differentiation of scar and hibernating myocardium. Generally, the myocardium with rest thallium uptake greater than 50% is thought to be viable myocardium. Occasionally, additional increased uptake over 10% on delayed thallium images is thought to be a hallmark of viable myocardium (Fig. 20.1) [14].

Several protocols can be used for the evaluation of myocardium using thallium myocardial SPECT, such as a rest-redistribution image or a stress-redistribution-reinjection image. The rest-redistribution protocol using thallium is mostly used for viability evaluation, and assesses rest blood flow and delayed redistribution simultaneously. The stress-redistribution-reinjection protocol can evaluate ischemia by stress-rest reversibility workup and viability by a reinjection technique.

The sensitivity and specificity of thallium SPECT to predict regional wall motion recovery after revascularization was reported to be 86% and 59%, respectively [9]. Relatively low specificity was thought to be the result of inclusion of the subendocardial infarction with thallium uptake lower than 50%.

Recently, myocardial SPECT with sestamibi or tetrofosmin has been used for the study of viability [15]. Sestamibi or tetrofosmin SPECT assesses the myocardium with preserved mitochondrial function, and subsequently viability using the fact that viable myocardium has preserved mitochondrial function. Generally speaking, the sensitivity of setamibi or tetrofosmin SPECT has inferior sensitivity to thallium SPECT for detection of viable myocardium. To reinforce the sensitivity, additional images following sublingual or intravenous nitrate administration can be obtained on sestamibi or tetrofosmin SPECT [16].

Assessment of Viability with FDG PET

FDG is an analog for glucose and enters the cytoplasm and undergoes the phosphorylation process which requires adenosine phosphate

(ATP). Because the phosphorylation process using ATP is conducted only in viable cells, and myocardium with FDG uptake can be regarded as viable myocardium. Myocardial FDG uptake is influenced by metabolic status, especially blood glucose and fatty acid level. Fatty acid metabolism is increased in the normal myocardium, while glucose is the main substrate in the ischemic myocardium [17]. For obtaining FDG images to assess viable myocardium, hyperinsulinemic-normal glucose level is most profit metabolic-hormonal status, which can be achieved by insulin clamp. However, because of the ease of accessibility, oral glucose intake is a preferred method in clinical practice [18]. Nicotinic acid derivatives such as acipimox inhibit peripheral lipolysis and indirectly increase myocardial glucose uptake. Acipimox can be used in performing myocardial FDG PET instead of using an insulin clamp [19].

The chronically hypoperfused myocardium can have severe hypoperfusion even in a rest state, thus, myocardial on SPECT can represent a persistent perfusion defect. In chronically hypoperfused myocytes, glycolysis is promoted to produce ATP, and therefore, FDG uptake on chronically hypoperfused myocardium shows greater FDG uptake than normal myocytes.

To obtain a more reliable result, it is recommended that myocardial perfusion be compared with myocardial FDG uptake. Myocardium with FDG uptake over 50% of the normal area is considered to be viable myocardium. The FDG uptake can be quantitatively assessed but semi-quantitative assessment comparing normal tissue is more widely used in the clinical setting.

FDG PET results can be classified into normal, viable myocardium, and scar tissue. Myocardial perfusion can be measured by myocardial perfusion PET using N-13 ammonia or Rb-82. Myocardial perfusion and glucose metabolism are preserved in normal myocardium, while myocardial perfusion and metabolism are impaired in scar tissue. In both cases myocardial perfusion and metabolism images look similar and are called matched lesions. In dysfunctioning viable myocardium, FDG uptake is preserved in the area of decreased perfusion assessed by N-13 ammonia or Rb-82 PET, which is called 'perfusion-metabolism mismatch' (Figs. 20.2 and 20.3). Perfusion-metabolism mismatch is a strong indicator for viable myocardium (Table. 20.2), and functional improvement is expected after revascularization [20, 21].

A meta-analysis summarizing 12 studies reported that the sensitivity and specificity of FDG PET in detecting viable myocardium were 93% and 58%, respectively [9]. Another study analyzing 12 FDG PET studies revealed that the left ventricular ejection fraction (LVEF) of patients with viable myocardium improved from 37% to 47%, while the LVEF of patients without viable myocardium showed no significant change at 39% to 40% [22].

Determining a treatment plan according to the presence of viable myocardium is an important prognostic factor. Data from a meta-analysis showed that the prognosis in viable myocardium was better in the revascularization group than in the medical treatment group, while the prognosis of nonviable myocardium was not different between the revascularization and the medical treatment group [23]. This result showed that the cardiovascular event rate can be decreased only in patients with viable myocardium by performing revascularization.

Conclusion

The assessment of viable myocardium is important in selecting patients who will benefit from revascularization. For patients with sufficient viable myocardium, revascularization is indicated, while patients with scar tissue should be treated medically. Myocardial perfusion SPECT and FDG PET are established methods with good diagnostic performance in assessing viable myocardium. Recently, advancements for tools such as SPECT/CT and PET/CT allow combining of anatomic information from CT angiography and functional information from SPECT or PET. The combined information of anatomic and functional information is expected to improve diagnostic accuracy in viability workup and to play a role in determining a treatment plan.

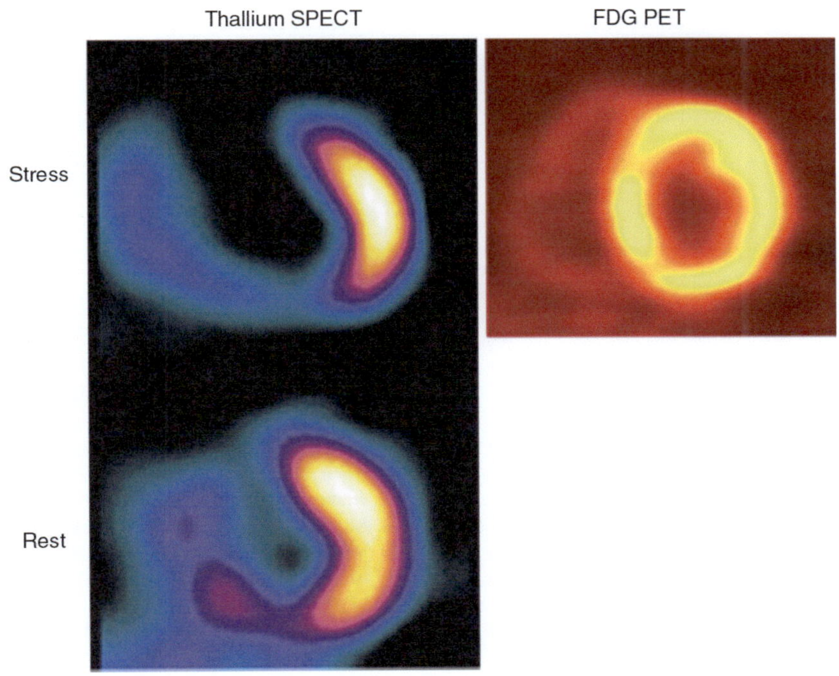

Fig. 20.2 Thallium-201 and ^{18}F-FDG PET images of viable myocardium. Severe perfusion decrease was noted on anterior, septum, and inferior wall on short axis of thallium SPECT. However FDG uptake was preserved on corresponding areas, suggestive of viable myocardium

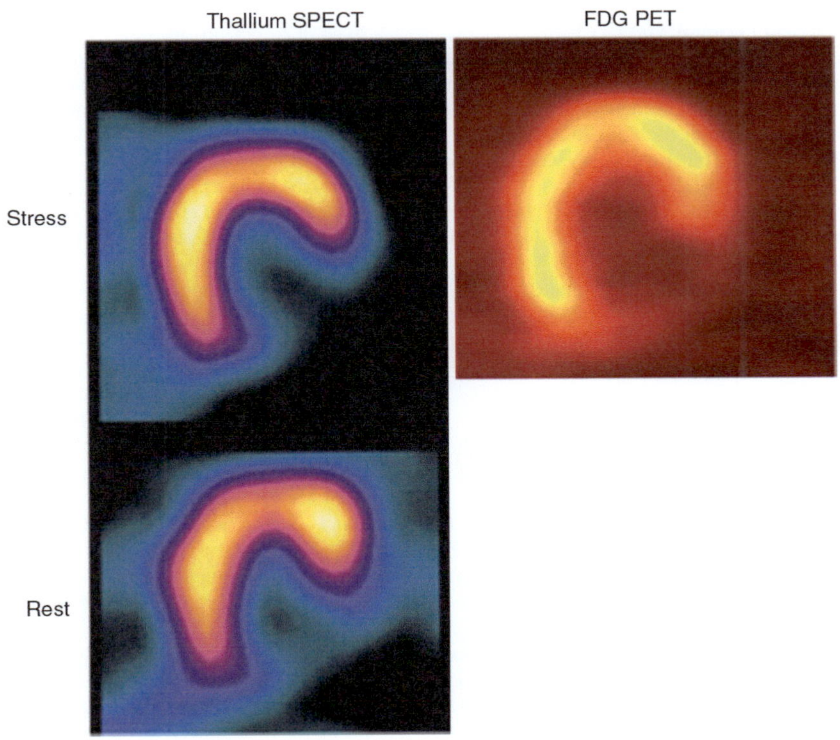

Fig. 20.3 Thallium-201 and ^{18}F-FDG PET images of scarred myocardium. Severe perfusion defect was noted in inferior and inferolateral wall on short axis of thallium SPECT. FDG PET showed matched defect, suggestive of scarred myocardium

Table 20.2 Interpretation of myocardial perfusion and glucose metabolism images

Diagnosis	Myocardial perfusion	Glucose metabolism (FDG)	Presence of viable myocardium
Normal (matched)	Normal	Normal	Present
Scar (matched)	Decreased	Decreased	Absent
Ischemia (stunning/ hibernation)	Decreased	Normal or increased	Present

References

1. Challapalli S, Bonow RO, Gheorghiade M. Medical management of heart failure secondary to coronary artery disease. Coron Artery Dis. 1998;9:659–74.
2. Alderman EL, Corley SD, Fisher LD, Chaitman BR, Faxon DP, Foster ED, Killip T, Sosa JA, Bourassa MG. Five-year angiographic follow-up of factors associated with progression of coronary artery disease in the Coronary Artery Surgery Study (CASS) CASS Participating Investigators and Staff. J Am Coll Cardiol. 1993;22(4):1141–54.
3. Schinkel AF, Poldermans D, Vanoverschelde JL, Elhendy A, Boersma E, Roelandt JR, et al. Incidence of recovery of contractile function following revascularization in patients with ischemic left ventricular dysfunction. Am J Cardiol. 2004;93:14–7.
4. Maes A, Flameng W, Nuyts J, Borgers M, Shivalkar B, Ausma J, et al. Histological alterations in chronically hypoperfused myocardium. Correlation with PET findings. Circulation. 1994;90:735–45.
5. Rahimtoola SH. The hibernating myocardium. Am Heart J. 1989;117:211–21.
6. Braunwald E, Kloner RA. The stunned myocardium: prolonged, postischemic ventricular dysfunction. Circulation. 1982;66:1146–9.
7. Bolli R. Myocardial 'stunning' in man. Circulation. 1992;86(6):1671–91.
8. Vanoverschelde JL, Melin JA. The pathophysiology of myocardial hibernation: current controversies and future directions. Prog Cardiovasc Dis. 2001;43: 387–98.
9. Bax JJ, van der Wall EE, Harbinson M. Radionuclide techniques for the assessment of myocardial viability and hibernation. Heart. 2004;90(Suppl 5):v26–33.
10. Bax JJ, Poldermans D, Elhendy A, Boersma E, Rahimtoola SH. Sensitivity, specificity, and predictive accuracies of various noninvasive techniques for detecting hibernating myocardium. Curr Probl Cardiol. 2001;26:147–86.
11. Bax JJ, Maddahi J, Poldermans D, Elhendy A, Cornel JH, Boersma E, et al. Sequential (201)Tl imaging and dobutamine echocardiography to enhance accuracy of predicting improved left ventricular ejection fraction after revascularization. J Nucl Med. 2002;43(6): 795–802.
12. Samady H, Elefteriades JA, Abbott BG, Mattera JA, McPherson CA, Wackers FJ. Failure to improve left ventricular function after coronary revascularization for ischemic cardiomyopathy is not associated with worse outcome. Circulation. 1999;100:1298–304.
13. Marwick TH, Zuchowski C, Lauer MS, Secknus MA, Williams J, Lytle BW. Functional status and quality of life in patients with heart failure undergoing coronary bypass surgery after assessment of myocardial viability. J Am Coll Cardiol. 1999;33:750–8.
14. Dilsizian V, Bonow RO. Current diagnostic techniques of assessing myocardial viability in patients with hibernating and stunned myocardium. Circulation. 1993;87:1–20.
15. Bonow RO, Dilsizian V. Thallium-201 and technetium-99 m-sestamibi for assessing viable myocardium. J Nucl Med. 1992;33:815–8.
16. Sciagrà R, Pellegri M, Pupi A, Bolognese L, Bisi G, Carnovale V, Santoro GM. Prognostic implications of Tc-99 m sestamibi viability imaging and subsequent therapeutic strategy in patients with chronic coronary artery disease and left ventricular dysfunction. J Am Coll Cardiol. 2000;36:739–45.
17. King LM, Opie LH. Glucose delivery is a major determinant of glucose utilisation in the ischemic myocardium with a residual coronary flow. Cardiovasc Res. 1998;39:381–92.
18. Gropler RJ. Methodology governing the assessment of myocardial glucose metabolism by positron emission tomography and fluorine 18-labeled fluorodeoxyglucose. J Nucl Cardiol. 1994;1:S4–14.
19. Knuuti MJ, Yki-Järvinen H, Voipio-Pulkki LM, Mäki M, Ruotsalainen U, Härkönen R, et al. Enhancement of myocardial [fluorine-18]fluorodeoxyglucose uptake by a nicotinic acid derivative. J Nucl Med. 1994;35:989–98.
20. Bax JJ, Patton JA, Poldermans D, Elhendy A, Sandler MP. 18-Fluorodeoxyglucose imaging with positron emission tomography and single photon emission computed tomography: cardiac applications. Semin Nucl Med. 2000;30:281–98.
21. Di Carli MF, Davidson M, Little R, Khanna S, Mody FV, Brunken RC, et al. Value of metabolic imaging with positron emission tomography for evaluating prognosis in patients with coronary artery disease and left ventricular dysfunction. Am J Cardiol. 1994; 73:527–33.

22. Maddahi J, Schelbert H, Brunken R, Di Carli M. Role of thallium-201 and PET imaging in evaluation of myocardial viability and management of patients with coronary artery disease and left ventricular dysfunction. J Nucl Med. 1994;35:707–15.

23. Allman KC, Shaw LJ, Hachamovitch R, Udelson JE. Myocardial viability testing and impact of revascularization on prognosis in patients with coronary artery disease and left ventricular dysfunction: a meta-analysis. J Am Coll Cardiol. 2002;39:1151–8.

21 Atherosclerosis

Jin-Chul Paeng

Atherosclerosis is a condition where arteries harden following the formation of atheroma in the vessel wall. As a result of atherosclerosis, the lumen of arteries narrows and blood flow to the subtended organ is restricted. Angina and transient ischemic attack are clinical manifestations from atherosclerosis of coronary or cerebral arteries. However, a graver consequence of atherosclerosis is thromboembolism of the end organs, such as cerebral infarct, myocardial infarct, or unstable angina. Thromboembolism is caused by rupture of atherosclerotic plaques in the critical arteries.

In the US, heart disease, including coronary artery disease, is the most common cause of death and cerebrovascular disease is the third most common cause. Additionally, based on a worldwide survey, coronary and cerebrovascular diseases are included in the three most common causes of death. Therefore, atherosclerosis is one of the most intriguing fields of medical imaging. In nuclear medicine, myocardial or cerebral perfusion imaging has been used for the assessment of hemodynamic changes caused by atherosclerosis. While perfusion imaging can provide information on the hemodynamic significance of an atherosclerotic lesion and a patient's prognosis, direct imaging of atherosclerosis is required for lesion localization and selection of treatment target. Conventional coronary angiography (CAG) and computed tomography (CT) CAG are the types of imaging methods used for atherosclerosis because they visualize the presence of atherosclerotic narrowing. However, evaluation of the simple presence of atherosclerotic plaques or resultant vascular narrowing has limited clinical significance because atherosclerosis is only a predisposing factor for fatal complications of thromboembolism, such as myocardial or cerebral infarct. Atherosclerosis is observed in 85% of the elderly population who are older than 50 years, and even 1 of 6 adolescents present with atherosclerosis [1]. However, all do not result in fatal complications. Furthermore, in many cases of myocardial infarct, culprit lesions of coronary artery thrombosis do not show critical arterial narrowing [2]. As a result, the first manifestation of coronary artery disease is fatal myocardial infarct or sudden cardiac death in 62% of male and 42% of female patients without preceding ischemic symptoms caused by chronic atherosclerosis [3]. Therefore, 'active-forming', 'rupture-prone', or 'vulnerable' plaque should be discriminated from other 'stable' plaques.

In the imaging of pathophysiologically significant atherosclerotic plaque, ^{18}F-fluorodeoxyglucose (FDG) positron emission tomography (PET) is now type of established method. In this chapter we will review pathogenesis of atherosclerosis, and various PET imaging methods targeting atherosclerotic plaques will be discussed with focus on FDG PET.

J.-C. Paeng, M.D., Ph.D. (✉)
Department of Nuclear Medicine, Seoul National University Hospital, Seoul 110-744, South Korea
e-mail: paengjc@snu.ac.kr

E.E. Kim et al. (eds.), *Clinical PET and PET/CT: Principles and Applications*,
DOI 10.1007/978-1-4419-0802-5_21,

Pathogenesis and Imaging Targets

Lipid is the most important component of atherosclerosis, and lowering of the circulating lipid (triglyceride or cholesterol) has been the major treatment targeting atherosclerosis [4, 5]. While hyperlipidemia remains an important contributor to the pathogenesis of atherosclerosis, recent interest has been directed on inflammation. Currently, atherosclerosis is considered a kind of chronic inflammation triggered by hyperlipidemia.

Low density lipoprotein (LDL) is critical in the initiation of atherosclerosis, which can diffuse through arterial endothelium. Although deposited LDL may involute spontaneously, it is prone to oxidization in the vessel wall because it is isolated from circulating antioxidants [6, 7]. LDL is converted to minimally modified LDL (mmLDL), oxidized LDL (oxLDL), and glycated LDL by oxidation. oxLDL is a powerful evoker of inflammation by stimulating endothelial cells (EC) and macrophage through CD14 and toll-like receptors [8, 9], when even mmLDL can stimulate EC. Following inflammatory stimulation, vascular EC express adhesion molecules such as selectin (CD62) and vascular cell adhesion molecule (VCAM)-1 [10], which are necessary for rolling or attachment of circulating leukocytes for migration into the inflammatory site. Recruited monocytes and derived macrophages release proteases such as matrix metalloproteinase (MMP) and cathepsin for easier cell migration in the inflammatory tissue [11, 12]. In addition, expression of scavenger receptors on macrophage is so enhanced that macrophage can engulf LDL derivatives through receptor-mediated endocytosis. Lipid-laden macrophages are called 'foam cells'. Macrophages also release critical cytokines such as tumor necrosis factor-α and interleukin (IL)-1β to amplify inflammation.

While atherosclerosis is initially pathologically characterized by foam cells, the progression of atherosclerosis is characterized by deposition of fibrous tissue. In this phase, atheroma is loosened by several proteases, and vascular smooth muscle cells (SMC) migrate into the loosened atheroma. The SMC produce extracellular matrix-filling materials such as collagen. Although various cytokines function via this process, IL-18, interferon (IFN)-γ, and CD40L are critical because they affect most of the inflammation-involved cells including the EC, macrophage, T-cell, SMC, and platelet. Therefore, there are drugs targeting these cytokines under development for atherosclerosis.

Neoangiogenesis and apoptosis in plaque are also results of inflammation and contribute to the progression of atherosclerosis [13]. Newly developed vessels in a plaque function as portals for leukocytes to migrate into the plaque, and thus, enhance inflammation. Moreover, the vessels are so fragile as to result in hemorrhage, by which plaque enlarges abruptly and thrombin is generated. Thrombin is another activator for inflammation-involved cells. Apoptosis of the inflammation-involved cells is a routine process in inflammation and is evidence of active inflammation.

Fatal complications of atherosclerosis occur when atherosclerotic plaque ruptures. The rupture of plaque is also caused by an inflammatory process in the plaque. IFN-γ, released by helper T-cells, inhibits collagen production through SMC. Furthermore, IL-1 and CD40L promote release of collagenase and MMP from macrophage [14]. The process induces thinning, erosion, and even disruption of the fibrous cap. Disruption of the fibrous cap results in the contact of blood with the highly thrombogenic plaque, and thus, is followed by rapid thrombus formation. Thrombus with a thin stalk can cause fatal complications such as acute coronary syndrome and cerebral infarct.

As described above, inflammation plays a key role in the entire process of atherosclerosis, including initiation, progression, and rupture. Therefore, most molecular imaging for vulnerable plaque has been targeted at inflammation. In nuclear medicine, various imaging probes labeled with gamma ray-emitting radioisotopes have been developed. They target each of the inflammatory processes, including oxLDL accumulation [15–17], glycated end-product accumulation [18], monocyte recruitment [19, 20], proteolytic enzyme activation [21, 22], SMC proliferation [23–25], platelet accumulation [26–29], neoangiogenesis [30–32], apoptosis [33–37], cytokine activation [38], and scavenger receptor activation [39, 40], etc. Many imaging probes have also been reported for PET and target platelet accumulatioin [41–43], choline metabolism [44, 45], MMP activation [46], macrophage accumulation [47], neoangiogenesis [48], and enhanced VCAM-1 expression [49]. However, FDG PET has been reported most often in atherosclerosis imaging, probably because FDG is an easily accessible radiotracer. There are also considerable clinical data from human studies for FDG PET as an imaging modality for atherosclerosis.

Atherosclerosis Imaging Using FDG PET

Mechanism

FDG accumulation in atherosclerotic plaques has been reported for about a decade [50, 51]. It is well known that FDG is accumulated in inflammatory lesions and FDG accumulation in atherosclerosis is regarded as a marker for active inflammation in the plaque, and therefore, for rupture-prone vulnerable plaque. FDG accumulation in inflammatory lesions is a result of activation of various inflammation-involved cells, mainly macrophage. Although some researchers reported nonspecific accumulation of FDG in calcified plaque [52], others observed close correlation of FDG accumulation with lesional macrophage. In rabbit atherosclerosis models, FDG uptake was closely correlated with distribution and density of macrophage in the plaques [53–56]. Additionally, FDG uptake on preoperative PET in human studies showed close correlation with distribution of CD68-positive macrophages in the specimens from endarterectomy [50, 57, 58]. With regard to other inflammation markers, FDG uptake was most closely correlated with CD68-positive cells in an endarterectomy specimen, although it has weaker correlation with other markers such as cathepsin K, MMP-9, and IL-18 in the specimen [59].

Clinical Implication

FDG PET in atherosclerosis is expected to be an imaging modality for vulnerable plaque, and subsequently, a marker for risk stratification and therapeutic efficacy monitoring. Selection of a treatment target is also an expected role of the imaging. For this purpose, FDG uptake should be correlated with inflammatory activity and prognosis.

FDG uptake is closely correlated with local inflammatory activity as described above. It is also correlates well with systemic inflammatory markers of serum MMP-1 and leukocyte count [60], although some researchers reported no definite correlation of FDG uptake with other inflammatory markers such as IL-18, fibrinogen, or C-reactive protein (CRP) [61]. This result suggests that FDG uptake can be a surrogate marker for systemic, or at least local, vascular inflammatory activity in atherosclerosis. In another study, FDG uptake was directly correlated with plaque disruption in a rabbit model fed with a high-cholesterol diet [55].

FDG uptake increases with increasing risk factors for fatal atherosclerotic diseases. It correlates with waist circumference, hypertension, carotid intima-media thickness, serum high-density lipoprotein, and CRP, all of which are significant risk factors for myocardial or cerebral infarct [62]. In that study, FDG uptake increased with increasing numbers of risk factors for metabolic syndrome. Another study reported similar results that FDG uptake correlates with risk factors such as smoking, age, hypertension, and hypercholesterolemia [63]. Although in regard to the risk factor of aging, a report stated that age does not affect FDG uptake in the vessels [51], while most other studies reported the correlation between them [63–65].

Calcification in major arteries detected on CT is direct evidence of atherosclerosis irrespective of inflammatory activity, and is an independent risk factor in the case of coronary artery involvement. However, it was repeatedly reported that calcification on CT does not correlate with FDG uptake on PET [51, 61, 66, 67]. This is reasonable because calcified plaque is regarded as rather stable, because FDG is accumulated mainly in active inflammatory lesions. As a result, FDG uptake was reported to be a better predictor of vascular events than calcified plaque detected on CT, although both were significant predictors [68]. In the correlation with MRI, FDG uptake was observed in atherosclerosis with necrotic lipid core [69].

Currently, some researchers have adopted FDG PET as an established imaging tool to assess inflammatory activity of atherosclerotic plaque [70, 71]. Moreover, therapeutic efficacy of anti-atherosclerotic drugs can be assessed using FDG PET. Probucol, an antioxidant, was reported to reduce FDG uptake of atherosclerotic plaques in a hypercholesterolemic rabbit model. The assessment of the efficacy of vitamin B or simvastatin, one of the main drugs used for atherosclerosis, were also reported using FDG PET [72, 73]. The application of FDG PET in therapeutic efficacy monitoring is a promising field for FDG PET in atherosclerosis.

Methods

The reproducibility of FDG PET in atherosclerosis was reportedly rather high when FDG PET was performed in the same patients and the uptake was assessed as standardized uptake value (SUV) with an interval of 2 weeks [74, 75] or with a longer-term interval [76]. However, selection of an adequate parameter on FDG PET is not as simple a problem for atherosclerosis as it is for cancer, where the maximal SUV is usually used. Among the reported studies on FDG PET of atherosclerosis, some researchers adopted maximal SUV for lesions [60, 61, 67, 68], while others adopted mean SUV for vessels of interest [62, 65, 74]. Theoretically, maximal SUV that represents maximal inflammatory activity will show better correlation with the vulnerability of a specific plaque. In another aspect, however, mean SUV may be a marker for the summed burden of a patient's whole vulnerable plaques, because it represents averaged total inflammatory activity. With this concept, some researchers have suggested a parameter of 'atherosclerosis burden' that is calculated by multiplying SUV with the volume of segmented vessel wall. The selection of parameter on FDG PET should be discreetly determined according to the purpose of the study.

The recent trend of combined imaging will be very useful in atherosclerosis imaging. The combined imaging modalities of PET and MRI can obtain synergistic information regarding the characteristics of a specific plaque [69] because each assesses a different aspect of plaque. Furthermore, newly developed atherosclerosis imaging probes for MRI and CT can be validated by combined imaging using FDG PET [77, 78]. MRI can also be used for partial volume correction of PET images [79] because most of the vessels are so small that they cannot avoid partial volume effect. However, myocardial FDG uptake is also a nasty problem in addition to the small size of coronary arteries, and some researchers have reported on a method for suppression of cardiac FDG uptake using a special diet of low carbohydrate and high fat [80, 81].

Arteritis Imaging Using FDG PET

Arteritis is usually observed in rheumatologic disorders, unless the patient has grafted vessels, stents, or some other form of vascular intervention. Takayasu's arteritis and giant cell arteritis are the most common types seen. As is in other inflammatory conditions, FDG PET can be used for the imaging of arteritis. There are many case reports in the literature that have reported significant FDG uptake in Takayasu's arteritis or giant cell arteritis. The role of FDG PET in arteritis is as a marker for inflammatory activity and to show the distribution of involved arteries. Although some researchers reported that FDG uptake in arteritis lesions is not directly correlated with other inflammatory markers [82], others have reported that FDG PET is correlated well with inflammatory activity by showing that FDG uptake in arteritis lesions decreased after treatment [83]. Therefore, more data are required to define an adequate parameter for inflammatory activity in arteritis using FDG PET.

References

1. Tuzcu EM, Kapadia SR, Tutar E, et al. High prevalence of coronary atherosclerosis in asymptomatic teenagers and young adults: evidence from intravascular ultrasound. Circulation. 2001;103:2705–10.
2. Hackett D, Davies G, Maseri A. Pre-existing coronary stenoses in patients with first myocardial infarction are not necessarily severe. Eur Heart J. 1988;9:1317–23.
3. Murabito JM, Evans JC, Larson MG, et al. Prognosis after the onset of coronary heart disease. An investigation of differences in outcome between the sexes according to initial coronary disease presentation. Circulation. 1993;88:2548–55.
4. Scandinavian Simvastatin Survival Study Group. Randomised trial of cholesterol lowering in 4444 patients with coronary heart disease: the Scandinavian Simvastatin Survival Study (4S). Lancet 1994;344: 1383–9.
5. The Long-Term Intervention with Pravastatin in Ischaemic Disease (LPID) Study Group. Prevention of cardiovascular events and death with pravastatin in patients with coronary heart disease and a broad range of initial cholesterol levels. The Long-Term Intervention with Pravastatin in Ischaemic Disease (LIPID) Study Group. N Engl J Med 1998;339:1349–57.
6. Kruth HS. Sequestration of aggregated low-density lipoproteins by macrophages. Curr Opin Lipidol. 2002;13:483–8.
7. Skalen K, Gustafsson M, Rydberg EK, et al. Subendothelial retention of atherogenic lipoproteins in early atherosclerosis. Nature. 2002;417:750–4.
8. Glass CK, Witztum JL. Atherosclerosis. The road ahead. Cell. 2001;104:503–16.
9. Miller YI, Chang MK, Binder CJ, et al. Oxidized low density lipoprotein and innate immune receptors. Curr Opin Lipidol. 2003;14:437–45.
10. Cybulsky MI, Iiyama K, Li H, et al. A major role for VCAM-1, but not ICAM-1, in early atherosclerosis. J Clin Invest. 2001;107:1255–62.
11. Amorino GP, Hoover RL. Interactions of monocytic cells with human endothelial cells stimulate monocytic metalloproteinase production. Am J Pathol. 1998;152:199–207.
12. Mason DP, Kenagy RD, Hasenstab D, et al. Matrix metalloproteinase-9 overexpression enhances vascular smooth muscle cell migration and alters remodeling in the injured rat carotid artery. Circ Res. 1999;85:1179–85.
13. Moulton KS, Heller E, Konerding MA, et al. Angiogenesis inhibitors endostatin or TNP-470 reduce intimal neovascularization and plaque growth in apolipoprotein E-deficient mice. Circulation. 1999; 99:1726–32.
14. Sukhova GK, Schonbeck U, Rabkin E, et al. Evidence for increased collagenolysis by interstitial collagenases-1 and -3 in vulnerable human atheromatous plaques. Circulation. 1999;99:2503–9.
15. Iuliano L, Signore A, Vallabajosula S, et al. Preparation and biodistribution of 99m technetium labelled oxidized LDL in man. Atherosclerosis. 1996;126:131–41.
16. Tsimikas S, Palinski W, Halpern SE, et al. Radiolabeled MDA2, an oxidation-specific, monoclonal antibody, identifies native atherosclerotic lesions in vivo. J Nucl Cardiol. 1999;6:41–53.
17. Shaw PX, Horkko S, Tsimikas S, et al. Human-derived anti-oxidized LDL autoantibody blocks uptake of oxidized LDL by macrophages and localizes to atherosclerotic lesions in vivo. Arterioscler Thromb Vasc Biol. 2001;21:1333–9.
18. Tekabe Y, Li Q, Rosario R, et al. Development of receptor for advanced glycation end products-directed imaging of atherosclerotic plaque in a murine model of spontaneous atherosclerosis. Circ Cardiovasc Imag. 2008;1:212–9.
19. Virgolini I, Muller C, Fitscha P, et al. Radiolabelling autologous monocytes with 111-indium-oxine for reinjection in patients with atherosclerosis. Prog Clin Biol Res. 1990;355:271–80.
20. Kircher MF, Grimm J, Swirski FK, et al. Noninvasive in vivo imaging of monocyte trafficking to atherosclerotic lesions. Circulation. 2008;117:388–95.
21. Schafers M, Riemann B, Kopka K, et al. Scintigraphic imaging of matrix metalloproteinase activity in the arterial wall in vivo. Circulation. 2004;109:2554–9.
22. Fujimoto S, Hartung D, Ohshima S, et al. Molecular imaging of matrix metalloproteinase in atherosclerotic lesions: resolution with dietary modification and statin therapy. J Am Coll Cardiol. 2008;52: 1847–57.
23. Narula J, Petrov A, Bianchi C, et al. Noninvasive localization of experimental atherosclerotic lesions with mouse/human chimeric Z2D3 F(ab′)2 specific for the proliferating smooth muscle cells of human atheroma Imaging with conventional and negative charge-modified antibody fragments. Circulation. 1995;92:474–84.
24. Carrio I, Pieri PL, Narula J, et al. Noninvasive localization of human atherosclerotic lesions with indium 111-labeled monoclonal Z2D3 antibody specific for proliferating smooth muscle cells. J Nucl Cardiol. 1998;5:551–7.
25. Johnson LL, Schofield LM, Weber DK, et al. Uptake of 111In-Z2D3 on SPECT imaging in a swine model of coronary stent restenosis correlated with cell proliferation. J Nucl Med. 2004;45:294–9.
26. Minar E, Ehringer H, Dudczak R, et al. Indium-111-labeled platelet scintigraphy in carotid atherosclerosis. Stroke. 1989;20:27–33.
27. Moriwaki H, Matsumoto M, Handa N, et al. Functional and anatomic evaluation of carotid atherothrombosis. A combined study of indium 111 platelet scintigraphy and B-mode ultrasonography. Arterioscler Thromb Vasc Biol. 1995;15:2234–40.
28. Mitchel J, Waters D, Lai T, et al. Identification of coronary thrombus with a IIb/IIIa platelet inhibitor radiopharmaceutical, technetium-99m DMP-444: a canine model. Circulation. 2000;101:1643–6.

29. Gawaz M, Konrad I, Hauser AI, et al. Non-invasive imaging of glycoprotein VI binding to injured arterial lesions. Thromb Haemost. 2005;93:910–3.
30. Sadeghi MM, Krassilnikova S, Zhang J, et al. Detection of injury-induced vascular remodeling by targeting activated alphavbeta3 integrin in vivo. Circulation. 2004;110:84–90.
31. Lee KH, Jung KH, Song SH, et al. Radiolabeled RGD uptake and alphav integrin expression is enhanced in ischemic murine hindlimbs. J Nucl Med. 2005;46: 472–8.
32. Hua J, Dobrucki LW, Sadeghi MM, et al. Noninvasive imaging of angiogenesis with a 99mTc-labeled peptide targeted at alphavbeta3 integrin after murine hindlimb ischemia. Circulation. 2005;111:3255–60.
33. Kolodgie FD, Petrov A, Virmani R, et al. Targeting of apoptotic macrophages and experimental atheroma with radiolabeled annexin V: a technique with potential for noninvasive imaging of vulnerable plaque. Circulation. 2003;108:3134–9.
34. Kietselaer BL, Reutelingsperger CP, Heidendal GA, et al. Noninvasive detection of plaque instability with use of radiolabeled annexin A5 in patients with carotid-artery atherosclerosis. N Engl J Med. 2004;350:1472–3.
35. Johnson LL, Schofield L, Donahay T, et al. 99mTc-annexin V imaging for in vivo detection of atherosclerotic lesions in porcine coronary arteries. J Nucl Med. 2005;46:1186–93.
36. Isobe S, Tsimikas S, Zhou J, et al. Noninvasive imaging of atherosclerotic lesions in apolipoprotein E-deficient and low-density-lipoprotein receptor-deficient mice with annexin A5. J Nucl Med. 2006; 47:1497–505.
37. Sarai M, Hartung D, Petrov A, et al. Broad and specific caspase inhibitor-induced acute repression of apoptosis in atherosclerotic lesions evaluated by radiolabeled annexin A5 imaging. J Am Coll Cardiol. 2007; 50:2305–12.
38. Annovazzi A, Bonanno E, Arca M, et al. 99mTc-interleukin-2 scintigraphy for the in vivo imaging of vulnerable atherosclerotic plaques. Eur J Nucl Med Mol Imag. 2006;33:117–26.
39. Elmaleh DR, Narula J, Babich JW, et al. Rapid noninvasive detection of experimental atherosclerotic lesions with novel 99mTc-labeled diadenosine tetraphosphates. Proc Natl Acad Sci USA. 1998;95: 691–5.
40. Tepe G, Duda SH, Meding J, et al. Tc-99m-labeled endothelin derivative for imaging of experimentally induced atherosclerosis. Atherosclerosis. 2001;157:383–92.
41. Yano Y, Budinger TF, Ebbe SN, et al. Gallium-68 lipophilic complexes for labeling platelets. J Nucl Med. 1985;26:1429–37.
42. Elmaleh DR, Fischman AJ, Tawakol A, et al. Detection of inflamed atherosclerotic lesions with diadenosine-5′,5‴-P1, P4-tetraphosphate (Ap4A) and positron-emission tomography. Proc Natl Acad Sci USA. 2006;103:15992–6.
43. Schulz C, Penz S, Hoffmann C, et al. Platelet GPVI binds to collagenous structures in the core region of human atheromatous plaque and is critical for atheroprogression in vivo. Basic Res Cardiol. 2008;103: 356–67.
44. Matter CM, Wyss MT, Meier P, et al. 18F-choline images murine atherosclerotic plaques ex vivo. Arterioscler Thromb Vasc Biol. 2006;26:584–9.
45. Kato K, Schober O, Ikeda M, et al. Evaluation and comparison of 11C-choline uptake and calcification in aortic and common carotid arterial walls with combined PET/CT. Eur J Nucl Med Mol Imag. 2009; 36:1622–8.
46. Breyholz HJ, Wagner S, Levkau B, et al. A 18F-radiolabeled analogue of CGS 27023A as a potential agent for assessment of matrix-metalloproteinase activity in vivo. Q J Nucl Med Mol Imag. 2007;51:24–32.
47. Nahrendorf M, Zhang H, Hembrador S, et al. Nanoparticle PET-CT imaging of macrophages in inflammatory atherosclerosis. Circulation. 2008;117:379–87.
48. Laitinen I, Saraste A, Weidl E, et al. Evaluation of alphavbeta3 integrin-targeted positron emission tomography tracer 18F-galacto-RGD for imaging of vascular inflammation in atherosclerotic mice. Circ Cardiovasc Imag. 2009;2:331–8.
49. Nahrendorf M, Keliher E, Panizzi P, et al. (18)F-4V for PET-CT imaging of VCAM-1 expression in atherosclerosis. JACC Cardiovasc Imag. 2009;2:1213–22.
50. Rudd JH, Warburton EA, Fryer TD, et al. Imaging atherosclerotic plaque inflammation with [18F]-fluorodeoxyglucose positron emission tomography. Circulation. 2002;105:2708–11.
51. Tatsumi M, Cohade C, Nakamoto Y, et al. Fluorodeoxyglucose uptake in the aortic wall at PET/CT: possible finding for active atherosclerosis. Radiology. 2003;229:831–7.
52. Laitinen I, Marjamaki P, Haaparanta M, et al. Non-specific binding of [18F]FDG to calcifications in atherosclerotic plaques: experimental study of mouse and human arteries. Eur J Nucl Med Mol Imag. 2006;33:1461–7.
53. Ogawa M, Ishino S, Mukai T, et al. (18)F-FDG accumulation in atherosclerotic plaques: immunohistochemical and PET imaging study. J Nucl Med. 2004;45:1245–50.
54. Zhang Z, Machac J, Helft G, et al. Non-invasive imaging of atherosclerotic plaque macrophage in a rabbit model with F-18 FDG PET: a histopathological correlation. BMC Nucl Med. 2006;6:3.
55. Aziz K, Berger K, Claycombe K, et al. Noninvasive detection and localization of vulnerable plaque and arterial thrombosis with computed tomography angiography/positron emission tomography. Circulation. 2008;117:2061–70.
56. Davies JR, Izquierdo-Garcia D, Rudd JH, et al. FDG-PET can distinguish inflamed from non-inflamed plaque in an animal model of atherosclerosis. Int J Cardiovasc Imag. 2010;26:41–8.

57. Tawakol A, Migrino RQ, Bashian GG, et al. In vivo 18F-fluorodeoxyglucose positron emission tomography imaging provides a noninvasive measure of carotid plaque inflammation in patients. J Am Coll Cardiol. 2006;48:1818–24.
58. Font MA, Fernandez A, Carvajal A, et al. Imaging of early inflammation in low-to-moderate carotid stenosis by 18-FDG-PET. Front Biosci. 2009;14:3352–60.
59. Graebe M, Pedersen SF, Borgwardt L, et al. Molecular pathology in vulnerable carotid plaques: correlation with [18]-fluorodeoxyglucose positron emission tomography (FDG-PET). Eur J Vasc Endovasc Surg. 2009;37:714–21.
60. Wu YW, Kao HL, Chen MF, et al. Characterization of plaques using 18F-FDG PET/CT in patients with carotid atherosclerosis and correlation with matrix metalloproteinase-1. J Nucl Med. 2007;48:227–33.
61. Rudd JH, Myers KS, Bansilal S, et al. Relationships among regional arterial inflammation, calcification, risk factors, and biomarkers: a prospective fluorodeoxyglucose positron-emission tomography/computed tomography imaging study. Circ Cardiovasc Imag. 2009;2:107–15.
62. Tahara N, Kai H, Yamagishi S, et al. Vascular inflammation evaluated by [18F]-fluorodeoxyglucose positron emission tomography is associated with the metabolic syndrome. J Am Coll Cardiol. 2007;49:1533–9.
63. Wasselius J, Larsson S, Sundin A, et al. Assessment of inactive, active and mixed atherosclerotic plaques by 18F-FDG-PET; an age group-based correlation with cardiovascular risk factors. Int J Cardiovasc Imag. 2009;25:133–40.
64. Yun M, Jang S, Cucchiara A, et al. 18F FDG uptake in the large arteries: a correlation study with the atherogenic risk factors. Semin Nucl Med. 2002;32:70–6.
65. Bural GG, Torigian DA, Chamroonrat W, et al. FDG-PET is an effective imaging modality to detect and quantify age-related atherosclerosis in large arteries. Eur J Nucl Med Mol Imag. 2008;35:562–9.
66. Ben-Haim S, Kupzov E, Tamir A, et al. Changing patterns of abnormal vascular wall F-18 fluorodeoxyglucose uptake on follow-up PET/CT studies. J Nucl Cardiol. 2006;13:791–800.
67. Wasselius JA, Larsson SA, Jacobsson H. FDG-accumulating atherosclerotic plaques identified with (18)F-FDG-PET/CT in 141 patients. Mol Imag Biol. 2009;11:455–9.
68. Rominger A, Saam T, Wolpers S, et al. 18F-FDG PET/CT identifies patients at risk for future vascular events in an otherwise asymptomatic cohort with neoplastic disease. J Nucl Med. 2009;50:1611–20.
69. Silvera SS, Aidi HE, Rudd JH, et al. Multimodality imaging of atherosclerotic plaque activity and composition using FDG-PET/CT and MRI in carotid and femoral arteries. Atherosclerosis. 2009;207(1): 139–43.
70. Arauz A, Hoyos L, Zenteno M, et al. Carotid plaque inflammation detected by 18F-fluorodeoxyglucose-positron emission tomography. Pilot study. Clin Neurol Neurosurg. 2007;109:409–12.
71. Tahara N, Kai H, Nakaura H, et al. The prevalence of inflammation in carotid atherosclerosis: analysis with fluorodeoxyglucose-positron emission tomography. Eur Heart J. 2007;28:2243–8.
72. Tahara N, Kai H, Ishibashi M, et al. Simvastatin attenuates plaque inflammation: evaluation by fluorodeoxyglucose positron emission tomography. J Am Coll Cardiol. 2006;48:1825–31.
73. Potter K, Lenzo N, Eikelboom JW, et al. Effect of long-term homocysteine reduction with B vitamins on arterial wall inflammation assessed by fluorodeoxyglucose positron emission tomography: a randomised double-blind, placebo-controlled trial. Cerebrovasc Dis. 2009;27:259–65.
74. Rudd JH, Myers KS, Bansilal S, et al. (18) Fluorodeoxyglucose positron emission tomography imaging of atherosclerotic plaque inflammation is highly reproducible: implications for atherosclerosis therapy trials. J Am Coll Cardiol. 2007;50:892–6.
75. Rudd JH, Myers KS, Bansilal S, et al. Atherosclerosis inflammation imaging with 18F-FDG PET: carotid, iliac, and femoral uptake reproducibility, quantification methods, and recommendations. J Nucl Med. 2008;49:871–8.
76. Wasselius J, Larsson S, Jacobsson H. Time-to-time correlation of high-risk atherosclerotic lesions identified with [(18)F]-FDG-PET/CT. Ann Nucl Med. 2009;23:59–64.
77. Okane K, Ibaraki M, Toyoshima H, et al. 18F-FDG accumulation in atherosclerosis: use of CT and MR co-registration of thoracic and carotid arteries. Eur J Nucl Med Mol Imag. 2006;33:589–94.
78. Hyafil F, Cornily JC, Rudd JH, et al. Quantification of inflammation within rabbit atherosclerotic plaques using the macrophage-specific CT contrast agent N1177: a comparison with 18F-FDG PET/CT and histology. J Nucl Med. 2009;50:959–65.
79. Izquierdo-Garcia D, Davies JR, Graves MJ, et al. Comparison of methods for magnetic resonance-guided [18-F]fluorodeoxyglucose positron emission tomography in human carotid arteries: reproducibility, partial volume correction, and correlation between methods. Stroke. 2009;40:86–93.
80. Williams G, Kolodny GM. Retrospective study of coronary uptake of 18F-fluorodeoxyglucose in association with calcification and coronary artery disease: a preliminary study. Nucl Med Commun. 2009;30:287–91.
81. Wykrzykowska J, Lehman S, Williams G, et al. Imaging of inflamed and vulnerable plaque in coronary arteries with 18F-FDG PET/CT in patients with suppression of myocardial uptake using a low-carbohydrate, high-fat preparation. J Nucl Med. 2009;50:563–8.
82. Arnaud L, Haroche J, Malek Z, et al. Is (18) F-fluorodeoxyglucose positron emission tomography scanning a reliable way to assess disease activity in Takayasu arteritis? Arthritis Rheum. 2009;60:1193–200.
83. Kobayashi Y, Ishii K, Oda K, et al. Aortic wall inflammation due to Takayasu arteritis imaged with 18F-FDG PET coregistered with enhanced CT. J Nucl Med. 2005;46:917–22.

Esophageal, Gastric, and Pancreatic Cancers

22

Chang Woon Choi, Tomio Inoue,
Nobukazu Takahashi, and E. Edmund Kim

Esophageal Cancer

Esophageal cancer is a leading cause of cancer mortality worldwide. Complete resection of esophageal cancer and adjacent malignant lymph nodes is the only potentially curative treatment. Accurate preoperative staging and assessment of therapeutic response after neoadjuvant therapy are crucial in determining the most suitable therapy and avoiding inappropriate attempts at curative surgery.

The diagnosis of esophageal cancer is confirmed by endoscopy and histopathologic examination. The major purposes of imaging in esophageal cancer are to distinguish between locoregional and systemic disease, to assess response to chemotherapy or chemoradiotherapy, and to identify recurrence of cancer.

Endoscopic ultrasonography (EUS) is the best modality for determining the depth of tumor invasion and presence of regional lymph node involvement. Combined use of fine-needle aspiration and EUS can improve assessment of lymph node involvement. Computed tomography (CT) is recommended for initial imaging after confirmation of malignancy at pathologic analysis, primarily to rule out unresectable or distant metastatic disease. Positron emission tomography (PET) is useful for assessment of distant metastases but is not appropriate for detecting and staging primary tumors. PET may also be helpful in restaging after neoadjuvant therapy because it allows identification of early response to treatment and detection of interval distant metastases. Each imaging modality has its own advantages and disadvantages; therefore, CT, EUS, and PET should be considered complementary modalities for preoperative staging and therapeutic monitoring of patients with esophageal cancer.

Fluorodeoxyglucose (FDG) PET adds clinically useful information to the information already obtained by standard means (mainly CT and EUS) throughout the different phases of clinical patient management: (1) At initial diagnosis: PET detects the most frequently distant lymph node involvement and organ metastases compared with conventional diagnostics, allowing a

C.W. Choi, M.D., Ph.D. (✉)
Research Institute of Radiological and Medical Sciences, Korea Institute of Radiological and Medical Sciences, Seoul 139-706, South Korea
e-mail: cwchoi@kcch.re.kr

T. Inoue, M.D., Ph.D. • N. Takahashi, M.D., Ph.D.
Department of Radiology, Yokohama City University Graduate School of Medicine, 3-9 Pukuura, Kanazawa-ku, Yokohama 236-0004, Japan
e-mail: tomioi@yokohama-cu.ac.jp

E.E. Kim, M.D.
M.D. Anderson Cancer Center, The University of Texas, 1515 Holcombe Blvd, Box 0059, Houston, TX 77030, USA
e-mail: ekim@mdanderson.org

E.E. Kim et al. (eds.), *Clinical PET and PET/CT: Principles and Applications*,
DOI 10.1007/978-1-4419-0802-5_22, © Springer Science+Business Media New York 2013

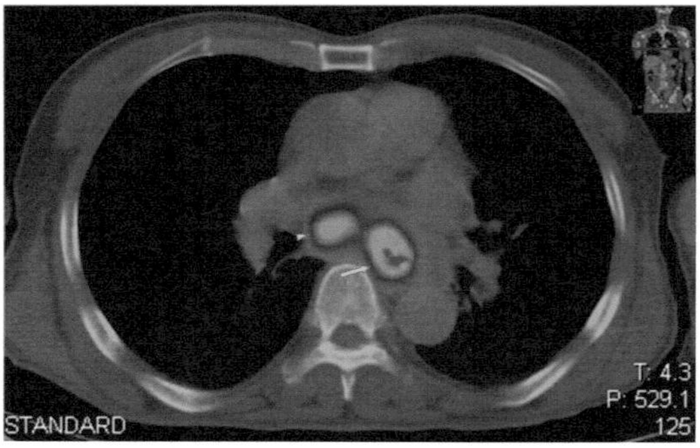

Fig. 22.1 Midesophageal cancer with lymph node metastasis on a PET/CT combined image: selected transverse PET/CT image of the midchest shows a markedly increased uptake of ^{18}F-FDG in the esophagus (*arrows*) and periesophageal lymph node. *Bigger arrow and arrowhead* in Fig.22.1

more accurate selection of the most appropriate treatment. (2) During chemotherapy: semiquantitative FDG PET allows early identification of nonresponding patients. Indeed, the metabolic response as measured by serial FDG PET can be used to predict the clinical and histopathologic response. Moreover, the PET response seems to be related to overall and disease-free survival. (3) After treatment: FDG PET allows accurate assessment of the residual tumor load. (4) During follow-up: FDG PET allows accurate detection and restaging of recurrent disease [1].

Staging

Accurate diagnosis of the extent and number of lymph node metastases is important for the management of patients with esophageal cancer because it relates to patients prognosis. The diagnositic accuracy and specificity of FDG PET for detection of regional lymph node metastases are relatively high, 82% and 90%, respectively (Fig. 22.1).

Depending on the applied standard of reference, the sensitivity of CT and FDG PET for detection of regional lymph node metastases are approximately 50% [2, 3]. The sensitivity of FDG PET and CT was not so high because of the existence of microscopic metastasis. Either intense FDG uptake in the primary lesions or physiologic FDG uptake in the myocardium and stomach may also obscure the tracer uptake in the metastatic lesion of adjacent lymph nodes. The detection of lymph node metastases, such as supraclavicular and infraclavicular lymph nodes in the border zone area between the cervical region and upper mediastinum, was difficult using CT in some cases of esophageal cancer, for which FDG PET could help with the visual interpretation of lymph node metastases on CT images. A skip metastasis beyond the adjacent lymph node area is a characteristic phenomenon of metastasis from esophageal cancer. If the range of the field of view of CT or MRI was not sufficient to observe skip lesions, whole-body FDG PET would be helpful in their detection. FDG PET, CT, and EUS are probably equivalent in tumor node metastasis staging accuracy when used independently.

Metastases from esophageal cancer are frequently found in the liver, lungs, and bones.

Monitoring Therapeutic Effect

Assessment of tumor response by FDG PET has been shown to correlate with histopathologic tumor regression and patient survival. Furthermore, quantitative measurements of tumor FDG uptake may predict histopathologic tumor response and patient outcome as early as 2 weeks after initiation of preoperative chemotherapy (Fig. 22.2).

Wieder et al. [4] investigated the time course of tumor glucose utilization in patients with esophageal cancer undergoing preoperative chemoradiotherapy. They measured the standard uptake value (SUV) of primary lesions prior to beginning therapy, 2 weeks after the initiation of chemoradiotherapy, and immediately preoperatively. Mean SUV at each point was 9.3, 5.7, and 3.3, respectively. The decrease in tumor SUV from baseline to day 14 was 44% in patients with histopathologic response, whereas it was 21% in patients without histopathologic response.

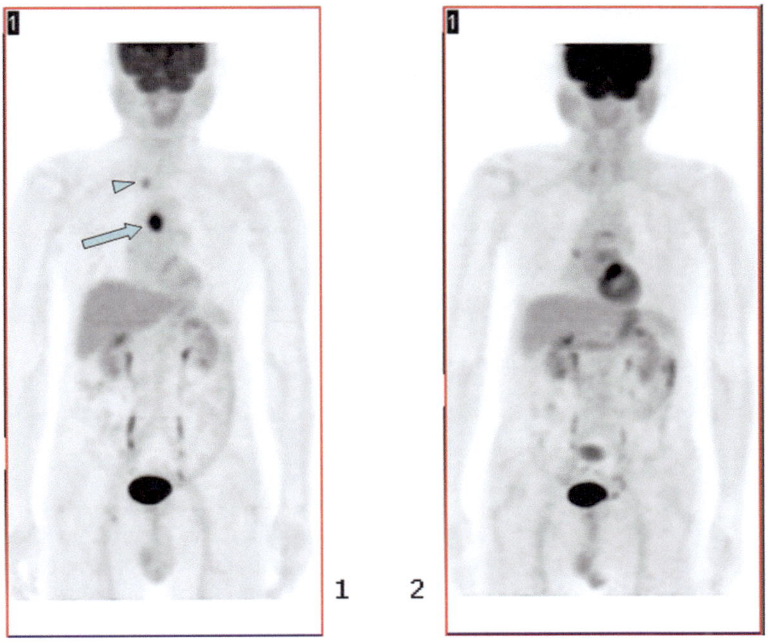

Fig. 22.2 (**a**) Esophageal cancer (*arrow*) with right mediastinal lymph node metastasis (*arrowhead*), (**b**) improved esophageal cancer after radiation therapy

These results suggested that FDG PET may be used for early identification of nonresponding tumors and therapy modification.

Rebollo Aquirre et al. [5] reviewed the literature analyzing the utility of FDG PET in the evaluation of neoadjuvant therapy response assessment. Ranges of sensitivity, specificity, positive predictive value, and negative predictive value for primary tumor response assessment were 27.3–93.3%, 41.7–95.2%, 70.8–93.3%, and 71.4–93.5%, respectively, and for N restaging they were 16.0–67.5%, 85.7–100%, 33–100%, and 91.7–93.3%, respectively. This result indicates that FDG PET is the promising imaging modality for neoadjuvant therapy response assessment in esophageal cancer and that prospective randomized multicenter trials with standardized protocols are needed. The accuracy for correct identification of recurrence in esophageal cancer is higher for FDG PET than for CT.

Gastric Cancer

Gastric cancer is the fourth most common cancer worldwide with approximately 930,000 new cases and 700,000 deaths per year. A cure can only be achieved by radical resection including an adequate lymphadenectomy. However, prognosis remains poor and cancer recurrence rates are high because of lymph node metastases. The main diagnostic tool to use for patients with suspected gastric cancer is an endoscope. FDG PET studies have been widely used in oncology diagnosis, but rarely in the diagnosis of gastric cancer. One reason could be that physiologic FDG uptake in the stomach is observed frequently and its contour of the tracer uptake is variable making it impossible to differentiate from gastric cancer [6]. The physiologic gastric uptake of FDG may partly be the result of smooth muscle activity [7], but the detail mechanism is still unknown.

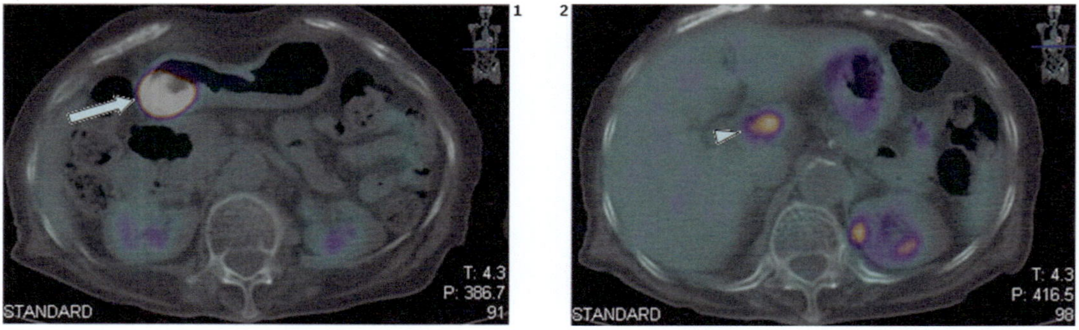

Fig. 22.3 (**a**) Gastric cancer (*arrow*), (**b**) lymph node metastasis (*arrowhead*)

Staging

Accurate assessment of lymph node status is important for appropriate treatment planning and determining prognosis in patients with gastric cancer. For the evaluation of lymph node metastasis, CT and FDG PET studies can be used (Fig. 22.3), although the sensitivity of these imaging modalities are low. The low sensitivity of PET and CT was insufficient to allow decision making for the extent of lymphadenectomy.

Although FDG PET is not an appropriate first-line diagnostic procedure in the detection of gastric cancer, and is not helpful in tumor staging, it may play a valuable role in the detection of distant metastases such as those of the liver, lungs, adrenal glands, ovaries, and skeleton. FDG PET may also be helpful in the follow-up of patients undergoing chemotherapy as it allows the identification of early response to treatment. Nevertheless, the combined use of CT and PET can be helpful in preoperative staging of gastric cancer and in the therapeutic monitoring of affected patients. Yoshioka et al. [8] reported that FDG PET exhibited whole lesions in 42 gastric cancer patients with a sensitivity of 71%, specificity of 74%, and accuracy of 73%. Uptake was high for the primary lesions, liver, lymph node, and lung metastases, but low for bone metastases, peritonitis, and pleuritis carcinomatoses.

The diagnosis of intra-abdominal dissemination in patients with gastric cancer is important for determining the indication for surgical resection. Nodules in the intra-abdominal cavity can be seen on FDG PET images, but the differentiation from physiologic intestinal FDG uptake is difficult. This diagnostic dilemma can be resolved by with a combined PET/CT technique.

Monitoring Therapeutic Effect

Use of FDG PET or combined PET/CT for the evaluation of gastric cancer recurrence after curative resection is useful in patients with recurrent gastric cancer, especially when recurrence is suspected in the clinical setting.

A multicenter study has confirmed the usefulness of FDG PET for suspected recurrent gastric cancer. The study evaluated 92 patients, of which 46 patients were suspected of recurrence by other imaging modalities (Group A), 19 patients were suspected of recurrence by tumor markers (Group B), and 27 underwent PET evaluation without evidence of recurrence (Group C). Recurrence of gastric cancer was confirmed in 31 patients (67%) in Group A, in 11 patients (58%) in Group B, and in 2 patients (7%) in Group C [9].

Ott et al. [10] investigated the predictability of FDG PET for responder to neoadjuvant

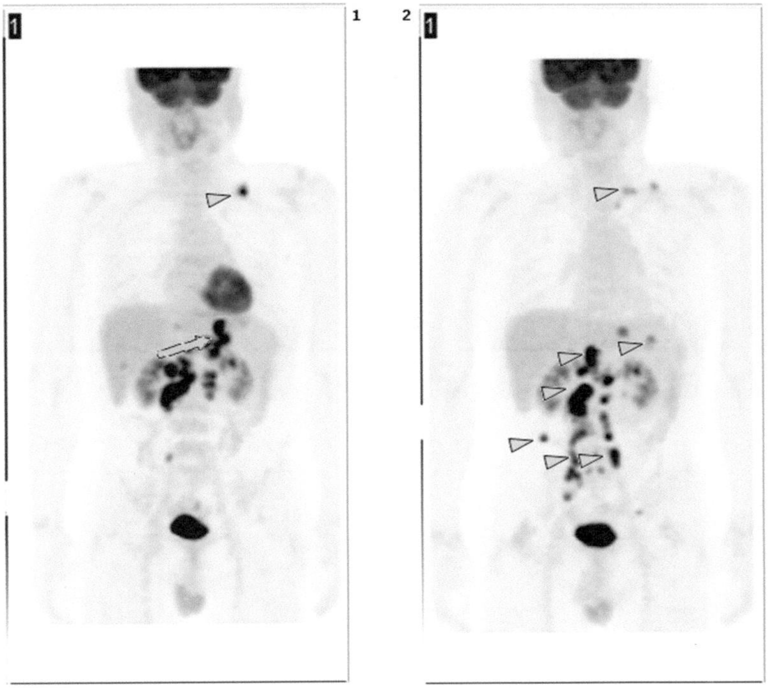

Fig. 22.4 (**a**) Gastric cancer with regional lymph node metastases (*arrow*) and left supraclavicular lymph node metastasis (*arrowhead*), (**b**) improved gastric cancer after chemotherapy, but newly developed multiple lymph node metastases (*arrowheads*)

chemotherapy in patients with gastric cancer. They conducted FDG PET examinations on patients with advanced gastric cancer at baseline and 14 days after initiation of cisplatinum-based polychemotherapy. When a reduction of tumor FDG uptake by more than 35% was used as a criterion for subsequent tumor response, the positive and negative predictive values of FDG PET for histopathologic response were 77% and 86%, respectively (Fig. 22.4).

Pancreatic Cancer

Patients with pancreatic cancer continue to have poor prognosis, with a 5-year survival rate of less than 5%. Surgery is the only treatment that offers a potential cure, but only 15–20% of patients are candidates for surgery. Although the morbidity and mortality of pancreas surgery has decreased during recent years, the long-term outcome of patients with pancreatic cancer remains poor. This poor outcome is generally attributed to a relatively chemotherapy-resistant disease and undetected metastases at the time of surgery. The preoperative diagnosis of primary pancreatic adenocarcinoma remains challenging, even for experienced clinicians. FDG PET is a novel imaging modality that takes advantage of selective FDG uptake and retention by malignant cells (Fig. 22.5).

FDG PET is one of the imaging modalities expected to improve the diagnostic accuracy for pancreatic tumors especially for differentiation between benign and malignant diseases. Generally, FDG PET reveals a high uptake of primary and metastatic lesions of pancreatic

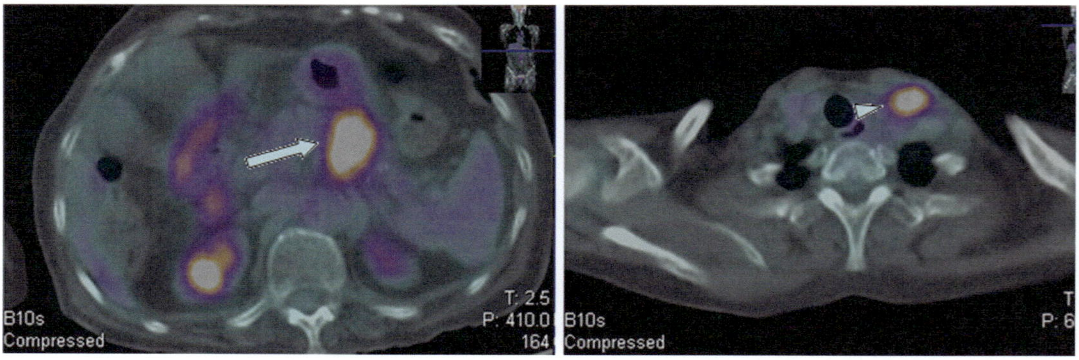

Fig. 22.5 (**a**) Pancreas tail cancer (*arrow*), (**b**) lymph node metastasis (*arrowhead*)

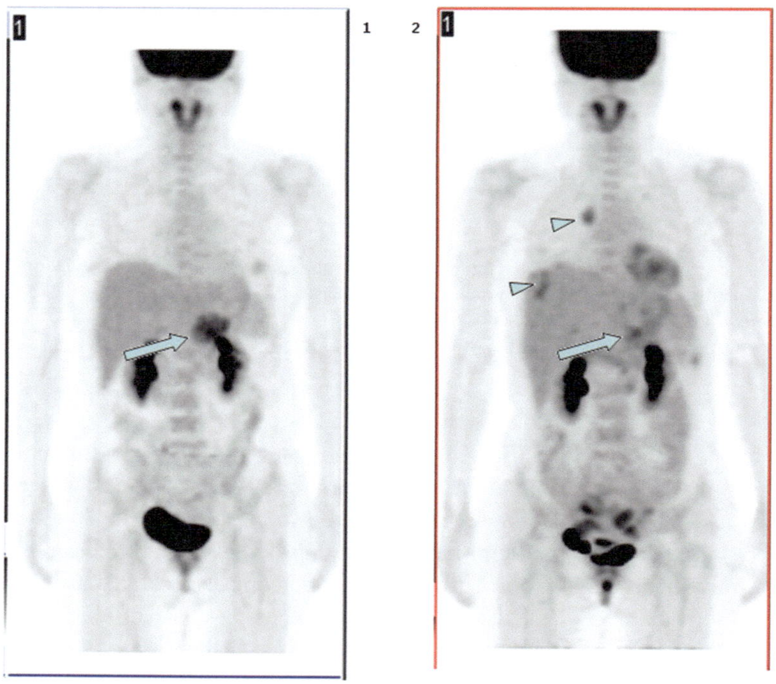

Fig. 22.6 (**a**) Pancreatic cancer (*arrow*), (**b**) improved pancreatic cancer after radiation therapy (*arrow*), but newly developed metastases in the liver and lung (*arrowheads*)

cancer (Fig. 22.6), while a lower FDG uptake shows benign pancreatic lesions such as chronic pancreatitis. Overexpression of glucose transporter (GLUT) and increased permeability of tumor vessels contribute to increased FDG uptake in pancreatic cancer. GLUT-1, a subtype of GLUT, is especially overexpressed in pancreatic cancer [11, 12].

Diagnosis of Primary Pancreatic Cancer

Because the normal pancreas has low glucose utilization, the focal areas of increased FDG uptake in the pancreas can be easily visualized. However, there is a limitation on FDG PET in the differentiation of pancreatic cancer from benign pancreatic diseases such as chronic pancreatitis and benign pancreatic cysts. In the case of chronic pancreatitis, a postinflammatory mass formulating pancreatitis mimics a malignant pancreatic disease. It is difficult to have an accurate differential diagnosis between the two diseases. The utility of FDG PET for differential diagnosis between benign and malignant disease was reported in a comparative study using CT [13–15], with the sensitivity and specificity of FDG PET ranging from 85% to 100%, and from 77% to 88%, respectively. Overall accuracy ranged from 85% to 95%. Gambhir et al. [16] reported that the weighted average sensitivity and specificity were 94% and 90%, compared with 82% and 75% for CT, respectively. These diagnostic results of FDG PET were superior to those of CT.

Objective interpretation of FDG PET in oncology is based on the semiquantitative index of FDG uptake in lesions (e.g., SUV). Several studies reported that the average SUV in pancreatic cancer was higher than that of benign pancreatic disease [13–15]. A lesion with an SUV of greater than 5.0 is likely to be malignant, while a lesion with an SUV of less than 2.5 is likely to be benign. However, we must keep in mind that the distribution of SUVs overlaps between benign and malignant lesions. A relatively lower specificity of FDG PET may be caused by the FDG uptake in inflammatory cells.

Early detection of pancreatic cancer is still difficult despite the recent development of imaging technology such us multi-detector CT, fast spin-echo MRI, and Doppler sonography. Overall detection sensitivity of PET and PET/CT varies between 90% and 95% and specificity from 82% to 100% for the diagnosis of pancreatic cancer, whereas for staging, sensitivity data vary from 61% to 100% and specificity data from 67% to 100% [17]. Although FDG PET can exhibit the biomorphologic information needed to identify the disease early, it is not acceptable as a screening tool for pancreatic cancer.

Staging

The identification of primary tumor extent and regional lymph node metastasis with FDG PET alone is not clinically sufficient because of a lack of spatial resolution. Physiologic intestinal FDG uptake and an intense FDG uptake in the primary lesion obscure the faint FDG uptake in the adjacent small lymph node lesions. The preoperative evaluation of resectability for pancreatic cancer fails to identify up to 25% of patients who are unfortunately found to be unresectable during surgical exploration. The combined imaging modalities of CT and FDG PET will aid in the interpretation of tumor extent and regional lymph node metastasis. PET/CT increased the sensitivity (87%) for detection of metastatic disease when combined with standard CT. In invasive cancer, PET/CT changed the management of 11% of patients. PET/CT should be considered in the initial workup of patients with potentially resectable pancreatic lesions [18].

The major advantage of FDG PET on staging has been its ability to identify distant metastases. The liver is the organ most commonly affected followed by the lungs and the bone marrow. FDG PET is useful in distinguishing metastatic hepatic lesions from pancreatic cancer. The sensitivity for detecting hepatic metastasis is about 70%. Significant intrahepatic cholestasis can be a cause of false-positive findings. In certain cases of pancreatic cancer, metastatic lesions in the liver that are invisible with CT and MRI could be visible with FDG PET.

Monitoring Therapeutic Effect

FDG PET is useful for the clinical follow-up and diagnosis of recurrent disease in patients with colorectal cancer and head/neck cancer because a good prognosis in patients with these cancers requires long-term follow-up after initial treatment. On the other hand, recurrent or metastatic lesions in patients with pancreatic cancer occur earlier than in patients with colorectal and head/neck cancers. There are few reports describing the utility of FDG PET for the detection of recurrent disease in patients with pancreatic cancer. Ruf et al. [19] reported that in 31 patients with suspected recurrent disease, 96% of local recurrences were detected with FDG PET compared with 23% with CT or MRI. The use of FDG PET may be useful for the detection of recurrent lesions after initial surgical treatment because postsurgical scars, which interfere the accurate diagnosis of recurrent disease on CT or MRI, may show faint or no FDG uptake.

The change of tumor FDG uptake derived from PET imaging before and after treatment can be used as an index for monitoring therapeutic effect. Patients with higher FDG uptake in pancreatic tumors tend to have a poor prognosis. Nakada et al. [20] compared the survival of 37 patients with high and low FDG SUVs using a mean SUV threshold of 3. In their study, high SUV correlated with shorter survival, and multivariate analysis of survival showed the SUV to be an independent prognostic factor in the inoperable group.

References

1. Salavati A, Basu S, Heidari P, et al. Impact of fluorodeoxyglucose PET on the management of esophageal cancer. Nucl Med Commun. 2009;30(2):95–116.
2. Kato H, Kuwano H, Nakajima M, et al. Comparison between positron emission tomography and computed tomography in the use of the assessment of esophageal carcinoma. Cancer. 2002;94:921–8.
3. Yoon YC, Lee KS, Shim YM, et al. Metastasis to regional lymph nodes in patients with esophageal squamous cell carcinoma: CT versus FDG PET for presurgical detection prospective study. Radiology. 2003;227(3):764–70.
4. Wieder HA, Brucher BL, Zimmermann K, et al. Time course of tumor metabolic activity during chemoradiotherapy of esophageal squamous cell carcinomas and response to therapy. J Clin Oncol. 2004;22(5):900–8.
5. Rebollo Aguirre AC, Ramos-Font C, Villegas Portero R, et al. 18F-fluorodeoxiglucose positron emission tomography for the evaluation of neoadjuvant therapy response in esophageal cancer: systematic review of the literature. Ann Surg. 2009;250(2):247–54.
6. Shreve PD, Anzai Y, Wahl RL. Pitfalls in oncologic diagnosis with FDG-PET imaging: physiologic and benign variants. Radiographics. 1999;19:61–77.
7. Cook GJR, Fogelman I, Maisey M. Normal physiological and benign pathological variants of 18-fluoro-2-deoxyglucose positron emission tomography scanning: potential for error in interpretation. Semin Nucl Med. 1996;24:308–14.
8. Yoshioka K, Yamaguchi K, Kubota K, et al. Evaluation of 18F-FDG PET in patients with advanced, metastatic or recurrent gastric cancer. J Nucl Med. 2003;44(5):690–9.
9. Nakamoto Y, Togashi K, Kaneta T, et al. Clinical value of whole-body FDG-PET for recurrent gastric cancer: a multicenter study. Jpn J Clin Oncol. 2009;39(5):297–302.
10. Ott K, Becker K, Stahl A, et al. Prediction of response to preoperative chemotherapy in gastric carcinoma by metabolic imaging: results of a prospective trial. J Clin Oncol. 2003;21(24):4604–10.
11. Higashi T, Tamaki N, Honda T, et al. Expression of glucose transporters in human pancreatic tumors compared with increased FDG accumulation in PET study. J Nucl Med. 1997;38:1337–44.
12. Reske SN, Grillenberger KG, Glatting G, et al. Overexpression of glucose transporter 1 and increased FDG uptake in pancreatic carcinoma. J Nucl Med. 1997;38:1344–8.
13. Inokuma T, Tamaki N, Torizuka T, et al. Evaluation of pancreatic tumors with positron emission tomography and F-18 fluorodeoxyglucose: comparison with CT and US. Radiology. 1995;195:345–52.
14. Delbeke D, Rose DM, Chapman WC, et al. Optimal interpretation of FDG-PET in the diagnosis, staging and management of pancreatic carcinoma. J Nucl Med. 1999;40:1784–91.
15. Zimny M, Bares R, Fass J, et al. Fluorine-18 fluorodeoxyglucose positron emission tomography in the differential diagnosis of pancreatic carcinoma: a report of 106 cases. Eur J Nucl Med. 1997;24–29:678–82.
16. Gambhir SS, Czernin J, Schwimmer J, et al. A tabulated summary of the FDG PET literature. J Nucl Med. 2001;42(Suppl 5):1S–93.
17. Pakzad F, Grobes AM, Ell PJ. The role of positron emission tomography in the management of pancreatic cancer. Semin Nucl Med. 2006;36(3):248–56.
18. Farma JM, Santillan AA, Melis M, et al. PET/CT fusion scan enhances CT staging in patients with pancreatic neoplasms. Ann Surg Oncol. 2008;15(9):2465–71.
19. Ruf J, Lopez Schirmeister HH, Oettle H, et al. Detection of recurrent pancreatic cancer: comparison of FDG-PET with CT/MRI. Pancreatology. 2005;5:266–72.
20. Nakada B, Nishimura S, Ishikawa T, et al. Prognostic predictive value of 18F-fluorodeoxyglucose positron emission tomography for patients with pancreatic cancer. Int J Oncol. 2001;19:53–8.

Hepatobiliary and Small Bowel Cancers

23

Byung-Tae Kim and E. Edmund Kim

General Considerations

Cancers of the liver can materialize in the parenchymal cells in hepatocellular cancers or from the intrahepatic bile ducts in cholangiocarcinomas, or they can metastasize from other organ tumors.

Hepatocellular Carcinoma

Hepatocellular carcinoma (HCC) is the most common cancer in the world in males, especially in the Far East Asian and sub-Saharan African countries, where the annual incidence is up to 500 cases per 100,000 population. In the US and Western Europe, it is less common; however, the annual incidence in the US has increased from 1.4 per 100,000 in the time period from 1976–1980 to 2.4 per 100,000 in the time period from 1991–1995 [1]. HCC is up to four times more common in men than in women. The incidence peaks in the fifth to sixth decades of life in Western countries but in one to two decades earlier in regions of Asia and Africa that have a high prevalence of HCC. The principal reason for the high incidence rates in parts of Asia and Africa is the frequency of chronic infection with hepatitis B or C viruses, which is an important risk factor. The incidence HCC is about 100-fold higher in individuals with evidence of hepatitis B virus infection than it is in noninfected controls. Any agent or factor that contributes to chronic, low-grade liver cell damage and mitosis causes hepatocyte DNA to become more susceptible to genetic alterations. In addition to chronic viral hepatitis, alcoholic liver disease, α_1-antitrypsin deficiency, hemochromatosis, tyrosinemia, and aflatoxin Bi are other risk factors for HCC.

Because HCC has a less specific clinical appearance, early diagnosis is difficult. The determination of serum levels of α-fetoprotein (AFP) and ultrasonography are suitable diagnostic or monitoring methods for patients with known risk factors. Only biopsy and histologic examination of suspected liver lesions can provide definitive diagnosis and grading of HCC. Imaging procedures to detect liver tumors include ultrasonography, computed tomography (CT), magnetic resonance imaging (MRI), hepatic artery angiography, and

B.-T. Kim, M.D., Ph.D. (✉)
Department of Nuclear Medicine, Sungkyunkwan University, School of Medicine Samsung Medical Center, Seoul, 135-710, South Korea
e-mail: btkimnm@skku.edu

E.E. Kim, M.D., M.S.
Departments of Nuclear Medicine and Diagnostic Radiology, The University of Texas MD Anderson Cancer Center and Medical School, 1515 Holcombe Blvd, Box 0059, Houston, TX 77030, USA

Graduate School of Convergence Science and Technology, Seoul National University, Seoul, South Korea
e-mail: ekim@mdanderson.org

E.E. Kim et al. (eds.), *Clinical PET and PET/CT: Principles and Applications*,
DOI 10.1007/978-1-4419-0802-5_23, © Springer Science+Business Media New York 2013

technetium scans. Ultrasonography is frequently used to screen high-risk populations and should be the first imaging modality of choice if HCC is suspected; it is less costly than CT and MRI and is relatively sensitive, detecting most tumors larger than 3 cm in diameter. Helical CT and MRI scans with contrast agents are being used with increasing frequency and show higher sensitivity. Percutaneous liver biopsy can be diagnostic if the sample is taken from the area localized by ultrasonography or CT. Because these tumors tend to be hypervascular, percutaneous biopsies should be performed with caution.

Staging of HCC is based on tumor size (<50% or ≥50% of the liver), ascites (absent or present), bilirubin (<3 or ≥3 mg/dL), and albumin (<3 or ≥3 g/dL) to establish Okuda stages I, II, or III. The Okuda system predicts clinical course better than the American Joint Cancer Committee tumor node metastasis classification system. The natural history of each stage without treatment is stage I, 8 months; stage II, 2 months; and stage III, less than 1 month.

Most patients die within 1 year of diagnosis. Anorexia and cachexia of malignancy are the most frequent causes of death. Although few patients have a resectable tumor because of underlying cirrhosis or distant metastases at the time of diagnosis, surgical resection offers the only chance for cure. Common sites of metastases are the lung, brain, bone, and adrenal gland. In patients at high risk for the development of HCC, screening programs have been initiated to identify small tumors at the time that they are still resectable. Because 20–30% of patients with early HCC do not have elevated levels of circulating AFP, screening using ultrasonography is recommended.

Liver transplantation can be considered as therapeutic option, but tumor recurrence and metastasis are major obstacles. Other approaches include hepatic artery embolization and chemotherapy, alcohol or radiofrequency ablation via ultrasound-guided percutaneous injection, and cryoablation. In patients with resectable tumors, polyprenoic acid (a retinoic acid formulation) and intra-arterial ^{131}I-labeled lipiodol have been reported to reduce the rate of recurrence.

A combined occurrence of HCC and cholangiocellular carcinoma has been noted. Fibrolamellar HCC is an important variant, and can be found in younger patients without liver cirrhosis.

Cholangiocellular Carcinoma

Cholangiocellular carcinoma (CCC) originates from the intra- or extrahepatic bile duct, with adenocarcinoma of the extrahepatic ducts being more common. There is a slight male preponderance (60%), and incidence peaks in the fifth to seventh decades of life. Apparent predisposing factors include some chronic hepatobiliary parasitic infestations, congenital anomalies with ectactic ducts, sclerosing cholangitis and chronic ulcerative colitis, and occupational exposure to possible biliary tract carcinogens (nitrosamines, aflatoxins). CCC lesions can be diffuse or nodular. Nodular lesions often arise at the bifurcation of the common bile duct (Klatskin tumors) and are usually associated with a collapsed gallbladder, a finding that mandates cholangiography to view proximal hepatic ducts.

The diagnosis is most frequently made by cholangiography following ultrasound demonstration of dilated intrahepatic bile ducts. Any focal strictures of the bile ducts should be considered malignant until proved otherwise. Endoscopic cholangiography permits obtaining specimens for cytology and insertion of stents for biliary drainage. In some cases, survival of 1–2 years is possible. Approximately 20% of patients have surgically resectable tumors, but 5-year survival is only 10–30%. The high recurrence rate limits the value of liver transplantation. Photodynamic therapy (intravenous hematoporphyrin with cholangioscopically delivered light) has been used with promising early results.

Metastatic Tumor

Metastatic tumor of the liver is common. Its size, high rate of blood flow, double perfusion by the hepatic artery and portal vein, and its Kupffer cell filtration function combine to make it the next most common site of metastases after the lymph nodes. In the US, the incidence of metastatic carcinoma is at least 20 times greater than that of primary carcinoma. At autopsy, hepatic metastasis was seen to occur in 30–50% of patients who died from malignant disease. Virtually all types of neoplasms, except those primarily in the brain, may metastasize to the liver. The most common primary tumors are those of the gastrointestinal tract, lung, and breast, as well as melanomas. Less common are metastases from tumors of the thyroid, prostate, and skin.

Most patients with hepatic metastases present with symptoms of only the primary tumor, and the asymptomatic hepatic involvement is discovered in the course of clinical evaluation. Evidence of metastatic invasion of the liver in any patient with a primary malignancy, especially of the lung, gastrointestinal tract, or breast, should be actively sought before resection of the primary lesion. An elevated level of alkaline phosphatase or a mass apparent on ultrasound, CT, or MRI examination of the liver may provide a presumptive diagnosis. Blind percutaneous needle biopsy of the liver results in a positive diagnosis of metastatic disease in only 60–80% of cases with hepatomegaly and elevated alkaline phosphatase levels. Serial sectioning of specimens (with two or three repeated biopsies) or cytologic examination of biopsy smears may increase the diagnostic yield by 10–15%. The yield is increased when biopsies are guided by ultrasonography or CT, or obtained during laparoscopy.

Most metastatic carcinomas respond poorly to all forms of treatment, which is usually only palliative. Rarely can a single, large metastasis be removed surgically. Systemic chemotherapy may slow tumor growth and reduce symptoms, but it does not alter the prognosis. Chemoembolization, intrahepatic chemotherapy, and alcohol or radiofrequency ablation may provide palliation.

Small Bowel Carcinoma

Small bowel carcinomas are rare, and most primary malignancies of the small bowel are of neuroendocrine origin. Special radiopharmaceuticals have been developed for positron emission tomography (PET) imaging of somatostatin-receptor positive tissue because FDG PET is less suitable for the investigation of neuroendocrine tumors, and the agent being most commonly used for this purpose is ^{68}Ga-DOTATOC [2]. The small bowel is a potential site for metastatic carcinoma and sarcoma. Although sarcomas are very heterogeneous, fluorodeoxyglucose (FDG) PET can be used to differentiate sarcomas from benign tumors of the small bowel and also distinguish between high- and low-grade sarcomas with good results [3].

Positron Emission Tomography

Although many articles have been published on the usefulness of FDG PET for metastatic cancers of the liver, only a few were reported for primary liver tumors. In 1982, Fukuda et al. [4] reported increased uptake of fluorine-18-fluoro-2-deoxyglucose (FDG), which is a glucose analog that competes with glucose at transport sites on the cell membrane and in intracellular enzymatic pathways, in the transplantable ascitic hepatoma (AH109A) cells by autoradiography. Yonekura et al. [5] also reported a continuous increase of FDG uptake in metastatic liver tumors from colon carcinoma compared with decrease of FDG uptake in normal liver tissues. In 1985, Paul et al. [6] imaged HCC after FDG injection using the Anger camera, and Nagata et al. [7] reported successful imaging of recurrent HCC and lymph node metastasis using dedicated whole-body FDG PET. The metabolism of FDG in HCC was described by Okazumi et al. [8] using a dynamic PET scanning method and hexokinase activity measurement. In their study, the rate of glucose inflow from the plasma into the cells was lower for the tumors than that for the surrounding liver tissue, and the rate of phosphorylation by hexokinase was significantly increased in malignant tumors.

In general, glycolysis and glucose utilization are increased in malignant tumors. FDG competes with glucose for phosphorylation by the enzyme hexokinase to FDG-6-phosphate. Phosphohexose isomerase, the enzyme involved in the next step of the glycolytic pathway, cannot act on phosphorylated FDG. The glucose-6-phosphatase, which catalyzes the dephosphorylation of FDG-6-phosphate, is relatively scant in malignant cells. Thus, there is more FDG trapped in malignant tumor cells than in normal cells.

In the normal liver, the concentration of glucose-6-phosphatase is high and may clear FDG faster. The differences in the hexokinase/glucose-6-phosphatase ratios and metabolic activity of normal and malignant liver tissue result in visibly increased FDG accumulation in HCC and metastatic tumors on FDG PET images.

Well-differentiated HCC may retain the properties of normal hepatocytes, and the enzyme activities of the glycolytic pathway resemble those of normal hepatocytes. A decrease in differentiation increases glycolytic enzymes and decreases glucose-6-phosphatase levels. The kinetic rate constants and uptake values are significantly higher in poorly differentiated HCC compared with those with higher differentiation. The glucose-6-phosphatase/hexokinase ratios of low-grade HCC have been found to be significantly higher than of high-grade HCC. This enzyme activity can be obtained from the rate constants using compartment models in dynamic FDG PET and has proven to be useful in the characterization of the tumor and monitoring of the therapeutic effect. Tumor size, morphology, vascularity, or lipiodol deposits do not influence the quantitative evaluation of viability by glucose metabolism.

Okazumi et al. [8] categorized HCC into three types depending on the pattern of accumulation 60 min after FDG injection: type 1, greater tumor FDG accumulation compared with surrounding liver tissue; type 2, nearly the same degree of accumulation as the surrounding liver tissue; type 3, less accumulation than the surrounding liver tissue. In their study of 20 patients with HCC, type 1 tumors were found in 11 patients (55%), type 2 tumors in six patients (30%), and type 3 tumors in three patients (15%). Three patients with CCC and 10 patients with metastatic liver cancer showed greater tumor FDG accumulation than surrounding liver tissue (corresponding to type 1 HCC).

Torizuka et al. [9] evaluated the metabolic activity of HCC after transarterial chemoembolization therapy in 30 patients using the tumor-to-nontumor standard uptake value (SUV) ratio and correlated it with the extent of tumor necrosis. They found that increased or similar FDG uptake (SUV ratio $\geq$0.6) suggests viable residual tumor, whereas decreased or absent FDG uptake (SUV ratio <0.6) indicates effective therapy (necrosis occurred in more than 90% of tumor tissue).

The results of these studies are important in understanding the pathophysiology of primary liver tumors, but study using dynamic FDG PET impractical because of its difficulty in performing as a common clinical study.

In 1998, Delbeke et al. [10] evaluated the usefulness of static whole-body FDG PET in the differentiation of benign and malignant hepatic lesions. Their prospective blinded-comparison clinical cohort study included 110 patients with hepatic lesions that were 1 cm or larger on screening CT. Confirmatory diagnosis was obtained by biopsy or surgery. Sixty-six liver metastases from adenocarcinoma and primary sarcoma and eight from CCC showed increased FDG uptake (SUV, >3.5; lesion-to-background ratio, >2), whereas only 16 of 23 HCCs had increased FDG uptake. Seven of 23 patients with HCC had poor FDG uptake. All 23 benign hepatic lesions, except for three abscesses, had poor uptake (SUV, <3.5; lesion-to-background ratio, <2). One of three abscesses had definitely increased FDG uptake and the others had equivocal uptake. These findings support the results of the studies by Okazumi et al. and Torizuka et al.

Trojan et al. [11] performed whole-body and regional FDG PET on 14 consecutive patients with HCC and compared the results with ultrasonography, contrast-enhanced helical CT, histologic grading, p53 protein expression, and serum AFP level. Increased FDG uptake of seven patients with HCC were indistinguishable from surrounding normal liver tissue in the other seven patients. Patients with increased FDG uptake had larger tumors and higher serum AFP levels than those with indistinguishable FDG uptake from normal tissue. Seven of eight moderately or poorly differentiated HCCs clearly had increased FDG uptake, whereas none of six well-differentiated HCCs were detected. The tumors in patients with strong p53 expression had increased FDG uptake. In this study, tumor size (>5 cm), differentiation, and serum AFP level were major predictors of tumor visualization on FDG PET. It was concluded that static FDG PET was not a useful modality in the early diagnosis of HCC, but was superior to other imaging methods for detection of extrahepatic spread.

To evaluate the diagnostic usefulness of FDG PET, Iwata et al. [12] used it in 48 HCCs, 5 CCCs, 20 metastatic tumors, 2 hemangiomas, and 3 focal nodular hyperplasias. The SUV ratios of multiple HCCs were significantly higher than those of single HCCs. They also compared the SUV and SUV ratio with the Child-Turcotte classification score and the Cancer of the Liver Italian Program score. Shiomi et al. [13] assessed the usefulness of FDG PET for predicting outcome in 48 patients with HCC. The tumor volume doubling time correlated significantly with SUV ratio but did not correlate with SUV. The cumulative survival rates of the patients with an SUV ratio greater than 1.5 were significantly lower than those of the patients with an SUV ratio below 1.5. On regression analysis using the Cox proportional hazards model, the SUV ratio and tumor number were significantly related to survival.

In 1999, Koyama et al. [14] acquired PET two sets of images (at 1 and 2 h) after FDG injection in 11 patients with 18 HCCs and 4 patients with 15 metastatic liver tumors. Tumor-to-nontumor ratios and tumor-to–soft-tissue ratios on 2-h images were significantly higher than those on 1-h images, whereas nontumorous liver tissue-to-soft-tissue ratios were not significantly different and showed no constant tendency.

Morikawa et al. [15] demonstrated increased FDG uptake on pretreatment PET in a patient with HCC, decreased FDG uptake after treatment, and re-increase on follow-up, which turned out to be a recurrence. They suggested that FDG PET might be useful in the evaluation of therapy response and recurrence monitoring for HCC.

Although many of the authors mentioned found that CCC usually showed increased FDG uptake compared with surrounding normal liver tissue, the number of cases was not large enough to analyze statistically. Kluge et al. [16] studied the usefulness of FDG PET for the detection and staging of CCC in 26 adenocarcinomas of the biliary tree, eight benign lesions of the bile ducts, and 20 controls. Twenty-four of 26 CCCs were positive, and all benign lesions as well as 18 of 20 controls were negative. Evaluation by visual means and tumor-to-nontumor ratios were equally accurate, whereas evaluation by SUV revealed lower accuracy. For the detection of metastatic lesions of CCC, FDG PET detected 7 of 10 distant metastases and only 2 of 15 regional or hepatoduodenal lymph node metastases. These findings suggest that FDG PET can be helpful for the detection of distant metastasis but not for the detection of regional lymph node involvement in CCC patients.

Keiding et al. [17] attempted to noninvasively detect CCC with FDG PET in patients with primary sclerosing cholangitis (PSC), which predisposes to CCC. Nine patients with PSC, six patients with PSC and CCC, and five controls were included in their study. In each of the PSC plus CCC patients, from two to seven hot spots (increased FDG uptake compared with surrounding liver tissue) were seen. No hot spot was seen in the other two groups. The net metabolic clearances (from Gjedde-Patlak plotting) of FDG in CCCs were significantly higher than in those of the other two groups. Thus, FDG PET may be useful in the detection of CCC during follow-up of patients with PSC.

Some authors found that FDG PET was more accurate than CT and could obtain additional information in detecting hepatic metastases [18–20]. The reported accuracy ranged between 93% and 98%. False-positive results can occur in marked intrahepatic cholestasis, abscess, and lung basal metastases [21], and false-negative results can be achieved when the metastatic lesion is small (<1 cm in diameter). The usefulness or diagnostic accuracy of metastatic hepatic tumors is described in the chapters on primary tumors. Other radiopharmaceuticals, such as ^{13}N-ammonia [22] and

^{11}C-ethanol [23, 24], have been tested in trials to detect liver tumors, but their use is not yet proved practical.

FDG PET/CT can be of definite value for investigating indeterminate hepatic lesions. FDG uptake in hepatic lesions that are also detectable by CT is highly suggestive of malignancy. FDG PET/CT has also demonstrated its usefulness for monitoring response to local palliative treatments such as thermal tumor ablation, and yielded better results than PET alone in the identification of residual or recurrent tumor following radiofrequency ablation [25]. PET/CT can further improve the detection of recurrent colorectal carcinoma and can increase staging accuracy from 78% with PET alone to 89% with PET/CT [26].

Outlook

The number of studies on FDG PET in primary hepatobiliary tumors was too small to establish clear indications. This was probably a result of relatively low sensitivity, but FDG PET can be used in the differentiation of malignant hepatic lesions from benign lesions, prediction of prognosis by noninvasive grading of differentiation, and the detection of distant metastases. Nevertheless, further studies are necessary for determining the exact role of FDG PET in the evaluation and management of patients with hepatobiliary tumors.

References

1. Dienstag JL, Isselbacher K. Tumors of the liver and biliary tract. In: Braunwald E, Fauci AS, Kasper DL, Hauser SL, Longo DL, Jameson JL, editors. Harrison's principles of internal medicine. 15th ed. New York: McGraw-Hill; 1998. p. 588–91.
2. Kowalski J, Henze M, Schuhmacher J, Macke HR, Hofmann M, Haberkorn U. Evaluation of positron emission tomography imaging using ^{68}Ga-DOTA-D Phe(1)-Tyr(3)-Octreotide in comparison to ^{111}In-DTPAOC SPECT. First results in patients with neuroendocrine tumors. Mol Imag Biol. 2003;5(1):42–8.
3. Bastiaannet E, Groen H, Jager PL, et al. The value of FDG PET in the detection, grading and response to therapy of soft tissue and bone sarcomas: a systemic review and meta-analysis. Cancer Treat Rev. 2004;30(1):83–101.
4. Fukuda H, Matsuzawa T, Abe Y, et al. Experimental study for cancer diagnosis with positron-labeled fluorinated glucose analogs: [18F]-2-fluoro-2-deoxy-D-mannose: a new tracer for cancer detection. Eur J Nucl Med. 1982;7:294–7.
5. Yonekura Y, Benua RS, Brill AB, et al. Increased accumulation of 2-deoxy-2-[^{18}F]fluoro-D-glucose in liver metastases from colon carcinoma. J Nucl Med. 1982;23:1133–7.
6. Paul R, Ahonen A, Roeda D, Nordman E. Imaging of hepatoma with 18F-fluorodeoxyglucose. Lancet. 1985;1(8419):50–1.
7. Nagata Y, Yamamoto K, Hiraoka M, et al. Monitoring liver tumor therapy with [^{18}F]FDG positron emission tomography. J Comput Assist Tomogr. 1990;14:370–4.
8. Okazumi S, Isono K, Enomoto K, et al. Evaluation of liver tumors using fluorine-18-fluorodeoxyglucose PET: characterization of tumor and assessment of effect of treatment. J Nucl Med. 1992;33:333–9.
9. Torizuka T, Tamaki N, Inokuma T, et al. Value of fluorine-18-FDG-PET to monitor hepatocellular carcinoma after interventional therapy. J Nucl Med. 1994;35:1965–9.
10. Delbeke D, Martin WH, Martin PS, et al. Evaluation of benign vs malignant hepatic lesions with positron emission tomography. Arch Surg. 1998;133:510–6.
11. Trojan J, Schroeder O, Raedle J, et al. Fluorine-18 FDG positron emission tomography for imaging of hepatocellular carcinoma. Am J Gastroenterol. 1999;94:3314–9.
12. Iwata Y, Shiomi S, Sasaki N, et al. Clinical usefulness of positron emission tomography with fluorine-18-fluorodeoxyglucose in the diagnosis of liver tumors. Ann Nucl Med. 2000;14:121–6.
13. Shiomi S, Nishiguchi S, Ishizu H, et al. Usefulness of positron emission tomography with fluorine-18-fluorodeoxyglucose for predicting outcome in patients with hepatocellular carcinoma. Am J Gastroenterol. 2001;96:1877–80.
14. Koyama K, Okamura T, Kawabe J, et al. The usefulness of ^{18}F-FDG PET images obtained 2 hours after intravenous injection in liver tumor. Ann Nucl Med. 1999;16:169–76.
15. Morikawa H, Shiomi S, Sasaki N, et al. Hepatocellular carcinoma monitored by F-18 fluorodeoxyglucose positron emission tomography after laparoscopic microwave coagulation therapy. Clin Nucl Med. 1999;24:536–8.
16. Kluge R, Schmidt F, Caca K, et al. Positron emission tomography with [^{18}F]fluoro-2-deoxy-D-glucose for diagnosis and staging of bile duct cancer. Hepatology. 2001;33:1029–35.
17. Keiding S, Hansen SB, Rasmussen HH, et al. Detection of cholangiocarcinoma in primary sclerosing cholangitis by positron emission tomography. Hepatology. 1998;28:700–6.

18. Gupta N, Bradfield H. Role of positron emission tomography scanning in evaluating gastrointestinal neoplasms. Semin Nucl Med. 1996;26:65–73.
19. Imbriaco M, Akhurst T, Hilton S, et al. Whole-body FDG-PET in patients with recurrent colorectal carcinoma. A comparative study with CT. Clin Positron Imag. 2003;3:107–14.
20. Vitola JV, Delbeke D, Sandler MP, et al. Positron emission tomography to stage suspected metastatic colorectal carcinoma to the liver. Am J Surg. 1996;171:21–6.
21. Frohlich A, Diederichs CG, Staib L, et al. Detection of liver metastases from pancreatic cancer using FDG PET. J Nucl Med. 1999;40:250–5.
22. Hayashi N, Tamaki N, Yonekura Y, et al. Imaging of the hepatocellular carcinoma using dynamic positron emission tomography with nitrogen-13 ammonia. J Nucl Med. 1995;26:254–7.
23. Dimitrakopoulou-Strauss A, Gutzler F, Strauss LG, et al. PET-Studien mit C-11-Athanol bei der intratumoralen therapie von hepatozellularen karzinomen. Radiology. 1996;36:744–9.
24. Dimitrakopoulou-Strauss A, Strauss LG, et al. Pharmacokinetic imaging of ^{11}C ethanol with PET in eight patients with hepatocellular carcinomas who were scheduled for treatment with percutaneous ethanol injection. Radiology. 1999;211:681–6.
25. Rosenbaum SJ, Stergar H, Antoch G, Veit P, Bockisch A, Kuhl H. Staging and follow-up of gastrointestinal tumors with PET/CT. Abdom Imag. 2006;31(1):25–35.
26. Cohade C, Osman M, Leal J, Wahl RL. Direct comparison of ^{18}F-FDG PET and PET/CT in patients with colorectal carcinoma. J Nucl Med. 2003;44(11):1797–803.

24 Colorectal Cancer

Hirofumi Shibata, Ukihide Tateishi, and Tomio Inoue

Introduction

Approximately 13% new cases of colorectal cancer are diagnosed in the US every year, and approximately 70% of these patients undergo a radical surgical resection of primary lesions, but only two thirds are cured. About one third of patients who undergo curative surgical resection of the primary lesion have a recurrence after the initial treatment [1]. After the initial surgical colorectal cancer resection, the accurate and early detection of potentially resectable metastatic tumors localized in the liver and lung is important in patient management. In cases of rectal cancer and sigmoid colon cancer, important also is the detection of pelvic recurrence that is amenable to resection with curative intent during the course of clinical follow-up after initial surgical treatment [2]. Diagnosis of recurrence and the appropriate selection of patients for surgery are difficult because of the low sensitivity of computed tomography (CT) for early metastasis. Scar formation after resection of rectal cancer, which mimics local recurrence on CT and magnetic resonance imaging (MRI) can make it difficult to accurately diagnose local recurrence. More accurate preoperative restaging using fluorodeoxyglucose (FDG) positron emission tomography (PET) would reduce the frequency of surgery for nonresectable recurrence, and a more sensitive form of detecting tumor recurrence may increase the rate of resectability at restaging.

H. Shibata (✉) • U. Tateishi, M.D., Ph.D.
Department of Radiology, Yokohama City University School of Medicine, Yokohama 236-0004, Japan
e-mail: hiroshibata34@yahoo.co.jp; utateish@yokohama-cu.ac.jp

T. Inoue, M.D., Ph.D.
Department of Radiology, Yokohama City University School of Medicine, 3-9 Pukuura, Kanazawa-ku, Yokohama 236-004, Japan
e-mail: tomioi@yokohama-cu.ac.jp

Staging

In stage 0, abnormal cells are found in the innermost lining of the colon. These abnormal cells can become cancer and spread into nearby normal tissue. Stage 0 is also called carcinoma in situ. In stage I, cancer has formed and spread beyond the innermost tissue layer of the colon wall to the middle layers. Stage I colon cancer is also referred to as Dukes A colon cancer. Stage II colon cancer is divided into stage IIA and stage IIB. Stage IIA: Cancer has spread beyond the middle tissue layers of the colon wall or has spread to nearby tissues around the colon or rectum. Stage IIB: Cancer has spread beyond the colon wall into nearby organs and/or through the peritoneum. Stage II colon cancer is also referred to as Dukes B colon cancer. Stage III colon cancer is divided into stage IIIA, stage IIIB, and stage IIIC. Stage IIIA: Cancer has spread from the innermost tissue layer of the colon wall to the middle layers and has spread to as many as three lymph nodes. Stage IIIB: Cancer

E.E. Kim et al. (eds.), *Clinical PET and PET/CT: Principles and Applications*,
DOI 10.1007/978-1-4419-0802-5_24, © Springer Science+Business Media New York 2013

has spread to as many as three nearby lymph nodes and has spread: beyond the middle tissue layers of the colon wall; or to nearby tissues around the colon or rectum; or beyond the colon wall into nearby organs and/or through the peritoneum. Stage IIIC: Cancer has spread to four or more nearby lymph nodes and has spread to or beyond the middle tissue layers of the colon wall, to nearby tissues around the colon or rectum, or to nearby organs and/or through the peritoneum. Stage III colon cancer is also referred to as Dukes C colon cancer. In stage IV, cancer may have spread to nearby lymph nodes and has spread to other parts of the body, such as the liver or lungs. Stage IV colon cancer is also referred to as Dukes D colon cancer.

For rectal cancer in stage 0, abnormal cells are found in the innermost lining of the rectum. The abnormal cells can become cancer and spread into nearby normal tissue. Stage 0 is also called carcinoma in situ. In stage I, cancer has formed and spread beyond the innermost lining of the rectum to the second and third layers and involves the inside wall of the rectum, but has not spread to the outer wall of the rectum or outside the rectum. Stage I rectal cancer is also referred to as Dukes A rectal cancer. In stage II, cancer has spread outside the rectum to nearby tissue, but it has not spread into the lymph nodes (small, bean-shaped structures found throughout the body that filter substances in a fluid called lymph and help fight infection and disease). Stage II rectal cancer is also referred to as Dukes B rectal cancer. In stage III, cancer has spread to nearby lymph nodes, but it has not spread to other parts of the body. Stage III rectal cancer is also referred to as Dukes C rectal cancer. In stage IV, cancer has spread to other parts of the body, such as the liver, lungs, or ovaries. Stage IV rectal cancer is also referred to as Dukes D rectal cancer.

Differential Diagnosis and Preoperative Staging

Preoperative staging with imaging modalities is usually limited because most patients will benefit from colectomy to prevent intestinal obstruction and bleeding. The extent of the disease can be evaluated during surgery with peritoneal exploration and excision of pericolonic and mesenteric lymph nodes. Performing an FDG PET examination preoperatively may be helpful if the detection of distant metastases will cancel surgery in patients with increased surgical risk.

The utility of FDG PET for initial preoperative staging in patients with colorectal cancer has not been established. Nabi et al. reported 100% sensitivity, 43% specificity, 90% positive predictive value, and 100% negative predictive value for FDG PET in the detection of primary colorectal cancer [3]. Yasuda et al. reported that 14 of 59 patients (24%) with colorectal adenoma had positive results on FDG PET [4]. In cases of colonic adenoma larger than 13 mm in diameter, sensitivity was 90%. The sensitivity of FDG PET for lesions localized in the ascending colon, descending colon, and cecum appeared to be higher than that of other sites because of less motion artifact by fixation.

Both FDG and CT had a poor sensitivity (29%) for detecting local lymph node involvement. FDG PET was, however, superior to CT for detecting hepatic metastases with a sensitivity of 88% and specificity of 100%, compared with 38% and 97%, respectively, for CT [3]. These data were confirmed in the studies by Mukai et al. and Kantorova et al. [6] who reported that FDG PET changed the treatment modality in 8% of patients and the extent of surgery in 13%.5, 6

Using PET/CT for staging caused a change in stage to occur in 26 patients (31%) as opposed to conventional imaging . Twelve patients (14%) were upstaged (change in N stage, 7; change in M stage, 4; change in N and M stages, 1), and 14 patients (17%) were downstaged (change in N stage, 10; change in M stage, 3; change in N and M stages, 1). Using PET/CT altered management intent in seven patients (8%) (curative to palliative, 6; palliative to curative, 1). Management was altered in ten patients (12%) [7]. Accuracy of PET/CT was evaluated as a lesion-based analysis. PET/CT detected 15 more intra-abdominal metastatic lesions than abdominopelvic CT (liver, 5; peritoneal seeding, 3; lateral pelvic node, 2; para-aortic node, 1; spleen, 1; synchronous cancer in stomach, 1; synchronous lesion in colon, 1). The sensitivity of FDG PET for the diagnosis of primary lesions and local lymph node metastases at initial diagnosis and initial preoperative staging is of limited clinical importance. Relative to PET alone, PET/CT has been reported to improve colorectal carcinoma staging up to 11% [8]. PET/CT images can detect more lesions than PET or CT; however, this would only be clinically relevant if the additional lesions change the tumor node metastasis system stage and cause change in patient management to occur. Although only a few studies have evaluated the performance of [18F]-FDG PET during the initial staging of colorectal carcinoma [6, 9], it is possible to hypothesize that PET/CT can be more effective in primary colorectal carcinoma because it provides both functional and anatomic data.

Diagnosis of Recurrence

Overall sensitivity of FDG PET imaging is in the range of 90% and specificity is higher than 70%, both superior to CT in detecting recurrent or metastatic colorectal carcinoma (Fig. 24.1). A meta-analysis of 11 clinical reports and 577 patients determined that the sensitivity and specificity of FDG PET for detecting recurrent colorectal cancer were 97% and 76%, respectively [10]. The accuracy, sensitivity, and specificity of FDG PET for the detection of local recurrent tumors were greater than 90% [10]. Ito et al. compared findings of FDG PET and MRI with histopathologic findings, and found that FDG PET could differentiate a scar from local recurrent tumor [11]. False-negative results on T2-weighted images on which the lesion is not shown as a high intense area, may be a result of the pathologic characteristic of recurrence as fibrotic changes with less tumor cell density. Abouzied et al. assessed the usefulness of FDG PET in 79 patients, including 55 colorectal patients with rising tumor markers and negative or inconclusive conventional imaging modalities, and FDG PET was able to elucidate the lesion responsible for the rising tumor markers in 59 of 79 patients (75%), and to guide appropriate patient management [12].

Flangen et al. reported the use of FDG PET in 22 patients with unexplained elevation of serum carcinoembryonic antigen (CEA) level after resection of colorectal carcinoma, and no abnormal findings on conventional workup, including CT [13]. Sensitivity and specificity of FDG PET for tumor recurrence were 100% and 71%, respectively. Valk et al. reported a sensitivity of 93% and a specificity of 92% in a similar group of 18 patients [14]. In both studies, PET correctly determined tumor in two thirds of patients with rising CEA levels and negative CT scans.

Direct comparison of CT and FDG PET in a total of 306 patients showed overall sensitivity of 95% for FDG PET and 66% for CT for all sites of recurrence [10–13]. Sensitivity for detection of hepatic recurrence was 95% and 83% for PET and CT, respectively, and for pelvic recurrence, 97% and 63%, respectively. FDG PET seems to be a more sensitive imaging modality than CT, especially in the abdomen and pelvis where approximately one third of the sites that were true positive using FDG PET were false negative using CT. Other studies have compared the accuracy of FDG PET and CT for detection of hepatic metastases[14–18]. Overall, FDG PET was more accurate than CT. A meta-analysis performed to compare noninvasive imaging methods (sonography, CT, MRI, and FDG PET) for the detection of hepatic metastases from colorectal, gastric, and esophageal cancers demonstrated that at an equivalent specificity of 85%, FDG PET had the highest sensitivity at 90% compared with 76% for MRI, 72% for CT, and 55% for sonography [19].

Delbeke et al. [17] compared PET and conventional CT to CT portography, which is more invasive than conventional CT and FDG PET. Diagnostic accuracy for hepatic recurrence of FDG PET was more accurate than CT or CT portography (92%, 78%, and 80%, respectively). The sensitivity of CT portography for hepatic recurrence was higher than that of FDG PET (97% vs. 91%), but FDG PET had a much higher specificity for hepatic recurrence [17]. In a recent prospective study on the clinical impact of ^{18}F-FDG in patients with suspected recurrence of colorectal cancer [17], the management plan for

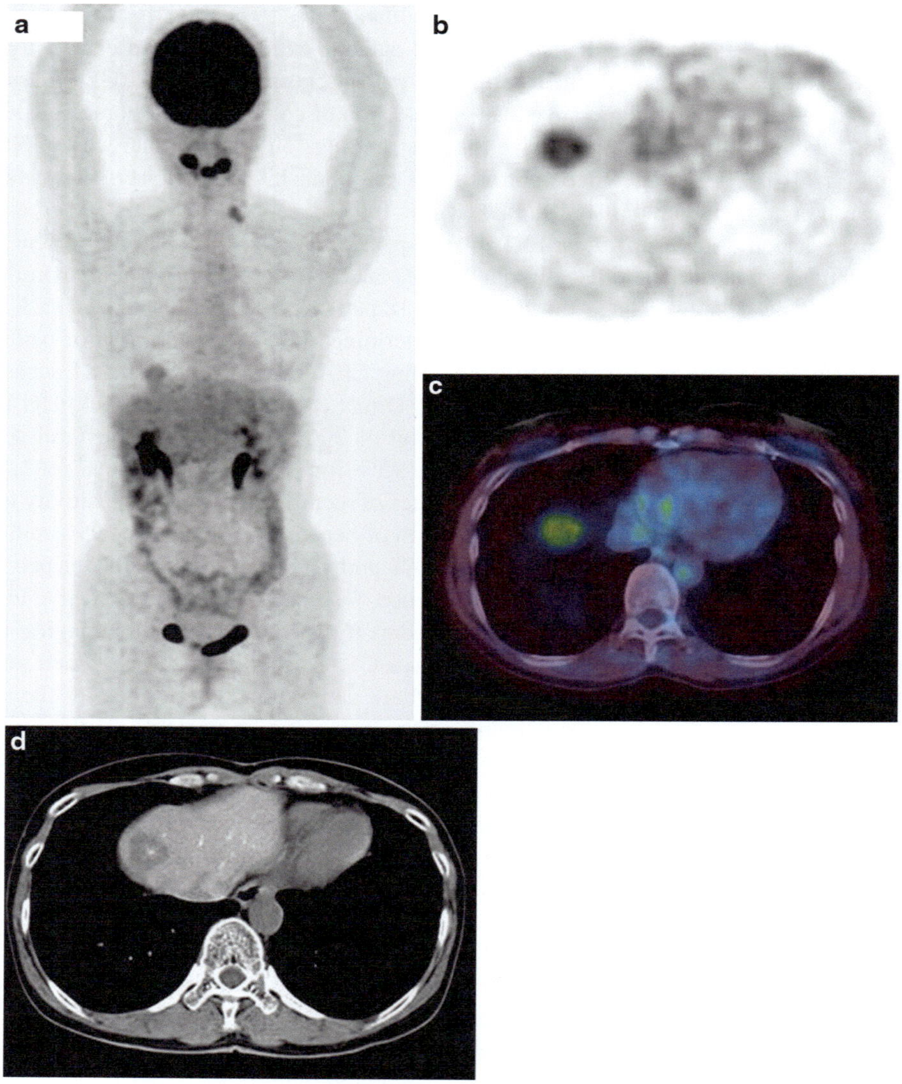

Fig. 24.1 (**a–d**) A 55-year-old woman with previously treated colon carcinoma. Whole-body PET maximum-intensity-projection (MIP) image reveals multiple abnormal uptake including the left supraclavicular node and suprahepatic lesion (**a**). Co-registered PET/CT reveals mislegistration of intrahepatic metastasis that was described as suprahepatic lesion on MIP image (**b–d**)

54 of 102 patients (53%) was altered as a direct result of unexpected PET findings, and planned surgery was canceled in 26 of 43 patients (60%) with incremental PET findings.

In a meta-analysis of the literature, FDG PET imaging changed the management of 102 of 349 patients (29%) [12]. FDG PET imaging detects unsuspected metastases in 13–36% of patients and has a clinical impact on 14–65% [12]. In the study by Delbeke et al., because of PET findings, surgical management was altered in 28% of patients (one third by initiating surgery, two thirds by avoiding surgery) [17]. In a survey-based study of 60 referring oncologists, surgeons, and generalists, FDG PET performed at initial staging had a major impact on the

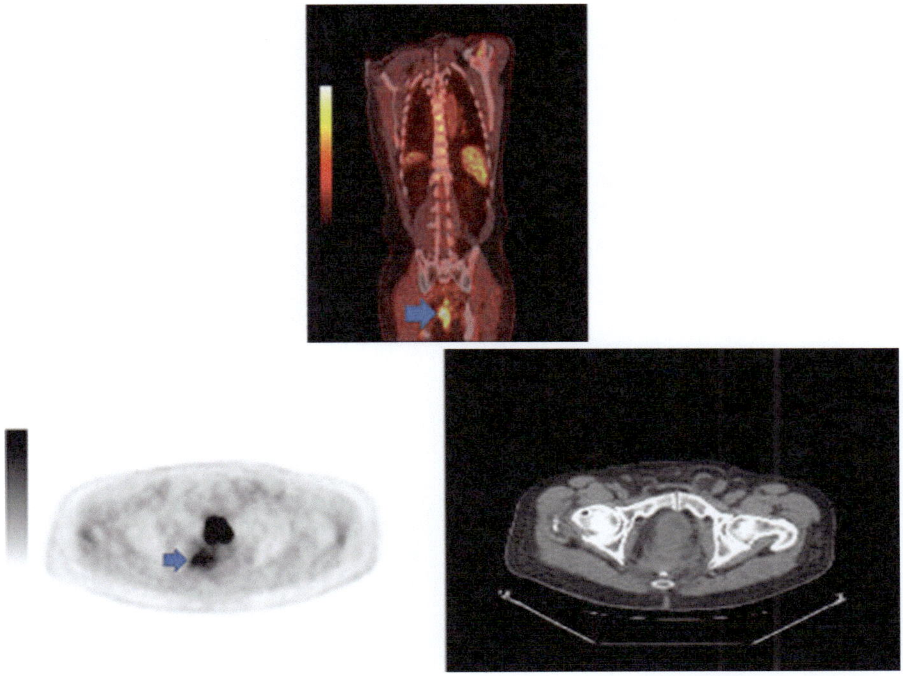

Fig. 24.2 Coronal ^{18}F-FDG PET/CT image (*top*) of the axial body shows a focal area of moderately increased activity in the rectum (*arrow*). Axial PET image (*left lower*) of the pelvis shows a focal area of slightly increased activity in the rectum (*arrow*). Noncontrasted CT image (*right lower*) of the pelvis at the same level shows a thickening of the rectal wall after radiation therapy. Biopsy showed a recurrent rectal cancer

management of patients with colorectal cancer and contributed to a change of clinical stage in 42% (80% upstaged, 20% down-staged) and a change in the clinical management in over 60% of patients [20–27].

The results of PET/CT had an impact on the management of 28 of 204 patients (14%); 7 of 28 patients with a change in treatment management had colorectal cancer representing 20% of patients (8 of 34) with gastrointestinal tumors [28]. Selzner et al. compared contrast-enhanced CT and noncontrast-enhanced PET/CT in 76 patients referred for restaging prior to resection of hepatic metastases [29]. For detection of hepatic metastases, contrast-enhanced CT and noncontrast-enhanced PET/CT had similar sensitivities of 95% and 91%, respectively. However, for the evaluation of patients with a prior hepatic resection, PET/CT had a superior specificity of 100% compared with 50% for contrast-enhanced CT. For local recurrence, PET/CT had a superior sensitivity of 93% compared with 53% for contrast-enhanced CT. A similar conclusion was reached for extrahepatic metastases with a sensitivity of 89% for PET/CT compared with 64% for contrast-enhanced CT. PET/CT had an impact on the management of 21% of patients. False-negative PET/CT results were seen for small lesions less than 5 mm and in some patients who had undergone chemotherapy in the month prior to PET/CT. Another study reported that recurrence and/or metastasis were confirmed in 56 of 68 patients during clinical follow-up after PET/CT imaging. The sensitivity of PET/CT diagnosis of colorectal cancer recurrence and/or metastasis was 94.6%, and the specificity was 83.3% (Fig. 24.2). The positive predictive value was 96.4% and the negative predictive value was 76.9%. PET/CT imaging detected one or more occult malignant lesions in eight cases where abdominal/pelvic CT and/or ultrasonography showed negative findings, and also detected more lesions than CT or ultrasonography did in 17 of 56 patients (30.4%). Recurrence and/or metastasis were detected in 22 of 24 cases (91.7%) with elevated serum CEA levels isomg FDG PET/CT imaging [30]. The major benefit of using FDG PET (PET/CT) may be avoiding inappropriate local therapies by documentation of widespread disease (Fig. 24.1).

Monitoring Therapy of Colorectal Carcinoma

Only a few studies have reported on the issue of PET criteria for defining response to treatment in comparison with clinical and pathologic response criteria. The specificity of PET/CT in the detection of neoadjuvant response has generally ranged between 70% and 80%, which is much higher than the performance of any other imaging modality [31].

Findlay et al. reported that responders could be discriminated from nonresponders after 4–5 weeks of chemotherapy by measuring FDG uptake before and during therapy [32]. Guillem et al. demonstrated that FDG PET imaging performed before and 4–5 weeks after completion of preoperative radiation, and 5-fluorouracil- based chemotherapy had the potential to assess pathologic response [33]. It was subsequently demonstrated that FDG PET imaging could predict long-term outcome after a median follow-up of 42 months [34]. The mean percentage decrease in SUV_{max} was 69% for patients free of recurrence and 37% for patients with recurrence. Currently, FDG PET/CT appears to be the best diagnostic tool for predicting the response to neoadjuvant chemoradiation therapy in locally advanced rectal cancer.

Conclusion

PET/CT has a significant impact on the management of patients with primary colorectal cancer. PET/CT specificity in the detection of neoadjuvant response is much better than that of any other imaging modality. Further evaluation is required to assess the impact of PET/CT on the outcome of patients with colorectal cancer and to explore the additional prognostic information that can be obtained by functional imaging.

References

1. August TA, Ottow RT, Sugarbaker PH. Clinical perspectives on human colorectal cancer metastases. Cancer Metastasis. 1984;3:303–24.
2. Turk PS, Wanebo HJ. Results of surgical treatment of nonhepatic recurrence of colorectal carcinoma. Cancer. 1993;72:4267–77.
3. Nabi AH, Doerr RJ, Lamonica DM, et al. Staging of primary colorectal carcinomas with F-18 fluorodeoxyglucose whole-body PET: correlation with histopathologic and CT findings. Radiology. 1998;206:755–60.
4. Yasuda S, Fuji H, Nakahara T, et al. F-18 FDG-PET detection of colonic adenoma. J Nucl Med. 2001; 42:989–92.
5. Mukai M, Sadahiro S, Yasuda S, et al. Preoperative evaluation by whole body 18F-fluorodeoxyglucose positron emission tomography in patients with primary colorectal cancer. Oncol Rep. 2000;7:85–7.
6. Kantorova I, Lipska L, Belohlavek O, et al. Routine 18F_FDG PET pre-operative staging of colorectal cancer: comparison with conventional staging and its impact on treatment decision making. J Nucl Med. 2003;44:1784–8.
7. Davey K, Heriot AG, Mackay J, et al. The impact of 18-fluorodeoxyglucose positron emission tomography-computed tomography on the staging and management of primary rectal cancer. Dis Colon Rectum. 2008;51:997–1003.
8. Cohade C, Osman M. Direct comparison of sup 18F-FDG PET and PET/CT in patients with colorectal carcinoma. J Nucl Med. 2003;44:1797–803.
9. Heriot AG, Hicks RJ, Drummond EG, et al. Does positron emission tomography change management in primary rectal cancer? A prospective assessment. Dis Colon Rectum. 2004;47:451–8.
10. Huebner RH, Park KC, Shepherd IE, et al. A meta-analysis of the literature for whole-body FDG PET detection of colorectal cancer. J Nucl Med. 2000; 41:1177–89.
11. Ito K, Kato T, Tadokoro M, et al. Recurrent rectal cancer and scar: differentiation with PET and MR imaging. Radiology. 1992;182:549–52.
12. Abouzied I, Zubeldia JM, Nabi RA. Role of F-18 fluorodeoxyglucose positron emission tomography in the detection of occult recurrent carcinoma presenting with rising tumor markers. J Nucl Med. 2002;43:23.
13. Flangen FL, Dehdashi FD, Gunbiyi OA, et al. Utility of FDG-PET for investigating unexplained plasma CEA elevation in patients with colorectal cancer. Ann Surg. 1998;227:319–23.

14. Valk PE, Abella-Columna E, Haseman MK, et al. Whole-body PET imaging with F-18-fluorodeoxyglucose in management of recurrent colorectal cancer. Arch Surg. 1999;134:503–11.
15. Schiepers C, Penninckx F, De Vadder N, et al. Contribution of PET in the diagnosis of recurrent colorectal cancer: comparison with conventional imaging. Eur J Surg Oncol. 1995;21:517–22.
16. Vitola V, Delbeke D, Sandler MP, et al. Positron emission tomography to stage metastatic colorectal carcinoma to the liver. Am J Surg. 1996;171:21–6.
17. Delbeke D, Vitola I, Sandler MP, et al. Staging recurrent metastatic colorectal carcinoma with PET. J Nucl Med. 1997;38:1196–201.
18. Ogunbiyi OA, Flanagan FL, Dehdashti F, et al. Detection of recurrent and metastatic colorectal cancer: comparison of positron emission tomography and computed tomography. Ann Surg Oncol. 1997;4: 613–20.
19. Kinkel K, Lu BM, et al. Detection of hepatic metastases from cancers of the gastrointestinal tract by using noninvasive imaging methods (US, CT, MRimaging, PET): a meta-analysis. Radiology. 2002;224(3): 748–56.
20. Beets G, Penninckx F, Schiepers C, et al. Clinical value of whole-body positron emission tomography with [18F]fluorodeoxyglucose in recurrent colorectal cancer. Br J Surg. 1994;81:1666–70.
21. Lai DT, Fulham M, Stephen MS, et al. The role of whole-body positron emission tomography with [18F]fluorodeoxyglucose in identifying operable colorectal cancer. Arch Surg. 1996;131:703–7.
22. Flamen P, Stroobants S, Van Cutsem E, et al. Additional value of whole body positron emission tomography with fluorine-18-2-fluoro-2deoxy-D-glucose in recurrent colorectal cancer. J Clin Oncol. 1999;17(3):894–901.
23. Imdahl A, Reinhardt MI, Nitzsche EU, et al. Impact of 18F-FDG positron emission tomography for decision making in colorectal cancer recurrences. Arch Surg. 2000;385(2):129–34.
24. Staib L, Schirrmeister H, Reske SN, et al. Is (18) F-fluorodeoxyglucose positron emission tomography in recurrent colorectal cancer a contribution to surgical decision making? Am J Surg. 2000;180(1):1–5.
25. Kalff Hicks R, Ware R. F-18 FDG PET for suspected or confirmed recurrence of colon cancer. A prospective study of impact and outcome. Clin Positron Imag. 2000;3:183.
26. Strasberg SM, Dehdashti F, Siegel BA, et al. Survival of patients evaluated by FDG PET before hepatic resection for metastatic colorectal carcinoma: a prospective database study. Ann Surg. 2001;233:320–1.
27. Ruers TJ, Langenhoff BS, Neeleman N, et al. Value of positron emission tomography with [F-18] fluorodeoxyglucose in patients with colorectal liver metastases: a prospective study. J Clin Oncol. 2002;20(2):388–95.
28. Bar-shalom R, Yefremov N, Guralnik L, et al. Clinical performance of PET/CT in the evaluation of cancer: additional value for diagnostic imaging and patient management. J Nucl Med. 2003;44:1200–9.
29. Selzner M, Hany TF, Wildbrett P, et al. Dose the novel PET/CT imaging modality impact on the treatment of patients with metastatic colorectal cancer of the liver? Ann Surg. 2004;204:1027–34.
30. Long-Bang C, Jin-Long T, Hai-Zhu S, et al. 18F-DG PET/CT in detection of recurrence and metastasis of colorectal cancer. World J Gastroenterol. 2007; 13(37):5025–9.
31. Carlo C, Lucia R, Paola AE, et al. Sequential FDG-PET/CT reliably predicts response of locally advanced rectal cancer to neo-adjuvant chemo-radiation therapy. Eur J Nucl Med Mol Imag. 2007;34:1583–93.
32. Findlay M, Young H, Cunningham D, et al. Noninvasive monitoring of tumor metabolism using fluorodeoxyglucose and positron emission tomography in colorectal cancer liver metastases: correlation with tumor response to fluorouracil. J Clin Oncol. 1996;14:700–8.
33. Guillem J, Calle J, Akhurst T, et al. Prospective assessment of primary rectal cancer response to preoperative radiation and chemotherapy using 18-fluorodeoxyglucose positron emission tomography. Dis Colon Rectum. 2000;43:18–24.
34. Guillem JG, Moore HG, Akhurst T, et al. Sequential preoperative fluorodeoxyglucose-positron emission tomography assessment of response to preoperative chemoradiation: a means for determining long term outcomes of rectal cancer. J Am Coll Surg. 2004;199:1–7.

Urologic Cancer

25

Tomio Inoue, Nobukazu Takahashi, Tetsuya Higuchi, and E. Edmund Kim

Positron emission tomography (PET) is a unique imaging modality with the capability of studying regional metabolism. ^{18}F-fluoro-deoxyglucose (FDG) is the most widely used tracer in the field of PET oncology. The clinical utility of oncology PET using FDG has been proven in the staging and restaging of malignant tumors such as those in the head/neck, lung, breast, and colorectal cancers, as well as malignant lymphoma and melanoma. In the field of urology, FDG PET has been evaluated for relevant malignancies with promising results in certain areas and disappointing results in others. At present, FDG PET is capable of visualizing urologic tumors and associated lymph nodes and distal metastatic sites. However, its use is severely limited by excretion of the most commonly used radioisotope via the urinary tract, making pelvic imaging particularly unrewarding. ^{11}C-choline, up-regulated in malignant cells, has shown potential usefulness in brain, prostate, and esophageal cancers with enhanced synthesis of membrane phospholipids. This chapter discusses the clinical usefulness of oncology PET in the field of urology, including renal cell, urinary bladder, and prostate cancer, as well as testicular tumors.

T. Inoue, M.D., Ph.D. (✉) • N. Takahashi, M.D., Ph.D.
Department of Radiology, Yokohama City University Graduate School of Medicine, 3-9 Pukuura, Kanazawa-ku, Yokohama 236-0004, Japan
e-mail: tomioi@yokohama-cu.ac.jp

T. Higuchi, M.D., Ph.D.
Department of Nuclear Medicine and Diagnostic Radiology, Gumma University School of Medicine, Maebashi 371-8511, Japan

E.E. Kim, M.D., M.S.
Departments of Nuclear Medicine and Diagnostic Radiology, The University of Texas MD Anderson Cancer Center and Medical School, 1515 Holcombe Blvd, Box 0059, Houston, TX 77030, USA

Graduate School of Convergence Science and Technology, Seoul National University, Seoul, South Korea
e-mail: ekim@mdanderson.org

Renal Cell Carcinoma

Renal cell cancers are responsible for 3% of all malignant tumors in adults, and males predominate in a 2:1 ratio. Clear cell type is the most common, accounting for 70–80%, with papillary (chromophilic, 10–15%), chromophobic (5–10%), and medullary (<1%) carcinomas accounting for much less. Approximately 5% of renal cell cancers develop a local recurrence in the tumor bed. The staging of renal cell cancer is based on the tumor node metastasis (TNM) classification (Table 25.1).

Few studies have to date reported on the imaging of renal cell carcinoma with PET or PET/CT. Most reports have dealt with the use of FDG, and other tracers such as ^{18}F-DOPA have become an object of clinical research. FDG accumulates with some cases of renal cell carcinoma. The accuracy of FDG PET for staging and management of renal cell carcinoma was reviewed by Khandani et al.

E.E. Kim et al. (eds.), *Clinical PET and PET/CT: Principles and Applications*,
DOI 10.1007/978-1-4419-0802-5_25, © Springer Science+Business Media New York 2013

Table 25.1 TNM classification and American Joint Committee on Cancer staging of renal cell cancer (revised in 2010)

T stage	
T0	No tumor
T1	<7 cm and limited to kidney 1a: <4 cm; 1b: 4–7 cm
T2	>7 cm and limited to kidney ; 2a: 7-10 cm; 2b: >10 cm
T3	Invasion of major veins, adrenal or perirenal fat within Gerota fascia; 3a: renal vein or perirenal fat; 3b: adrenal(s) or inferior vena cava below diaphragm; 3c: inferior vena cava above diaphragm
T4	Beyond Gerota fascia (including contiguous extension into the ipsilateral adrenal gland)
N stage	
N0	No regional node metastasis
N1	Regional node(s)
M stage	
M0	No distant metastasis
M1	Distant metastasis
AJCC stage	
Stage I	T1, N0, M0
II	T2, N0, M0
III	T3, N0, or T1-3, N1, M0
IV	T4, N2 or M1

[1], who addressed the utility of FDG-PET in the detection of primary and metastatic lesion of RCC comparing with CT. In regard to the diagnostic accuracy of FDG PET for restaging of renal cell carcinoma, Safei et al. [2] found that FDG PET classified the clinical stage correctly in 32 of 36 patients with advanced renal cell carcinoma (89%) and was incorrect for 4 patients (11%). The sensitivity and specificity of FDG PET were 87% and 100%, respectively. In 25 biopsied lesions with 20 malignant lesions and five benign lesions, PET correctly classified 21 of 25 (84%) (sensitivity, 88% ; specificity, 75%). Poggi et al. [3] reported a case of a minimally symptomatic intramedullary spinal cord metastasis, an uncommon and often diagnostically challenging lesion, which was confirmed by PET.

As mentioned above, FDG PET can be useful in characterizing anatomic lesions of unknown significance in patients with renal cell carcinoma. However, we need clinical results of larger patient numbers to establish the clinical utility of FDG PET in staging and restaging renal cell carcinoma.

^{11}C-acetate, as a metabolic substrate of beta-oxidation and a precursor of amino acid, fatty acid and sterol, has proved useful in detecting various malignancies. High-quality whole-body images could be obtained by using large doses (20 mCi) of ^{11}C-acetate. PET with ^{11}C-acetate can detect renal cell cancer. The advantages of ^{11}C-acetate are that it is less time consuming (the whole procedure can be completed within 45 min after injection), and it has no hyperglycemic effect and no sink phenomenon due to the high accumulation of radioactive tracer in the urinary tract. The disadvantages are increased uptake in the salivary glands, pancreas, and sometimes the bowels, which may cause either false-positive or false-negative results, and it is dependent on an on-site cyclotron.

Ureter Cancer

The primary lesions of urinary tract cancer cannot be clearly found using FDG PET because of the urinary excretion of radioactivity in the urinary tract. However, recurrent or advanced cases of ureter cancer are detected by FDG PET. The clinical usefulness of FDG PET in detecting ureter cancer has not been established.

Urinary Bladder Cancer

Bladder cancer accounts for 3% of all malignant tumors, and males are affected two to three times as often as are females. Approximately 95% of bladder cancers are urothelial carcinomas, and less common types are squamous cell carcinoma (<5%) and adenocarcinoma (<1%). Irrespective of the staging level being addressed, the available techniques uniformly have limitations, as well as advantages and disadvantages. A common shortcoming of computed tomography (CT) and magnetic resonance imaging (MRI) is a lack of specificity. The specificity of conventional imaging techniques is further compromised by attempts to increase sensitivity. As long as nonspecific anatomic changes are used as discriminating criteria, increases in diagnostic sensitivity can occur at the price of specificity.

Few data are available on FDG PET imaging of bladder cancer as a result of physiologic excretion of FDG via the bladder. It is hoped that advances in PET imaging will overcome the limitations of the currently available techniques. The significance of the limitations of a given imaging modality depends to some degree on whether the modality is being used for clinical decision making or for patient stratification in a clinical trial [4].

The detection of primary lesions of urinary bladder cancer is difficult because it is hampered by the urinary excretion of administered radiopharmaceuticals. From the viewpoint of pharmacokinetics of radiopharmaceuticals, ^{11}C-methionine or ^{11}C-choline is available for detecting primary bladder tumor. It is possible to visualize urinary bladder tumors larger than 1 cm in diameter with PET using ^{11}C-methionine, but the value of the method in the staging of the lesions is not superior to conventional methods [5].

Lymph node staging with FDG PET in patients with urinary bladder cancer is valuable in urologic oncology. Heicappell et al. [6] used FDG PET on eight patients with bladder cancer before pelvic lymph node dissection. The results of FDG PET were then compared with the histology of pelvic lymph nodes obtained at surgery. Lymph node metastases were detected by histopathologic examination in three patients with bladder cancer. At the sites with histologically proven metastases, increased FDG uptake suspicious of metastatic disease was found in two of three patients. These results suggest that FDG PET may be a valuable diagnostic tool in the staging of pelvic lymph nodes in bladder cancer.

Prostate Cancer

The prostate, seminal vesicles, and Cowper bulbourethral glands make up the accessory sex glands in the male and are extraperitoneally embedded in vascular connective tissue of the subperitoneal space. The base of the prostate abuts the bladder neck and encircles the urethra. The Denonvillier fascia lies between the anterior surface of the rectum and the posterior surface of the prostate. The prostate has a volume of approximately 4.5×4×3 cm and has three zones (inner periurethral, estrogen-dependent transitional, and testosterone-dependent outer zones). Prostate cancer is the most frequent cancer diagnosed in males and the second leading cause of male death from cancer. The diagnosis is based on palpable findings, prostate-specific antigen (organ but not tumor specific) values, endorectal ultrasound, and is confirmed by transrectal segmental biopsy. Reasons for referral imaging include tumor visualization and assessment of tumor extent. Tumor staging is based on the TNM classification (Table 25.2). Prostate cancer poses a diagnostic dilemma in regard to FDG PET for the detection of primary lesions, which may be blocked by the crosstalk from eliminated radioactivity in the urinary bladder. The detectability of FDG PET for metastatic bone lesions, which are common in prostate cancer, is inferior to that of a conventional bone scan.

PET with ^{11}C-choline and ^{11}C-acetate can be started at 5–10 min postinjection. Because there

Table 25.2 TNM classification of prostate cancer

T stage	
Tx	Cannot be assessed
T0	No tumor
T1	Not palpable or visible 1a: histologic tumor<5% tissue; 1b: >5%; 1c: tumor by systemic needle biopsy
T2	Within prostate 2a: < one half of one lobe; 2b: > one half of one lobe; 2c: both lobes
T3	Extend through capsule 3a: peristaltic issue or microscopic invasion of the bladder neck; 3b: seminal vesicles
T4	Invasion of bladder neck, pelvic muscles, rectum, or pelvic wall
N stage	
Nx	Cannot be assessed
N0	No regional node metastasis
N1	Metastasis in external (obturator), internal or presacral node
M stage	
M0	No distant metastasis
M1	Distant metastasis

is no elimination of the tracer in the urinary bladder during image data acquisition, the uptake of tracer in the prostate gland can be easily visualized. ^{11}C-choline is a metabolic tracer of phospholipids on the cell membrane; turnover is accelerated in the presence of cell proliferation, such as cancer cells [7]. The uptake of ^{11}C-choline in prostate cancer is higher than that of prostate hypertrophy [8], but there is some overlap between the tracer uptake in prostate cancer and that in benign disease. PET with ^{11}C-choline is also effective in detecting the metastatic lesions in intrapelvic lymph nodes [9]. However, in some cases, intestinal elimination of ^{11}C-choline restricts the detection of metastatic lesions in intrapelvic and intra-abdominal lymph nodes. Preliminary PET studies on patients with recurrent prostate cancer revealed uptake of ^{18}F-fluorocholine in the prostatic bed and also in metastatic lymph nodes [10]. Recently, hybrid PET/MRI has been developed and it is suggested that it may further improve identification and localization of significant primary prostate cancer [11]. In addition, application of newly developed 18F-FACBC is reported to have promising ability to detect primary and metastatic lesion of prostate cancer [12]

Testicular Cancer

Testicular cancer is a rare disease, representing only 1% of all cancers in males and is the most common cancer in the age group between 20 and 40 years; 40–50% of testicular tumors are seminoma and 50% are nonseminomatous cancers.

There is substantial uptake of FDG into the normal testis, which declines with age. The normal levels of FDG uptake in the testis relative to patient age should be considered in the interpretation of FDG scans of the inguinal and lower pelvic regions [13].

In restaging, a negative FDG PET result predicts fibrotic residual mass in seminomatous germ cell tumors. Moreover, it could be useful in predicting fibrotic residual mass in seminomatous germ cell tumors in those patients with no teratoma component in their primary tumor [14]. FDG PET is a clinically useful predictor of a viable tumor in postchemotherapy residuals of pure seminoma, especially those greater than 3 cm [15]. FDG PET is superior to CT for the assessment of residual tumors after chemotherapy of germ cell cancer and may thus have an increased effect on patient management. PET must be performed at least 2 weeks following completion of therapy. However, the possibility of false-positive PET findings as a result of reactive supradiaphragmatic inflammatory processes early after chemotherapy must be considered [16, 17].

Conclusion

FDG is the most commonly used PET radiopharmaceutical in assessing malignant tumors. However, urinary tract tumor assessment is restricted by the renal elimination of FDG. PET imaging using FDG offers no significant benefits over conventional imaging modalities for renal cell and bladder carcinomas. As a result of the low metabolic activity of prostate cancer, FDG PET does not differentiate adequately between adenoma and carcinoma, or detect local recurrence after radical prostatectomy with sufficient sensitivity.

PET using ^{11}C-choline and ^{11}C-acetate enables us to obtain pelvic images without radioactivity of eliminated tracer in the urinary tract. We can identify the radioactivity of primary lesions in the urinary bladder and prostate. Lymph node staging with FDG PET, specifically in bladder cancer, has been shown to have a potential clinical benefit. Further studies are required to determine the clinical value of retroperitoneal lymph node staging and recurrent disease detection in germ cell tumors. Encouraging early results have been obtained for the use of serial PET measurements to predict and assess therapy response to chemotherapy, which can also be valuable in urologic oncology. PET undoubtedly is capable of diagnosing malignancy in soft-tissue masses or lymph nodes before such changes become apparent on conventional cross-sectional imaging modalities (CT or MRI). Future accumulation of large studies related with PET/MRI and new PET tracer will enhance the development of clinical application of PET in the field of urology.

References

1. Khandani AH, Rathmell WK. Positron emission tomography in renal cell carcinoma: an imaging biomarker in development. Semin Nucl Med. 2012;42(4):221–30.
2. Safei A, Figlin R, Hoh CK, et al. The usefulness of F-18 deoxyglucose whole-body positron emission tomography (PET) for restaging of renal cell cancer. Clin Nephrol. 2002;57:56–62.
3. Poggi MM, Patronas N, Buttman JA, et al. Intramedullary spinal cord metastasis from renal cell carcinoma: detection by positron emission tomography. Clin Nucl Med. 2001;26:837–9.
4. See WA, Fuller JR. Staging of advanced bladder cancer. Current concepts and pitfalls. Urol Clin North Am. 1992;19:663–83.
5. Ahlstrom H, Malmstrom PU, Letocha H, et al. Positron emission tomography in the diagnosis and staging of urinary bladder cancer. Acta Radiol. 1996;37:180–5.
6. Heicappell R, Muller-Mattheis V, Reinhardt M, et al. Staging of pelvic lymph nodes in neoplasms of the bladder and prostate by positron emission tomography with 2-[(18)F]-2-deoxy-D-glucose. Eur Urol. 1999;36:582–7.
7. Hara T, Kosaka M, Kishi H. PET imaging of brain tumor with [methyl-^{11}C] choline. J Nucl Med. 1997;38:842–7.
8. Hara T, Kosaka N, Kishi H. PET imaging of prostate cancer using carbon-11-choline. J Nucl Med. 1998; 39:990–5.
9. Inoue T, Oriuchi N, Tomiyoshi K, et al. A shifting landscape: what will be next FDG in PET oncology? Ann Nucl Med. 2002;16:1–9.
10. DeGrado TR, Baldwin SW, Wang S, et al. Synthesis and evaluation of F-18 labeled choline analogs as oncologic PET tracers. J Nucl Med. 2001;42:1805–14.
11. Park H, Wood D, Hussain H, et al. Introducing parametric fusion PET/MRI of primary prostate cancer. J Nucl Med. 2012;53(4):546-51.
12. Schuster DM, Votaw JR, Nieh PT, et al. Initial experience with the radiotracer anti-1-amino-3-18F-fluorocyclobutane-1-carboxylic acid with PET/CT in prostate carcinoma. J Nucl Med. 2007;48(1):56-63.
13. Kitajima K, Nakamoto Y, Senda M, et al. Ann Nucl Med. 2007;21(7):405–10.
14. Spermon JR, De Geus-Oei LF, Kiemeney LA, et al. The role of (18)fluoro-2-deoxyglucose positron emission tomography in initial staging and restaging after chemotherapy for testicular germ cell tumours. BJU Int. 2002;89:549–56.
15. De Santis M, Bokemeyer C, Becherer A, et al. Predictive impact of 2-18-fluoro-2-deoxy-D-glucose positron emission tomography for residual postchemotherapy masses in patients with bulky seminoma. J Clin Oncol. 2001;19:3740–4.
16. Tsatalpas P, Beuthien-Baumann B, Kropp J, et al. Diagnostic value of F-18 FDG positron emission tomography for detection and treatment control of malignant germ cell tumors. Urol Int. 2002;68:157–63.
17. Cremerious U, Effert PJ, Adam G, et al. FDG PET for detection and therapy control of metastatic germ cell tumor. J Nucl Med. 1998;39:815–22.

Gynecologic Cancers

26

Seok-Ki Kim, Sung Eun Kim, June-Key Chung, and E. Edmund Kim

Introduction

Gynecologic cancers constitute approximately 20% of visceral cancers in women and are divided into three major types: ovarian, cervical, and endometrial cancers. The majority of gynecologic cancers require surgical removal, along with adjuvant radiotherapy or chemotherapy. The therapeutic option varies with the type and stage of cancer. Therefore, accurate staging is necessary for optimal treatment.

A variety of radiographic techniques are used for evaluating patients with suspected or diagnosed gynecologic malignancies. Unfortunately, morphologic imaging techniques are not optimal for diagnosis, staging, or identifying recurrent disease, when a specific tumor marker, such as serum CA-125, can hold some value for tracking status and heralding recurrence during postoperative patient management [1, 2].

The advent of positron emission tomography (PET) enables us to metabolically detect active gynecologic cancers with greater accuracy than anatomic imaging techniques. Furthermore, PET is more sensitive for the presence of active cancer than that determined by tumor markers, which, at present, are generally available [3]. Currently, most PET systems are installed as combined PET/computed tomography (CT) scanners that provide combined PET and CT images with acceptable precision. Anatomic information obtained from CT increases the usefulness of PET because the abdominopelvic cavity has complex spatial structures. As for other tumors, fluorine-18-fluorodeoxyglucose (^{18}F-FDG) is the most commonly used PET agent in gynecologic oncology today.

Ovarian Cancer

Ovarian carcinoma is the leading cause of death among women with gynecologic malignancies. There were 25,400 new reported cases of ovarian cancer, with 14,300 deaths attributed to this disease in the US in 1999 [4].

S.-K. Kim, M.D. (✉)
Department of Nuclear Medicine, National Cancer Center, Gyeonggi-do 410-769, South Korea
e-mail: skim@ncc.re.kr

S.E. Kim, M.D., Ph.D.
Department of Nuclear Medicine, Korea University College of Medicine, Guro Hospital, Seoul 152-703, South Korea
e-mail: seiong@korea.ac.kr

J.-K. Chung, M.D., Ph.D.
Department of Nuclear Medicine, Seoul National University College of Medicine, Seoul 110-744, South Korea
e-mail: jkchung@plaza.snu.ac.kr

E.E. Kim, M.D., M.S.
Departments of Nuclear Medicine and Diagnostic Radiology, The University of Texas MD Anderson Cancer Center and Medical School, 1515 Holcombe Blvd, Box 0059, Houston, TX 77030, USA

Graduate School of Convergence Science and Technology, Seoul National University, Seoul, South Korea
e-mail: kim@mdanderson.org

E.E. Kim et al. (eds.), *Clinical PET and PET/CT: Principles and Applications*,
DOI 10.1007/978-1-4419-0802-5_26,

Most ovarian tumors are first discovered when they are already in the advanced stage. Imaging techniques are relied on to identify the location of suspected lesions and to provide optimal treatment in the hope of reducing mortality. Ovarian cancer commonly seeds the peritoneal surfaces of the abdomen and pelvis and is often seen on the serosal and mesenteric surfaces of the large and small intestine, as well as the liver surface. The right and left hemidiaphragms are also common metastatic sites. Ovarian cancer recurs quite frequent despite successful implementation of cytoreductive surgery and chemotherapy, and 20–30% of early ovarian cancer and 50–75% of advanced ovarian cancer recurs although initial complete remission has taken place. Thus, exact diagnosis and early detection of recurrence are crucial to patient management. Ovarian cancer also has the potential to spread through the lymphatic vessels and commonly involves para-aortic lymph nodes without affecting the pelvic nodes. Ovarian cancer rarely metastasizes via the blood to the liver parenchyma, lungs, bones, or brain.

Although the disease usually spreads transperitoneally as tumor implant accompanying ascites, some tumor seedings are often not visible by conventional techniques such as sonography, CT, and MRI. The clinical requirements for PET imaging in patients with ovarian cancer are preoperative diagnosis and staging and differentiation between metastases and nonmalignant pathologic conditions. For pretreatment staging, FDG PET could be helpful in a limited patient group possessing high risks of ovarian cancer. Because it was recently discovered that PET/CT could provide additional anatomic information, PET/CT is expected to be used more for pretreatment staging than PET alone. In addition to staging, FDG PET could be useful for patients with a high suspicion of recurrence (i.e., rise of CA-125), especially in cases where conventional imaging techniques present no evidence of disease. FDG PET provides critical information for treatment planning such as recurrence site or pattern. FDG PET can evaluate treatment response early and show a close relationship with overall survival, although this has not been yet been determined using large scale clinical trials.

Differential Diagnosis of Adnexal Mass and Preoperative Evaluation

Although the CA-125 tumor marker is elevated in the majority of patients with advanced ovarian cancer, an established screening procedure for early detection of ovarian cancer is not yet available. A mass lesion of the ovary is usually detected during gynecologic examination, whereas imaging methods are necessary for evaluating the tumor status and spread. Chou et al. [5] reported a quite high diagnostic accuracy of about 90% for transvaginal color Doppler sonography, whereas the diagnostic roles of other imaging modalities have not been fully investigated. Grab et al. [6] compared diagnostic accuracy of sonography, MRI, and PET in the evaluation of adnexal masses. In a series with 101 patients, sonographic examination resulted in correct classification of 11 of 12 ovarian malignancies (sensitivity, 92%) but with a specificity of only 60%. With MRI and PET, specificities improved to 84% and 80% respectively, but sensitivities decreased. When all imaging modalities were combined, sensitivity and specificity were 92% and 85%, respectively, and accuracy was 86%. The combination of sonography with MRI and PET may improve accuracy in the differentiation of benign from malignant ovarian lesions. However, MRI, CT, and FDG PET have not been fully investigated in their role in the initial workup of all ovarian tumors. A study reported that ultrasonography, PET, and MRI were not helpful in selected women after the diagnosis of ovarian cancer [7]. However, Ju and Kim [8] reported that FDG PET/CT could be helpful in selected patients with clinically high suspicion of ovarian malignancy. They enrolled 101 patients according to CA-125 level, sonography finding, and menstrual status. In those patients, the sensitivity and specificity for ovarian cancer were 100% and 92.5%, respectively. FDG PET appeared to be more helpful in the differential diagnosis of solid ovarian mass rather than cystic ovarian mass.

The values and limitations of FDG PET in the diagnosis of suspected primary ovarian cancer have recently been detailed. It has been reported that most ovarian carcinomas show an increased

FDG uptake, whereas the borderline ovarian tumor shows mild FDG accumulation, which indicates the modest nature of borderline ovarian tumor [8]. Borderline ovarian tumor is one of the most important clinical disease entities, and prognosis is better than for other ovarian malignancy, although it might require laparotomy and surgical staging for diagnosis. However, low glucose metabolism of borderline tumors or early-stage ovarian cancers, together with high FDG uptake in inflammatory lesions, diminishes the sensitivity and specificity of FDG PET for the diagnosis of primary ovarian cancer [6].

Immunoscintigraphy has been thought to be the most specific imaging technique, however, it has not been accepted as a routine method for imaging. Krag [9] reported that in patients with ovarian cancer, immunoscinitigraphy had a sensitivity and specificity of 69% and 57%, respectively, for CT, 44% and 79%, respectively.

Preoperative Evaluation of Patients With a Pelvic Mass

The first report on FDG accumulation in ovarian cancer was by Hubner et al. [10]. They found a sensitivity of 93% and a specificity of 82% for assessing previous tumors. In the preoperative evaluation of patients with a pelvic mass, PET has been reported to have positive and negative predictive values (NPV) of 86% and 76%, respectively, for malignancy. Zimny et al. [11] evaluated FDG PET in 26 patients suspected of having ovarian cancer. Quantitative analysis revealed a mean standardized uptake value (SUV) of 6.8 ± 2.3 in primary ovarian carcinoma compared with 2.6 ± 1.2 in benign masses. The sensitivity, specificity, and diagnostic accuracy were 88%, 80%, and 85%, respectively.

FDG accumulation from an inflammatory lesion could cause additional issues in ovarian cancer, such as in other cancers. Schroder et al. [12] Reported on the preoperative detectability of FDG PET in ovarian carcinoma. With regard to metabolic differentiation of primary ovarian tumors, 24 of 28 the cases (85.8%) were correctly diagnosed using PET. The only false-positive findings resulted from an inflammatory adnexal mass, which illustrates the limitation of PET in distinguishing malignant from inflammatory processes (also showing an increased glucose metabolism). Römer et al. [13] conducted a study comprising 24 patients, four of 19 with a primary ovarian mass who had an inflammatory adnexal process, and showed an increased FDG uptake in all cases. Because of this fact, in their study, FDG PET showed a specificity of only 54%, whereas the sensitivity was 83%. Quantitative analysis of SUV, as recommended by the interdisciplinary consensus meeting, does not improve the diagnostic differentiation of inflammatory adnexal masses from malignant tumors.

Staging

Staging diagnosis is one of the major prognostic factors of ovarian cancer [14]. At diagnosis, approximately 70% of patients have tumors that have spread beyond the ovary and pelvis to the abdomen (stage III) or beyond (stage IV). Fewer than 20% of patients with advanced ovarian cancer (stage III and IV) live for 5 years after diagnosis [15]. CT and MRI are not reliable in evaluating tumor spread because lymph node metastases and smaller peritoneal implants can be missed.

At present, exploratory laparotomy is the "gold standard" in the staging of ovarian cancer. Staging laparotomy is required for histologic confirmation of the diagnosis, identification of tumor spread, and debulking of tumor masses prior to chemotherapy. Modern imaging techniques have been introduced for preoperative evaluation of the disease. Sonography, CT, and MRI, however, lack the potential for distinguishing benign reactive changes from cancer infiltration [16]. FDG PET can be clinically used for more complete staging of patients with primary or recurrent ovarian cancer.

Manuel et al. [17] evaluated the detectability of FDG PET prior to surgical exploration and correlated PET images with surgicopathologic findings in primary ovarian cancer. The sensitivity and specificity of FDG PET were 78% and

86%, respectively. On a region basis (the abdomen and pelvis were divided into five regions of interest) the sensitivity and specificity of PET were 43% and 92%, respectively, while CT or MRI was only 29% sensitive. PET is of limited value for the detection of microscopic seeding. A typical finding on FDG PET, in cases with peritoneal seeding, is diffused and increased uptake around the peritoneal pouch.

Extraperitoneal Metastasis

Another important strength of FDG PET is the ability of detecting distant metastasis. Although distant metastasis (except peritoneal spread) is not frequent in ovarian cancer, extraperitoneal involvement such as lymph node metastasis, and rarely solid organ metastasis, take place. In advanced cases, FDG PET could detect unexpected metastases to the supraclavicular lymph node or cardiophrenic lymph node. The clinical importance of this additional extraperitoneal metastasis remains to be clarified.

Recurrent Ovarian Carcinoma

To date, studies have focused on the role of FDG PET in patients with recurrent ovarian cancer. FDG PET can be helpful in detecting small recurrent lesions in patients in whom posttherapeutic alterations in anatomy may make it difficult to interpret conventional imaging studies. In recent reports [18–20], FDG PET was superior to conventional CT or MRI for detecting recurrent disease. The sensitivity was 83–91% versus 45–91%, and specificity was 66–93% versus 46–84% for PET and CT/MRI, respectively [18].

Posttreatment Surveillance Without the Evidence or Suspicion of Recurrence

Second-look laparotomy, defined as "a systematic surgical reexploration in asymptomatic patients who have no clinical evidence of tumor following initial surgery and completion of a planned program of chemotherapy for ovarian cancer" has been widely used to assess response to chemotherapy in clinical trials and standard management of ovarian cancer [21]. However, the second-look laparotomy does not affect survival. In patients with advanced disease, as many as 50% with negative results on second-look laparotomy following combination chemotherapy, have experienced a subsequent recurrence. This discouraging statistic suggests that, (1) even a thorough exploration does not reveal microscopic residuals in many patients, and (2) this group of patients should be strongly considered for adjuvant chemotherapy.

PET has been evaluated as a substitute for second-look surgery in ovarian cancer patients with a complete clinical, radiographic, and serologic response following primary surgery and chemotherapy [22]. Casey et al. [23] studied the role of PET with second-look laparotomy in seven patients. PET scans were consistent with the presence of tumors in all six patients with residual cancer, even though serum ovarian tumor markers remained below the normal threshold in three of the patients at the time of scanning. Whole-body PET would provide a sensitive noninvasive "second-look method" with little patient discomfort, with reasonably fast patient throughput and at a reasonable cost.

Although PET cannot rule out microscopic persistent or recurrent disease, a negative scan provides prognostic information. It has been demonstrated that patients with a longer relapse-free interval have a higher likelihood of benefiting from surgery. Furthermore, the response rate to re-treatment increases with the duration of the treatment-free interval. Patients with a 6-month treatment-free interval have potentially platinum-sensitive disease and patients with a treatment-free interval of longer than 24 months have the greatest likelihood of benefiting from re-treatment. Zimny et al. [24] reported that the median relapse-free interval was 20 months for negative PET scans compared with only 6 months for positive scans. Chung et al. [25] showed that the median duration of survival was 29.6 months with the second-look laparotomy and 30.9 months after PET ($p > 0.05$) in patients on who PET was performed or second-look laparotomy after primary chemotherapy.

In comparing FDG PET with second-look laparotomy, the sensitivity for small residual lesions of FDG PET was not as sensitive as for second-look laparotomy [26, 27]. Therefore, we do not have enough evidence to recommend FDG PET as routine substitute for second-look laparotomy. The value of second-look laparotomy seems questionable in the aspects of safety and survival gain; and FDG PET is noninvasive and could evaluate unexpected extraperitoneal distant metastasis simultaneously. Therefore, FDG PET could be considered as a substitute for second-look laparotomy.

Cases With High Risk or Suspicion of Recurrence

FDG PET can more accurately detect recurrent lesions in the setting of suspicious recurrence is clinically high, such as unexplained high CA-125 levels, whereas the accuracy of FDG PET seems to be lower in the cases of low suspicious recurrence. The high accuracy of FDG PET with the addition of CA-125 suggests that this combination may have a significant role in the management of patients with ovarian cancer. The most appropriate biopsy site can be localized by PET prior to tissue changes detected by CT or MRI [18]. In a study by Zimny et al. [24] with 106 scans obtained from 54 patients, the overall sensitivity and specificity for detecting recurrent ovarian cancer were 83% and 83%, respectively. However, the diagnostic accuracy assessed by receiver operating characteristic analysis varied between the subgroups of patients enrolled in the study. PET was more accurate in patients with suspected recurrence with a diagnostic accuracy of 93% and sensitivity of 94% compared with 71% and 65% in patients judged as clinically free of disease [19]. More importantly, the analysis of patients with rising tumor marker CA-125 and negative or nondiagnostic findings of conventional imaging revealed a sensitivity of 96% with only one false-negative result [20]. In a report by Nakamoto et al. [26] on a patient-based analysis, overall sensitivity, specificity, and accuracy of conventional imaging modalities were 73%, 75%, and 73%, respectively, and these rates improved to 92%, 100%, and 94%, respectively, by considering both conventional imaging modalities and PET findings. Although FDG PET is useful in a setting of high CA-125, FDG PET alone might be more accurate than CA-125. The sensitivity and specificity of CT or MRI were 0.68 (range, 0.49–0.83) and 0.58 (range, 0.33–0.80), whereas those of CA-125 were 0.81 (range, 0.62–0.92) and 0.83 (range, 0.58–0.96), and those of FDG PET were 0.90 (range, 0.82–0.95) and 0.86 (range, 0.67–0.96) [19, 20].

Corresponding to the studies where the old PET scanner was used, many studies using newly developed PET/CT scanners were reported to show the same clinical effectiveness as the PET scanner [28–31] evaluated the lesion detectability and effectiveness in patients with recurrent ovarian cancer and compared CT with combined PET/CT. PET/CT identified additional lesions compared with CT in 12 or 15 patients (80%) and changed the management course in 11 of 15 patients (73%). The sensitivity, specificity, and accuracy using PET/CT in recent studies ranges from 88.2%–93.3%, 71.4%–96.9%, and 85.4%–91.2%, respectively [29, 32, 33].

Peritoneal Carcinomatosis

PET is of limited value for the detection of microscopic seeding. Typical findings of FDG PET in cases with peritoneal seeding are diffused increased uptake around the peritoneal pouch. However, it is sometimes difficult to differentiate abnormal uptake form the normal uptake pattern. Special attention is required to differentiate peritoneal seeding from increased bowel activity. Zimny et al. [11] reported that the sensitivity, specificity, and diagnostic accuracy were 50%, 95% and 80%, respectively, for evaluating peritoneal metastases. In other words, PET misses poorly localized microscopic spread disease [26]. Schroder et al. [12] reported that the sensitivity of FDG PET for the detection of peritoneal carcinomatosis was 72%, which is somewhat lower, but still higher than the 45% achieved with CT. MRI also is not a great improvement over CT because most metastases in the mesentery and the small intestine remain undetected by both methods.

FDG PET imaging of the abdomen and pelvis can be difficult because of the physiologic bowel uptake and bladder activity and the lack of anatomic landmarks. A new combined PET/CT scanning technique provides combined PET and CT images without the problem of organ motion, temporal differences, and patient positioning [31]. Although CT imaging compared with PET/CT might not be optimal for diagnostic aim, PET/CT obtains more anatomic information over CT, and is more advantageous than PET, especially in lesions with complex peritoneal location. PET/CT seems to be helpful in some types of ovarian cancers with moderate FDG accumulation, mucinous ovarian cancer, because CT could depict easily the FDG void cystic portion of mucinous portion of the tumor. But its utility for peritoneal carcinomatosis remains to be investigated [12, 34, 35].

Treatment Response Monitoring, Clinical Impact on Patient Management, and Cost Effectiveness

FDG PET is used for prediction for treatment response in ovarian cancer [36, 37]. As mentioned in the previously, FDG PET could be used as a substitute for the second-look laparotomy in patients with risk for surgery and can subsequently impact the clinical pathway.

FDG PET is helpful in detecting and staging recurrent ovarian cancer when applied in selecting the most appropriate treatment and avoiding second-look surgeries using the Monte Carlo simulation analysis [38, 39]. Assumptions in the management pathway were: (1) a PET-positive scans led to either laparoscopy or laparotomy, followed by chemotherapy (true-positive PET) or follow-up (false-positive PET); (2) a PET-negative scan resulted in continued follow-up (true-negative PET) or laparotomy (false-negative PET); and, (3) a laparotomy led to chemotherapy or follow-up. The number of unnecessary laparotomies was reduced from 70% to 5% using PET to manage the diagnostic evaluation. Cost savings per patient ranged from $1,941 to $11,766. Therefore, FDG PET can reduce unnecessary invasive staging procedures and management with PET in place of second-look surgery would yield substantial cost savings to the patient. Early detection of recurrence also could have a positive impact on cost effectiveness [38]. FDG PET could have an impact on the patient management pattern. As a result of FDG PET findings, the treatment management was changed in 24.7% to 58% of patients with ovarian cancer [26, 29, 30, 39].

FDG PET and CA-125 were compared as predictors to chemotherapy [39] with FDG PET being superior to CA-125 in prediction after chemotherapy. FDG PET could predict the effect of chemotherapy using pre- and postchemotherapy FDG PET imaging and was more accurate than the routinely used CA-125. More importantly, FDG PET following chemotherapy was related to survival, although CA-125 was not.

Indications in Ovarian Cancers

Initial Evaluation and Staging of Ovarian Tumor

There is no evidence for the usage of differential diagnosis of ovarian tumor, although FDG PET could be used for clinically and serologically suspicious ovarian tumor.

Although FDG PET alone has not been used routinely as a preoperative staging tool, it is useful combining CT and FDG PET in preoperative staging where PET/CT could be an optimal tool. Because initially advanced ovarian cancer has a possibility of extrapelvic or extra-abdominal metastatic lesion, FDG PET could be helpful.

Surveillance After Initial Treatment

FDG PET is recommended in cases with a high risk of recurrence, where CA-125 increased without explanatory lesions. Additionally, it is strongly recommended if other conventional imaging has a negative result. It is also recommended in patients with low risk, and if second-look laparotomy is planned, FDG PET should be considered as a noninvasive substitute, especially in inoperable cases.

Limitation in Ovarian Cancers

Distinguishing Malignant From Benign Lesions

The limitation of FDG PET is distinguishing malignant from inflammatory processes, which also show an increased glucose metabolism [17].

False-positive results for corpus luteum cyst, ovarian endometriosis, and gestational pouch were reported with a focally raised FDG uptake [14].

Type of Tumor

False-positive results were seen in benign serous cyst adenoma, endometriosis, and endometrioma, and false-negative PET results observed in a mesothelioma and a borderline serous tumor [8].

Tumor Size

Lesions smaller than 1 cm are quite difficult to identify not only because of the relatively poor spatial resolution but also the longer acquisition time of PET. Count recovery from small lesions may not be sufficient because of peristalsis of the alimentary tract and respiratory movement during image acquisition. Thus, even if PET findings are negative, small lesions may sometimes be detected by second-look laparotomy. However, follow-up patients typically receive chemotherapy for recurrence and systemic metastasis. Small lesions that cannot be detected on PET scans can be sensitive to drugs, while larger lesions are resistant to drugs because of possible penetration barriers. Therefore, if FDG PET reveals highly accumulated lesions remaining in a patient even after repeated chemotherapy, resection would be recommended. If PET findings are negative, chemotherapy can be proposed because some small lesions may remain. Thus, PET can be useful for therapeutic decision making [26].

Nonpathologic (Physiologic) Uptake

Physiologic uptakes in the stomach, colon, ureter, and bladder are sometimes difficult to differentiate from pathologic lesions. Such accumulation can mask abnormal uptake because of tiny disseminated lesions [26]. The combination of hydration, administration of a diuretic such as furosemide, and use of a Foley catheter with a drainage bag is an effective method of reducing physiologic uptake in the kidneys, ureter, and bladder, although reducing physiologic uptake in the colon is difficult [40].

The use of SUVs and SUV ratio can be helpful in the distinction between physiologic bowel activity and ovarian cancer metastatic to the bowel serosa. Manuel et al. [17] suggested that SUV and SUV ratio (cut-off value of 3.0 for SUV and 1.75 for SUV ratio) were significantly higher in cases of cancer metastasis to the bowel than those with no evidence of bowel metastases.

11C Methionine PET

Tumor imaging in the pelvis can be problematic because normal excreted activity in the urine may interfere with tumor identification. An essential amino acid, methionine, labeled with ^{11}C, has been found to be a valuable tracer for metabolic imaging of human cancer. High uptake of ^{11}C methionine may correlate with poor histologic grade of differentiation and high cell proliferation, which suggests that tissue uptake of methionine may reflect the biologic aggressiveness of cancer [41].

Lapela et al. [41] showed that it is possible to separate poorly differentiated from well-differentiated tumors. They tried to differentiate benign and malignant ovarian tumors. They reported that benign or borderline malignant tumors did not accumulate ^{11}C methionine, whereas all carcinomas had significant uptakes. The mean SUV of the primary carcinoma was 7.0 ± 2.2, and the mean Ki was 0.14 min^{-1}.

We found that ^{11}C methionine PET can be used to differentiate physiologic uptake of FDG from true lesion [42]. In a series of 16 gynecologic cancers, the higher diagnostic accuracy of the methionine PET (sensitivity = 80% [4/5 cases], specificity = 100% [11/11 cases], and accuracy = 94% [15/16 cases]) than that of FDG PET (sensitivity = 40% [2/5 cases], specificity = 91% [10/11 cases], accuracy = 75% [12/16 cases]) was found for the detection of the recurrent gynecologic cancer in the pelvic region postoperatively.

Cervical Cancer

Uterine cervix carcinoma is estimated to be the second most frequently diagnosed cancer in women worldwide. Although the overall mortality from cervical cancer has decreased because of early detection and treatment of preinvasive disease, the mortality of invasive cervical cancer has not changed in the last 30 years.

The treatment and prognosis of invasive cervical cancer are determined by the stage of disease, volume of the primary tumor, grade of tumor, and presence of lymph node metastasis. Cross-sectional imaging modalities such as CT and MRI have proved to be useful for evaluating morphologic risk factors such as tumor size, depth of stromal invasion, stage of disease, and lymph node metastasis. An overall staging accuracy of 58–88% has been reported, but a low sensitivity of 44% was found. Neither tumor size nor early parametrial invasion can be evaluated reliably. MRI is now considered to be the most accurate imaging method for evaluation of tumor size and parametrial invasion. An overall staging accuracy of 80–92% has been shown, whereas 50% sensitivity for nodal metastasis is similar to that with CT [43].

Tumor volume can be overestimated as a result of paralesional edema. Small parametrial invasion and lymph node metastasis could be missed and tumor invasion or spread could be underestimated.

Preoperative Staging: Lymph Node Staging

Patients with an early stage of cervical cancer without lymph node metastasis are considered surgical candidates, whereas radiotherapy is often the preferred treatment when lymph node metastases are present [44]. Uterine cervical cancer metastasizes in a predictable pattern. The tumor usually spreads sequentially from the primary cervical lesion to the pelvic, para-aortic, and supraclavicular lymph nodes, and then ultimately to nonnodal distant metastatic sites such as the lung, liver, and bone. Metastasis to para-aortic lymph nodes in the absence of pelvic nodal metastasis is exceptionally uncommon [44, 45]. The status of lymph node metastasis is an important prognostic factor and crucial to creating a treatment plan. Conventional modalities such as CT and MRI have been used for noninvasive testing for lymph node staging.

Several reports have compared FDG PET with CT and surgical staging for detecting lymph node metastasis in patients with cervical cancer. Sugawara et al. [46] reported an 86% sensitivity of FDG PET for pelvic and para-aortic lymph node metastasis, as compared with a 57% sensitivity of CT in a study of 21 patients with cervical cancer with stages 1B to 4A. Grigsby et al. [47] reported that FDG PET detects abnormal lymph node regions more often than does CT. In 101 patients, CT demonstrated abnormally enlarged pelvic lymph nodes in 20 (20%) and para-aortic lymph nodes in seven (7%) of the 101 patients. PET demonstrated abnormal FDG uptake in pelvic lymph nodes in 67 (67%), in paraaortic lymph nodes in 21 (21%), and in supraclavicular lymph node in eight (8%) of the 101 patients. FDG PET could depict unexpected lesions that CT could not.

Reinhardt et al. [48] reported that node staging resulted in sensitivities of 91% with FDG PET and 73% with MRI and specificities of 100% with PET and 83% with MRI, respectively. The positive predictive value (PPV) of PET was 100%, and that of MRI was 67%. The metastatic involvement of lymph node sites was identified on PET with a PPV of 90%, and on MRI it was 64% ($p<0.05$). Earlier, Narayan et al. also reported similar results for accuracy (PET, 85% vs. MRI, 75%) [49]. A study by Williams et al. [50] reported the different result with others, but their study protocol of PET appeared suboptimal.

Para-aortic lymph nodes are out of the irradiation field in standard pelvic radiation treatment of uterine cervical cancer. If para-aortic lymph node metastasis is suspected, the irradiation of the para-aortic area is needed. The sensitivity and specificity of CT and MRI for para-aortic lymph node metastasis are not satisfactory. Rose et al. [51] reported a sensitivity and specificity of 75% and 92%, respectively, for FDG PET in depiciting para-aortic lymph node metastasis in patients with more advanced stages (2B to 4A) before surgical staging lymphadenectomy. They observed a higher sensitivity of FDG PET for pelvic (100%) than for para-aortic (75%) lymph node metastases. Although the accuracy of FDG PET for para-aortic lymph node is not satisfactory, it seems to be the most accurate noninvasive method for assessing para-aortic status. Generally, FDG PET is a reliable alternative to conventional imaging for lymph node staging in patients with cervical cancer.

Recurrence

The recurrence rate of uterine cervical cancer is reported to be 6.5% following surgery and 26.2% after radiation therapy alone. About half of all cases of recurrent uterine cervical cancer are confined to the pelvic cavity, but some cases show metastatic lesions in the lymph nodes, lung, bone, and liver.

Radiologic studies such as intravenous renography, ultrasonography, CT and MRI are used to detect recurrent cervical cancer. It is difficult, however, for these imaging modalities to differentiate recurrent tumor from postoperative or radiation fibrosis, and to detect normal-sized metastatic lymph nodes and extrapelvic metastases. PET is effective in differentiating recurrence from scar tissue, and, in addition, can be used to obtain whole-body images to detect recurrence that was not clinically suspected.

Park et al. [52] reported the accuracy of CT and PET in the diagnosis of recurrent uterine cervical cancer in 36 patients. The sensitivity, specificity, and accuracy of CT were 78%, 83%, and 81%, respectively, while for PET, the corresponding figures were 100%, 94% ($p=0.0339$), and 97% ($p=0.0244$), respectively. Sun et al. [53] reported the sensitivity and specificity of 90% and 100%, respectively, with FDG PET in evaluation of recurrent ovarian cancer. PET could detect 7.9% of early recurrence in patients with clinically NED status.

Diagnostic accuracy of recent research using PET/CT is superior to PET (92.3% vs. 78.8%) [22, 26]. Sensitivity, specificity, and accuracy of the most recent study were 90.3%, 81.0%, 86.5%, respectively, and patient treatment plans changed following PET/CT in 23.1% of patients [54].

Treatment Response

Nakamoto et al. [55] reported a high sensitivity of FDG PET in monitoring therapeutic response of cervical cancer. In that study, FDG PET was performed prior to therapy and at a mean of 4.6 months after radiation in 20 patients with histologically proved uterine cervical cancer who were undergoing a "curative" course of radiation. FDG PET is a sensitive tool for detecting active cervical cancer following radiation therapy. The sensitivity, specificity, and accuracy were 100%, 60%, and 70%, respectively. With regard to the relatively low specificity, it is well known that FDG also accumulates in inflammatory foci, which can lead to false-positive findings.

Although PET would not completely replace monitoring of tumors using these modalities, this noninvasive technique could have a greater role for screening patients during follow-up because of its high sensitivity.

Prognosis

Grigsby et al. [47] reported that the findings on PET are a better predictor of survival than those on CT in patients with carcinoma of the cervix. The 2-year progression-free survival, based solely on para-aortic lymph node status, was 64% in CT-negative and PET-negative patients, 18% in CT-negative and PET-positive patients, and 14% in CT-positive and PET-positive patients ($p<0.0001$). A multivariate analysis demonstrated that the most significant prognostic factor for progression-free survival was the presence of positive para-aortic lymph nodes as detected using PET ($p=0.025$). Pinkus et al. [56] evaluated the prognostic value of FDG PET in patients with cervical cancer using a simple visual analysis of primary tumor characteristics (scoring of heterogeneity, size, shape, and lymph node involvement). Only 8% of patients with a good prognosis by PET died, while 76% of patients with a poor prognosis by PET died within 2 years. The study extended the value of FDG PET in cervical cancer patients, powerfully separating patients who have an excellent prognosis from those with a poor prognosis who may require more aggressive initial treatment.

In a study of the prognostic value of SUV on FDG PET, squamous cell type uterine cervix cancer with high glucose metabolic activity results in a poor outcome. The survival of the high peak SUV group (> 13) was worse than the low peak SUV group (< 13). Two-year survival rates were 76.0% and 92.3% for the high and low peak SUV groups, respectively [57].

Indications in Cervical Cancers

(1) FDG PET is recommended for recurrent cervical cancer.
(2) FDG PET is recommended for lymph node staging for initial workup.

FDG PET is a more sensitive and specific noninvasive test for lymph node staging in pelvic and para-aortic lymph nodes than other conventional imaging. FDG PET could depict unexpected distant metastatic lesion in some advanced cases. This could potentially change the treatment plan.

(3) FDG PET could be helpful in the prediction of the prognosis and treatment effect but additional research is needed.

Limitations

Substantially increased uterine vascularity was generally observed in the secretory and menstrual phases using radionuclide imaging. In vivo FDG uptake could be altered by blood flow, transport, and hexokinase activity, therefore, FDG uptake in a normal uterus could be altered by the menstrual cycle phase. Preclinical studies have shown that FDG uptake in an estrogen-stimulated uterus is significantly greater than if no stimulation is present. Recently, a case of intrauterine accumulation of FDG during menstruation was reported [58].

Other Gynecologic Cancers

Endometrial Cancer

Endometrial cancer is one of the most common gynecologic malignancies and is predominant in postmenopausal women. Clinically, many endometrial cancers are found during the early stage of cancer because of clinical signs and symptoms such as vaginal bleeding, where the prognosis is known to be good. However, a considerable number of patients with advanced and relapsed disease reveal a poor prognosis.

As of yet, there is not sufficient data to validate the usefulness of FDG PET in detecting endometrial cancer. However, several studies have shown promising results that FDG PET is sensitive and specific in detection of recurrent or metastatic lesions. Nakahara et al. [59] reported on a case of endometrial cancer. FDG PET revealed heterogeneous and marked accumulation in the endometrium. Belhocine et al. [60] reported that feasibility of FDG PET for detecting early recurrence in endometrial cancer in 14 patients who showed no evidence of disease following treatment. Of the 14 patients, FDG PET diagnosed recurrence in two patients, where one of the two patients had a PET finding of enlarged hypermetabolic abdominal focus, although CT showed a negative result. The second patient had a single focus of hypermetabolic activity on the liver and a focal hypodensity in the same location on CT. Therefore, PET can be a useful method for detecting early recurrence in patients with endometrial cancer who showed no evidence of disease on conventional follow-up.

Uterine Sarcoma

FDG PET was useful in the diagnosis of sarcoma even though SUV was low. Umesaki et al. [61]

reported the cases of five sarcomas and evaluated the effectiveness of FDG PET for the diagnosis of uterine sarcoma in comparison with other diagnostic methods. PET examinations were 100% positive for the five sarcomas; MRI was 80% positive (four of five cases), and sonography was 40% positive (two of five cases). The mean SUV of the sarcomas was 4.5 ± 1.3.

Vulvar Cancer

Cohn et al. [62] undertook a prospective pilot study on the performance of FDG as a method for detection of groin metastases from vulvar cancer. Fifteen patients underwent PET prior to exploration of 29 groins. On a patient-by-patient basis, PET had a sensitivity of 80%, specificity of 90%, PPV of 80%, and NPV of 90% in demonstrating metastases. On a groin-by-groin basis, PET had a sensitivity of 67%, specificity of 95%, PPV of 86%, and NPV of 86%. The results of PET were relatively insensitive in predicting lymph node metastasis, and a negative study is not a reliable surrogate for a pathologically negative groin. However, the high specificity of PET suggests that it is useful in planning radiation therapy as an adjunct to lymphatic mapping and sentinel lymph node dissection.

References

1. Soper JT. Radiographic imaging in gynecologic oncology. Clin Obstet Gynecol. 2001;44:485–94.
2. Vardi J, Tadros G, Foemmel R, Shebes M. Plasma lipid-associated sialic acid and serum CA125 as indicators of disease status with ovarian cancer. Obstet Gynecol. 1989;73:379–83.
3. Gupta NC, Frank AR, Casey MJ. FDG PET imaging for post-treatment evaluation of patients with genitourinary malignancies. J Nucl Med. 1992;33:829.
4. Landis SH, Murray T, Bolden S, Wingo PA. Cancer statistics. CA Cancer J Clin. 1999;49:8–31.
5. Chou CY, Chang CH, Yao BL, et al. Color Doppler ultrasonography and serum CA125 in the differentiation of benign and malignant ovarian tumors. J Clin Ultrasound. 1994;22:491–6.
6. Grab D, Flock F, Stohr I, Nussele K. Classification of asymptomatic adnexal masses by ultrasound, magnetic resonance imaging, and positron emission tomography. Gyncol Oncol. 2000;77:454–9.
7. Kawahara K, Yoshida Y, Kurokawa T, et al. Evaluation of positron emission tomography with tracer 18-fluorodeoxyglucose in addition to magnetic resonance imaging in the diagnosis of ovarian cancer in selected women after ultrasonography. J Comput Assist Tomogr. 2004;28:505–16.
8. Ju W, Kim SC. Discrepancy between magnetic resonance and 18F-fluorodeoxyglucose positron emission tomography imaging in a case of borderline ovarian tumor. Int J Gynecol Cancer. 2007;17:1031–3. Epub 2007 Mar 26.
9. Krag DN. Clinical utility of immunoscintigraphy in managing ovarian cancer. J Nucl Med. 1993;34: 545–8.
10. Hubner KF, McDonald TW, Niethammer JG, et al. Assessment of primary and metastatic ovarian cancer by positron emission tomography using 2-[^{18}F]deoxyglucose. Gynecol Oncol. 1993;51:197–204.
11. Zimny M, Schroder W, Wolters S, et al. 18F-fluorodeoxyglucose PET in ovarian carcinoma: methodology and preliminary results. Nuklearmedizin. 1997;36:228–33.
12. Schroder W, Zimny M, Rudlowski C, et al. The role of 18F-fluoro-deoxyglucose positron emission tomography in diagnosis of ovarian cancer. Int J Cancer Oncol. 1999;9:117–22.
13. Romer W, Avril N, Dose J, et al. Metabolische Charakterisierung von Ovarialtumoren mit der Positronen-Emissions-Tomographie und F-18 Fluordeoxyglukose. Rofo. 1997;166:62–8.
14. Omura GA, Bradhy MF, Homesley HD, et al. Long-term follow-up and prognostic factor analysis in advanced ovarian carcinoma: the Gynecologic Oncologic Group experience. J Clin Oncol. 1991;9: 1138–50.
15. Ozols RF. Chemotherapy of ovarian cancer. In: De Vita VT, Hellman S, Rosenberg SA, editors. Cancer: principles and practice of oncology, Updates, vol. 1. 2nd ed. Philidelphia: N.B. Lippincott; 1988. p. 1–12.
16. Bragg DG, Hricak H. Imaging in gynecologic malignancies. Cancer. 1993;71:1648–51.
17. Manuel M, Holschneider CH, Williams CM, et al. Correlation of FDG PET scans with surgicopathologic findings in ovarian cancers. J Nucl Med. 2002;43:29.
18. Delbeke D, Martin WH. Positron emission tomography imaging in oncology. Radiol Clin North Am. 2001;39:883–917.
19. Torizuka T, Nobezawa S, Kanno T, et al. Ovarian cancer recurrence: role of whole-body positron emission tomography using 2-[fluorine-18]-fluoro-2-deoxy-D-glucose. Eur J Nucl Med. 2002;29:797–803.
20. Yen R-F, Sun S-S, Shen Y-Y, et al. Whole-body positron emission tomography with ^{18}F-fluoro-2-deoxyglucose for the detection of recurrent ovarian cancer. Anticancer Res. 2001;21:3691–4.
21. Barter J, Barnes W. Second-look laparotomy. In: Rubin S, Sutton G, editors. Ovarian cancer. New York: McGraw-Hill; 1993. p. 269–300.
22. Rose PG, Faulhaber P, Miraldi F, et al. Positron emission tomography for evaluating a complete clinical

response in patients with ovarian or peritoneal carcinoma: correlation with second-look laparotomy. Gynecol Oncol. 2001;82:17–21.
23. Casey MJ, Gupta NC, Muths CK. Experience with positrom emission tomography (PET) scans in patients with ovarian cancer. Gynecol Oncol. 1994;53:331–8.
24. Zimny M, Siggelkow W, Schroder W, et al. 2-[Fluorine-18]-fluoro-2-deoxy-D-glucose positron emission tomography in the diagnosis od recurrent ovarian cancer. Gynecol Oncol. 2001;83:310–5.
25. Chung J-K, Kang SB, Kim MH, et al. The role of 18F-FDG PET in patients with advanced epithelial ovarian carcinoma as a substitute for second-look operation. J Nucl Med. 2002;43:282.
26. Nakamoto Y, Saga T, Ishimori T, et al. Clinical value of positron emission tomography with FDG for recurrent ovarian cancer. AJR AM J Roentgeol. 2001;176:1449–54.
27. Karlan BY, Hoh C, Tse N, et al. Whole-body positron emission tomography with (fluorine-18)-2-deoxyglucose can detect metastatic carcinoma of the fallopian tube. Gynecol Oncol. 1993;49:383–8.
28. Mangili G, Picchio M, Sironi S, Viganò R, Rabaiotti E, Bornaghi D, Bettinardi V, Crivellaro C, Messa C, Fazio F. Integrated PET/CT as a first-line re-staging modality in patients with suspected recurrence of ovarian cancer. Eur J Nucl Med Mol Imaging. 2007;34:658–66. Epub 2006 Dec 20.
29. Chung HH, Kang WJ, Kim JW, Park NH, Song YS, Chung JK, Kang SB, Lee HP. Role of [^{18}F]FDG PET/CT in the assessment of suspected recurrent ovarian cancer: correlation with clinical or histological findings. Eur J Nucl Med Mol Imaging. 2007;34:480–6. Epub 2006 Nov 7.
30. Simcock B, Neesham D, Quinn M, Drummond E, Milner A, Hicks RJ. The impact of PET/CT in the management of recurrent ovarian cancer. Gynecol Oncol. 2006;103:271–6. Epub 2006 Apr 19.
31. Blodgett TM, Meltzer CC, Townsend DW, et al. PET/CT in restaging patients with ovarian carcinoma. J Nucl Med. 2002;43:310.
32. Nanni C, Rubello D, Farsad M, et al. (18)F-FDG PET/CT in the evaluation of recurrent ovarian cancer: a prospective study on forty-one patients. Eur J Surg Oncol. 2005;31:792–7.
33. García-Velloso MJ, Jurado M, Ceamanos C, Aramendía JM, Garrastachu MP, López-García G, Richter JA. Diagnostic accuracy of FDG PET in the follow-up of platinum-sensitive epithelial ovarian carcinoma. Eur J Nucl Med Mol Imaging. 2007;34:1396–405. Epub 2007 Feb 21.
34. Drieskens O, Stroobants S, Gysen M, et al. Positron emission tomography with FDG in the detection of peritoneal and retroperitoneal metastases of ovarian cancer. Gynecol Obstet Invest. 2003;55:130–4.
35. Turlakow A, Yeung HW, Salmon AS, et al. Peritoneal carcinomatosis: role of (18)F-FDG PET. J Nucl Med. 2003;44:1407–12.
36. Baum RP, Przetak C. Evaluation of therapy response in breast and ovarian cancer patients by positron emission tomography (PET). Q J Nucl Med. 2001; 45:257–68.
37. Smith GT, Hubner KF, McDonald T, et al. Cost analysis of FDG PET for managing patients with ovarian cancer. Clin Positron Imaging. 1999;2:63–70.
38. Smith GT, Hubner KF, McDonald T, et al. Avoiding second-look surgery and reducing costs in managing patients with ovarian cancer by applying F-18-FDG PET. Clin Positron Imaging. 1998;1:263.
39. Soussan M, Wartski M, Cherel P, Fourme E, Goupil A, Le Stanc E, Callet N, Alexandre J, Pecking AP, Alberini JL. Impact of FDG PET-CT imaging on the decision making in the biologic suspicion of ovarian carcinoma recurrence. Gynecol Oncol. 2008;108:160–5. Epub 2007 Oct 24.
40. Miraldi F, Vesselle H, Faulhaber PF, et al. Elimination of artifactual accumulation of FDG in PET imaging of colorectal cancer. Clin Nucl Med. 1998;23:3–7.
41. Lapela M, Leskinen-Kallio S, Varpula M, et al. Metabolic imaging of ovarian tumors with carbon-11-methioninre: a PET study. J Nucl Med. 1995;36: 2196–220.
42. Jeong HJ, Chung J-K, Paeng JC, et al. Usefulness of ^{11}C methionine PET in the pelvic region for evaluation of recurrent gynecologic cancer in postoperative state. J Nucl Med. 2002;43:283.
43. Hricak H, Yu KK. Raiology in invasive cervical cancer. AJR AM J Roentgeol. 1996;167:1101–8.
44. Eifel PJ, Berek JS, Thigpen JT. Cancer of the cervix, vagina, and vulva. In: De Vita VT, Hellman S, Rosenberg SA, editors. Cancer: principles and practice of oncology. 5th ed. Philidelphia: Lippincott-Raven; 1433. p. 1478–997.
45. Morice P, Sabourin JC, Pautier P, et al. Isolated paraaortic node involvement in stage IB/II cervical carcinoma. Eur J Gynaecol Oncol. 2000;21:123–5.
46. Sugawara Y, Eisbruch A, Kosuda S, et al. Escaluation of FDG PET in patients with cervical cancer. J Nucl Med. 1999;40:1125–31.
47. Grigsby PW, Siegel BA, Dehdashti F. Lymph node staging by positron emission tomography in patients with carcinoma of the cervix. J Clin Oncol. 2001; 19:3745–9.
48. Reinhardt MJ, Ehritt-Braun C, Vogelgesang D, et al. Metastatic lymph nodes in patients with cervical cancer: detection with MR imaging and FDG PET. Radiology. 2001;218:776–82.
49. Narayan K, Hicks RJ, Jobling T, et al. A comparison of MRI and PET scanning in surgically staged loco-regionally advanced cervical cancer: potential impact on treatment. Int J Gynecol Cancer. 2001;11:263–71.
50. Williams AD, Cousins C, Soutter WP, et al. Detection of pelvic lymph node metastases in gynecologic malignancy: a comparison of CT, MR imaging, and positron emission tomography. AJR AM J Roentgeol. 2001;177:343–8.
51. Rose PG, Adler LP, Rodriguez M, et al. PET for evaluating paraaortic nodal metastasis in locally advanced cervical cancer before surgical staging: a surgico-pathologic study. J Clin Oncol. 1999;17:41–5.

52. Park DH, Kim KH, Park SY, et al. Diagnosis of recurrent uterine carvical cancer: computed tomography versus positron emission tomography. Korean J Radiol. 2000;1:51–5.
53. Sun SS, Chen TC, Yen RF, et al. Value of whole-body ^{18}F-fluoro-2-deoxyglucose positron emission tomography in the evaluation of recurrent cervical cancer. Anticancer Res. 2001;21:2957–62.
54. Chung HH, Jo H, Kang WJ, Kim JW, Park NH, Song YS, Chung JK, Kang SB, Lee HP. Clinical impact of integrated PET/CT on the management of suspected cervical cancer recurrence. Gynecol Oncol. 2007;104:529–34. Epub 2006 Oct 16.
55. Nakamoto Y, Eisbruch A, Achtyes ED, et al. Prognostic value of positron emission tomography using F-18-fluorodeoxyglucose in patients with cervical cancer undergoing radiotherapy. Gynecol Oncol. 2002;84:289–95.
56. Pinkus E, Miller TR, Grisby PW. Improved prognostic value of FDG PET in patients with cervical cancer using a simple visual analysis of tumor characteristics. J Nucl Med. 2002;43:28.
57. Jang HJ, Lee KH, Kim YH, et al. The role of FDG PET for predicting prognosis in squamous cell type uterine cervical carcinoma patients. J Nucl Med. 2002;43:28.
58. Yasuda S, Ide M, Takagi S, Shohtsu A. Intrauterine accumulation of F-18 FDG during menstruation. Clin Nucl Med. 1997;22:793–4.
59. Nakahara T, Fujii H, Ide M, et al. F-18 FDG uptake in endometrial cancer. Clin Nucl Med. 2001;26:82–3.
60. Belhocine TZ, Bolle KS, Willems-Foidart J. Usefulness of ^{18}F-FDG PET in the post-therapy surveillance of endometrial carcinoma. J Nucl Med. 2002;43:118–9.
61. Umesaki N, Tanada T, Miyama M, et al. Positron emission tomography 18F-fluorodeoxyglucose of uterine sarcoma: a comparison with magnetic resonance imaging and power doppler imaging. Gynecol Oncol. 2001;80:372–7.
62. Cohn DE, Dehdashti F, Gibb RK, et al. Prospective evaluation of positron emission tomography for the detection of groin node metastases from vulva cancer. Gynecol Oncol. 2002;85:179.

Lymphoma

27

E. Edmund Kim and Franklin C.L. Wong

The term *lymphoma* identifies two distinct groups of tumors: Hodgkin's disease (HD) and non-Hodgkin's lymphoma (NHL). Since the late 1970s, significant progress has been made in the elucidation of the pathogenesis of NHL as a clonal malignant expansion of B or T cells. B lymphocytes are generated in the bone marrow as a result of a multistep differentiation process. On entering the germinal center (GC), B cells activate into centroblasts, proliferate, and mature into centrocytes. Cells that have exited the GC have two fates: differentiation into either plasma cells or into memory B cells. Based on the absence or presence of somatic immunoglobulin (Ig) hypermutation, B-cell NHL can be grouped into two broad histogenetic categories: One derived from pre-GC B cells and devoid of Ig mutations (mantle cell lymphoma, chronic lymphocytic leukemia/small lymphocytic lymphoma), and the other derived from B cells that have transited through the GC and harbor Ig mutations (follicular lymphoma, lymphoplasmacytoid lymphoma, mucosa-associated lymphoid tissue lymphoma, diffuse large cell lymphoma, Burkitt's lymphoma). The pathogenesis of lymphoma represents a multistep process involving the progressive and clonal accumulation of multiple genetic lesions affecting proto-oncogenes and tumor suppressor genes. The genome of lymphoma cells is relatively stable and is characterized by few nonrandom chromosomal abnormalities, commonly represented by chromosomal translocations. A new classification, called the Revised European-American Lymphoma, was created in the early 1990s to establish definitions for distinct lymphomatous diseases, based on morphologic, clinical, immunophenotypic, and molecular genetic features (Table 28.1).

Lymphomas are the third most common childhood malignancy and account for approximately 10% of cancers in children [1]. Approximately two thirds of the lymphomas diagnosed in children are NHL, but the remainder are HD. The three major histologic categories of NHL in children are lymphoblastic lymphoma, small noncleaved cell (Burkitt's) lymphoma, and large cell lymphoma. In adults, Burkitt's and lymphoblastic lymphoma are rare, but follicular center cell lymphoma predominates. The age of Hodgkin's incidence is bimodal, with a first peak in adults 20–30 years old and a second peak in late adulthood.

E.E. Kim, M.D., M.S. (✉)
Departments of Nuclear Medicine and Diagnostic Radiology, The University of Texas MD Anderson Cancer Center and Medical School, 1515 Holcombe Blvd, Box 0059, Houston, TX 77030, USA

Graduate School of Convergence Science and Technology, Seoul National University, Seoul, South Korea
e-mail: ekim@mdanderson.org

F.C.L. Wong, M.D., Ph.D., J.D.
Departments of Nuclear Medicine and Neurooncology, The University of Texas MD Anderson Cancer Center, Houston, TX 77030, USA
e-mail: fwong@mdanderson.org

E.E. Kim et al. (eds.), *Clinical PET and PET/CT: Principles and Applications*,
DOI 10.1007/978-1-4419-0802-5_27, © Springer Science+Business Media New York 2013

Most patients present with rapidly enlarging neck and mediastinal lymphadenopathy. Cough, wheezing, or shortness of breath and facial swelling are frequent complaints. Other presenting sites include cervical nodes, Waldeyer's ring, cutaneous lesions, bone marrow, and single or multiple bone disease.

It was predicted that in 2002 there would be 60,900 new cases of lymphoma (7,000 HD and 53,900 NHL) diagnosed in the UA, and that 25,800 people (1,400 HD and 24,400 NHL) would die from this diagnosis [2]. NHL accounts for 5% of new cancers in men and 4% of new cancers in women each year in the US, and is responsible for 5% of deaths [3]. The median age at NHL diagnosis was 65 years, and NHL incidence increases with age and peaks in the 80–84-year age group. There has been a striking increase in NHL incidence rates over the past four decades, with NHL being more common in males. The overall mortality rate for NHL has decreased significantly in the past 25 years [4]. The 5-year survival rate is approximately 90% for children with early-stage NHL and 70% for those with advanced-stage disease [4].

The phases of patient management include obtaining an adequate biopsy for an accurate diagnosis, a careful history and physical examination, appropriate laboratory studies, imaging studies, and, possibly, further biopsies to determine stage accuracy and to plan therapy. Treatment choices include no initial therapy, radiotherapy, cytotoxic chemotherapy, a variety of new biologic therapies, and hematopoietic stem cell transplantation.

The purpose of laboratory studies is to aid in determining the prognosis (e.g., lactate dehydrogenase [LDH], β_2-microglobulin, albumin) and identifying abnormalities in other organ systems that might complicate therapy (e.g., renal or hepatic dysfunction). Almost all patients should have a bone marrow aspirate and biopsy performed. Patients with follicular lymphoma have bone marrow involvement approximately 50% of the time, while it is seen in approximately 15% of patients with diffuse large B-cell lymphoma [5].

Diagnosis and Staging of Lymphoma

The goal of the initial evaluation of a patient with lymphoma is to provide information that allows intelligent planning of therapy, imparting the prognosis to the patient, and making possible comparisons between patients in clinical trials. The studies to accomplish these goals can be aimed at identifying sites of involvement, characteristics of the patient, or characteristics of the lymphoma that predict treatment outcome.

The Ann Arbor staging system was developed for patients with HD and identifies anatomic sites of involvement by lymphoma type (Table 27.1). Patients are also subcategorized by the presence of unexplained fevers, night sweats, or weight loss (Table 27.2).

Although chest radiography is abnormal in less than 50% of patients, identification of hilar or mediastinal adenopathy, parenchymal lesions, or pleural effusions provides an easy method for reevaluation. Computed tomography (CT) can identify both nodal and extranodal sites of involvement for monitoring the response to therapy. Magnetic resonance imaging (MRI) is useful in identifying bone, bone marrow, and central nervous system (CNS) involvement. However, it has not yet been accepted as a substitute for bone marrow biopsy. Nuclear bone scans can sometimes be useful in patients who present with or develop back pain. Gallium scans are more often used as part of the staging evaluation, and they are more likely to be positive in patients with aggressive diffuse large B-cell lymphoma than in more indolent follicular lymphoma. Gallium avidity at midtreatment cycle or at the end of treatment is associated with a much higher relapse rate than seen in patients who have negative results on gallium scan [6, 7]. After a patient has received three or four cycles of the planned treatment regimen, or at the completion of the entire regimen, they should be reevaluated to determine response to therapy. Patients who have a complete response are more likely to be cured than patients who have achieved only a partial response. Documenting complete remission is particularly important because salvage treatment

Table 27.1 Groups of malignant lymphoma based on World Health Organization classification

B cell	T cell
Indolent (low risk)	
Chronic lymphocytic leukemia, lymphocytic lymphoma	Large granular lymphocytic leukemia, T and NK
Lymphoplasmacytic lymphoma, Waldenström disease	Mycosis fungoides, Sezary syndrome
Hairy cell leukemia	Chronic T cell leukemia/lymphoma (HTLV+)
(Splenic) Marginal zone lymphoma	
Nodal and extranodal MALT B cell lymphoma	
Follicular center lymphoma, grade I or II	
Aggressive (intermediate risk)	
Prolymphocytic leukemia	Prolymphocytic leukemia
Plasmacytoma, multiple myeloma	Peripheral T cell lymphoma, unspecified
Mantle cell lymphoma	Angioimmunoblastic T cell lymphoma
Follicular center lymphoma, grade III	Angiocentric lymphoma
Diffuse large cell B cell lymphoma	Intestinal T cell lymphoma
Primary mediastinal large B cell lymphoma	Anaplastic large cell lymphoma (T and null cell)
High grade B cell lymphoma, Burkitt-like	
Very aggressive (high risk)	
Precursor B lymphoblastic lymphoma/leukemia	Presursor T lymphoblastic lymphoma/leukemia
Burkitt lymphoma, acute B cell leukemia	
Plasma cell leukemia	
Hodgkin's disease	

Table 27.2 Ann Arbor staging system

Stage	Findings
I	Single lymph node region or single extralymphatic organ or site (IE)
II	Two or more lymph node regions on the same side of diaphragm or localized extralymphatic organ or site (IIE)
III	Lymph node regions on both sides of diaphragm or localized extralymphatic organ or site (IIIE) or spleen (IIIS) or both (III SE)
IV	Diffuse one or more extralymphatic organs with or without lymph node involvement

Modifiers base on constitutional symptoms (>38°, night sweat, >10% BW loss in 6 m)
A, not present, *B*, present symptoms (subcategory indicators)

such as high-dose therapy and marrow transplantation can sometimes cure disease in patients who fail to respond to initial therapy. In sites of bulky disease, masses do not always completely regress. This does not necessarily mean that patients will have persisting lymphoma. Biopsy can be difficult under such circumstances and is not always accurate. If the patient was known to have a positive gallium or fluorodeoxyglucose (FDG) uptake at the onset of treatment, normal results of that scan, despite a residual mass, raise the possibility that only residual fibrous tissue is present.

Positron emission tomography (PET) offers the unique capability of revealing metabolic activity throughout the body. Increased glucose metabolism is a basic biochemical hallmark of tumor cells, and the glucose analog FDG is transported, phosphorylated, and metabolically trapped in malignant cells [7, 8]. L-[methyl-^{11}C] methionine (MET) is another widely used tumor-seeking tracer for PET. Methionine is an essential amino acid needed for protein and polyamine synthesis, and is also involved in transsulfuration and transamination reactions. Furthermore, methionine acts as a precursor for S-adenosylmethionine, which is the predominant biologic methyl group donor [9]. Methionine metabolism is altered in cancer cells, and the accumulation of MET in malignant tumors is principally caused by its enhanced transport across the plasma membrane of tumor cells. Leskinen-Kallio et al. [10] found that MET uptake was increased both in high- and low-grade NHL, whereas FDG was found to be superior to MET in distinguishing high-grade from other grade tumors. Rodriguez et al. [11] also concluded that FDG uptake was associated with malignancy grade, but no relationship was found between MET uptake and malignancy grade.

Nodal staging is instrumental, but not the only factor, in defining the treatment strategy for a patient with HD or NHL. The histologic type, presence of B symptoms such as weight loss, fever or night sweats, age, extent of disease, extranodal manifestations, and serum level of LDH are also important prognostic factors. However, nodal staging is the major factor differentiating limited from advanced disease. Advanced disease is best managed by aggressive chemotherapy, but involved field radiotherapy, possibly combined with a short course of chemotherapy, is often curative for limited disease. Nodes smaller than 10 mm are usually considered to be free of disease. However, normal-sized nodes may contain tumor cells, whereas enlarged nodes may show only immunoreactive cells.

FDG and MET seem to accumulate avidly in both high- and low-grade lymphomas, and the total number of discrepant findings in individual lymph node sites (15/178) on CT and PET was similar to those on FDG and MET [12]. The avid physiologic accumulation of MET in the liver, pancreas, intestine, and bone marrow concealed a group of pathologic lymph nodes detected by FDG and CT. On the other hand, MET was superior to FDG in detecting mediastinal disease in the patient with diabetes. FDG and MET are known to accumulate in inflammatory tissue, although MET probably accumulates to a lesser extent [13]. The small size of the lesion is probably the major reason for false-negative findings. The central location, together with lack of attenuation correction, may have further affected lesion detectability in the para-aortic area. Attenuation correction has not been shown to improve overall sensitivity for tumor detection either with conventional filtered back-projection reconstruction or new iterative reconstruction methods. The advantages of attenuation correction and sophisticated image reconstruction may manifest in easier image interpretation and better anatomic localization. Attenuation correction also makes possible the elimination of reconstruction artifacts and the quantification of tracer uptake. In current clinical practice, the detection of lymphoma in small abdominal nodes can pose a problem. Unfortunately, the current method for PET does not resolve this challenge completely. Further clinical studies are warranted using combined PET/CT, which has been suggested to be a more useful diagnostic tool in cancer patients than PET alone [14]. Overall, PET shows a greater number of positive lesions than does CT, and rigorous histologic verification of all suspected findings in patients with lymphoma is difficult because of possible multiorgan involvement in deeply situated sites.

The bone scan has been used traditionally in the evaluation of bone involvement in lymphoma. Findings are characterized by relatively discrete uptake of tracer, and the sensitivity in detecting bone metastases using diphosphonate molecules results from the early osteoblastic reaction. Osteolytic lesions that are commonly encountered in NHL often escape scintigraphic detection. Radiography is mainly used to exclude false-positive findings on bone scans. The Ga 67 scan is of limited usefulness in detecting skeletal involvement of lymphoma. Lymphomatous infiltration of skeletal structures may occur as a result of both hematogenous spread of the disease and direct invasion from adjacent involved tissues. Even localized lymphomatous infiltration of bone marrow is considered evidence of generalized disease, whereas scintigraphic or radiologic findings of an isolated osseous lesion are thought to be local disease. FDG PET was suitable for identifying osseous involvement in malignant lymphoma with a high positive predictive value and was thereby more sensitive and specific than bone scan [15]. A potential limitation of FDG for assessing malignant osseous lesions may be its physiologic accumulation in bone marrow. In untreated patients, this accumulation is generally quite homogeneous, and is comparatively low with standard uptake value (SUV) levels of 0.7–1.3. On the other hand, in areas of lymphomatous involvement, despite large differences depending on the degree of malignancy, FDG uptake is high, with SUVs of 3.5–31.0 (median 8.5) [15, 16].

Human immunodeficiency virus (HIV) is neutrotrophic and is involved in the pathogenesis of several of the neurologic syndromes, including HIV encephalopathy and progressive dementia. The CNS may also be involved with opportunistic infections or malignancies associated with progressive immunosuppression. The opportunistic infection that most commonly involves the CNS in patients with acquired immune deficiency syndrome (AIDS) is *Toxoplasma gondi*. This infection may produce a diffuse meningoencephalitis or cause focal lesions. Imaging studies such as CT and MRI are used to detect treatable complications of HIV infection such as toxoplasmosis or lymphoma and may often reveal focal or multifocal ring-enhanced lesions. However, without histopathologic confirmation, a specific diagnosis can be difficult. It is not possible to differentiate CNS lymphoma from toxoplasmosis in the HIV-infected individual on the basis of CT or MRI findings because of the similarity in the appearance of the lesions. FDG PET was able to accurately differentiate between a malignant (lymphoma) and nonmalignant etiology for CNS lesions [17]. Both qualitative visual inspection of the images as well as semiquantitative analysis using count density ratios revealed similar results. It was concluded that FDG PET can be useful in the management of AIDS patients with CNS lesions because high FDG uptake most likely represents a malignant process that should be biopsied for confirmation rather than treated presumptively as infectious.

Assessment of Lymphoma Therapy Using ^{18}F-FDG-PET

Accurate evaluation of therapeutic response is of vital importance in the management of patients with lymphoma [18]. The main endpoint of chemotherapy is achieving complete remission which is associated with a longer progression-free survival and potential cure than is partial remission. The definition of complete remission is usually based on anatomic imagings that may be unable to differentiate viable tumor from posttreatment changes such as scarring or fibrosis. Residual abnormalities that occur after therapy are usually considered to represent persistent lymphoma; however, only a maximum of 10–20% of residual masses was reported to be positive for lymphoma at the completion of treatment [19]. Thus, there was no difference in the CT-documented response rates and the size of residual masses between patients who experience disease relapse and those who remain disease free [20]. CT does not consistently distinguish between dividing tumor cells and posttherapy fibrosis. Patients with aggressive NHL have positive CT findings in approximately 50% of cases after chemotherapy, and long-term follow-up shows that only 50% or fewer of those with positive CT findings have disease relapse or other evidence of residual tumor [21]. CT is a poor predictor of clinical outcome after treatment of aggressive NHL, and a posttherapy CT positive for NHL does not indicate that the time to progression for that patient will be significantly different from that for a patient with normal CT findings [20]. Although MRI provides better morphologic details than does CT when contrast material is not used, the low sensitivity rate (45%) showed that MRI was not ideal for predicting outcome [22]. The Ga-67 scan has also been reported to be an independent predictor of outcome after one to two cycles of chemotherapy [21]. Nevertheless, the Ga-67 scan is less efficacious than ^{18}F-FDG PET for intra-abdominal tumors, and may be less sensitive in detecting disease in some instances of aggressive lymphoma or HD [23].

Over the past few years, a large body of evidence has confirmed the potential role of ^{18}F-FDG PET, including both dedicated and coincidence PET systems, in the monitoring of lymphomas [24]. Although a change in ^{18}F-FDG uptake at multiple early times during chemotherapy has been described, this change was only marginally predictive of outcome [25]. The response to neoadjuvant chemotherapy has been characterized as one of the most important prognostic factors. It has been recently found that ^{18}F-FDG PET has a high prognostic value for evaluation of therapy as early as after one cycle of chemotherapy in aggressive NHL and HD [26]. After the completion of chemotherapy, although there was a statistically significant difference between patients with ^{18}F-FDG PET-negative findings and patients with ^{18}F-FDG PET-positive findings, ^{18}F-FDG PET results were not as good a predictor of long-term outcome. ^{18}F-FDG PET findings following the completion of chemotherapy yielded a significantly lower sensitivity and negative predictive value than did findings after the first cycle. Resolution of therapy-induced anatomic changes on CT or MRI usually lags behind tumor cell mortality.

Various reports have shown the effectiveness of ^{18}F-FDG PET in the posttreatment evaluation of lymphomas. ^{18}F-FDG PET was found to be superior to the Ga-67 scan in accurately detecting disease sites in aggressive NHL and HD, with a sensitivity of 100% and 80.3%, respectively [23]. Furthermore, ^{18}F-FDG PET has a higher diagnostic and prognostic value than CT in the posttreatment evaluation of lymphomas [27]. Thus, ^{18}F-FDG PET has become the most helpful noninvasive modality in differentiating tumor recurrence from fibrosis when CT shows a residual mass [26]. Positive ^{18}F-FDG PET results after one cycle of chemotherapy reflect the metabolic activity of potentially resistant clones that, although responding to chemotherapy, do so more slowly than do those homogeneously sensitive tumor cells. Negative ^{18}F-FDG PET results after the first cycle were highly suggestive of long-term remission, whereas negative results after the completion of chemotherapy were less accurate. ^{18}F-FDG PET after the first cycle of chemotherapy remains far more predictive of outcome than later use of ^{18}F-FDG PET.

I 131 anti-B1 (CD 20) radioimmunotherapy (RIT) has been recognized as a promising approach for treatment of NHL. It is sometimes difficult to differentiate posttherapeutic scar tissue from viable residual tissue on CT, potentially leading to incorrect management of patients. Baseline tumor glucose metabolism (SUV) did not predict the response of NHL to treatment, and SUV at 1–2 months after RIT correlated well with the ultimate best response of NHL to RIT. The decreases in SUV in responders were almost parallel to the decreases in tumor size measured by CT [28]. Metabolic changes with radiation therapy appear to be more gradual than those after chemotherapy.

Studies on the initial staging and restaging of lymphomas have shown a definite benefit with higher sensitivity (93–98%) in detection of lymph nodal involvement using FDG PET/CT, compared with 61–87% sensitivity using contrast-enhanced CT. The specificity of PET/CT was 99–100%, compared with 85–91% using contrast-enhanced CT [29]. PET/CT also provides significantly better exclusion of lymphomatous involvement when compared with contrast-enhanced CT alone. Additionally, PET/CT did not result in false-positive findings with regard to lung and bone involvement [30]. It has been reported that PET/CT can provide information on long-term prognosis after only two to four cycles of induction chemotherapy [31]. One study investigated the clinical diagnostic necessity of PET/CT after only two or four cycles of induction chemotherapy and concluded that PET/CT would have reduced the diagnostic imaging costs over the course [32]. The diagnostic value of low-dose CT in the setting of PET/CT is currently the subject of scientific studies. It has been indicated that low-dose CT acquisitions may be adequate for the staging and restaging of lymphoma [33].

Conclusion

Three principal opportunities for FDG PET to optimize the management of HD and NHL can be defined: in improving the accuracy of initial staging, in defining response to treatment, and in refining follow-up after completion of treatment. In low-grade lymphoma, FDG PET appears to be of less value, frequently failing to demonstrate disease seen on conventional imaging [34]. Functional imaging with FDG PET may have an important role in the management of lymphoma, enabling more precise and accurate tailoring of treatment to the true disease status of the patient, both at presentation and subsequently during and after completion of first-line treatment.

References

1. Sandlund JT, Downing JR, Crist WM. Non-Hodgkin's lymphoma in childhood. N Engl J Med. 1996;334:1238–41.
2. Jemal A, Thomas A, Murray T, et al. Cancer statistics. CA Cancer J Clin. 2002;52:23–47.
3. Newton R, Ferlay J, Beral V, et al. The epidemiology of non-Hodgkin's lymphoma: comparison of nodal and extranodal sites. Int J Cancer. 1997;72:923–7.
4. Glass AG, Karnell LH, Menck HR. The national cancer data base report on non-Hodgkin's lymphoma. Cancer. 1997;80:2311–20.
5. Weisenburger D. The International Lymphoma Study Group classification of non-Hodgkin's lymphoma: pathology findings from a large multicenter study. Mod Pathol. 1997;10:136A.
6. Larcos G, Farlow DC, Antico VF, et al. The role of high dose Ga-67 scintigraphy in staging untreated patients with lymphoma. Austr N Z J Med. 1994;24:5–8.
7. Tatsumi M, Kitayama H, Sugahara H, et al. Whole-body hybrid PET with F-18 FDG in the staging of non-Hodgkin's lymphoma. J Nucl Med. 2001;42:601–8.
8. Carr R, Barrington S, Madam B, et al. Detection of lymphoma in bone marrow by whole-body positron emission tomography. Blood. 1998;91:3340–6.
9. Finkelstein JD, Martin JJ. Methionine metabolism in mammals. J Biol Chem. 1986;26:1582–7.
10. Leskinen-Kallio S, Ruotsalainem U, Någren K, et al. Uptake of C-11 methionine and fluorodeoxyglucose in non-Hodgkin's lymphoma: a PET study. J Nucl Med. 1991;32:1211–8.
11. Rodriguez M, Rehn S, Ahlstrom H, et al. Predicting malignancy grade with PET in non-Hodgkin's lymphoma. J Nucl Med. 1995;36:1790–6.
12. Sutinen E, Jyrkio S, Varpula M, et al. Nodal staging of lymphoma with whole-body PET: comparison of C-11 methionine and FDG. J Nucl Med. 2000;41:1980–8.
13. Kubota R, Kubota K, Yamada S, et al. Methionine uptake by tumor tissue: a microautoradiographic comparison with FDG. J Nucl Med. 1995;36:484–92.
14. Charion M, Beyer T, Kinahan PE, et al. Whole-body FDG PET and CT imaging of malignancies using a combined PET/CT scanner. J Nucl Med. 1999;40:256.
15. Moog F, Kotzerke J, Reske SN. FDG-PET can replace bone scintigraphy in primary staging of malignant lymphoma. J Nucl Med. 1999;40:1407–13.
16. Lapela M, Leskinen-Kallio S, Minn H, et al. Increased glucose metabolism in untreated non-Hodgkin's lymphoma: a study with PET and F-18 FDG. Blood. 1995;9:3522–7.
17. Hoffman JM, Waskin HA, Schifter T, et al. FDG-PET in differentiating lymphoma from nonmalignant central nervous system lesions in patients with AIDS. J Nucl Med. 1993;34:567–75.
18. DeVita VT, Cannelos GP. The lymphomas. Semin Hematol. 1999;36:84–94.
19. Surbone A, Longo DL, DeVita VL, et al. Residual abdominal masses in aggressive non-Hodgkin's lymphoma after combination chemotherapy; significance and management. J Clin Oncol. 1988;6:1832–7.
20. Janicek M, Kaplan W, Neuberg D, et al. Early restaging gallium scans predict outcome in poor prognosis patients with aggressive non-Hodgkin's lymphoma treated with high-dose CHOP chemotherapy. J Clin Oncol. 1997;15:1631–7.
21. Front D, Bar-Shalom R, Mor M, et al. Aggressive non-Hodgkin's lymphoma: early prediction of outcome with Ga-67 scintigraphy. Radiology. 2000;214:253–7.
22. Hill M, Cunningham D, MacVicar D, et al. Role of magnetic resonance imaging in predicting relapse in residual masses after treatment of lymphoma. J Clin Oncol. 1993;11:2273–8.
23. Kostakoglu L, Leonard JP, Coleman M, et al. Comparison of F-18 fluorodeoxyglucose PET and Ga-67 scintigraphy in evaluation of lymphoma. J Clin Oncol. 2000;19:10a.
24. Mikhaeel NG, Timothy AR, Hain SF, O'Doherty MJ. F-18 FDG PET for the assessment of residual masses on CT following treatment of lymphomas. Ann Oncol. 2000;11:147–50.
25. Romer W, Hanauske A, Ziegler S, et al. Positron emission tomography in non-Hodgkin's lymphoma: assessment of chemotherapy with fluorodeoxyglucose. Blood. 1998;91:4464–71.
26. Kostakoglu L, Coleman M, Leonard JP, et al. PET predicts prognosis after 1 cycle of chemotherapy in aggressive lymphoma and Hodgkin's disease. J Nucl Med. 2002;43:1018–27.
27. Jerusalem G, Beguin Y, Fassotte MF, et al. Whole-body PET using F-18 FDG for post-treatment evaluation in Hodgkin's disease and non-Hodgkin's lymphoma has

higher diagnostic and prognostic value than classical CT scan imaging. Blood. 1999;94:429–33.
28. Torizuka T, Zasadny KR, Kison PV, et al. Metabolic response of non-Hodgkin's lymphoma to I-131 anti-B1 radioimmunotherapy: evaluation with FDG PET. J Nucl Med. 2000;41:999–1005.
29. Hernandez-Maraver D, Hernandez-Navarro F, Gomez-Leon N, et al. Positron emission tomography/computed tomography: diagnostic accuracy in lymphoma. Br J Haematol. 2006;135(3):293–302.
30. Schaefer NG, Strobel K, Taverna C, Hany TF. Bone involvement in patient with lymphoma: the role of FDG-PET/CT. Eur J Nucl Med Mol Imag. 2007;34(1):60–7.
31. Querellou S, Valette F, Bodet-Milin C, et al. FDG-PET/CT predicts outcome in patients with aggressive non-Hodgkin's lymphoma and Hodgkin's disease. Ann Hematol. 2006;85(11):759–67.
32. Strobel K, Schaefer NG, Renner C, et al. Cost-effectiveness therapy remission assessment in lymphoma patients using 2-F-18 fluor-2-deoxy-D-glucose positron emission tomography/computed tomography: is an end of treatment exam necessary in all patients? Ann Oncol. 2007;18(4):658–64.
33. Schaefer NG, Hany TF, Taverna C, et al. Non-Hodgkin's lymphoma and Hodgkin's disease: coregistered FDG PET and CT at staging and restaging- do we need contrast-enhanced CT? Radiology. 2004;232(2):823–9.
34. Hoskin PJ. FDG PET in the management of lymphoma: a clinical perspective. Eur J Nucl Med. 2002;29:449–51.

Melanoma, Myeloma, and Sarcoma 28

E. Edmund Kim and Franklin C.L. Wong

Cutaneous melanoma is a readily curable tumor, with 85% of diagnosed patients enjoying long-term survival following simple surgical excision. There has been a steady increase in melanoma incidence over the past century. In the United States, melanoma is diagnosed in at least 54,200 people a year, approximately 15 in 100,000 [1]. Disseminated melanoma is a devastating illness with limited effective treatment options, prompting the evolution of efforts designed to identify metastatic disease early and to develop novel biologic therapies. The application of immunotherapy has so far provided benefit to only a small percentage of patients. In the majority of patients with metastatic disease, many of whom are young, the chemotherapy or biologic therapy is unsuccessful.

Melanomas are the most common (70%) primary intraocular malignancy in Caucasians, and they arise from uveal melanocytes residing in the uveal stroma and originating from the neural crest. The precise anatomic origin of ocular melanomas was unspecified in approximately 25% of cases, and 73% of the tumors arose within the globe (mainly from the choroid). Uveal melanoma, similarly to retinitis pigmentosa, may not constitute a single disease but consist of an assortment of maladies with multiple genetic origins that simply culminate in a limited phenotype. In contrast to a phenotype associated with cell death, uveal melanoma is characterized by uncontrolled proliferation. Lymphatic spread has not been demonstrated, as would be expected from the absence of lymphatics in the eye in contrast to cutaneous melanomas. Hematogenous metastasis to the liver is frequent, and plasminogen activator as well as epidermal growth factor may play a role in the occurrence and progression of metastases.

Many aspects of melanoma treatment such as sentinel node dissection, isolated limb perfusion, and cytotoxic or biologic (or both) therapies remain controversial and inconclusive. No lack of effective alternatives has allowed the implementation and evolution of new treatments because no systemic therapy has yet been shown to significantly prolong survival. The identification of tumor rejection antigens recognized by CD4 and CD8 T cells as well as prognostically significant roles of antibody response to melanoma antigens has spawned a renaissance of immunotherapy. Cutaneous and ocular melanomas differ in their systemic symptoms, metastatic patterns, and susceptibility to treatments.

E.E. Kim, M.D., M.S. (✉)
Departments of Nuclear Medicine and Diagnostic Radiology, The University of Texas MD Anderson Cancer Center and Medical School, Houston, TX 77030, USA

Graduate School of Convergence Science and Technology, Seoul National University, Seoul, South Korea
e-mail: ekim@mdanderson.org

F.C.L. Wong, M.D., Ph.D., J.D.
Departments of Nuclear Medicine and Neurooncology, The University of Texas MD Anderson Cancer Center, Houston, TX 77030, USA
e-mail: fwong@mdanderson.org

E.E. Kim et al. (eds.), *Clinical PET and PET/CT: Principles and Applications*,
DOI 10.1007/978-1-4419-0802-5_28,

Multiple myeloma is the major plasma cell tumor and represents a spectrum of diseases characterized by clonal proliferation and accumulation of immunoglobulin-producing cells that are terminally differentiated B cells. The spectrum includes clinically benign conditions such as monoclonal gammopathy of unknown significance (MGUS); indolent conditions such as Waldenström's macroglobulinemia; the more common malignant entity, plasma cell myeloma, a disseminated B-cell malignancy; and a more aggressive form, plasma cell leukemia, with circulating malignant plasma cells in the blood. It is a relatively uncommon malignancy in the US. Among hematologic malignancies, it constitutes 10% of tumors and ranks as the second most frequently occurring cancer after non-Hodgkin lymphoma. Approximately 14,600 new patients were diagnosed in 2003 [1]. Its incidence has slowly increased in the US and increases with advancing age. Clinical manifestations are the results of a variety of pathogenic mechanisms, including cytokine production, effect of the tumor mass itself, deposition of the M protein, suppression of T- and B-cell functions, and occasionally autoimmune disorders.

In the US, the incidence of soft-tissue sarcoma is approximately 7,800 new cases per year [1]. A little more than 50% of these new patients will die of the disease. It is clear that soft-tissue sarcoma diagnosed at an early stage is eminently curable by wide en bloc resection, but when diagnosed at the time of extensive local or metastatic disease, it is rarely curable. Soft-tissue sarcomas can occur in any site throughout the body. Almost 50%appear in the extremities, with two thirds of extremity lesions occurring in the lower limbs, and 30% intra-abdominally divided equally between visceral and retroperitoneal lesions. Soft-tissue tumors generally are categorized according to the normal tissue they mimic. Although most soft tissues arise from embryonic mesoderm, tumors of the peripheral nervous system (ectoderm), and some tumors of uncertain histogenesis are included as soft-tissue tumors that can be benign or malignant. The ratio of benign to malignant tumors is more than 100:1. Unlike carcinomas, sarcomas do not demonstrate in situ changes, nor does it appear that sarcomas originate from benign soft-tissue tumors except for malignant peripheral nerve sheath tumor in patients with neurofibromatosis. Sarcomas are characterized by local invasiveness. Lymph node metastases are uncommon, with the exception of selected cell types usually associated with childhood sarcoma. Most sarcomas metastasize hematogenously, and the clinical behavior is determined by anatomic location, grade, and size, rather than by specific histologic pattern.

Malignant tumors arising from the skeletal system are rare. Osteosarcoma and Ewing's sarcoma, the two most common bone tumors, occur mainly during childhood and adolescence. Other mesenchymal (spindle cell) tumors such as malignant fibrous histiocytoma (MFH) are less common. Today, limb-sparing surgery is routine, and adjuvant chemotherapy dramatically increases overall survival.

Diagnosis and Staging

Identification of features that may mark lesions suspicious for melanoma can be simply recalled by using the minemonic ABCDE: asymmetry, borders that are irregular or diffuse, color variegation, diameter larger than 5 mm, and enlargement or evolution. Bleeding and ulceration occur in 10% of localized melanomas and in 54% of late melanomas, and is a poor prognostic finding. Suspicious lesions with irregular raised surfaces, ulceration, bleeding, variegations, or recent changes in color or size should have a full-thickness excisional biopsy performed on them.

The staging of cutaneous melanoma involves segregation by local, regional, or distant disease and strongly correlates with survival. The most important staging information is the Breslow depth, presence of ulceration, and nodal status. Stages I and II designate early (low-risk) and later (intermediate-risk) tumors, respectively. Distant metastases define stage IV disease, whereas regional lymph node metastases (N1 or N3) define stage III disease (Table 28.1).

Asymptomatic patients with T1 lesions do not appear to benefit from any diagnostic imaging.

Table 28.1 Tumor node metastasis staging of malignant melanoma with 5-year survival rates

T stage				
T1	a: <1 mm thickness, no ulcer; b: <1 mm thickness with ulcer			
T2	a: 1–2 mm thickness, no ulcer; b: 1–2 mm thickness with ulcer			
T3	a: 2–4 mm thickness, no ulcer; b: 2–4 mm thickness with ulcer			
T4	a: >4 mm thickness, no ulcer; b: >4 mm thickness with ulcer			
N stage				
N1	a: 1 microscopic node metastasis; b: 1 macroscopic node metastasis; c: 1 in-transit or satellite node metastasis			
N2	a: 2–3 microscopic nodal metastases.; b: 2–3 macroscopic nodal metastases; c: 2–3 in-transit or satellite nodal metastases			
N3	Metastases in>4 nodes, or matted or in-transit or satellite regional nodes			
M stage				
M1	a: Distant metastases in skin, subcutaneous tissue, distant node with normal LDH			
	b: Lung metastasis with normal LDH			
	c: Metastases in all other visceral sites with normal LDH, or any distant metastasis with abnormal LDH			
Stage				*5-year survival rate (%)*
0	Tis	N0	M0	–
IA	T1a	N0	M0	95
IB	T1b/2a	N0	M0	90
IIA	T2b/3a	N0	M0	78
IIB	T3b/4a	N0	M0	65
IIC	T4b	N0	M0	45
IIIA	Any Ta	N1a/2a	M0	67
IIIB	Any Tb	N1a/2a	M0	52
	Any Ta	N1b/2b,c	M0	54
IIIC	Any Tb	N1b/2b,c	M0	26
	Any T	N3	M0	27
IV	Any T	Any N	M1a	19
	Any T	Any N	M1b	7

A chest radiograph is obtained in patients with stage IB or greater. Liver function tests, especially lactate dehydrogenase (LDH), and radiologic tests such as brain magnetic resonance imaging (MRI) and body computed tomography (CT) are indicated in stages III and IV disease or otherwise symptomatic patients. Advances in imaging techniques have improved the ability to identify and localize primary and metastatic melanomas. Lymphoscintigraphy can provide valuable assistance in localizing sentinel lymph node(s) for biopsy, and it is particularly helpful for tumor locations with variable lymphatic drainage. Imaging using technetium (Tc-99m) sestamibi, Tc-99m tetrafosmin, and I-123 iodobenzamide (for melanotic melanomas) show promise, and Tc-99m sestamibi appears a reasonably inexpensive substitute for whole-body positron emission tomography (PET) with ^{18}F-fluorodeoxyglucose (FDG) in staging melanoma.

The diagnosis of choroidal and ciliary body melanomas has reached a high degree of accuracy at eye centers by utilizing clinical examination, sonography, and fluorescein angiography. No biopsy is performed. The most commonly encountered conditions mimicking melanoma include a choroidal nevi, peripheral disciform degeneration, congenital hypertrophy of the retinal pigment epithelium, and choroidal hemangioma. Ocular sonography is more sensitive than MRI or CT for the detection of extraocular extension of choroidal malignant melanoma [2].

Sonography and fluorescein angiography combined are useful in patient follow-up. The usefulness of radioactive phosphorus (^{32}P) in determining malignancy remains controversial, and radioimmunoscintigraphy using Tc-99m monoclonal antibodies are still too preliminary to be reliable diagnostic tools [3]. Metastatic workup should be performed with liver enzyme measurement and CT or sonography. Although it is known that the detection of melanoma cells in blood cannot automatically be presumed as a definite sign for the presence of metastatic disease, polymerase chain reaction might help in interpreting the result of conventional markers for metastasis in the future [4].

Because patients with myeloma present with a variety of symptoms, the diagnosis of myeloma is quite often delayed. An older patient with unexplained back or bone pain, infection, anemia, or renal insufficiency should be screened for myeloma. The evaluation includes a hemogram, serum and urine protein electrophoresis and immunofixation, quantitative immunoglobulin levels, urinary protein excretion in 24 h, bone marrow aspiration and biopsy, and complete skeletal radiographic survey. Radiography shows early-phase osteopenia, and lytic punched out lesions with increasing tumor burden. Bone scans are seldom positive because of the predominant osteolytic activity. Measurement of bone mineral density is useful for the therapeutic response. MRI provides a better assessment of tumor burden, and more than 95% of patients with myeloma show MRI abnormalities [5]; one third have focal lesions, and another one third have heterogenous marrow. A focal marrow plasmacytoma can be analyzed using CT-guided fine-needle aspiration allowing cytologic diagnosis. MRI and CT do not readily distinguish between active disease and scar tissue, necrosis, bone fracture, or benign disease. Traditional staging depends heavily on the extent of disease evident on a radiologic bone survey.

The presence of soft-tissue sarcoma is almost invariably suggested by the development of a mass. The mass is usually large, often painless, and may be associated with an episode of injury by the patient. The focus of the clinical evaluation is to determine the likelihood of a benign or malignant soft-tissue tumor, the involvement of muscular or neurovascular structures, and the ease with which biopsy or subsequent excision can be obtained. Accurate diagnosis requires adequate and representative biopsy of the tumor, and the tissue must be well fixed and well stained.

The most useful immunohistochemical markers are the intermediate filaments such as keratin and S-100. Cytogenetic analyses reveal clonal chromosome alterations in the majority of sarcomas [6]. The three most common histopathologic subtypes of soft-tissue sarcoma are MFH, liposarcoma, and leiomyosarcoma. The most common extremity sarcomas are liposarcoma, MFH, tendosynovial sarcoma, and fibrosarcoma. Most retroperitoneal sarcomas are liposarcomas or leiomyosarcomas. The most frequently encountered chest wall sarcomas are desmoids, liposarcomas, and myogenic sarcomas. Virtually all gastrointestinal sarcomas were previously classified as leiomyosarcomas or leiomyoblastomas. It is now recognized that many gastrointestinal sarcomas do not express markers of myogenic differentiation and are better classified as gastrointestinal stromal tumors, or, if they exhibit neural differentiation, gastrointestinal autonomic nerve tumors. The pattern of recurrence is intra-abdominal, including hepatic metastasis [7]. Leiomyosarcoma is the most common type of genitourinary sarcoma and arises in the bladder, kidney, or prostate. Rhabdomyosarcoma arising in paratesticular tissues is a disease seen in young men. Approximately 10–15% of all sarcomas occur in children. The majority of pediatric patients have small cell sarcomas, including embryonal rhabdomyosarcoma, Ewing's sarcoma, and primitive neuroectodermal tumor. There have been significant changes in the staging of soft-tissue sarcoma. The new staging system (Table 28.2) includes both size and depth, and the criteria of the Hajdu staging system are tumor size, location and grade (Table 28.3). Size is a continuous variable, and the decision to divide tumors into less than 5 cm or greater than or equal to 5 cm is arbitrary. Stage IB (low-grade, large superficial tumors) is uncommon, as is stage IIC (high-grade, large superficial tumors). Depth

Table 28.2 The new staging system for soft-tissue sarcoma

Stage	Description
IA (G1, T1, M0)	Low-grade intracompartmental lesion without metastasis
IB (G1, T2, M0)	Low-grade extracompartmental lesion, without metastasis
IIA (G2, T1, M0)	High-grade intracompartmental lesion without metastasis
IIIA (G1 or G2, T1, M1)	Intracompartmental lesion, any grade, with metastasis
IIIB (G1, or G2, T2, M1)	Extracompartmental lesion, any grade, with metastasis

Table 28.3 Hajdu staging for soft-tissue tumors

Stage	Grade	Size (cm)	Location
0	G1	<5	Superficial
IA	G2/G3	<5	Superficial
IB	G1	<5	Deep
IC	G1	>5	Superficial
IIA	G2/G3	<5	Deep
IIB	G2/G3	>5	Superficial
IIC	G1	>5	Deep
III	G2/G3	>5	Deep

is of less value when incorporated with other prognostic factors such as size. Stage IV disease from lymph node metastasis is rare.

For early recurrence, grade seems predominant, whereas for late recurrence, size assumes a progressively more important role. Whether or not age should be a determinant in a staging system is as yet unclear. It does appear that the early and the late stages of disease are similar in both children and adults, but the intermediate-stage lesions have a better prognosis in children [8]. Site appears to be a significant factor in survival. Patients with retroperitoneal sarcoma can and do die of local recurrence, an uncommon event in extremity lesions. The intra-abdominal visceral leiomyosarcomas still maintain a high metastatic rate as the primary cause of death.

Radiographic evaluation combined with the clinical history and histologic examination is necessary for accurate diagnosis of bone sarcoma. A bone tumor is evaluated by five radiographic parameters: anatomic site, border, bone destruction, matrix formation, and periosteal reaction. Benign tumors have round, smooth, well-circumscribed borders without cortical destruction or periosteal reaction. Malignant lesions have irregular, poorly defined margins with bone destruction and wide area of transition with periosteal reaction. The surgical staging system developed by Enneking and colleagues [9] is based on the grade (G), location (T), and lymph node involvement as well as metastasis (M). MRI and CT, combined with nuclear bone scans and angiography, allow the physician to develop a three-dimensional construct of the local tumor area before surgery and thereby formulate a detailed surgical approach. MRI is most accurate for determining the intraosseous extent of tumor. Angiography is performed only if the primary tumor is in the vicinity of the major vascular structures. CT and MRI are equally accurate in evaluating cortical changes. MRI is superior to CT for detecting muscle involvement in the knee, pelvis, and shoulder [10].

PET in Melanoma, Myeloma, and Sarcoma

The accurate staging and surveillance of melanomas remain difficult, and a range of conventional structural imaging modalities are often used on patients with melanoma. Functional imaging using Ga-67 citrate has restricted its regular use to relatively few centers because of its inconvenience of multiple imaging sessions. Ga-67 scanning in melanoma is predicated on the avidity of tumor uptake, most likely mediated by transferring receptor expression. Its utility in the management of patients with malignant melanoma has shown a sensitivity of greater than 80% and a specificity of 90% [11,12]. The use of FDG in the management of patients with malignancy has recently been implemented. FDG tumor uptake is related to the nonspecific increase in glucose transporters seen in many malignant processes, and malignant melanoma appears to have a particularly high avidity for this metabolic marker [13]. Comparison of Ga-67 citrate, single photon emission computed tomography (SPECT), and FDG PET has been made in 121 patients with melanoma with high clinical risk of occult metastatic disease [12]. PET correctly identified more disease than Ga-67 SPECT in 14 cases, including three incidental primary tumors, and showed true-negative results in three additional patients with abnormal Ga-67 SPECT. There were six patients with true-positive Ga-67 SPECT results in whom FDGPET showed false-negative findings. FDG PET provided incremental diagnostic information compared with Ga-67 SPECT in 17 of 23 patients, while Ga-67 SPECT provided incremental information compared with PET in 6 of 23 cases ($p=0.035$). It was concluded that FDG PET provides incremental and clinically important information in approximately 10% of patients at a low incremental cost, which, combined with greater patient convenience and lower radiation dosimetry, makes FDG PET the functional imaging technique of choice for the evaluation of suspected metastatic melanoma. Recognition of small-volume disease is a potential limitation of both FDG PET and Ga-67 SPECT. For deep lesions, the higher spatial resolution of PET may offer a relative advantage. The combination of FDG PET and CT improves diagnostic capability by combining the ability of CT to detect small lung metastases with the high sensitivity of FDG PET in detecting intra-abdominal tumors.

The efficacy of FDG PET in the diagnosis of involved lymph node basins was good [14]. Sensitivity was 95% (35/37); specificity, 84% (16/19); accuracy, 91% (51/56); positive predictive value, 92% (35/38); and negative predictive value, 89% (16/18). Metastases were shown histologically in 114 of 657 surgically removed lymph nodes. FDG PET detected 100% of metastases that were larger than10 mm, 83% of metastases that were 6–10 mm in size, and 23% of metastases less than or equal to 5 mm. Moreover, FDG PET had high sensitivity (≥93%) only for metastases with more than 50% lymph node involvement or with capsular infiltration. The sensitivities of whole-body PET and planar coincidence scintigraphy in 55 patients with melanoma with 108 lesions were 89% and 18%, respectively [15]. The tumor to background activity contrast was generally lower in planar coincidence scintigraphy than in PET, and the decrease in planar coincidence scintigraphy detection was found in lesions smaller than 22 mm in diameter. Pretreated melanoma lesions can cause diagnostic problems at restaging if the FDG uptake is low and equivalent to the surrounding tissue. Therefore, a new radiopharmaceutical that can provide further information about a lesion is needed. Tyrosine is a well-known amino acid used for melanin formation. It is transported into the cells and transformed to dihydroxyphenylalanine (DOPA). The phenoloxidase is responsible for the complete conversion of DOPA to melanin. 6-[^{18}F]-fluoro-L-dopa (FDOPA) uptake was enhanced in 14 of 22 metastatic lesions (64% sensitivity). FDG uptake was 1.5-fold higher than FDOPA uptake in 18 of 22 metastases from melanoma, whereas FDOPA uptake was 1.5-fold higher than FDG uptake in two patients with hepatic metastases. FDOPA can help to identify viable melanoma metastases in patients with negative FDG findings and thus may help in the selection of patients who would benefit from further treatment [16].

A reliable whole-body technique with both functional and morphologic information is necessary to identify the extent and activity of multiple myeloma for staging arid monitoring treatments. Ninety-eight PET scans using ^{18}F-FDG were obtained in 66 patients with myeloma, with 25 patients having two or more scans, and compared with clinical and staging information including MRI and CT scans [17]. Negative PET findings reliably predicted stable MGUS. Conversely, 16 previously untreated patients with active myeloma all had focal or diffusely positive scan findings; four (25%) had negative full radiologic surveys, and another four had focal extramedullary diseases that were confirmed by biopsy or other imaging modalities. Persistent positive PET findings after therapy predicted early relapse. In 13 of 16 patients (81%) with relapsing myeloma, new sites were identified using PET. PET also was helpful in identifying focal recurrent disease in six patients with nonsecretory or hyposecretory myeloma.

Soft-tissue sarcomas are a heterogeneous group of tumors that arise from tissue of mesenchymal origin and are characterized by infiltrative local growth and hematogenous metastases. Morphologic imaging modalities are used for the assessment of tumor location, form, size, infiltration of the surrounding tissue, and presence of satellite metastases. FDG PET visualized soft-tissue sarcomas, indicated the grade of malignancy, and detected local recurrence [18]. The data reported in the literature indicate a high sensitivity (>90%) but a lower specificity (65–88%) in the detection of soft-tissue sarcomas. The false-negative results in patients with suspected soft-tissue lesions are in low-grade tumors which have low FDG uptake. False-positive results may be caused by inflammatory lesions, previous irradiation with scar tissue, and fibrolipoma [19]. The standard uptake value (SUV) has been helpful in the diagnosis of high-grade tumors. The limitation of the SUV is the differentiation of low-grade sarcomas or at least a subset of low-grade soft-tissue tumors because sarcomas are histologically heterogeneous. Depending on histology and phosphorylation, FDG uptake can be different for the various histologic subtypes. The use of several kinetic parameters obtained from the dynamic FDG data provides more information about FDG pharmacokinetics than SUV of a single acquisition. The transport constant k_1 is primarily a parameter for the transport capacity of FDG, and the rate constant k_3 is associated with the phosphorylation rate of the radiopharmaceutical.

The blood volume in a tumor tissue is a parameter that modulates the uptake of the tracer. Therefore, the use of the vascular fraction of a target volume is another parameter that may improve the diagnostic accuracy. In addition to compartment analysis, the fractal dimension may help to quantify heterogeneity. All of these parameters can be influenced by the size and shape of a tumor as well as the resolution of imaging system. Pixels at the center of the tumor may have higher values, whereas the values may decrease for pixels located toward the edge of the tumor. However, this effect is generally modulated by the inhomogeneous distribution of FDG within the malignancy because of differences in blood supply, viability, and other factors. The SUV and the fractal dimension seemed to be helpful for the grade II and the grade III classification versus lipoma and scar [20]. According to the data, the FDG turnover in lipomas is more deterministic than in tumors and in scars. Because of large overlap of SUVs between the different grading groups, the comparison of the mean SUV may not be useful in the individual patient. The FDG metabolic rate according to the graphic Patlak method was comparable with the one calculated with the transport rates of the two-tissue compartment [21]. The metabolic rate of FDG could distinguish high-grade sarcomas from benign lesions but not low-grade tumors. With 92% accuracy for the prediction of grade III tumors but a low prediction for all other groups when only the SUV was used [20], the differentiation of inflammatory lesions from tumor tissue, especially grade III tumors, can be a problem. However, an inflammatory lesion has low prevalence and can often be diagnosed using clinical criteria and laboratory values.

Another problem is the differentiation of scar tissue and tumor recurrence, which is a biologic problem and concerns primarily irradiated patients. Nonspecific repair processes lead to an enhanced FDG uptake, although radiation therapy usually is performed at least 3 months before the use of FDG PET. Interestingly, one abscess with high uptake of FDG and enhanced tissue perfusion did not accumulate ^{11}C-aminoisobutyric acid [22]. The amino acids can be advantageous, with clear signal showing only the transport capacity of the tumor and no further metabolic steps. A direct comparison of FDG PET and FDG PET/CT for detection of recurrent melanoma showed that both studies had significantly higher sensitivity (100%) and specificity (99%) than noncontrast CT (67% and 92%, respectively) [23]. Another advantage of PET/CT is that the entire body can be scanned in a single examination, which is especially beneficial in patients with multiple morbidities. The detection of distant metastasis can spare patients the ordeal of costly and unnecessary surgeries. Downstaging after a successful treatment also reduces costs by ruling out the need for further therapy.

References

1. Jemal A, Murray T, Samuels A, et al. Cancer statistics, 2003. CA Cancer J Clin. 2003;53:5–26.
2. Scott IU, Murray TG, Hughes JR. Evaluation of imaging techniques for detection of extraocular extension of choroidal melanoma. Arch Ophthalmol. 1998; 116:897–901.
3. Modorati G, Brancato R, Paganelli G, et al. Immunoscintigraphy with three step monoclonal pretargeting technique in diagnosis of uveal melanoma: preliminary results. Br J Ophthalmol. 1994;78:19–24.
4. Haynie GD, Shen TT, Gragoudas ES, et al. Flow cytometric analysis of peripheral blood lymphocytes in patients with choroidal melanoma. Am J Ophthalmol. 1997;124:357–61.
5. Kusumoto S, Jinnai I, Itoh K, et al. Magnetic resonance imaging patterns in patients with multiple myeloma. Br J Hematol. 1997;99:649–54.
6. Fletcher J, Kozakewich H, Hoffer F, et al. Diagnostic relevance of clonal chromosome aberrations in malignant soft tissue tumors. N Engl J Med. 1991;324: 436–41.
7. Conlon K, Casper E, Brennan M. Primary gastrointestinal sarcomas: analysis of prognostic variables. Ann Surg Oncol. 1995;2:26–30.
8. Laluaglia M, Heller G, Ghavimi F, et al. The effect of age at diagnosis on outcome in rhabdomyosarcoma. Cancer. 1994;73:109–14.
9. Enneking WF, Spanier SS, Goodman MA. A system for the surgical staging of musculoskeletal sarcoma. Clin Orthop. 1980;153:106–9.
10. Bloem JL, Taminian AHM, Euldenink F, et al. Radiologic staging of primary bone sarcoma: MRI, scintigraphy, angiography and CT correlated with pathologic examination. Radiology. 1988;169:805–11.
11. Kagan R, Witt T, Bines S, et al. Gallium-67 scanning for malignant melanoma. Cancer. 1998;61:272–4.
12. Kaiff V, Hicks RJ, Ware RE, et al. Evaluation of high-risk melanoma: comparison of F-18 FDG PET and high-dose Ga-67 SPECT. Eur J Nucl Med. 2002;29:506–15.
13. Tyler DS, Onaitis M, Kherani A, et al. Positron emission tomography scanning in malignant melanoma. Cancer. 2000;89:1019–25.
14. Crippa F, Leutner M, Belli F, et al. Which kinds of lymph node metastases can FDG PET detect? A clinical study in melanoma. J Nucl Med. 2000;41:1491–4.
15. Steinert HC, Voellmy DR, Trachsel C, et al. Planar coincidence scintigraphy and PET in staging malignant melanoma. J Nucl Med. 1998;39:1892–7.
16. Dimitrakopoulou-Strauss A, Strauss LG, Burger C. Quantitative PET studies in pretreated melanoma patients: a comparison of 6-[F-18] fluoro-L-dopa with F-18 FDG and O-15 water using compartment and noncompartment analysis. J Nucl Med. 2001;42: 248–56.
17. Diuie BGM, Waxman AD, D'Agnolo A, et al. Whole-body F-18 FDG-PET identifies high-risk myeloma. J Nucl Med. 2002;43:1457–63.
18. Schwarzbach M, Dimitrakopoulou-Strauss A, Willeke F, et al. Clinical value of F-18 FDG-PET imaging in soft tissue sarcomas. Ann Surg. 2000;231:380–6.
19. Strauss LG. F-18 deoxyglucose and false-positive results: a major problem in the diagnostics of oncological patients. Eur J Nucl Med. 1996;23:1409–15.
20. Dimitrakopoulou-Strauss A, Strauss LG, Schwarzbach M, et al. Dynamic F-18 PET-FDG studies in patients with primary and recurrent soft tissue sarcomas: impact on diagnosis and correlation with grading. J Nucl Med. 2001;42:713–20.
21. Eary JF, Mankoff DA. Tumor metabolic rates in sarcoma using FDG-PET. J Nucl Med. 1998;39:250–4.
22. Schwarzbach M, Wideke F, Dimitrakopoulou-Strauss A, et al. Functional imaging and detection of local recurrence in soft tissue sarcomas by PET. J Nucl Med. 1998;39:250–4.
23. Iagaru A, Quon A, Johnson D, Gambhir SS, McDougall IR. 2-Deoxy-2-F-18 fluor-D-glucose positron emission tomography/computed tomography in the management of melanoma. Mol Imaging Biol. 2007;9(1):50–7.

Carcinoma of Unknown Primary

29

Gi-Jeong Cheon

Introduction

Carcinoma of unknown primary (CUP) represents the group of heterogeneous tumors, which can be defined as the presence of histologically proven metastatic disease and unidentified site of origin at the time of diagnosis in spite of comprehensive diagnostic workup [1]. CUP tumors are not infrequently encountered in oncologic practice. The incidence of CUP tumors in oncologic patients is 0.5–7% at the time of the initial diagnosis [2, 3] and its prevalence is between 3% and 15% [4]. Frequent first settings for the metastatic lesions are lymph nodes (37%); of these, 31% are located in the head and neck region, which is the most common site for metastases of unknown origin [5, 6]. CUP tumors present metastatic dissemination patterns that are different from those observed in oncologic conditions with known primary tumors: (1) Short symptomatic prediagnostic interval exists before the clinical presentation; (2) CUP tumor becomes symptomatic at the time of metastatic disseminations; (3) the most frequent primary sites in patients with CUP tumors do not include the several most common primary tumors in the general population; (4) no specific metastatic location has been consistently associated with a specific primary tumor site [7]. These aspects make it difficult to locate the primary tumor, which is one of the most important factors for establishing the most effective treatment [8].

The management of these tumors presents considerable challenges to the treating physicians because therapeutic decisions are often determined by the nature of the primary tumors and failure to detect the primary tumors impedes optimization of treatment planning and may negatively influence patient prognosis [1, 6]. Five-year survival rates for patients with CUP tumors vary greatly between 6% and 70% and largely determined by histology and location of metastases [9, 10]. Patients with undifferentiated tumors and adenocarcinomas have a poorer prognosis than those with squamous cell carcinomas [6]. Cervical metastases offer a better prognosis than metastases in the lung or liver [5]. It was reported that median survival of patients with CUP tumors was approximately 1 year, but a median survival of 23 months was described for patients with CUP tumors and identified primary sites, which was subsequently treated with a specific therapy [11]. This suggested that early detection of the primary lesion enables a rational approach to treatment and can significantly change the prognosis of patients with CUP tumors [12].

The primary tumor is detected in less than 40% of patients by conventional diagnostic procedures, frequently, only after having performed

G.-J. Cheon, M.D. (✉)
Molecular Imaging Research Center, Korea Institute of Radiological and Medical Sciences (KIRAMS), Department of Nuclear Medicine, Korea Cancer Center Hospital, Nowon-gu, Seoul 139-706, South Korea
e-mail: larry@kcch.re.kr

E.E. Kim et al. (eds.), *Clinical PET and PET/CT: Principles and Applications*,
DOI 10.1007/978-1-4419-0802-5_29, © Springer Science+Business Media New York 2013

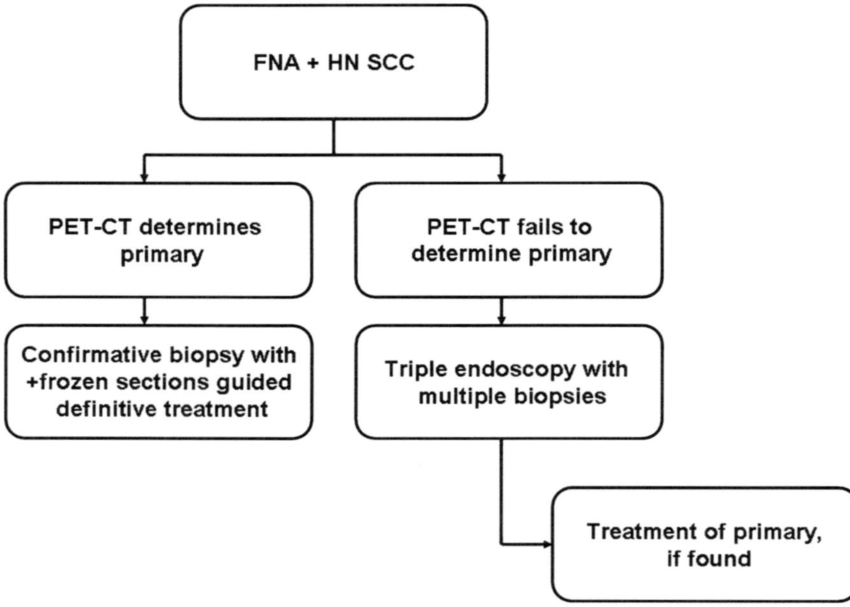

Fig. 29.1 PET/CT in patients with unknown primary head and neck cancer. *FNA* fine-needle aspiration, *HN* head and neck, *SCC* squamous cell carcinoma (Courtesy by Fleming and Johansen [45])

many examinations, which are often nonconclusive and generate discomfort for the patient as well as a high economic cost [3, 4]. It is clear, therefore, that it is becoming increasingly necessary to use new diagnostic tools and concepts to uncover occult primary tumors even if these do not yet play a role in routine diagnostic work (Fig. 29.1) [6].

Positron emission tomography (PET) using fluorodeoxyglucose (FDG) has become the preferred imaging modality in the diagnosis and management of many different types of cancers [13]. As most malignant tumors have a high glucose metabolism compared with normal tissue, a high tumor-to-background contrast can be achieved on FDG PET imaging, which is frequently of benefit when screening for the unknown primary tumors [6]. Combined PET/CT has proved superior to CT or PET alone in detecting primary and metastatic cancer [14]. In the case of head and neck malignancy, FDG PET/CT can detect overall malignant lesions with a sensitivity of 91–98%, a specificity of 92–93%, and an accuracy from 72% to 94% [13–15]. As a result of the relatively good prognosis of patients with CUP tumors located in the head and neck and the expected favorable cost effectiveness, research examining the use of FDG PET in CUP tumors in the head and neck region has been published [6, 14, 15]. However, the use of FDG PET is still limited because of its availability and relative high cost, and is not established as a clinical benefit in this area [6].

General Diagnostic Procedure

Although the therapeutic response and prognosis of patients with CUP tumors are generally poor, it is dependent on the cancer types or origins. Generally, patients with undifferentiated tumors and adenocarcinomas have a poorer prognosis than those with squamous cell carcinomas [6]. As some cancers (breast, ovarian, prostatic, and thyroid) have a specific treatment, metastases from those specific cancers offers a better prognosis

Table 29.1 Diagnostic procedure performed in patients with CUP syndrome presenting with cervical lymph node metastases

Sonography of neck and abdomen
Panendoscopy (oropharynx, larynx, nasopharynx, hypopharynx)
Fine-needle biopsy of suspicious lymph node
Chest radiography; mammography; CT and/or MRI of head, neck, and thorax
Bone scintigraphy
Stool for occult blood, urinalysis, blood count, erythrocyte sedimentation rate
Serum analysis (electrolyte, liver function test, amylase, phosphatase, etc.)
Tumor markers (PSA, hCG, AFP, CEA, CA125, etc.)

and therapeutic response [11]. However, as the median survival of patients with CUP syndrome is short, the remainder of the life of the patient should not be passed in an endless round of fruitless diagnostic studies causing discomfort and frustration [6].

Basic investigation for patients with CUP tumors and cervical lymph node metastases include patient history documentation, physical examination with inspection and palpation of the oropharynx; endoscopy of the nasopharynx and hypopharynx; laryngoscopy; sonography of the neck, thyroid, and abdomen; and serology (Table 29.1) [16]. The most important aspect of the workup of a patient with CUP tumor is the evaluation of the tissue obtained at biopsy. If fine needle aspiration cytology is insufficient for diagnostic certainty, excision biopsy is recommended for histologic diagnosis [17, 18]. In poorly differentiated tumors, immunohistochemical, cytogenetic, and molecular biologic studies can be extremely useful in identifying sarcomas, germ cell tumors, lymphomas, neuroendocrine carcinomas, and other tumors for which diagnosis would suggest a more specific therapeutic approach. Because in most situations, no single antibody is specific enough to identify the primary site with certainty, a battery of immunohistochemistry testing is often used and sometimes valuable in locating tumor characteristics such as thyroglobulin, cytokeratines, S-100 antigen, prostatic specific antigen, estrogen receptor, etc., which can lead to histologic tumor identification [19].

Radiography and/or computed tomography (CT) of the thorax are essential and CT/magnetic resonance imaging (MRI) of the abdomen is highly recommended in case of adenocarcinoma [6]. Endoscopy of the upper aerodigestive tracts with systematic biopsies should be performed for all patients with CUP tumors of the cervical lymph nodes. Often, serum tumor markers such as prostate-specific antigen (PSA), thyroglobulin, β-human chorionic gonadotropin (β-hCG), α-fetoprotein (AFP), carcinoembryonic antigen (CEA), etc., are helpful in indicating the primary site of CUP tumors, but they are nonspecific for tumor localization in most case [20], and additional diagnostic procedures of asymptomatic organs, such as contrast enemas of the bowel or urogenital tract, mammography, thyroid scan, or endoscopy of other tracts, are of a little diagnostic value [6].

Positron Emission Tomography

CUP tumor represents a heterogeneous group of metastatic tumors for which no primary site can be detected following a thorough medical history, careful clinical examination, and extensive diagnostic workup [1]. Attempts to identify the primary tumor in patients with CUP tumors are often time consuming, expensive, and ultimately unsuccessful [1, 6].

PET imaging of increased glucose metabolism using FDG has been found to be of value in patients with CUP tumors in spite of the rather unspecific metabolic processes involved. Because most malignant tumors have a high glucose metabolism compared with normal tissue, a high tumor-to-background contrast can be achieved on FDG PET imaging, which is frequently of benefit when screening for unknown primary tumors [6]. In 1994, studies that evaluated the usefulness of PET with ^{18}F-FDG in detecting the primary origin in patients with CUP tumors began to be reported [21]. The reason was that the technique's capacity to noninvasively detect different tumor types in the whole body a single examination [22]. Most studies report that ^{18}F-FDG PET detects the primary tumor in

Table 29.2 Diagnostic performance of FDG PET/CT in primary tumor detection

Study and year	Primary tumor detection rate (%)	Sensitivity (%)		Specificity (%)	
		Value	95% CI	Value	95% CI
Fencl et al. 2007 [25]	22	55	38–70	75	62–85
Nassenstein et al. 2007 [26]	28	100	74–100	85	69–94
Fleming et al. 2007 [27]	73	94	73–99	100	61–100
Bruna et al. 2007 [28]	38	93	70–99	77	57–90
Wartski et al. 2007 [29]	34	93	69–99	73	48–89
Ambrosini et al. 2006 [30]	53	100	84–100	95	76–99
Fakhry et al. 2006 [31]	32	70	40–89	75	47–91
Pelosi et al. 2006 [32]	35	83	66–93	87	73–94
Nanni et al. 2005 [33]	57	100	76–100	89	57–98
Freudenberg et al. 2005 [34]	57	86	60–96	100	65–100
Gutzeit et al. 2005 [35]	33	88	66–97	89	73–96
Pooled estimate[a]	37	84	78–88	84	78–89

[a]Adapted from Kwee and Kwee [24]

approximately 40% of cases in which negative results were found using conventional diagnostic procedures [8]. Because of the high sensitivity and specificity of ^{18}F-FDG PET for tumor detection, if the primary tumor is not located using ^{18}F-FDG PET, it is not detected during follow-up in most cases [22, 23].

In a meta-analysis, Kwee and Kwee [24] reviewed previous reports systematically [25–35] and described the detection of unknown primary tumors on FDG PET (Table 29.2). Their results indicated that overall, FDG PET/CT was able to detect 37% of primary tumors in patients with CUP tumors, and sensitivity and specificity were reasonably high (both 84%). In their meta-analysis, lung cancer and oropharyngeal and pancreatic carcinoma were the most frequently detected primary tumors using FDG PET/CT (33%, 16%, and 5%, respectively). The most commonly reported locations of false-positive FDG PET results were in the lung and oropharynx (both 15%). Causes of false-positive results may be a result of FDG uptake in benign conditions with increased glycolysis, high physiologic FDG uptake, and artifacts of attenuation correction. False-negative FDG PET results were found most often in breast cancer (27%). They suggested that the reasons of false-negative PET results in breast cancer could be attributed to the small size (<1 cm), slow growth, and low grade of malignancy with low or no FDG uptake, which could be overlooked on FDG PET.

Seve et al. [36] performed a meta-analysis and reported similar findings in detection rate of FDG PET (41%; range, 24%–63%). FDG PET detected 17% more tumors than were identified using CT, but there were no tumors that were detected only by CT. PET/CT was able to detect more primary tumors than either of the other imaging modalities. They reported that six studies [23, 37–41] provided data on changes in treatment planning in response to additional information provided by FDG PET scans. In 42 of 121 patients (34.7%) from those studies, a therapeutic change was attributed to FDG PET findings, that is, either to the detection of the primary tumor and/or to the detection of previously unknown metastases. In 32 of those 42 patients who had an unknown primary tumor identified, the treatment strategy changed from CUP chemotherapy to specific therapy for the tumor site, whereas the detection of unknown distant metastases (10 of 42) led to a transition from curative to palliative intent. However, no study formally has assessed the contribution of FDG PET with survival in patients with CUP tumors [36]. Although Mantaka et al. [40] reported better survival in patients who were diagnosed using PET, survival was not altered by discovery of the primary tumors in the other study [37].

FDG PET was sensitive for the detection of primary tumor and, in approximately 41% of patients, revealed tumors that had gone undetected by other modalities [36]. Whole-body FDG PET also detected previously unrecognized regional or distant metastases in approximately 37% of patients. FDG PET exhibits high overall sensitivity for detection of unknown primary. However, a relatively low rate of primary site detection of CUP was found in the reported data [21–26, 36], although FDG PET had higher sensitivity and specificity than any other imaging modalities. The reasons for the relatively low rates of primary site detection can be attributed to the following facts: (1) the biologic features of the primary tumor can be different from those of the tumor cells in the nodal regions (metastases may have higher uptake levels of FDG than in the primary); (2) the primary lesion is usually small, making it difficult to find, especially in anatomically complicated areas; and (3) the primary tumor can disappear after seeding the metastasis because its angiogenic incompetence leads to marked apoptosis and cellular turnover, or it may have regressed spontaneously [12].

The role of FDG PET is limited in slowly growing tumors such as well-differentiated neuroendocrine tumors, compared with the most common malignancies of CUP tumor, namely adenocarcinoma, squamous cell carcinoma, and poorly differentiated carcinoma. In case of neuroendocrine tumors, tumor-specific tracers in addition to FDG can be used to detect the primary site and assess stage [42, 43]. Prasad et al. [43] performed receptor PET/CT using Ga-68-DOTA-NOC for the detection of undiagnosed primary sites of neuroendocrine tumors. Among 59 patients with documented neuroendocrine tumors and unknown primary, Ga-68-DOTA-NOC localized the primary site in 35 patients (59%), which was superior to In-11 octreotide scan (39%) as well as CT alone (20%). Although only a limited number of studies [42–44] have been published dealing with CUP of pathologically identified specific tumors such as neuroendocrine tumor, PET imaging with a specific radiotracer including peptide receptor, monoclonal antibody, or other kinds of tumor-specific targeting agents can play a role in the management of patients with a certain specific tumors.

Conclusion

FDG PET/CT has been successfully used for the detection of CUP tumors, identifying the primary lesions in 22–73% of patients (average, 37%) with a negative diagnostic workup [25–35]. The detection of primary tumors in patients with CUP tumor is important for several reasons, including finding a potentially treatable tumor and allowing therapy to be targeted as appropriately as possible [36]. Early identification of the primary tumor is a fundamental prerequisite for changing a patient's prognosis and prolonging survival [11]. Prognosis increases considerably for patients with CUP syndrome and curable tumor node metastasis staging, if the primary tumor is found before the start of therapy [6]. Furthermore, FDG PET is useful for defining prognosis, because the prognosis depends on the tumor burden and stage of the disease.

FDG PET is an important diagnostic tool for exploration for unknown primary tumors and offers high sensitivity and whole-body imaging in a single test. Therefore, FDG PET should be considered in the early stage of diagnostic workup, prior to routinely performed morphologic imaging modalities [45]. On the other hand, it should be realized that FDG PET/CT is an expensive examination, and false-positive findings may result in unnecessary additional invasive diagnostic procedures which have associated morbidities and costs [36]. No systematic study has been performed to determine the incidence and clinical course of CUP tumors. The additive value of FDG PET and its cost effectiveness for patients with CUP tumors should be further investigated.

References

1. Pavlidis N. Forty years experience of treating cancer of unknown primary. Acta Oncol. 2007;46:592–601.
2. Abbruzzese JL, Abbruzzese MC, Hess KR, et al. Unknown primary carcinoma: natural history and

prognostic factors in 657 consecutive patients. J Clin Oncol. 1994;12:1272–80.
3. Daugaard G. Unknown primary tumours. Cancer Treat Rev. 1994;20:119–47.
4. Abbruzzese JL, Abbruzzese MC, Lenzi R, et al. Analysis of a diagnostic strategy for patients with suspected tumors of unknown origin. J Clin Oncol. 1995;13:2094–103.
5. Lefebvre JL, Coche-Dequent B, Van Ton J, et al. Cervical lymph nodes from unknown primary tumors in 190 patients. Am J Surg. 1990;160:443–6.
6. Scheidhauer K, Avril N, Bonkowsky VM. Carcinoma of unknown primary. In: Wieler HJ, Coleman RE, editors. PET in clinical oncology. Heidelberg: Springer; 2000. p. 169–76.
7. Leinard RJ, Nystrom JS. Diagnostic evaluation of patients with carcinoma of unknown primary tumor site. Semin Oncol. 1993;20:244–50.
8. Delgado-Bolton RC, Fernandez-Perez C, Gonzalez-Mate A, et al. Meta-analysis of the performance of ^{18}F-FDG PET in primary tumor detection in unknown primary tumors. J Nucl Med. 2003;44:1301–14.
9. Altman E, Cadmann E. An analysis of 1539 patients with cancer of unknown primary site. Cancer. 1986;57:120–4.
10. Smith PE, Krements ET, Chapman W. Metastatic cancer without a detectable primary site. Am J Surg. 1967;113:633–7.
11. Raber MN, Faintuch J, Abbruzzese JL, et al. Continuous infusion of 5-fluorouracil, etoposide, and cisplatin in patients with metastatic carcinoma of unknown primary origin. Ann Oncol. 1991;2:519–20.
12. Dong M, Zhao K, Lin X, et al. Role of fluorodeoxyglucose-PET versus fluorodeoyglucose PET/computed tomography in detection of unknown primary tumor: a meta-analysis of the literature. Nucl Med Commun. 2008;29:791–802.
13. Endo K, Oriuchi N, Higuchi T, et al. PET and PET/CT using ^{18}F-FDG in the diagnosis and management of cancer patients. Int J Clin Oncol. 2006;11:286–96.
14. Branstetter BF, Blodgett TM, Brun T, et al. Head and neck malignancy: is PET/CT more accurate than PET or CT alone? Radiology. 2005;235:580–6.
15. Syed R, Bomanji JB, Nagabhushan N, et al. Impact of combined ^{18}F-FDG PET/CT in head and neck tumors. Br J Cancer. 2005;92:1046–50.
16. Leonard RJ, Nystrom JS. Diagnostic evaluation of patients with carcinoma of unknown primary site. Semin Oncol. 1993;20:244–50.
17. Van der Brekel MPM, Castelijins JA, Steel H, et al. Modern imaging techniques and ultrasound-guided aspiration cytology for the assessment of neck node metastasis A prospective comparative study. Eur Arch Otorhinolaryngol. 1993;250:11–7.
18. Wang RC, Goepfert H, Barber AE, et al. Unknown primary squamous cell carcinoma metastatic to the neck. Arch Otolaryngol Head Neck Surg. 1990;116:1388–93.
19. Hainsworth JD, Wright EP, Johnson DH, et al. Poorly differentiated carcinoma of unknown primary site: clinical usefulness of immunoperoxidase staining. J Clin Oncol. 1991;9(11):1931–8.
20. Panza N, Lombardi G, Rosa M, et al. High serum thyroglobulin levels, diagnostic indicators in patients with unknown primary sites. Cancer. 1987;60: 2233–6.
21. Rege S, Maass A, Chaiken L, et al. Use of positron emission tomography with fluorodeoxyglucose in patients with extracranial head and neck cancers. Cancer. 1994;73:3047–58.
22. Bohuslavizki KH, Klutmann S, Kroger S, et al. FDG PET detection of unknown primary tumors. J Nucl Med. 2000;41:816–22.
23. Lassen U, Daugaard G, Eigtved A, et al. ^{18}F-FDG whole body positron emission tomography (PET) in patients with unknown primary tumors (UPT). Eur J Cancer. 1999;35:1076–82.
24. Kwee TC, Kwee RM. Combined FDG-PET/CT for the detection of unknown primary tumors: systemic review and meta-analysis. Eur Radiol. 2009;19: 731–44.
25. Fencl P, Belohlavek O, Skopalova M, et al. Prognostic and diagnostic accuracy of [^{18}F]FDG-PET/CT in 190 patients with carcinoma of unknown primary. Eur J Nucl Med Mol Imaging. 2007;34:1783–92.
26. Nassenstein K, Veit-Haibach P, Stergar H, et al. Cervical lymph node metastases of unknown origin: primary tumor detection with whole-body positron emission tomography/computed tomography. Acta Radiol. 2007;23:1–8.
27. Fleming AJ, Smith SP, Paul CM, et al. Impact of [^{18}F]-2-fluorodeoxyglucose-positron emission tomography/computed tomography on previously untreated head and neck cancer patients. Laryngoscope. 2007;117: 1173–9.
28. Bruna C, Journo A, Netter F, et al. On the interest of PET with ^{18}FFDG in the management of cancer of unknown primary (CUP). Med Nucl. 2007;31:242–9.
29. Wartski M, Le Stanc E, Gontier E, et al. In search of an unknown primary tumor presenting with cervical metastases: performance of hybrid FDG-PET-CT. Nucl Med Commun. 2007;28:365–71.
30. Ambrosini V, Nanni C, Rubello D, et al. ^{18}F-FDG PET/CT in the assessment of carcinoma of unknown primary origin. Radiol Med. 2006;111:1146–55.
31. Fakhry N, Barberet M, Lussato D, et al. Role of [^{18}F]-FDG PET-CT in the management of the head and neck cancers. Bull Cancer. 2006;93:1017–25.
32. Pelosi E, Pennone M, Deandreis D, et al. Role of whole body positron emission tomography/computed tomography scan with ^{18}F-fluorodeoxyglucose in patients with biopsy proven tumor metastases from unknown primary site. Q J Nucl Med Mol Imaging. 2006;50:15–22.
33. Nanni C, Rubello D, Castellucci P, et al. Role of ^{18}F-FDG PET-CT imaging for the detection of an unknown primary tumor: preliminary results in 21 patients. Eur J Nucl Med Mol Imaging. 2005;32:589–92.
34. Freudenberg LS, Fischer M, Antoch G, et al. Dual modality of ^{18}F-fluorodeoxyglucose positron emission

tomography/computed tomography in patients with cervical carcinoma of unknown primary. Med Princ Pract. 2005;14:155–60.
35. Gutzeit A, Antoch G, Kühl H, et al. Unknown primary tumors: detection with dual-modality PET/CT – initial experience. Radiology. 2005;234:227–34.
36. Seve P, Billotey C, Broussolle C, et al. The role of 2-deoxy-2-[F-18]fluoro-D-glucose positron emission tomography in disseminated carcinoma of unknown primary site. Cancer. 2007;106:292–9.
37. Kole A, Niewey O, Bruim J, et al. Detection of known occult primary tumors using position emission tomography. Cancer. 1998;82:1160–6.
38. Kolesnikov-Gauthier H, Levy E, Merlet P, et al. FDG PET in patients with cancer of an unknown primary. Nucl Med Commun. 2005;26:1059–66.
39. Lonneux M, Reffad A. Metastases from unknown primary tumor. PET-FDG as initial diagnostic procedure? Clin Positron Imaging. 2000;3:137–41.
40. Mantaka P, Baum RP, Hertel A, et al. PET with 2-[F-18]- fluoro-2-deoxy-D-glucose (FDG) in patients with cancer of unknown primary (CUP): influence on patients' diagnostic and therapeutic management. Cancer Biother Radiopharm. 2003;18:47–58.
41. Scott CL, Kudaba I, Stewart JM, Hicks RJ, Rischin D. The utility of 2-deoxy-2-[F-18]fluoro-D-glucose positron emission tomography in the investigation of patients with disseminated carcinoma of unknown primary origin. Mol Imaging Biol. 2005;7:236–43.
42. Ambrosini V, Tomassetti P, Rubello D, et al. Role of ^{18}F-dopa PET/CT imaging in the management of patients with ^{111}In-pentetreotide negative GEP tumors. Nucl Med Commun. 2007;28:473–7.
43. Prasad V, Ambrosini V, Hommann M, et al. Detection of unknown primary neuroendocrine tumours (CUP-NET) using ^{68}Ge-DOTA-NOC receptor PET/CT. Europ J Nucl Med Mol Imag. 2010;37:67–77. doi:10.1007/s00259-009-1205-y.
44. Ambrosini V, Tomassetti P, Castellucci P, et al. Comparison between ^{68}Ge-DOTA-NOC and ^{18}F-DOPA PET for the detection of gastro-entero-pancreatic and lung neuro-endocrine tumours. Eur J Nucl Med Mol Imaging. 2008;35:1431–8.
45. Fleming AJ, Johansen ME. The clinician's expectations from the use of positron emission tomography/computed tomography scanning in untreated and treated head and neck cancer patients. Curr Opin Otolaryngol Head Neck Surg. 2008;16:127–34.

^{18}F-FDG Positron Emission Tomography in the Evaluation of Infectious and Inflammatory Diseases

30

Kyung-Han Lee and June-Key Chung

Introduction

Positron emission tomography (PET) with fluorine-18 fluoro-2-deoxy-D-glucose (FDG) is a powerful diagnostic tool that detects cells with enhanced glucose utilization. While this imaging technique is most widely applied for cancer disease, FDG is not a tumor-specific probe but is also avidly accumulated by inflammatory cells. Owing to this property, in the appropriate settings, FDG PET can also be applied in detecting and characterizing a variety of infectious and inflammatory diseases, which includes diseases caused by infections from bacteria, mycobacteria, virus, and fungi, as well as many noninfectious inflammatory processes.

In patients with infectious diseases, computed tomography (CT) and magnetic resonance imaging (MRI) offers lesion delineation with excellent anatomic resolution and soft-tissue contrast [1]. However, such methods can be less specific, and difficulties often arise in differentiating active from indolent lesions in areas of previous surgical intervention. In such settings, radiolabeled leukocyte or gallium scintigraphy can provide valuable information regarding inflammatory activity and physiologic alterations associated with disease. Leukocyte scans, however, have several shortcomings, including the need for laborious preparation and risk of blood handling. Gallium scans have the disadvantage that results can only be obtained after several days of delay [2]. In addition, the diagnostic accuracy of these methods depends on the site of disease. For instance, gallium scans have decreased sensitivity for abdominal lesions resulting from substantial background uptake, and leukocyte scans have low sensitivity for spine infection.

FDG PET offers several advantages over conventional scintigraphic techniques for evaluating infectious diseases. Infectious lesions are imaged using high contrast because they show high FDG uptake amid low background activity [3]. Spatial resolution is superior to gamma cameras, and thereby allows better anatomic localization of regions with abnormal activity; this is particularly true for hybrid PET/CT systems. Furthermore, diagnostic results are available within approximately two hours. Other advantages of FDG PET include higher sensitivity for chronic and low-grade infections, applicability to patients with neutropenia, and minimal interference from metal implants. Combined, FDG PET is becoming increasingly accepted as a cost-effective and efficient modality, and an adjunct or alternative to other imaging

K.-H. Lee, M.D., Ph.D. (✉)
Department of Nuclear Medicine, Samsung Medical Center, Sungkyunkwan University, School of Medicine, Seoul 135-710, South Korea
e-mail: khnm.lee@samsung.com

J.-K. Chung, M.D., Ph.D.
Department of Nuclear Medicine, Seoul National University College of Medicine, Seoul 110-744, South Korea
e-mail: jkchung@plaza.snu.ac.kr

E.E. Kim et al. (eds.), *Clinical PET and PET/CT: Principles and Applications*,
DOI 10.1007/978-1-4419-0802-5_30, © Springer Science+Business Media New York 2013

modalities for the evaluation of infectious and inflammatory diseases.

The role of FDG PET in the diagnosis and evaluation of infectious diseases has rapidly expanded over the years. In general, the sensitivity of FDG PET in depicting infections compares favorably with other diagnostic modalities. It has shown to be highly useful in patients with suspected osteomyelitis, especially in chronic low-grade infections and in vertebral osteomyelitis. The sensitivity of FDG PET in prosthetic joint infections is also high, and while reported specificity varies, recognition of typical uptake patterns has been shown to diagnose infection with acceptable specificity. Furthermore, the body of evidence is growing for the utility of FDG PET in evaluating many other diseases, including vasculitis and fever of unknown origin, especially when a definite diagnosis is not achieved using other modalities.

FDG Uptake in Inflammatory Cells

The ability of FDG PET to image infectious and inflammatory foci is largely based on avid uptake of the tracer by infiltrating macrophages, neutrophils, and lymphocytes [4–7]. Active glucose utilization (and increased FDG uptake) occurs when such cells are activated by inflammatory stimuli, and the molecular mechanisms mediating this metabolic response are now being revealed. When phagocytic leukocytes come into contact with a stimulus, their oxygen consumption is dramatically increased in a phenomenon called the "respiratory burst". In this response, microbicidal radical oxygen species are generated through the assembly and activation of the multicomponent complex nicotinamide adenine dinucleotide phosphate (NADPH) oxidase. Oxygen consumed during this process is coupled to increased glucose catabolism through the hexose monophosphate shunt, which provides the cells with NADPH that acts as the electron donor to the oxidase. Thus, phagocytes activated by inflammatory stimuli exhibit a dramatic influx of glucose as an energy source required for high metabolic activity associated with chemotactic and phagocytic activities [8, 9].

Neutrophils comprise two thirds of the white blood cells in normal peripheral blood and constitute the prime part of our defense against various microorganisms. In the acute phase of bacterial infection, neutrophils are one of the first inflammatory responders recruited by chemotactic signals to the lesion site. The cells then internalize and kill the microbes with reactive oxygen species generated by consuming large amounts of oxygen and glucose through the process of respiratory burst. Tan et al. showed that neutrophils that are chemically activated with phorbol myristate acetate (PMA) significantly increase deoxyglucose uptake. This effect could be blocked by inhibition of either protein kinase C or tyrosine kinase, implicating that the process requires both signaling pathways [10]. Our group showed that PMA-stimulated neutrophil enhancement of FDG uptake is dependent on phosphatidyl inositol-3 kinase activity, a key signaling pathway through which insulin augments glucose metabolism [11]. Jones and colleagues demonstrated a temporal dissociation between stimulated respiratory burst activity and deoxyglucose uptake in neutrophils [12]. It was noted that priming without actual stimulation of respiratory burst was sufficient to enhance neutrophil glucose uptake, demonstrating that respiratory burst stimulation is not essential for the metabolic response [12]. More recently, Schuster and coworkers reported a linkage between lipopolysaccharide-stimulated neutrophil deoxyglucose uptake with p38 and hypoxia-inducible factor-1 pathways [13].

Monocyte-macrophages participate both in nonspecific innate immunity and in helping in the initiation of specific defense mechanisms, and are thus vital to the regulation and development of inflammation. Similarly to neutrophils, monocytes also robustly augment glucose uptake in response to inflammatory stimulators. Fukuzumi et al. showed that macrophages accelerate deoxyglucose uptake two- to three-fold in response to lipopolysaccharide stimulation [14]. Ahmed and coworkers showed in monocyte-macrophage cells that PMA-induced respiratory burst was accompanied by a 50% increase in deoxyglucose uptake, and that this required tyrosine kinase and

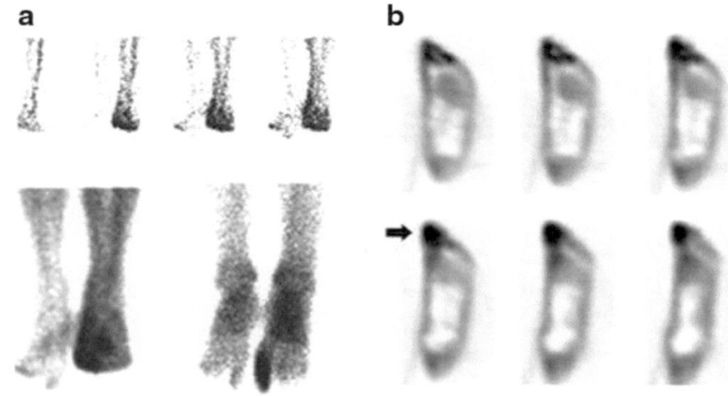

Fig. 30.1 (**a**) Three-phase bone scintigraphy scan of a diabetic patient with chronic osteomyelitis of the first toe shows focal increase in blood flow, pool, and delayed uptake. (**b**) PET demonstrates high focal FDG uptake in the chronic osteomyelitis lesion of the toe (*arrow*)

protein kinase C activity [9]. Using interferon-γ as the primer, our group demonstrated that enhancement of monocyte FDG uptake actually occurs during the priming process without the requirement of respiratory burst activation [15].

Augmentation of inflammatory cell glucose uptake by their activation appears to be largely mediated by up-regulation of glucose transporter function. PMA-stimulated glucose uptake in neutrophils was accompanied by 1.6- to 2.1-fold increases in transporter affinity for glucose [10]. Ahmed and coworkers showed that PMA-stimulated macrophage deoxyglucose uptake occurs through an increase in transporter affinity for glucose [9]. In T cell enriched lymphocytes, Chakrabarti et al. observed increases in Glut-1 levels that peaked at 48 h after stimulation by phytohemagglutinin [16]. Furthermore, enhancement of glucose uptake by lipopolysaccharide was accompanied by increased Glut-1 expression in macrophages [14] or translocation of the transporter from neutrophil interior to the cell surface [13].

In contrast to tumors that show gradual increase in FDG uptake for hours after injection, there are several reports that inflammatory lesions may gradually reduce their uptake levels after 60 min [6, 7]. Such findings can partly be explained by dephosphorylation of FDG-6-P in inflammatory cells because of significant levels of glucose-6-phosphatase [17]. Also, whereas false negative findings resulting from elevated blood glucose concentrations are a well-recognized problem for FDG PET imaging in tumor patients, there is some evidence that FDG uptake in infectious or inflammatory lesions is less affected by hyperglycemia compared with tumor tissue [18]. While this suggestion awaits further verification, the implication is of significant importance because infection imaging is often required in diabetes patients with suspected infection and poor blood glucose control such as detecting Charcot osteoarthropathy and osteomyelitis in the setting of complicated diabetic feet (Fig. 30.1).

Clinical Applications

Chronic Osteomyelitis

Osteomyelitis is an infection of the bone or bone marrow, most commonly caused by *Staphylococcus aureus*. Chronic osteomyelitis is a severe and sometimes incapacitating condition that is often recurring because it is difficult to treat definitely despite prolonged antibiotics and surgical débridement. The condition may result from inadequate treatment of acute osteomyelitis, from infection caused by trauma, iatrogenic causes or compound fractures, from infection with organisms such as *Myocobacterium tuberculosis*, or from contiguous spread from soft-tissues lesions. Unlike acute osteomyelitis, chronic osteomyelitis usually causes no acute constitutional symptoms and presents as a long-standing discharging sinus or chronic bone pain. Diagnosis can remain a clinical challenge because lesions are often reactivated after years of indolence, with uncharacteristic laboratory and radiologic features.

A variety of imaging techniques are available to assist in the diagnosis of chronic osteomyelitis. Plain radiographs can provide clues of osteolytic or sclerotic lesions but are more often equivocal. MRI is highly sensitive in detecting bone marrow changes and can provide detailed information regarding the extent and activity of the infectious process. However, MRI studies often show nonspecific findings and are of limited value in infections of small bones, diabetic or immune compromised patients, previous trauma, surgery, or preexisting marrow conditions. Three-phase bone scans are highly sensitive for detecting skeletal lesions but lack specificity for discerning infection. Gallium scans have better specificity but the accuracy in suspected osteomyelitis is only 70–80% [19], and false-positive results are seen in healing fractures or uninfected endoprostheses [20, 21]. Leukocyte scans have a reasonable accuracy for detecting chronic osteomyelitis. However, the false-negative rate can be relatively high, particularly in osteomyelitis of the axial skeleton where granulocytes are naturally present [22, 23]. In addition, it is sometimes difficult to differentiate between osteomyelitis and soft-tissue infections surrounding the bone using this method.

FDG PET has emerged as a promising imaging technique for evaluating infections of the soft tissues and the skeleton [24]. Figure 30.1 demonstrates three-phase bone scintigraphy and FDG PET images of a patient with chronic osteomyelitis in the foot. It appears that FDG PET is particularly useful in patients who are suspected of having chronic osteomyelitis but show negative findings on other imaging modalities or when infection of the axial skeleton is suspected. In an early prospective study of 31 patients, FDG PET could detect chronic osteomyelitis with a sensitivity of 100% and a specificity of 92% [25]. In another study of 51 patients with chronic osteomyelitis suspected in the peripheral or central skeleton, the sensitivity and specificity of FDG PET were 97–100% and 95%, respectively, compared with 86–92% and 77–82%, respectively, for combined bone scanning and antigranulocyte imaging [26]. de Winter et al. investigated 60 patients with suspected chronic musculoskeletal infection and found that FDG PET correctly identified all 25 cases with infection [27]. Of the four false-positive findings, two cases underwent surgery within 6 months. The sensitivities, specificities, and accuracies were 100%, 88%, and 93%, respectively, for the entire group, and 100%, 90%, and 94%, respectively, for patients with suspected infection of the central skeleton [27]. FDG PET is also sensitive in identifying chronic spondylitis from tuberculous infection [28, 29], and FDG uptake in these lesions appears to decrease or normalize with tuberculostatic treatment [30].

Because of its extremely high sensitivity, a negative PET study virtually rules out osteomyelitis [31]. This can be important when bone anatomy and structure have been altered by trauma, surgery, or soft-tissue infection, which makes diagnosis of chronic osteomyelitis difficult by radiologic modalities. Thus, FDG PET is highly useful in patients with suspected chronic osteomyelitis in whom bone anatomy has been altered (Fig. 30.2). In a recent study of 33 patients with suspected chronic osteomyelitis with trauma, FDG PET showed a sensitivity, specificity, and accuracy of 88%, 100%, and 90% for axial skeleton and 100%, 85%, and 91% for appendicular bone, respectively [32].

A recent study compared the accuracy of current imaging modalities in the diagnosis of chronic osteomyelitis by a systematic review and meta-analysis of 23 clinical studies [33]. Pooled data revealed FDG PET to be the most sensitive technique, with a sensitivity of 96% compared with 82% for bone scintigraphy, 61% for leukocyte scintigraphy, 78% for combined bone and leukocyte scintigraphy, and 84% for MRI. Pooled specificity was also highest for FDG PET at 91%, followed by leukocyte scintigraphy at 84%, and MRI at 77%, and lowest for bone scintigraphy at 25% [33].

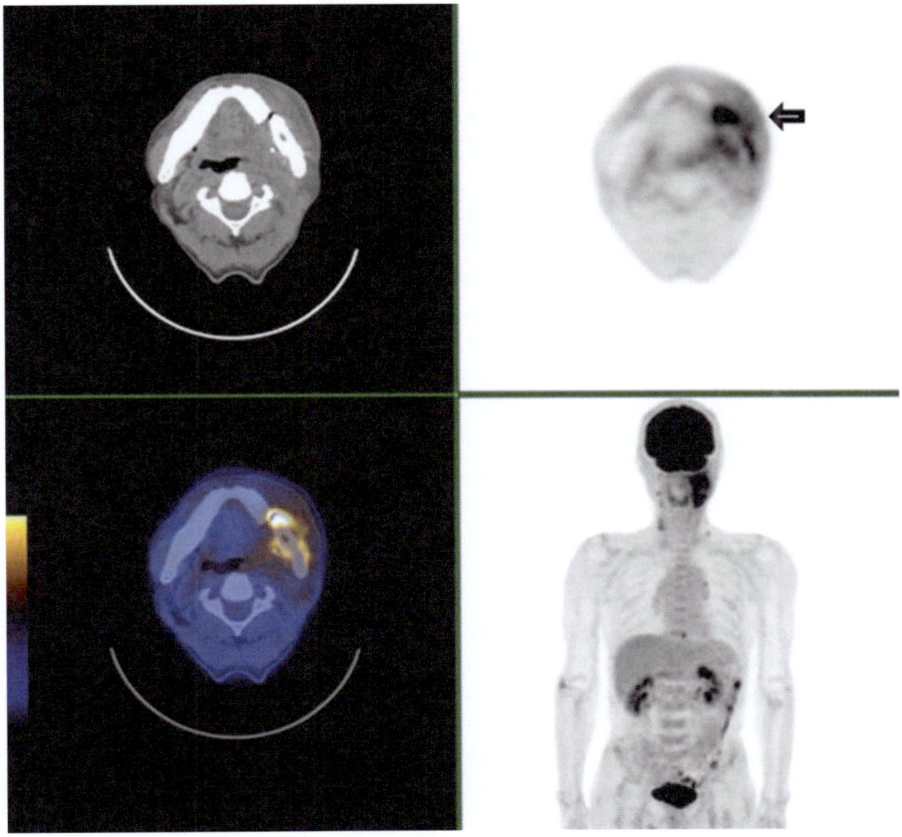

Fig. 30.2 FDG PET/CT scan of a patient who had undergone partial mandibulectomy with reconstruction showed focal increased FDG uptake on the left mandible (*arrow*). This lesion was later revealed to be caused by chronic osteomyelitis of the mandible around the surgical site

Limb Arthroplasty-Associated Infection

Arthroplasty is operative surgical procedure in which the arthritic or dysfunctional joint surface is artificially replaced or remodeled by surgical procedure. The most successful and common form of arthroplasty is the replacement of the arthritic joint with prosthesis to relieve pain, restore range of motion, and improve muscle strength and function. Total hip arthroplasty, for example, would replace an entire osteoarthritic hip joint with a prosthetic hip that includes both the acetabulum and the head and neck of the femur. Arthroplasty-related pain commonly occurs in patients after surgery, and because prosthesis infection is potentially dangerous, accurate differentiation between prosthesis infection and aseptic loosening is crucial in order to apply the correct treatment.

Multiple imaging modalities can be used for evaluating patients with painful arthroplasty. MRI has limited specificity caused by the presence of violated bone. Bone scintigraphy is highly sensitive and has a high negative predictive value, but lacks sufficient specificity to discern prosthesis infection from loosening [34]. A combination of a gallium scan with bone scan can improve specificity, but at the expense of a significant decrease in sensitivity [35, 36]. Leukocyte scintigraphy has better accuracy for diagnosing an infected prosthesis. A previous study of 143 patients who underwent reoperation for a loose or painful joint arthroplasty or a resection arthroplasty showed indium-111 leukocyte scans to have 77% sensitivity, 86% specificity, and 84% accuracy for predicting bone infection [37].

FDG PET offers an effective modality for detecting postarthroplasty infection. FDG PET, unlike CT or MRI, is not affected by the presence of metal implants, and is particularly useful in patients who have clinical and laboratory signs of infection but indistinct signs on bone scan and radiographs [38]. In an early study of 62 patients (74 prostheses) in whom infection was suspected, FDG PET showed 90% sensitivity, 89% specificity, and 90% accuracy for detecting hip prostheses infection [39]. In a recent meta-analysis that reviewed and analyzed five selected studies in the literature, FDG PET showed a pooled sensitivity of 83% and specificity of 87% for distinguishing between septic and aseptic loosening of hip prosthesis [40]. However, caution is necessary to avoid false-positive interpretation of nonspecific periprosthetic FDG activity that often persists for long periods compared with other bone procedures. As such, it has been suggested that positive results should be reserved for lesions with increased FDG uptake present along the interface between the prosthesis and bone [41].

In the study by Zhuang et al., FDG PET showed a lower specificity of 72% for detecting knee prostheses infection, although the sensitivity was 91% [39]. A somewhat lower specificity for FDG PET in detecting arthroplasty-related infection of the knee compared with the hip is confirmed by other studies. Van Acker et al. reported that in 21 patients, FDG PET demonstrated a sensitivity of 100% but lower specificity of 73% for detecting knee prostheses infection [42]. The diagnostic criteria for interpretation of FDG uptake in infections associated with knee prostheses are not yet as optimal as with hip prosthesis. Although the reason for relatively higher false-positive rates is not clear, artifacts introduced by attenuation correction of PET images may contribute [43]. FDG PET is highly useful for detecting infections associated with arthroplasty of the hips, and to a lesser extent in knee prosthesis.

Vasculitis

Vasculitis is a disorder characterized by inflammation of the blood vessels with diverse clinical manifestations that depend on size of involved vessels and organs affected by ischemia. Although some cases manifest with only symptoms and signs of systemic inflammation, varying degrees of presentation can range from mild morbidities to severe life-threatening multisystemic diseases. Different types of primary systemic vasculitis include giant cell arteritis, Takayasu arteritis, polyarteritis nodosa, Wegener's granulomatosis, and Kawasaki disease. As with any less than common disease, making a diagnosis or management decision in patients with vasculitis can be difficult [44]. Suppression of inflammation and preservation of vascular competence are the aims of treatment.

Doppler sonography, CT, and MRI allow a noninvasive approach to evaluating vasculitis, partially replacing angiography by allowing simultaneous evaluation of luminal and vascular wall changes [45]. Leukocyte scintigraphy allows visualization of focal areas of neutrophil accumulation as well as information regarding abnormal neutrophil kinetics in the lung and spleen [46]. It has also been found to be useful for detecting unsuspected sites of disease, help monitor disease activity, and is particularly superior to CT for detecting vasculitic involvement of the respiratory tract [47, 48]. However, leukocyte scans can have limited utility in vasculitic diseases that present as chronic inflammation with lower levels of neutrophil content.

FDG PET is increasingly recognized as a useful tool for evaluating inflammation of large vessels. FDG PET has been shown to identify a greater number of affected vascular regions in both giant cell arteritis and Takayasu's arteritis than morphologic imaging using MRI. Visual grading of vascular FDG uptake helps discriminate arteritis from atherosclerosis and therefore provides high specificity [49].

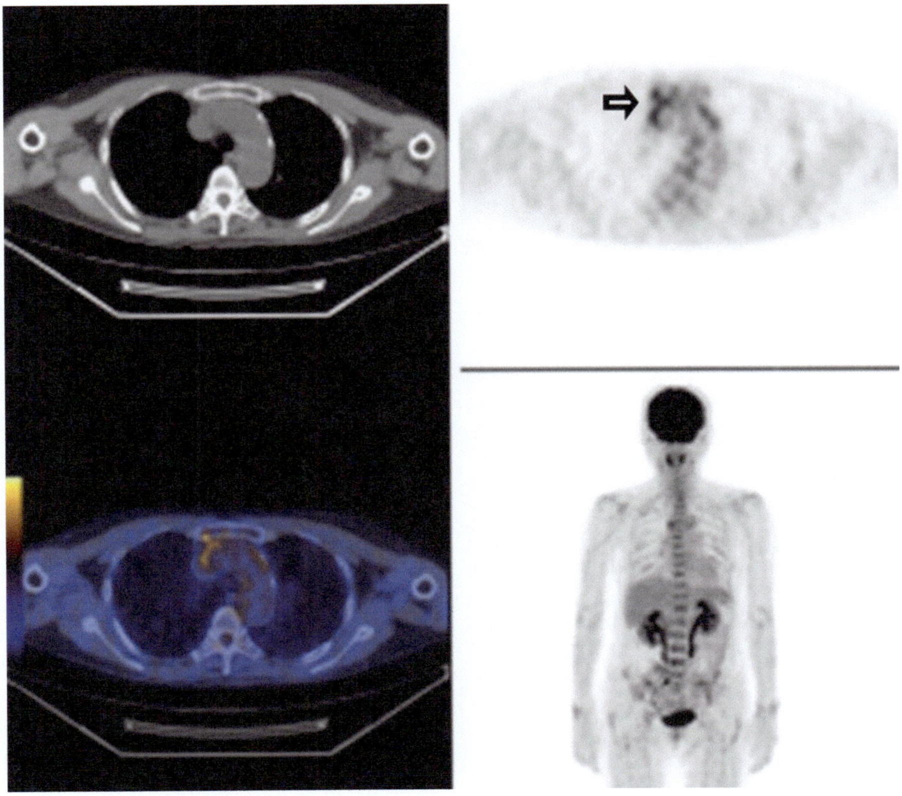

Fig. 30.3 FDG PET/CT scan of a 65-year-old female with unexplained fever for 4 weeks showed increased FDG uptake in the aortic arch (*arrow*; peak SUV, 3.2) and brachiocephalic artery. Clinical signs and symptoms improved with corticosteroid therapy under the diagnosis of giant cell arteritis

Giant cell arteritis and polymyalgia rheumatica show increased FDG uptake on affected vessel walls (Fig. 30.3) [50, 51]. Such increases in FDG have been shown to normalize after successful steroid therapy [52, 53], suggesting that FDG PET may aid in the evaluation of the extent, therapy response, and recurrence of these diseases. Takayasu's arteritis is a form of chronic large vessel vasculitis that mostly affects young females in Asian and Latin American regions. The disease mainly involves and causes stenosis or obstruction of the aorta and its main branches as well as the coronary and pulmonary arteries. Because signs and symptoms at the early stage are nonspecific, diagnosis is usually made at a relatively later stage. By demonstrating FDG accumulation on affected vessels, FDG PET has been shown to have potential to detect Takayasu's arteritis at an early phase, thus permitting early treatment and possible prevention of progression [54–56].

FDG PET can also provide information regarding disease activity and treatment response of large-vessel vasculitis [57]. Walter et al. examined the ability of FDG PET for assessing disease activity and extent in 26 patients with giant cell arteritis or Takayasu's arteritis. PET revealed abnormal uptakes in 18 cases, and showed a sensitivity of less than 50% in patients with low C-reactive protein (CRP) and erythrocyte sedimentation rate (ESR) levels and sensitivities of 95.5% and 80.7%, respectively, when CRP and ESR levels were high [58]. In another study, Otsuka et al. observed three cases of vasculitis with initial intense FDG uptake in the vessels that normalized after steroid therapy, correlating with normalization of laboratory data and symptomatic improvement [59]. These findings suggest FDG PET to be an effective technique for assessing the activity and the extent of large-vessel vasculitis.

The use of new combined PET/CT scanners provides additional anatomic information, thereby allowing the evaluation of disease activity and vessel morphology as well as the localization of the inflammatory process in the same session [60, 61]. Thus, FDG PET/CT may help in the diagnosis of systemic vasculitis when nonspecific symptoms and equivocal serology are presented; to define the distribution of inflammatory lesions; to monitor the response of inflammatory lesions to treatment; and to improve our understanding of the pathophysiology the disease.

Fever of Unknown Origin

Fever of unknown origin (FUO) is generally defined as recurrent fever of 38.3°C or greater lasting 2–3 weeks or longer, with uncertain diagnosis after appropriate evaluation. The three major categories of disease that accounts for FUO are infection, neoplasm, and noninfectious inflammatory disease. Routine diagnostic approaches include physical examination, thorough history taking, standardized laboratory tests, and simple imaging procedures. There is a need for more complex or invasive techniques, however, if routine diagnostic strategies fail.

Traditional scintigraphic imaging studies for FUO have been done with Ga-67 citrate, labeled leukocytes, and bone scintigraphy. Leukocyte scans have a high diagnostic accuracy in the detection of granulocytic pathology, but they are only of limited value in FUO because of the low prevalence of purulent processes in these cases [62]. Ga-67 citrate is taken up by acute or chronic granulomatous and autoimmune inflammations as well as various tumors, and is thus currently considered to be the tracer of choice in the diagnostic workup of FUO [63]. However, gallium scans have low image resolution, require delayed imaging, and physiologic intestinal distribution of gallium reduces its specificity for detecting abdominal lesions.

FDG PET has recently emerged as a useful alternative for scintigraphic evaluation of FUO. Because of its high sensitivity, FDG PET can be useful for detecting foci as an origin of fever in these patients. An example of a patient with FUO caused by large vessel vasculitis is shown in Figure 30.3. FDG PET has a particular advantage in that it is capable of detecting all three major categories of disease that account for FUO. This is a significant trait because infection actually accounts for only 20–40% of FUOs, with the remaining patients having tumors, collagen vascular disease, or noninfectious inflammation.

In an early study, Lorenzen et al. described FDG PET findings in 16 FUO patients with inconclusive conventional diagnostics [64]. Among 12 cases that showed nonphysiologic FDG accumulation, PET findings led to the final diagnosis in 11 cases. FDG PET was negative in two patients with rheumatic fever and in two patients in whom the origin of fever was unrevealed [64]. Blockmans et al. investigated FDG PET in 58 consecutive cases of FUO and found that 24 of 46 abnormal FDG PET scans were helpful for diagnosis, while 22 were noncontributory [65]. In a subgroup of 40 patients who had both FDG PET and gallium scintigraphy, each was helpful for diagnosis in 35% and 25%, respectively [65].

These earlier reports have subsequently been supported with prospective investigations. Kjaer and coworkers conducted a prospective study comparing the diagnostic value of FDG PET and indium-111 granulocyte scintigraphy in 19 patients with FUO [66]. The results showed sensitivities of 71% and 50%, and specificities of 92% and 46% for granulocyte scintigraphy and FDG PET, respectively. Their study showed superior diagnostic performance of granulocyte scintigraphy for detection of localized causes of FUO, and that high false-positive rates of FDG PET can lead to lower specificity [66]. In another prospective study, Buysschaert et al. performed FDG PET on 74 of 110 collected patients who fulfilled the criteria of classic FUO [67]. Abnormal FDG PET results were found in 53 cases in which 19 scans were helpful. A diagnosis was established in 31 of the 53 patients with an abnormal scan and in 8 of the 21 patients with a normal scan. Among the 39 patients with a final diagnosis, 49% of the scans were helpful [67]. A more recent multicenter prospective study was performed by Bleeker-Rovers et al. in an effort to validate the use of FDG PET as part of a structured diagnostic protocol in patients with FUO [68]. A structured diagnostic protocol including FDG PET was used on 70 recruited patients with FUO, and was found to be clinically helpful in 33% of cases. In that study, FDG PET contributed more often to the final diagnosis in patients with continuous than periodic fever, and was not helpful in patients with normal ESR and CRP [68].

With its current widespread availability, hybrid PET/CT scanners could facilitate the usefulness of FDG imaging in patients with FUO by allowing anatomic localization of increased uptake leading to better achievement of a final diagnosis. Federici et al. evaluated the value of FDG PET/CT in 14 hospitalized patients with FUO or unexplained prolonged inflammatory syndrome [69]. A diagnosis was reached in 88% and 50% of patients with abnormal and normal PET/CT findings, respectively. In this study, however, FDG PET/CT was essential for final diagnosis in only 23% of cases, suggesting its role as a second-level test, when conventional CT is normal or unable to discriminate active from silent lesions [69]. Keidar and coworkers performed a recent prospective study of FDG PET/CT in 48 consecutive patients with FUO [70]. FDG PET/CT detected suggestive foci of increased uptake in 27 patients, which was found to be correct in 22 cases. The identified underlying disease was infection in nine patients, inflammatory process in 10, and malignancy in three. All 21 patients with negative PET/CT had a systemic nonfocal infection or drug-induced fever, or showed spontaneous resolution of the febrile state [70]. A recent study investigated the value of FDG PET/CT using whole diagnostic contrast enhanced CT in FUO [71]. Among 48 patients, the cause was explained in 44 cases; 18 microbial infections, nine autoimmune inflammations, four noninfectious granulomatous diseases, eight malignancies, and five immunity disorders. In 46 cases, the PET/CT interpretation was correct. The cause was overlooked in one case, and uptake in atherosclerotic change was misinterpreted as vasculitis in another case. The reached sensitivity was 97% and specificity was 75% [71].

Although there is relatively limited data on the precise clinical role of FDG PET in FUO, available data indicate that it could play a role as a second-line procedure contributing to the final diagnosis in about one third to one half of patients. In the category of infectious diseases, focal abdominal-thoracic or soft-tissue infections, or chronic osteomyelitis can be diagnosed using FDG PET with a high degree of certainty. Negative findings using FDG PET essentially rule out orthopedic prosthetic infection. In noninfectious inflammation, FDG PET can detect large-vessel vasculitis and can visualize such diseases as inflammatory bowel disease and sarcoidosis. FDG PET is highly sensitive in detecting many diseases in the category of neoplasm, including lymphoma, colorectal cancer, and sarcoma. Because of favorable characteristics of FDG PET, conventional scintigraphic techniques can be replaced by FDG PET in institutions in where PET is available. Hybrid PET/CT scanners will improve the diagnostic impact of FDG imaging even further. Exactly how FDG PET/CT should be implemented into an evidence-based diagnostic algorithm for FUO will need to be resolved with the accumulation of additional prospective data analyzed without selection bias.

Inflammatory Bowel Disease

Intense colonic FDG uptake can be seen in such nonmalignant pathologic processes as acute enterocolitis (Fig. 30.4), pseudomembranous colitis, and inflammatory bowel disease (IBD) [72]. IBD is a group of diseases that cause inflammation in either or both small and large bowels. Crohn's disease and ulcerative colitis are the best-known forms. The chronicity and unpredictability of IBD makes it a difficult disease to treat; therefore, early

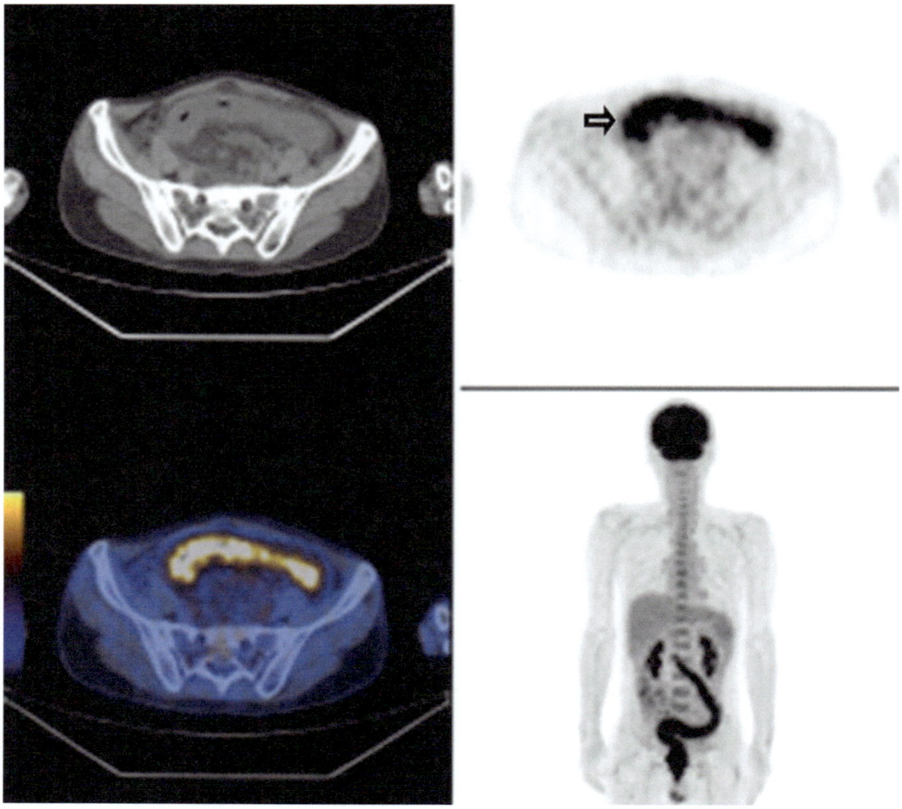

Fig. 30.4 A 57-year-old male who had a history of previous left hemicolectomy for colon cancer was admitted for abdominal pain and diarrhea. FDG PET/CT scan showed intense uptake (*arrow*; peak SUV, 8.6) in a long segment of the rectosigmoidal colon. The patient was diagnosed as having ischemic colitis by clinical workup

detection is essential in developing patient confidence and cooperation. Imaging techniques can aid in the diagnosis of IBD, a process that is essentially one of exclusion, as well as for determining disease activity, which can be clinically important for making appropriate treatment plans. Leukocyte scintigraphy is useful in evaluating the disease activity of IBD, but is time consuming and requires blood handling.

Active inflammatory lesions in Crohn's disease or ulcerative colitis have increased glucose consumption allowing visualization using FDG PET. PET studies in IBD include the incidental identification of IBD during studies performed for other indications, the evaluation of suspected IBD, and the assessment of known IBD. Thus, FDG PET can be used to identify active inflammation in IBD [73]. In an early study by Bicik et al., six patients with Crohn's disease or ulcerative colitis prospectively underwent endoscopy and FDG PET. PET showed high glucose uptake in histologically confirmed areas of inflammation, which was higher with clinically active disease [74]. Additionally, FDG PET was recently investigated for its findings in patients with quiescent ulcerative colitis in a remission state. Among 10 patients, four had increased FDG uptake in the colonic or ileal uptake despite negative endoscopic, histologic, and symptom assessment. This has important implications in the understanding of ulcerative colitis disease quiescence [75].

Children who are suspected of having IBD require particularly noninvasive diagnostic tools that depict localization and acuity of inflammation. FDG PET was shown to be a useful adjunct to colonoscopy and barium studies in 18 young patients with IBD and seven with nonspecific abdominal pain or diarrhea. The overall sensitivity of PET for detecting IBD was 81% and a specificity of 85%. On a segment-by-segment basis, PET correctly identified active disease in 76% of individual bowel segments, with a sensitivity and specificity of 71% and 81%, respectively [76]. In another study of 23 young patients with suspected IBD, FDG PET showed a sensitivity of 98%, specificity of 68%, and accuracy of 83% with histology as reference. FDG PET was even more reliable for the small bowel [77]. These studies indicate that high sensitivity and accuracy allows FDG PET to be an attractive noninvasive tool for depicting bowel inflammation in children and young patients.

PET/CT can provide structural information regarding FDG uptake sites that help identify regions of active inflammation in IBD with anatomic accuracy. This was demonstrated in a prospective study by Meisner et al. who performed FDG PET/CT on 12 patients experiencing exacerbation of IBD; seven with Crohn's disease and five with ulcerative colitis [78]. In ulcerative colitis patients, FDG activity was seen in 13 of 24 regions, and there was 96% correlation between FDG activity and clinical indicators of disease activity. In Crohn's disease patients, FDG activity was seen in 19 of 32 regions, and again, there was 81% correlation between FDG and clinical disease activity. These findings indicate that FDG PET/CT can be used to monitor inflammation activity in IBD [78]. The role of FDG PET/CT in patients with Crohn's disease for differentiating acute transmural inflammatory stenoses was also evaluated. FDG PET/CT was prospectively performed in 17 Crohn's disease patients scheduled to undergo surgical resection for obstructive symptoms. Of the 13 patients who underwent surgery, 12 had histopathologic correlation. Acute and chronic inflammation, fibrosis, and muscle hypertrophy were found in all patients. FDG uptake was higher in severe chronic inflammation and no patient with predominant fibrosis or muscle hypertrophy had a high uptake level. These findings indicate that FDG PET helps identify Crohn's disease patients with active inflammation and may provide helpful information in deciding surgery for patients with obstructive symptoms [79]. In a recent study, the ability of repeat FDG PET/CT for monitoring of improvement of disease activity with was investigated before and after successful medical therapy in five patients with moderately active IBD [80]. All patients showed significant clinical improvement. Repeat PET/CT showed a significant improvement in the total score of all segments from 32 pretreatment to 14 posttreatment. Of 11 pretreatment active segments, nine segments became inactive or displayed decreased activity. Thus, appropriate PET/CT quantification demonstrates decreased FDG uptake with successful treatment in active IBD and correlates with symptom improvement [80].

Available evidence to date indicates FDG PET as having excellent sensitivity for detecting active bowel inflammation in suspected or known IBD. It can be especially useful in children for early evaluation of suspected IBD who may not tolerate an invasive test such as colonoscopy. It also appears useful in known IBD patients for differentiating between inflammatory flares from noninflammatory processes. Furthermore, as the magnitude of FDG accumulation appears to correlate with disease activity, FDG PET can be a useful aid in long-term monitoring or assessment of therapeutic efficacy in patients with IBD. In view of the physiologic intestinal FDG activity seen in subjects without abdominal disease, however, it is probably important to avoid potential false-positive interpretations of bowel activity.

Pulmonary Infection and Inflammation

Active infection or inflammation in the lungs often displays high FDG uptake that can be difficult to differentiate from malignancy or metastases [81]. Pneumonia typically appears on FDG PET as segmental or lobar uptake lesions (Fig. 30.5) [82, 83]. Thus, FDG uptakes that are

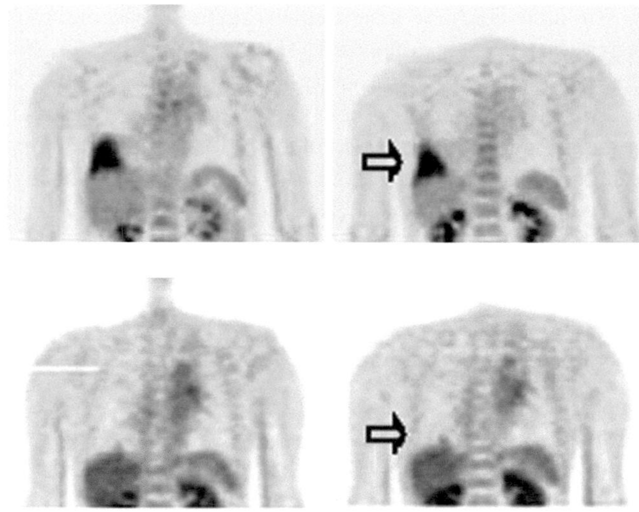

Fig. 30.5 (**a**) FDG PET in a case with acute bacterial pneumonia demonstrates intense segmental FDG uptake in the right lower lung (*arrow*). (**b**) FDG uptake normalized on follow-up examination after antibiotic therapy (*arrow*)

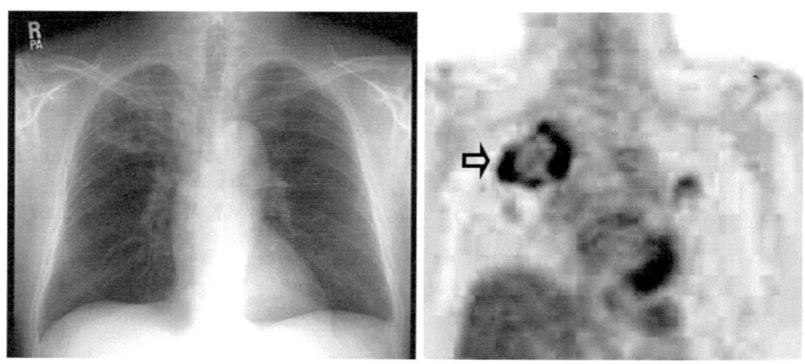

Fig. 30.6 (**a**) Chest radiograph of a patient undergoing evaluation of esophageal cancer showed active pulmonary tuberculosis in the right upper lung. (**b**) FDG PET scan demonstrates intense uneven FDG uptake in the lung lesion (*arrow*)

apical, segmental, or lobar in distribution can readily be identified as infectious lesions. The magnitudes of FDG in infectious lesions are generally lower than that of cancers. However, organizing bacterial pneumonia lesions often show substantially elevated uptake levels comparable with those of malignancies [84, 85].

Tuberculosis is an infectious disease caused primarily by *Myocbacterium tuberculosis* that usually attacks the lungs, although other parts of the body can be affected. Radiographs are relied on for diagnosis, as well as microscopic examination and culture of bodily fluids. In endemic regions, tuberculosis is a common cause for false-positive PET findings because lesions have robust FDG accumulation that mimics malignancy (Fig. 30.6) [86, 87]. FDG PET may show activities and extents of infection not demonstrable by chest radiographs or CT images, and may thus be useful in the assessment of disease activity of tuberculosis. In patients with known pulmonary tuberculosis, intense uptake of lung lesions on FDG PET indicates acute active and open stages [88]. FDG PET may also have the potential for monitoring response to antituberculosis treatment, where metabolic response could indicate clinical response and guide duration of antimicrobial therapy [89].

Pulmonary areas of high glycolysis rate can also reflect inflammatory activity of interstitial lung disease. A prospective study investigated FDG PET in 21 patients referred for lung biopsy because of diffuse interstitial lung disease. The results showed a tendency for the 14 patients with idiopathic pulmonary fibrosis to have higher FDG uptake levels, although this did not reach statistical significance [90]. In a more recent study, Umeda et al. applied dual-time-point FDG PET in 50 patients with idiopathic interstitial pneumonia, including 21 cases with idiopathic pulmonary fibrosis, 18 with nonspecific interstitial pneumonia, and 11 with cryptogenic organizing pneumonia [91]. Early FDG uptake value was higher for the organizing pneumonia group and the accuracy for distinguishing the group was sensitivity, specificity, and accuracy of 91%, 94% and 94%, respectively. Late FDG uptake values in the first two groups were significantly higher in patients with deteriorated pulmonary function after 1 year of follow-up [91]. These studies suggest that FDG uptake levels can be useful for the differential diagnosis and prediction of disease progression in patients with idiopathic interstitial pneumonia.

Sarcoidosis

Sarcoidosis is a chronic systemic disorder of unknown cause that most frequently affects the lung, although virtually any organ can be involved. Significant FDG uptake is observed in both thoracic lesions and lymphadenopathy from sarcoidosis [92–94]. Increased FDG uptake in the mediastinal lymph nodes affected by sarcoidosis is often comparable with malignant lymphoma or lymph node metastases [95], which can lead to false-positive interpretation as malignancy.

Gallium scintigraphy has been successfully used to diagnose and stage sarcoidosis. Comparison of the uptake of FDG and Ga-67 citrate was evaluated in 18 patients with pulmonary and extrapulmonary sarcoidosis. Gallium scan detected 17 of 21 pulmonary and 15 of 31 extrapulmonary sites, while FDG PET detected all 21 pulmonary and 28 of 31 extrapulmonary sites [96]. In another study of 24 patients with histologically proved thoracic sarcoidosis, gallium scan detected a total of 64 lesions with a mean of 2.6 lesions per patient, while FDG PET detected a total of 85 lesions with 3.5 lesions per patient. The interobserver variability showed a kappa value of 0.79 [97]. These studies indicate that FDG PET may allow a more accurate evaluation of thoracic and extrapulmonary sarcoidosis.

Brudin et al. measured regional glucose metabolism rates from FDG PET in seven patients with histologically proven sarcoidosis, which returned to normal in those patients treated with high-dose steroids [98]. Theirs was the first study to suggest that FDG PET could be useful for evaluating disease activity in sarcoidosis [98]. In a study evaluating longitudinal changes in FDG PET in a patient with pulmonary sarcoidosis receiving corticosteroid therapy, initial PET showed high FDG uptake in the hilar and mediastinal lymph nodes and a high focal uptake in the peripheral lungs. Although there was no significant change in FDG uptakes by treatment with inhaled corticosteroids, PET following treatment with systemic corticosteroids showed complete normalization of FDG uptake [99]. Braun et al. retrospectively evaluated FDG PET/CT findings in 20 consecutive patients with biopsy-proved sarcoidosis; 13 had thoracic sarcoidosis and seven had extrathoracic sarcoidosis [100]. As a result, the sensitivity of FDG PET/CT for localizing thoracic, sinonasal, and pharyngolaryngeal lesions was 100%, 100%, and 80%, respectively. Follow-up PET/CT was performed on five patients after corticosteroid treatment. Complete regression of all foci of pathologic tracer uptake was exhibited in two cases permitting corticosteroid withdrawal. Improvement of incomplete regression of mediastinopulmonary disease occurred in two patients, and disease progression was assessed in one patient [100]. A recent study correlated pre- and posttherapy FDG PET with standard disease activity parameters in 12 patients with refractory sarcoidosis during infliximab treatment. All patients showed clinical improvement by conventional parameters although in one case to only a minor degree. Symptoms improved in 11 of 12 patients although chest radiographic stages did not change. FDG PET revealed either improvement or normalization in 11 of 12 clinically responding patients. Peak standardized uptake value (SUV) decreased 55% overall but increased 34% in the patient with a limited response. Changes imaged using FDG PET during infliximab treatment in patients with sarcoidosis correlated with signs of clinical improvement to a considerate extent [101]. Aide et al. showed that a reduction in FDG uptake in response to 2 weeks of oral corticosteroids can also provide diagnostic information for discriminating sarcoidosis from cancer [102].

The imaging features of sarcoidosis are diverse and can be seen using a variety of imaging techniques. It is important for physicians in the imaging field to recognize the common imaging features and patterns of sarcoidosis in order to raise the possibility in the appropriate clinical setting. While PET does not currently appear to have a major role for diagnosing sarcoidosis, it can be useful for assessing inflammatory activity and treatment effects in known patients.

Acquired Immunodeficiency Syndrome

Human immunodeficiency virus (HIV) primarily infects and kills helper T cells, macrophages, and dendritic cells. Therefore, patients with acquired immunodeficiency syndrome (AIDS) whose helper T cell numbers decline below a critical level, cell-mediated immunity is lost, and the body becomes progressively more susceptible to opportunistic infections including cytomegalovirus, *Cryptococcus neoformans*, and tuberculosis. Malignancies are also increased including HIV-associated lymphoma as a result of Epstein-Barr virus, Kaposi's sarcoma-associated herpes virus, and anogenital cancer as a result of the human papilloma virus. Because of the variety of the types of infection that occur in patients with AIDS, it is essential to determine the nature of the underlying infection before effective therapy is instituted. FDG PET can be used to detect opportunistic infections and malignancies in AIDS patients. A major role of FDG PET is to detect the correct location for initiating further procedures such as biopsy, aspiration, or other diagnostic modalities. FDG PET has been shown to successfully localize infection sites caused by pseudomonas, mycobacteria, cryptococcal, and staphylococcal microorganisms in AIDS patients.

O'Doherty et al. evaluated FDG PET findings in 80 patients with AIDS and FUO, confusion, and/or weight loss [103]. Half-body PET performed on 57 patients had a sensitivity of 92% and a specificity of 94% for localization of focal pathology that needed treatment. Patients with a variety of infections had disease localized for appropriate biopsy or sampling, and nodal and extranodal sites were identified in 13 patients with lymphoma. Brain PET performed in 23 cases showed abnormalities in all 19 patients with MRI identified focal space occupying lesions103. Caution was required, however, so that lymph node uptake in patients with generalized lymphadenopathy were not mistaken for lymphoma. In a recent study using FDG PET/CT in AIDS patients suffering from FUO, results were abnormal and helpful for diagnosis in nine of 10 cases [104]. Tuberculosis infection was diagnosed in six patients; two cases had lymphoma and one had Kaposi's sarcoma. FDG PET/CT directly suggested sites for biopsy in six patients. The remaining single patient with normal PET/CT had drug-induced fever [104].

The incidence of primary central nervous system lymphomas [105] is increased several thousand-fold in AIDS patients, but differentiation from toxoplasmosis infection is difficult because both appear as ring-enhancing lesions. FDG PET can detect lymphomas with high sensitivity and can be separated from toxoplasmosis lesions that have lower FDG accumulation. Thus, FDG PET has been proposed to differentiate brain lymphoma and opportunistic infections in AIDS, and may obviate the need for brain biopsy in suspected patients [106–108].

Conclusion

FDG PET is rapidly evolving to becoming very sensitive for the detection and localization of a variety of infectious and inflammatory diseases. PET has theoretical and practical advantages over other scintigraphic methods such as leukocyte scan or gallium scintigraphy. It is becoming more and more evident that FDG PET imaging can play a major role in the evaluation of patients with suspected infection or inflammation, in whom other imaging modalities are inconclusive. PET has been shown to be particularly valuable in the evaluation of chronic osteomyelitis, infected prostheses, sarcoidosis, and fever of unknown origin. PET imaging used to detect and characterize infection and inflammation will increasingly contribute to our understanding of these disorders and may well become a major clinical indication in the day-to-day practice of medicine.

References

1. Ma LD, Frassica FJ, Bluemke DA, Fishman EK. CT and MRI evaluation of musculoskeletal infection. Crit Rev Diagn Imaging. 1997;38:535–68.
2. Alazraki NP. Radionuclide imaging in the evaluation of infections and inflammatory disease. Radiol Clin North Am. 1993;31:783–94.
3. Sugawara Y, Braun DK, Kison PV, Russo JE, Zasadny KR, Wahl RL. Rapid detection of human infections with fluorine-18 fluorodeoxyglucose and positron emission tomography: preliminary results. Eur J Nucl Med. 1998;25(9):1238–43.
4. Kubota R, Yamada S, Kubota K, Ishiwata K, Tamahashi N, Ido T. Intratumoral distribution of fluorine-18-fluorodeoxygolucose in vivo: high accumulation in macrophages and granulation tissues studies by microautoradiography. J Nucl Med. 1992;33:1872–980.
5. Ishimori T, Saga T, Mamede M, Kobayashi H, Higashi T, Nakamoto Y, Sato N, Konishi J. Increased ^{18}F-FDG uptake in a model of inflammation: Concanavalin A-mediated lymphocyte activation. J Nucl Med. 2002;43:658–63.
6. Yamada S, Kubota K, Kubota R, Ido T, Tamahashi N. High accumulation of fluorine-18-fluorodeoxyglucose in turpentine-induced inflammatory tissue. J Nucl Med. 1995;36:1301–6.
7. Nakamoto Y, Higashi T, Sakahara H, et al. Delayed FDG-PET scan for the differentiation between malignant and benign lesions. J Nucl Med. 1999; 36:1301–6.
8. Weisdorf DJ, Craddock PR, Jacob HS. Glycogenolysis versus glucose transport in human granulocytes: differential activation in phagocytosis and chemotaxis. Blood. 1982;60:888–93.
9. Ahmed N, Kansara M, Berridge MV. Acute regulation of glucose transport in a monocyte-macrophage cell line: Glut-3 affinity for glucose is enhanced during the respiratory burst. Biochem J. 1997;327: 369–75.
10. Tan AS, Ahmed N, Berridge MV. Acute regulation of glucose transport after activation of human peripheral blood neutrophils by phorbol myristate acetate, fMLP, and granulocyte-macrophage colony-stimulating factor. Blood. 1998;91:649–55.
11. Paik JY, Ko BH, Choe YS, Choi Y, Lee KH, Kim BT. PMA-enhanced neutrophil [^{18}F]FDG uptake is independent of integrin occupancy but requires PI3K activity. Nucl Med Biol. 2005;32:561–6.
12. Jones HA, Cadwallader KA, White JF, Uddin M, Peters AM, Chilvers ER. Dissociation between respiratory burst activity and deoxyglucose uptake in human neutrophil granulocytes: implications for interpretation of ^{18}F-FDG PET images. J Nucl Med. 2002;43:652–7.
13. Schuster DP, Brody SL, Zhou Z, Bernstein M, Arch R, Link D, Mueckler M. Regulation of lipopolysaccharide-induced increases in neutrophil glucose uptake. Am J Physiol Lung Cell Mol Physiol. 2007;292:L845–51.
14. Fukuzumi M, Shinomiya H, Shimizu Y, Ohishi K, Utsumi S. Endotoxin-induced enhancement of glucose influx into murine peritoneal macrophages via GLUT1. Infect Immun. 1996;64:108–12.
15. Paik JY, Lee KH, Choe YS, Choi Y, Kim BT. Augmented ^{18}F-FDG uptake in activated monocytes occurs during the priming process and involves tyrosine kinases and protein kinase C. J Nucl Med. 2004;45:124–8.
16. Chakrabarti R, Jung CY, Lee TP, Liu H, Mookerjee BK. Changes in glucose transport and transporter isoforms during the activation of human peripheral blood lymphocytes by phytohemagglutinin. J Immunol. 1994;152:2660–8.
17. Paik J-Y, Lee K-H, Byun S-S, Choe YS, Kim B-T. Usefulness of insulin to improve F-18 FDG labeling and retention for in vivo PET imaging of monocyte trafficking. Nucl Med Commun. 2002;23:551–7.
18. Zhuang HM, Cortés-Blanco A, Pourdehnad M, Adam LE, Yamamoto AJ, Martínez-Lázaro R, Lee JH, Loman JC, Rossman MD, Alavi A. Do high glucose levels have differential effect on FDG uptake in inflammatory and malignant disorders? Nucl Med Commun. 2001;22:1123–8.
19. Merkel KD, Brown ML, Dewanjee MK, Fitzgerald RH. Comparison of indium-labeled leukocyte imaging with sequential technetium-gallium scanning in the diagnosis of low-grade musculoskeletal sepsis. J Bone Joint Surg. 1985;67A:465–76.
20. Al-Sheik W, Sfakianakis GN, Mnaymneh W, Hourani M, Heal A, Duncan RC, Burnett A, Ashkar FS, Serafini AN. Subacute and chronic bone infections: diagnosis using In-111, Ga-67 and Tc-99 m MDP bone scintigraphy, and radiology. Radiology. 1985;155:501–6.
21. Plestro JP. The current role of gallium imaging in infection. Semin Nucl Med. 1994;24:128–41.

22. Datz FL. Indium-111 labeled leukocytes for the detection of infection: current status. Semin Nucl Med. 1994;24:92–109.
23. Palestro CJ, Kim CK, Swyer AJ, Vallabhajosula S, Goldsmith SJ. Radionuclide diagnosis of vertebral osteomyelitis: indium-111-leukocyte and technetium-99m-methylene diphosphonate bone scintigraphy. J Nucl Med. 1991;32(10):1861–5.
24. Stumpe KD, Dazzi H, Schaffner A, von Schulthess GK. Infection imaging using whole-body FDG-PET. Eur J Nucl Med. 2000;27:822–32.
25. Guhlmann A, Brecht-Krauss D, Suger G, Glatting G, Kotzerke J, Kinzl L, Reske SN. Chronic osteomyelitis: detection with FDG PET and correlation with histopathologic findings. Radiology. 1998;206(3): 749–54.
26. Guhlmann A, Brecht-Krauss D, Suger G, Glatting G, Kotzerke J, Kinzl L, Reske SN. Fluorine-18-FDG PET and technetium-99 m antigranulocyte antibody scintigraphy in chronic osteomyelitis. J Nucl Med. 1998;39(12):2145–52.
27. de Winter F, van de Wiele C, Vogelaers D, de Smet K, Verdonk R, Dierckx RA. Fluorine-18 fluorodeoxyglucose-position emission tomography: a highly accurate imaging modality for the diagnosis of chronic musculoskeletal infections. J Bone Joint Surg Am. 2001;83-A(5):651–60.
28. Schmitz A, Kalicke T, Willkomm P, Grunwald F, Kandyba J, Schmitt O. Use of fluorine-18 fluoro-2-deoxy-D-glucose positron emission tomography in assessing the process of tuberculous spondylitis. J Spinal Disord. 2000;13(6):541–4.
29. Ho AY, Pagliuca A, Maisey MN, Mufti GJ. Positron emission scanning with ^{18}F-FDG in the diagnosis of deep fungal infections. Br J Haematol. 1998;101: 392–3.
30. Kalicke T, Schmitz A, Risse JH, Arens S, Keller E, Hansis M, Schmitt O, Biersack HJ, Grunwald F. Fluorine-18 fluorodeoxyglucose PET in infectious bone diseases: results of histologically confirmed cases. Eur J Nucl Med. 2000;27:524–8.
31. Zhuang H, Duarte PS, Pourdehand M, Shnier D, Alavi A. Exclusion of chronic osteomyelitis with F-18 fluorodeoxyglucose positron emission tomographic imaging. Clin Nucl Med. 2000;25(4):281–4.
32. Hartmann A, Eid K, Dora C, Trentz O, von Schulthess GK, Stumpe KD. Diagnostic value of 18F-FDG PET/CT in trauma patients with suspected chronic osteomyelitis. Eur J Nucl Med Mol Imaging. 2007;34:704–14.
33. Termaat MF, Raijmakers PG, Scholten HJ, Bakker FC, Patka P, Haarman HJ. The accuracy of diagnostic imaging for the assessment of chronic osteomyelitis: a systematic review and meta-analysis. J Bone Joint Surg Am. 2005;87(11):2464–71.
34. Smith SL, Wastie ML, Forster I. Radionuclide bone scintigraphy in the detection of significant complications after total knee joint replacement. Clin Radiol. 2001;56(3):221–4.
35. Merkel KD, Brown ML, Fitzgerald Jr RH. Sequential technetium-99 m HMDP gallium-67 citrate imaging for the evaluation of infection in the painful prosthesis. J Nucl Med. 1986;27:1413–7.
36. Kraemer WJ, Saplys R, Waddell JP, Morton J. Bone scan, gallium scan, and hip aspiration in the diagnosis of infected total hip arthroplasty. J Arthroplasty. 1993;8(6):611–6.
37. Scher DM, Pak K, Lonner JH, et al. The predictive value of indium-111 leukocyte scans in the diagnosis of infected total hip, knee, or resection arthroplasties. J Arthroplasty. 2000;15:295–300.
38. Temmerman OP, Heyligers IC, Hoekstra OS, Comans EF, Roos JC. Detection of osteomyelitis using FDG and positron emission tomography. J Arthroplasty. 2001;16(2):243–6.
39. Zhuang H, Duarte PS, Pourdehnad M, Maes A, Van Acker F, Shnier D, Garino JP, Fitzgerald RH, Alavi A. The promising role of ^{18}F-FDG PET in detecting infected lower limb prosthesis implants. J Nucl Med. 2001;42(1):44–8.
40. Zoccali C, Teori G, Salducca N. The role of FDG-PET in distinguishing between septic and aseptic loosening in hip prosthesis: a review of literature. Int Orthop. 2009;33(1):1–5.
41. Zhuang H, Alavi A. F-18-fluorodeoxyglucose positron emission tomographic imaging in the detection and monitoring of infection and inflammation. Semin Nucl Med. 2002;32(1):47–59.
42. Van Acker F, Nuyts J, Maes A, Vanquickenborne B, Stuyck J, Bellemans J, Vleugels S, Bormans G, Mortelmans L. FDG-PET, ^{99m}Tc-HMPAO white blood cell SPET and bone scintigraphy in the evaluation of painful total knee arthroplasties. Eur J Nucl Med. 2001;28(10):1496–504.
43. Heiba SI, Luo JQ, Sadek S, Macalental E, Cacavio A, Rosen G, Abdel-Dayem HA. Attenuation correction induced artifact in F-18 FDG PET imaging following total knee replacement. Clin Positron Imaging. 2000;3:237–9.
44. Johnston SL, Lock RJ, Gompels MM. Takayasu arteritis: a review. J Clin Pathol. 2002;55(7):481–6.
45. Angeli E, Vanzulli A, Venturini M, Zoccai GB, Del Maschio A. The role of radiology in the diagnosis and management of Takayasu's arteritis. J Nephrol. 2001;14(6):514–24.
46. Peters AM. Nuclear medicine in vasculitis. Rheumatology. 2000;39:463–70.
47. Jonker N, Peters AM, Gaskin G, Pusey CD, Lavender JP. A retrospective study of granulocyte kinetics in patients with systemic vasculitis. J Nucl Med. 1992;33:491–7.
48. Reuter H, Wraight EP, Qasim FJ, Lockwood CM. Management of systemic vasculitis: contribution of scintigraphic imaging to evaluation of disease activity and classification. Q J Med. 1995;88:509–16.
49. Walter MA. [^{18}F]fluorodeoxyglucose PET in large vessel vasculitis. Radiol Clin North Am. 2007; 45(4):735–44.

50. Blockmans D, Maes A, Stroobants S, Nuyts J, Bormans G, Knockaert D, Bobbaers H, Mortelmans L. New arguments for a vasculitic nature of polymyalgia rheumatica using positron emission tomography. Rheumatology (Oxford). 1999;38(5): 444–7.
51. Blockmans D, Stroobants S, Maes A, Mortelmans L. Positron emission tomography in giant cell arteritis and polymyalgia rheumatica: evidence for inflammation of the aortic arch. Am J Med. 2000; 108(3):246–9.
52. Turlakow A, Yeung HW, Pui J, Macapinlac H, Liebovitz E, Rusch V, Goy A, Larson SM. Fluorodeoxyglucose positron emission tomography in the diagnosis of giant cell arteritis. Arch Intern Med. 2001;161(7):1003–7.
53. Blockmans D. The use of (^{18}F)fluoro-deoxyglucose positron emission tomography in the assessment of large vessel vasculitis. Clin Exp Rheumatol. 2003;21(6 Suppl 32):S15–22.
54. Hara M, Goodman PC, Leder RA. FDG-PET finding in early-phase Takayasu arteritis. J Comput Assist Tomogr. 1999;23(1):16–8.
55. Belhocine T, Blockmans D, Hustinx R, Vandevivere J, Mortelmans L. Imaging of large vessel vasculitis with ([18])FDG PET: illusion or reality? A critical review of the literature data. Eur J Nucl Med Mol Imaging. 2003;30(9):1305–13.
56. Webb M, Al-Nahhas A. Molecular imaging of Takayasu's arteritis and other large-vessel vasculitis with 18F-FDG PET. Nucl Med Commun. 2006; 27(7):547–9.
57. Steňová E, Mištec S, Povinec P. FDG-PET/CT in large-vessel vasculitis: its diagnostic and follow-up role. Rheumatol Int. 2010; 30(8):1111–4.
58. Walter MA, Melzer RA, Schindler C, Müller-Brand J, Tyndall A, Nitzsche EU. The value of [^{18}F]FDG-PET in the diagnosis of large-vessel vasculitis and the assessment of activity and extent of disease. Eur J Nucl Med Mol Imaging. 2005;32(6):674–81.
59. Otsuka H, Morita N, Yamashita K, Nishitani H. FDG-PET/CT for diagnosis and follow-up of vasculitis. J Med Invest. 2007;54(3–4):345–9.
60. Henes JC, Müller M, Krieger J, Balletshofer B, Pfannenberg AC, Kanz L, Kötter I. [^{18}F] FDG-PET/CT as a new and sensitive imaging method for the diagnosis of large vessel vasculitis. Clin Exp Rheumatol. 2008;26(3 Suppl 49):S47–52.
61. Kok J, Lin M, Patapanian H, Shingde M, Lin P, Chu J. [^{18}F]FDG PET/CT in the diagnosis of large vessel vasculitis. Intern Med J. 2009;39(4):267–9.
62. Meller J, Becker W. Nuclear medicine diagnosis of patients with fever of unknown origin. Nuklearmedizin. 2001;40(3):59–70.
63. Peters AM. The use of nuclear medicine in infections. Br J Radiol. 1998;71(843):252–61.
64. Lorenzen J, Buchert R, Bohuslavizki KH. Value of FDG PET in patients with fever of unknown origin. Nucl Med Commun. 2001;22(7):779–83.
65. Blockmans D, Knockaert D, Maes A, De Caestecker J, Stroobants S, Bobbaers H, Mortelmans L. Clinical value of [^{18}F]fluoro-deoxyglucose positron emission tomography for patients with fever of unknown origin. Clin Infect Dis. 2001;32(2):191–6.
66. Kjaer A, Lebech AM, Eigtved A, Højgaard L. Fever of unknown origin: prospective comparison of diagnostic value of ^{18}F-FDG PET and 111In-granulocyte scintigraphy. Eur J Nucl Med Mol Imaging. 2004; 31(5):622–6.
67. Buysschaert I, Vanderschueren S, Blockmans D, Mortelmans L, Knockaert D. Contribution of ([18])fluoro-deoxyglucose positron emission tomography to the work-up of patients with fever of unknown origin. Eur J Intern Med. 2004;15(3):151–6.
68. Bleeker-Rovers CP, Vos FJ, Mudde AH, Dofferhoff AS, de Geus-Oei LF, Rijnders AJ, Krabbe PF, Corstens FH, van der Meer JW, Oyen WJ. A prospective multi-centre study of the value of FDG-PET as part of a structured diagnostic protocol in patients with fever of unknown origin. Eur J Nucl Med Mol Imaging. 2007;34(5):694–703.
69. Federici L, Blondet C, Imperiale A, Sibilia J, Pasquali JL, Pflumio F, Goichot B, Blaison G, Weber JC, Christmann D, Constantinesco A, Andrès E. Value of ([18])F-FDG-PET/CT in patients with fever of unknown origin and unexplained prolonged inflammatory syndrome: a single centre analysis experience. Int J Clin Pract. 2010; 64(1): 55–60.
70. Keidar Z, Gurman-Balbir A, Gaitini D, Israel O. Fever of unknown origin: the role of 18F-FDG PET/CT. J Nucl Med. 2008;49(12):1980–5.
71. Ferda J, Ferdová E, Záhlava J, Matějovič M, Kreuzberg B. Fever of unknown origin: a value of ([18])F-FDG-PET/CT with integrated full diagnostic isotropic CT imaging. Eur J Radiol. 2010; 73(3): 518–25.
72. Tatlidil R, Jadvar H, Bading JR, Conti PS. Incidental colonic fluorodeoxyglucose uptake: correlation with colonoscopic and histopathologic findings. Radiology. 2002;224(3):783–7.
73. Spier BJ, Perlman SB, Reichelderfer M. FDG-PET in inflammatory bowel disease. Q J Nucl Med Mol Imaging. 2009;53(1):64–71.
74. Bicik I, Bauerfeind P, Breitbach T, von Schulthess GK, Fried M. Inflammatory bowel disease activity measured by positron-emission tomography. Lancet. 1997;350(9073):262.
75. Rubin DT, Surma BL, Gavzy SJ, Schnell KM, Bunnag AP, Huo D, Appelbaum DE. Positron emission tomography (PET) used to image subclinical inflammation associated with ulcerative colitis (UC) in remission. Inflamm Bowel Dis. 2009;15(5):750–5.
76. Skehan SJ, Issenman R, Mernagh J, Nahmias C, Jacobson K. ^{18}F-fluorodeoxyglucose positron tomography in diagnosis of pediatric inflammatory bowel disease. Lancet. 1999;354(9181):836–7.

77. Löffler M, Weckesser M, Franzius C, Schober O, Zimmer KP. High diagnostic value of ^{18}F-FDG-PET in pediatric patients with chronic inflammatory bowel disease. Ann N Y Acad Sci. 2006;1072:379–85.
78. Meisner RS, Spier BJ, Einarsson S, Roberson EN, Perlman SB, Bianco JA, Taylor AJ, Einstein M, Jaskowiak CJ, Massoth KM, Reichelderfer M. Pilot study using PET/CT as a novel, noninvasive assessment of disease activity in inflammatory bowel disease. Inflamm Bowel Dis. 2007;13(8):993–1000.
79. Jacene HA, Ginsburg P, Kwon J, Nguyen GC, Montgomery EA, Bayless TM, Wahl RL. Prediction of the need for surgical intervention in obstructive Crohn's disease by ^{18}F-FDG PET/CT. J Nucl Med. 2009;50(11):1751–9.
80. Spier BJ, Perlman SB, Jaskowiak CJ, Reichelderfer M. PET/CT in the evaluation of inflammatory bowel disease: studies in patients before and after treatment. Mol Imaging Biol. 2010; 12(1):85–8.
81. Bakheet SM, Saleem M, Powe J, Al-Amro A, Larsson SG, Mahassin Z. F-18 fluorodeoxyglucose chest uptake in lung inflammation and infection. Clin Nucl Med. 2000;25(4):273–8.
82. Jones HA, Clark RJ, Rhodes CG, Schofield JB, Krausz T, Haslett C. Positron emission tomography of ^{18}FDG uptake in localized pulmonary inflammation. Acta Radiol Suppl. 1991;376:148.
83. Goswami GK, Jana S, Santiago JF, Buyukdereli G, Salem SS, Heiba S, Abdel-Dayem HM. Discrepancy between Ga-67 citrate and F-18 fluorodeoxyglucose positron emission tomographic scans in pulmonary infection. Clin Nucl Med. 2000;25(6):490–1.
84. Kapucu LO, Meltzer CC, Townsend DW, Keenan RJ, Luketich JD. Fluorine-18-fluorodeoxyglucose uptake in pneumonia. J Nucl Med. 1998;39(7):1267–9.
85. Tateishi U, Hasegawa T, Seki K, Terauchi T, Moriyama N, Arai Y. Disease activity and ^{18}F-FDG uptake in organising pneumonia: semi-quantitative evaluation using computed tomography and positron emission tomography. Eur J Nucl Med Mol Imaging. 2006;33(8):906–12.
86. Bakheet SM, Powe J, Ezzat A, Rostom A. F-18-FDG uptake in tuberculosis. Clin Nucl Med. 1998;23(11):739–42.
87. Goo JM, Im JG, Do KH, Yeo JS, Seo JB, Kim HY, Chung JK. Pulmonary tuberculoma evaluated by means of FDG PET: findings in 10 cases. Radiology. 2000;216(1):117–21.
88. Yang CM, Hsu CH, Lee CM, Wang FC. Intense uptake of [F-18]-fluoro-2 deoxy-D-glucose in active pulmonary tuberculosis. Ann Nucl Med. 2003;17(5):407–10.
89. Hofmeyr A, Lau WF, Slavin MA. *Mycobacterium tuberculosis* infection in patients with cancer, the role of 18-fluorodeoxyglucose positron emission tomography for diagnosis and monitoring treatment response. Tuberculosis (Edinb). 2007;87(5):459–63.
90. Nusair S, Rubinstein R, Freedman NM, Amir G, Bogot NR, Izhar U, Breuer R. Positron emission tomography in interstitial lung disease. Respirology. 2007;12(6):843–7.
91. Umeda Y, Demura Y, Ishizaki T, Ameshima S, Miyamori I, Saito Y, Tsuchida T, Fujibayashi Y, Okazawa H. Dual-time-point ^{18}F-FDG PET imaging for diagnosis of disease type and disease activity in patients with idiopathic interstitial pneumonia. Eur J Nucl Med Mol Imaging. 2009;36(7):1121–30.
92. Gotway MB, Storto ML, Golden JA, Reddy GP, Webb WR. Incidental detection of thoracic sarcoidosis on whole-body ^{18}fluorine-2- fluoro-2-deoxy-D-glucose positron emission tomography. J Thorac Imaging. 2000;15(3):201–4.
93. Lewis PJ, Salama A. Uptake of fluorine-18-fluorodeoxyglucose in sarcoidosis. Nucl Med. 1994;35(10):1647–9.
94. Prabhakar HB, Rabinowitz CB, Gibbons FK, O'Donnell WJ, Shepard JA, Aquino SL. Imaging features of sarcoidosis on MDCT, FDG PET, and PET/CT. AJR Am J Roentgenol. 2008;190(3 Suppl):S1–6.
95. Krüger S, Buck AK, Mottaghy FM, Pauls S, Schelzig H, Hombach V, Reske SN. Use of integrated FDG-PET/CT in sarcoidosis. Clin Imaging. 2008;32(4):269–73.
96. Nishiyama Y, Yamamoto Y, Fukunaga K, Takinami H, Iwado Y, Satoh K, Ohkawa M. Comparative evaluation of ^{18}F-FDG PET and ^{67}Ga scintigraphy in patients with sarcoidosis. J Nucl Med. 2006; 47(10):1571–6.
97. Prager E, Wehrschuetz M, Bisail B, Woltsche M, Schwarz T, Lanz H, Sorantin E, Aigner RM. Comparison of ^{18}F-FDG and ^{67}Ga-citrate in sarcoidosis imaging. Nuklearmedizin. 2008;47(1):18–23.
98. Brudin LH, Valind SO, Rhodes CG, Pantin CF, Sweatman M, Jones T, Hughes JM. Fluorine-18 deoxyglucose uptake in sarcoidosis measured with positron emission tomography. Eur J Nucl Med. 1994;21(4):297–305.
99. Milman N, Mortensen J, Sloth C. Fluorodeoxyglucose PET scan in pulmonary sarcoidosis during treatment with inhaled and oral corticosteroids. Respiration. 2003;70(4):408–13.
100. Braun JJ, Kessler R, Constantinesco A, Imperiale A. 18F-FDG PET/CT in sarcoidosis management: review and report of 20 cases. Eur J Nucl Med Mol Imaging. 2008;35(8):1537–43.
101. Keijsers RG, Verzijlbergen JF, van Diepen DM, van den Bosch JM, Grutters JC. 18F-FDG PET in sarcoidosis: an observational study in 12 patients treated with infliximab. Sarcoidosis Vasc Diffuse Lung Dis. 2008;25(2):143–9.
102. Aide N, Allouache D, Ollivier Y, de Raucourt S, Switsers O, Bardet S. Early 2′-deoxy-2′-[18F]fluoro-D-glucose PET metabolic response after corticosteroid therapy to differentiate cancer from sarcoidosis and sarcoid-like lesions. Mol Imaging Biol. 2009;11(4):224–8.
103. O'Doherty MJ, Barrington SF, Campbell M, Lowe J, Bradbeer CS. PET scanning and the human immunodeficiency virus-positive patient. J Nucl Med. 1997;38(10):1575–83.

104. Castaigne C, Tondeur M, de Wit S, Hildebrand M, Clumeck N, Dusart M. Clinical value of FDG-PET/CT for the diagnosis of human immunodeficiency virus-associated fever of unknown origin: a retrospective study. Nucl Med Commun. 2009;30(1):41–7.
105. Flinn IW, Ambinder RF. AIDS primary central nervous system lymphoma. Curr Opin Oncol. 1996;8(5):37357–66.
106. Hoffman JM, Waskin HA, Schifter T, Hanson MW, Gray L, Rosenfeld S, Coleman RE. FDG-PET in differentiating lymphoma from nonmalignant central nervous system lesions in patients with AIDS. J Nucl Med. 1993;34(4):567–75.
107. Villringer K, Jager H, Dichgans M, Ziegler S, Poppinger J, Herz M, Kruschke C, Minoshima S, Pfister HW, Schwaiger M. Differential diagnosis of CNS lesions in AIDS patients by FDG-PET. J Comput Assist Tomogr. 1995;19(4): 532–6.
108. Heald AE, Hoffman JM, Bartlett JA, Waskin HA. Differentiation of central nervous system lesions in AIDS patients using positron emission tomography (PET). Int J STD AIDS. 1996;7(5): 337–46.

31 Positron Emission Tomography in Radiation Treatment

Sang-Moo Lim and E. Edmund Kim

In the era of image-guided radiation therapy, treatment plans require narrower tumor margins and more attention dedicated to the location and configuration of tumor for better outcomes. Traditional anatomy-based modalities such as plain radiographs, computed tomography (CT), sonography, and magnetic resonance imaging (MRI) that yield high spatial resolution and accurate anatomic localization, are essential for radiation therapy planning, but may significantly under- or overestimate the extent of the disease. Advances in medical imaging, such as portal imaging, ultrasound, cone-beam CT, positron emission tomography (PET), MRI, and new software and hardware systems demonstrate accurate staging, planning, and delivery in radiation therapy with high geometric precision. Functional imaging such as single-photon emission computed tomography (SPECT), PET/CT, and magnetic resonance spectroscopy (MRS) that permit the visualization of the biologic pathways of tumors, are being incorporated into the algorithm for the workup, management, and evaluation of treatment effects in the radiation oncology practice. PET/CT could provide biologic imaging information and modify the clinical staging and target definition from the anatomic imaging. In addition to the concept of gross tumor volume, clinical and planning target volume, biologic target volume and dose painting were introduced [1–3]. This chapter will focus on the role of PET/CT in the staging (sensitivity and specificity), target volume definition, and possible assessment of response to radiation treatment. Future possibilities of new radiotracers to evaluate hypoxia, proliferation, etc. will be discussed.

S.-M. Lim, M.D., Ph.D. (✉)
Department of Nuclear Medicine, Korea Institute of Radiological & Medical Sciences, Seoul 139-706, South Korea
e-mail: smlim328@kirams.re.kr

E.E. Kim, M.D., M.S.
Departments of Nuclear Medicine and Diagnostic Radiology, The University of Texas MD Anderson Cancer Center and Medical School, Houston, TX 77030, USA

Graduate School of Convergence Science and Technology, Seoul National University, Seoul South Korea
e-mail: ekim@mdanderson.org

Changes in the Staging and Target Volume by PET/CT

The use of PET/CT in radiation oncology treatment planning is a recent clinical research activity. It is clear that PET/CT is superior to CT for a variety of tumor sites, and 25–30% of patients will have alterations in their radiation treatment plan as a result of new findings on PET/CT [2–4]. Modern radiation treatment paradigm of using ever increasingly narrow margins requires greater precision in target volume delineation, and failure to do so can clearly increase the risk of marginal failure when using such highly conformal approaches such as intensity-modulated radiation

E.E. Kim et al. (eds.), *Clinical PET and PET/CT: Principles and Applications*,
DOI 10.1007/978-1-4419-0802-5_31,

therapy (IMRT) or imaging-guided radiation therapy. There is an abundance of data on PET and PET/CT systems on the diagnosis and staging of a variety of malignancies in the other chapters of this textbook.

Carcinoma of unknown primary (CUP) represents a heterogeneous group of tumors presenting remarkably without an identifiable origin that are seen in 2–5% of newly diagnosed cancer cases. Identification of the site of origin facilitates targeted management and in its absence often results in less than optimal outcomes. Greater than 41% of patients with CUP had an identifiable primary after fluorodeoxyglucose (FDG) PET. The overall sensitivity, specificity, and accuracy of PET in this setting were 92%, 82%, and 80%, respectively. Knowledge of the site of origin can refine the selection of radiation therapy techniques in this cohort of patients.

Contrast-enhanced MRI and CT remain the mainstay for the diagnosis and evaluation of primary and metastatic brain tumors. The role of FDG PET is relatively limited because of the rather high physiologic glucose metabolism of the normal brain parenchyma. However, the PET-avid areas were treated with a 10–20% higher dose without untoward toxicities. In brain tumor imaging, *O*-(2-^{18}F fluoroethyl)-L-tyrosine (FET) and L-[Methyl-^{11}C]methionine (MET) both have an advantage over FDG, as they do not accumulate in normal brain cells. FET PET reliably distinguished between posttreatment benign lesions and tumor recurrence. ^{18}F-fluorodeoxythymidine (FLT) has shown that uptake correlated to tumor grade with less effect from disruption of the blood brain barrier than FET. The ideal tracer for brain tumors is yet to be identified.

Head and neck tumors are surrounded by a multitude of sensitive and critical structures confined to a small area of the body, and necessitate narrow margins to minimize the risk of treatment-related toxicities. In the diagnosis and staging of head and neck cancers, PET/CT has been shown to have a higher sensitivity, specificity, and accuracy when compared with PET or CT alone for a variety of histologies, but limitation exists as a result of physiologic uptake of the radiotracer in normal tissues such as the lymphoid-bearing tissues (e.g., Waldeyer's ring), salivary glands, brown fat, vocal folds, and skeletal muscle. Over 70% of patients with head and neck cancers will present with locally advanced disease. The correct staging and evaluation will assist in tailoring therapy and avoid unnecessary interventions of therapeutic approaches. In patients with node negative (N0) head and neck cancers, 25–30%will have pathologically positive neck metastases. Several PET studies have shown that in small volume disease, the detection rate of PET ranges from 0% to 30%. This is not unexpected, however, because 40% of occult metastases are less than 1 cm, which is below the resolution for many of the older PET systems. On average, gross target volumes GTVs of the primary tumor based on CT were three times as large as volumes based on PET. Although there was no difference in volumes of individual lymph nodes, PET/CT detected a greater number of tumor-bearing nodes and revealed occult metastatic disease in several patients. Twenty-five percent of patients had a change in management because of changes noted on PET/CT. In the assessment of response to treatment, PET seems to offer an advantage in detecting persistent or recurrent disease with a sensitivity and specificity near 100% compared with 75% for CT or MRI. Early identification of residual or recurrent disease may provide the opportunity for early salvage therapies and avoid unnecessary surgical interventions [5–8].

In lung cancers, treatment is often complicated by associated atelectasis and/or consolidation. If a lung tumor causes atelectasis, it becomes extremely difficult to define the actual tumor using CT. In this situation, most radiation oncologists would, when in doubt, prefer to define a larger target volume and possibly encompass part of the atelectasis rather than risk missing part of the tumor with a smaller target volume. The result of this approach was further compromise of pulmonary function along with the associated increased risk of radiation-induced pneumonitis. The planning target volumes PTVs changed by up to 50% and improvement in GTV definitions were observed using PET/CT in non-small cell lung cancer. This can potentially result in a reduction of pulmonary toxicity by reducing the mean lung dose in patients currently eligible for high-dose radiotherapy. In primary lung cancer, the presence of mediastinal involvement dramatically alters the outcome in patients treated with multimodality therapy. In evaluating the mediastinum, the negative predicative value for PET is 90% although the positive predicative value remains less than optimal (80%). In patients who are PET-negative assessment of the mediastinum, elective irradiation of this area can be omitted safely. There are significant advantages to avoiding mediastinal irradiation when possible. These include the ability to escalate dose to the primary and reduction in the volume of normal tissue irradiated such as the esophagus, heart, and lung. Malignant mediastinal involvement can be missed in those patients with relatively high FDG uptake in the heart. Issues associated with organ motion by gating image acquisition and irradiation to the respiratory cycle are still being researched [9–12].

In esophageal cancers, the superior detection of distant metastases compared with conventional methods has resulted in the increasing role of PET/CT imaging in the initial staging, assessment of treatment response, and follow-up of patients. PET surpassed CT for locoregional lymph node staging, although its sensitivity rates are yet quite modest. Perhaps the greatest benefit of PET/CT in esophageal cancer is the identification of locoregional and distant metastatic disease with an incremental benefit of 20% over CT staging alone. Additionally, there is a decrease in the GTV with the addition of FDG PET information in 35% of patients, and an increase of 21% with modifications of the GTV that affected the planning treatment volume by 52%. These modifications also affected the percentage of total lung volume in 74% of the patients receiving 20 Gy, which may potentially affect treatment-related toxicities and treatment response. PET imaging may also differentiate responders to preoperative chemotherapy from nonresponders with adenocarcinomas of the esophagogastric junction. In addition, PET may reveal metastatic lymph nodes and lead to increases in the target volume that can significantly influence radiotherapy management. It may still, however, have some limited utility in assessing locoregional therapeutic response such as undetected residual microscopic disease or false-positive results due to inflammatory esophagitis and ulceration. The accuracy of PET/CT detection also can be improved in combination with other modalities such as endoscopy [13].

Among gynecologic cancers, PET and PET/CT are superior to CT alone in the staging of cervical cancer. For patients with pelvic and para-aortic metastases, extended-field radiation therapy (EFRT) offers a survival advantage. However, the toxicities associated with EFRT have historically limited its use in most cervical cancer patients, even in those with high-risk disease. Noninvasive approaches to staging such as PET/CT can help to select patients who can benefit from EFRT using PET/CT. A number of dosimetric publications have reported varying IMRT techniques to boost grossly involved para-aortic nodes. PET-guided IMRT planning was performed to determine if the pelvis could be treated with conventional anterior-posterior/posterior-anterior fields while treating the para-aortic nodes with IMRT. 59.4 Gy to PET-avid grossly involved para-aortic nodes could be achieved while delivering 50.4 Gy to the pelvis and limiting the dose to the small bowel, kidney, and spinal cord. Similarly, the use of FDG PET was shown to be feasible with cervical brachytherapy for monitoring sequential response and individualizing dose optimization. A complete response on PET was predictive of excellent survival (5-year survival, 92%) whereas partial response was predictive of poor survival (5-year survival, 46%). Of the patients with new sites of abnormal FDG uptake outside the treatment volume, none were alive at 5 years. In a small trial of patients with advanced ovarian cancer (stages III and IV) treated with neoadjuvant chemotherapy, PET response after the first and second cycle of chemotherapy clearly predicted the likelihood of survival with a median survival time of 38 months in responders and 23 months in nonresponders. Although radiation therapy is not routinely used for ovarian cancer, special indication may offer an opportunity for focal irradiation in patients who have completed consolidative chemotherapy after maximal surgical debulking. In such cases, focal residual masses or focal recurrences can be effectively managed with irradiation.

For patients with early stage of colorectal cancer (CRC), surgical management remains the standard of care. In patients with more advanced disease, preoperative chemoradiation therapy has been encouraged because of its reduced recurrence rate and toxicity. Nevertheless, nearly half of these patients will have recurrence within the first 3 years after treatment. The goal of posttreatment surveillance strategies is to detect early, small volume recurrent or metastatic deposits in the hope of maximizing the chances of survival. Because the majority of the recurrences are local and frequently amenable to surgery, it is vital that the precise location and extent of the relapse is well documented. Currently, diagnostic imaging strategies using CT are controversial in the surveillance of CRC. It is frequently difficult to differential scar tissue from recurrent disease, thus lowering the sensitivity and specificity of CT. MRI and PET can be used to augment surveillance programs in the posttreatment setting. Although MRI has been shown to be more valuable in detecting recurrent pelvic disease with higher sensitivity, specificity, and accuracy rates than CT, its use has not been supported as a substitute for CT in routine surveillance and should be selectively used. Studies evaluating the utility of PET/CT in the detection of recurrence in CRC appeared to suggest a high sensitivity for detecting the primary tumor but a relative insensitivity of PET and PET/CT in detecting regional lymph node metastases in rectal cancer despite a high specificity of nearly 96%. However, PET/CT was found to be more useful in the identification of distant metastatic sites such as the liver or lung. PET/CT seems to be superior in the restaging of CRC and for surveillance strategies after definitive therapies. This added benefit of PET/CT clearly can influence surgical decision making, better stratifying candidates for resection and identifying those who are more appropriately treated with alternate approaches, including palliation. FDG/PET detected unsuspected disease in 25% of patients considered to have resectable hepatic metastasis by conventional staging. In addition, they demonstrated that FDG PET screening was associated with excellent postresection 5-year overall survival for patients undergoing resection. In planning for radiation therapy, an increase in the size of the GTV in 50% of their cases leading to a 20% increase in the size of the PTV compared with volumes based on CT alone was reported. PET/CT in radiation treatment planning for rectal cancer produced greater uniformity between observers' definition of the GTV based on combined PET/CT compared with CT alone. The area of greatest enhancement was in the definition of nodal disease potentially leading to few marginal misses.

The management of both Hodgkin lymphoma (HL) and non-Hodgkin's lymphomas with radiation has undergone a dramatic evolution in the last decade from first-line comprehensive therapy in some cases to adjuvant therapy after chemotherapy in most stages, currently. Results of a number of prospective trials continue to confirm the contribution of focal consolidative radiation therapy in bulky and advanced disease. Staging of HL is carried out by a variety of invasive and noninvasive modalities. Improved accuracy in staging lymphomas with PET/CT over conventional anatomic imaging has made functional imaging a cornerstone in this disease entity. Because most lymphomas are highly FDG-avid, the ability of PET/CT to show anatomy and metabolism is the ideal modality for early assessment of response and routine surveillance. Therefore, it is essential to have a pretreatment FDG PET study to assess residual masses accurately and early monitoring of response to the treatment. Several researchers have been investigating the role of PET/CT in the early assessment of response to chemotherapy before treatment completion [14, 15]. Such important data could help stratify and identify patients who may benefit from more tailored treatments based on response, perhaps after one or two cycles of therapy. Although the appropriate therapy change has not yet been established, high-risk patient subsets can be reliably identified. FDG PET has also been a useful tool for assessing initial staging, response to therapy, and follow-up of children diagnosed with lymphoma. FDG PET imaging was performed before and after the first cycle of therapy predicts outcome in diffuse large cell and HL. PET-negative scans after the first cycle portended a sustained complete response with a median follow-up at 28 months. PET seems to have a prognostic value in patients undergoing bone marrow transplantation as well, where a positive FDG PET scan after salvage chemotherapy and prior to autologous stem cell transplantation is indicative of an extremely poor prognosis. Certainly, the ability of FDG PET to better differentiate between viable tumor and fibrosis has proved valuable for response assessment after completion of therapy and as a prognostic marker early during treatment. With respect to radiation treatment planning, field reductions, which are the modern equivalents of the so called involved node radiotherapy, are now routinely used for the standard approach to radiation therapy. As a result, precise anatomic delineation of lymphoma involvement becomes increasingly important. In this scenario, PET is rapidly being introduced, providing better definition of the involved field because of its higher accuracy for nodal and organ staging than CT. The radiation field was altered based on PET information. However, FDG PET and PET/CT have a greater tendency toward upstaging HD patients that will relate to larger RT volumes trend as well.

Stereotactic radiosurgery and body radiosurgery/radiotherapy are special applications of stereotactic techniques to radiation therapy. The key concept behind these applications is the use of specialized localization techniques coupled with limited tumor margins to tumors treated with very high doses in a limited number of fractions. Precise target delineation is very critical in this instance. Failure to accurately define the tumor in most instances results in treatment failure or greater worrisome compromise of nearby critical structures given the high dose per fraction. For brain metastases treated with radiosurgery, FDG PET augmented MRI evaluation for the examination of tumor radionecrosis versus tumor progression. Linac-based hypofractionated stereotactic body radiation therapy was performed for the liver, lung tumors and recurrent, unresectable, previously irradiated squamous cell carcinoma of the head and neck without significant toxicity. The impact of PET/CT in treatment planning can be of great clinical significance in dose escalation approaches to further minimize in-field failures [16].

Identification of GRV With PET

CT is the reference imaging modality for radiation treatment planning, however, CT images lack contrast between soft-tissue structures and tumor extension. Compared with CT, MRI has shown to be more accurate in evaluating soft tissue and can be more sensitive for bone invasion of head and neck tumors, but it also has its limitations, such as geometric distortions at field-of-view edges, and artifacts at interfaces of bone and air.

FDG PET can identify the primary tumor in head and neck cancer more accurately than conventional imaging. FDG PET missed a small superficial tumor and misinterpreted a floor of mouth tumor for a tongue tumor. Comparing the role of co-registered CT, MRI, and FDG PET in delineating the primary tumor, PET was closest to depicting the true tumor volume, although all three imaging modalities (in addition to PET) failed to identify a small fraction (approximately 10%) of the macroscopic tumor, mainly superficial mucosal extension [17–20].

Application of radiopharmaceuticals other than FDG (Fig. 31.1) that depict different characteristics of tumor cells may also play a role in accurate tumor definition (e.g., amino acid-based radiopharmaceuticals FET and MET). In brain tumor imaging, FET and MET both have an advantage over FDG, as they do not accumulate in normal brain cells. When comparing FET PET with FDG/PET and CT in patients with head and neck cancer, both FET PET and FDG PET were superior to CT in the detection of tumor. FET PET showed no uptake in physiologic and inflammatory tissue, resulting in a higher specificity for tumor detection than FDG PET. A drawback of FET PET was a

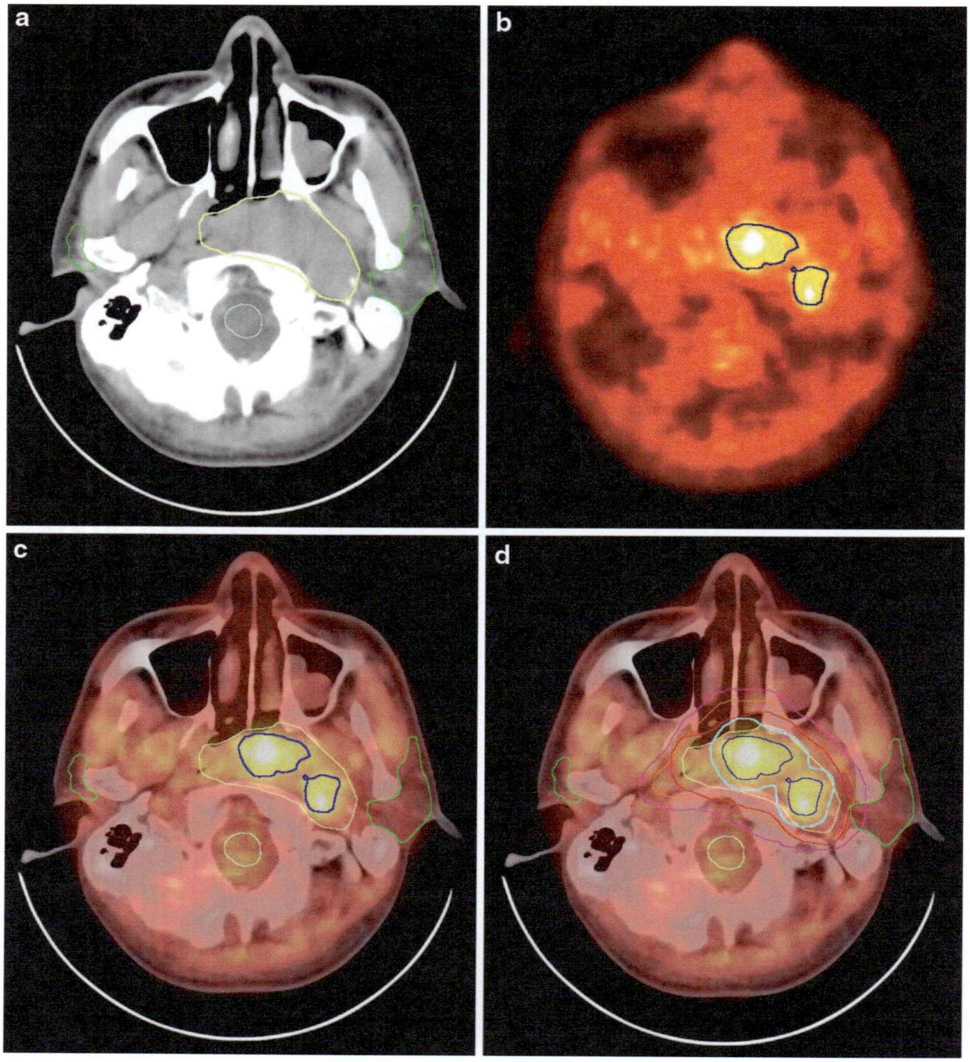

Fig. 31.1 An example of delineation of the GTV and the corresponding HTV with a T/C ratio of 1.3 from ^{18}F-FMISO PET/CT data. (**a**) GTV in a CT axial image. (**b**) $HTV_{1.3}$ in a ^{18}F-FMISO PET axial image. (**c**) GTV and $HTV_{1.3}$ delineated together from ^{18}F-FMISO PET/CT data. (**d**) PTV for each tumor volume. *GTV* gross tumor volume, *HTV* hypoxic tumor volume, *PTV* planning target volume, *T/C* tumor-to-cerebellum ratio

lower sensitivity, caused by a relatively low tumor uptake compared with FDG PET. MET PET images in patients with brain tumors were investigated by correlating MET uptake with histologic examination of stereotactic biopsies. Solid parts of brain tumors as well as brain tissue with infiltrating tumor cells were detected with high sensitivity (87%) and specificity (89%). In target volume definition of meningioma patients with skull-base tumors, MET PET is superior in defining tumor infiltration in the surrounding structures compared with CT/MRI. Furthermore, MET PET significantly decreased the interobserver variability in tumor delineation as compared with CT/MRI-based delineation [13].

Interobserver Variability in Target Volume Definition

Interobserver variability of radiation target volume definition is a widely recognized problem. In laryngeal cancer for example, target definition using only CT leads to significant inter- and intraobserver variations in delineation of the GTV [21]. When imaging modalities become more accurate, the interobserver variability will decrease. A reduction in the interobserver variability is seen by incorporating FDG PET/CT data into the treatment planning [13, 17–20]. A reduction in the mean volume difference was reported when FDG PET was incorporated into the CT-based GTV definition of various solid tumors. This was associated with a reduction of the standard deviation from 38.6 to 14.4 cm^3. When analyzing target definition of 22 patients with no-small cell lung cancer by 11 observers, the amount of disagreement was reduced from 45% (CT-based) to 18% (PET/CT-based).

Thresholding in GTV Definition

Studies comparing GTV definition using FDG PET (GTVpet) and T1-weighted contrast-enhanced MRI (GTVmri) in high-grade astrocytomas consistently showed that GTVpet was smaller than GTVmri [22, 23]. Similar studies comparing GTVpet to delineation using CT or MRI (GTVct/mri) have been performed in head and neck cancer. Results show either no difference between GTVs or that GTVpet was significantly smaller than GTVct/mri. A reason for this might be that the optimal way to delineate a tumor on PET is not clearly defined, resulting in variations in the methods for defining GTVpet. In clinical nuclear medicine, PET studies are usually interpreted qualitatively, while in radiation oncology a more quantitative approach is necessary as edge detection is required for tumor contouring. PET images can be interpreted by visual assessment only (GTVvis) or by choosing thresholds (i.e., segmenting a lesion on the basis of a given level of radioactivity) [22]. The threshold could be any fixed cut-off of the standardized uptake value, and some investigators choose a cut-off of 2.5 (GTV2.5). Thresholds are more commonly defined as a fixed percentage of the maximum tumor activity, for example 40% (GTV40%), or adaptive threshold based on the signal-to-background ratio (GTVucl). This method aims to incorporate specific PET imaging properties by deriving a mathematical function from phantom measurements of objects of various sizes under various signal-to-background conditions. The choice of a tool for target volume definition based on PET images is far from trivial.

Intratumoral Biologic Characteristics

Tumor hypoxia is a strong contributor to radiation resistance. Kaanders et al. correlated the hypoxic fraction measured by staining tumor biopsies with pimonidazole, an exogeneous hypoxia marker, with locoregional tumor control after radiotherapy of advanced head and neck cancer. Tumor control inversely correlated with the hypoxic fraction [24]. Various treatment modifications are available to counteract hypoxia induced radioresistance: irradiating during hyperoxic gas breathing under normobaric or hyperbaric conditions, adding a hypoxic cell sensitizer (nimorazole) or a hypoxic cytotoxin (tirapazamine), or increasing the radiation dose. To various extents these modifications lead to increased toxicity. Because not every patient benefits from these treatment intensifications, careful selection of patients is necessary, and PET could be of value as a predictive tool. For imaging of tumor hypoxia, both imidazole- and nonimidazole-containing agents have been developed. Imidazole-containing radiopharmaceuticals are [^{18}F] fluoromisonidazole (FMISO) and [^{123}I] iodoazomycin arabinoside. Nonimidazole tracers are ^{99m}Tc 4,9-diaza-3,3,10,10- tetramethyldodecan-2,11-dione-dioxime (^{99m}Tc HL91) and ^{64}Cu-diacetyl-bis(*N*-4-methylthiosemicarbazone) (^{64}Cu-ATSM) [23]. Hypoxia can be transient due to structural and functional abnormalities of the tumor microvessels. These abnormalities cause disturbances in the blood supply leading to temporal shutdown of vessels. Therefore, areas identified as 'normoxic' could be 'hypoxic' at a different time point. These changes occur at the microregional level and little is known about the sensitivity of PET scanning for such changes. Irradiation itself can cause rapid changes in oxygenation and perfusion. Even if the information obtained by functional imaging correlates with a relevant tumor characteristic, and even if that characteristic has an impact on clinical decision making on treatment selection, one must be aware that the temporal stability of the imaged data may be limited.

Another tumor characteristic associated with radioresistance is tumor cell proliferation, especially in squamous cell carcinomas that can be counteracted by shortening the overall treatment time, which has been shown to be effective in several randomized clinical trials. Because this is also treatment intensification, PET could possibly help in selecting patients by identifying highly proliferating tumors, and thereby spare those patients who are not likely to benefit from the increased toxicity. Cell proliferation can be identified by labeling DNA precursors, such as thymidine or deoxyuridine, that are incorporated in DNA replication during the S phase of cycling cells. Clinical studies show a correlation between FLT uptake and the Ki-67 labeling index [25].

Epidermal growth factor receptor (EGFR) inhibition is another strategy to counteract tumor cell proliferation. EGFR plays a key role in cellular proliferation of head and neck cancer. The amount of EGFR expression in tumor biopsies could reliably be used to select the dose fractionation scheme that had the greatest chance of benefiting the patient. Adding an EGFR-inhibitor (cetuximab) to the radiation treatment in a randomized clinical trial resulted in increased tumor control with only limited increase of toxicity. New radiopharmaceuticals are developed in the preclinical phase to quantify tumor EGFR expression with PET (e.g., Ga-68-EGF and Zr-89- cetuximab).

Concept of Dose Painting

The concept of dose painting is to visualize tumor subvolumes with a potential resistance to irradiation and to paint some additional dose onto that volume [26, 27]. This was applied in a pilot study demonstrating an IMRT plan where a subvolume of the oropharyngeal tumor, identified by increased ^{64}Cu-ATSM retention, received an extra dose of 10 Gy. Despite the dose escalation in this dose painting exercise, the parotid glands could still be adequately spared with this high-precision IMRT technique (Fig. 31.2). At the level of the tumor microenvironment, it is conceivable that new cells formed in the proliferating cell compartment push older cells away from the blood vessels resulting in a gradual depletion of oxygen and nutrients. Tumor cells in the hypoxic compartment would be pushed further down the oxygen gradient and eventually die of oxygen deficiency and starvation. This 'pattern of hypoxia' is measured in micrometers and therefore cannot be detected by in vivo imaging techniques such as PET because of limited spatial resolution, as PET images hypoxia at a more global level. Furthermore, the radiation dose delivery also has a certain resolution. Given these limitations, dose painting will most likely only be feasible with subvolumes greater than 0.5 cm^3. PET imaging would then need to identify subvolumes within the tumor with a larger-than-average content of hypoxic cells [23, 24].

Conclusion

Integrating biologic or molecular information of tumors into radiation oncology might help in deciding not only where, but also how, radiation therapy should be delivered. The addition of functional imaging to the standard anatomically based target volume definition has already shown significant advantages, especially when images are co-registered. The reduction of interobserver variability is obvious and can increase the stan-

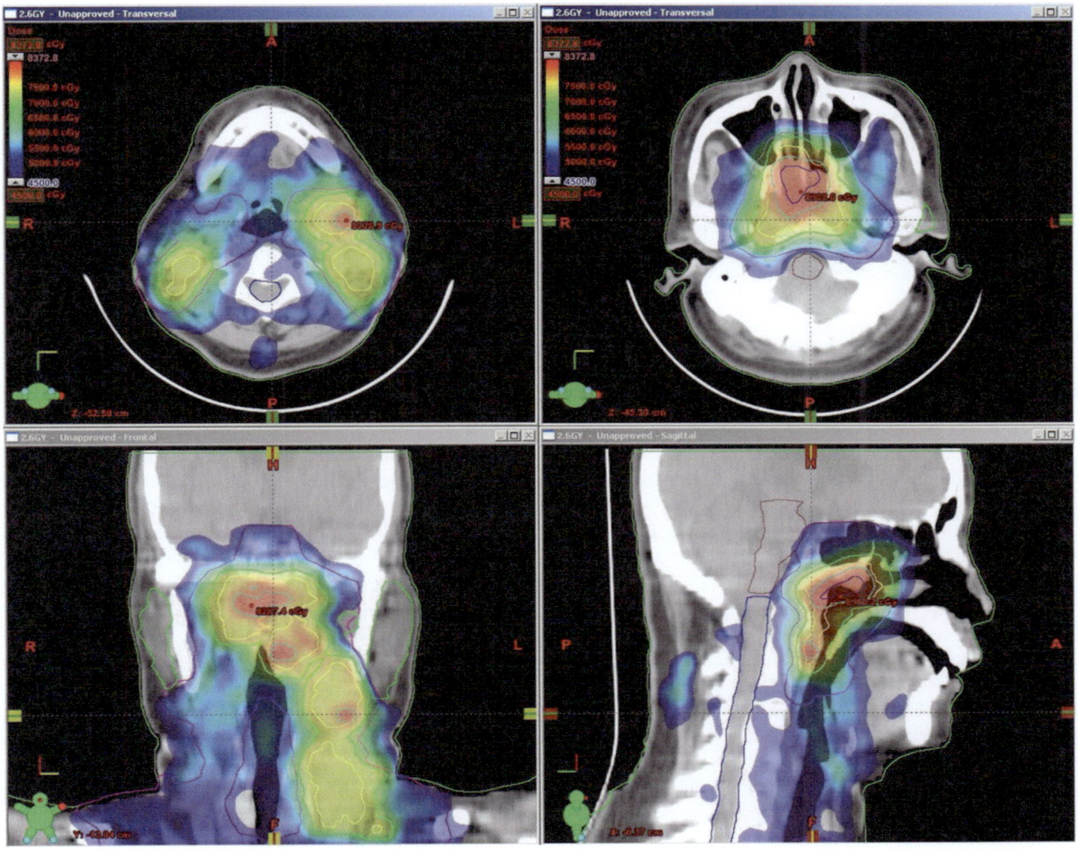

Fig. 31.2 Example of a ^{18}F-FMISO PET/CT-guided IMRT plan for a nasopharyngeal carcinoma patient. Dose-painting strategies derived from simultaneous integrated boost (SIB)-IMRT are displayed as color washes of dose distribution

dard of care for all patients, not only by reducing geographically missing parts of the cancer, but also by reducing the irradiated volume of normal tissues and organs at risk. As more studies validating the various functional imaging properties become available, more treatment-related decisions (dose painting, shortening overall treatment time, adding a sensitizer) will need to be tested in clinical trials. The goals are challenging and clear. First, to enlarge the therapeutic window by increasing the tumor control probability and decreasing the normal tissue complication probability; second, to develop predictive assays that can serve as selection tools for patients that are likely to benefit from intensified treatments.

References

1. Schinagl DAX, Kaanders JHAM, Oyen WJG. From anatomical to biological target volumes: the role of PET in radiation treatment planning. Cancer Imaging. 2006;6:S107–16.
2. Grosu AL, Piert M, Weber WA, Jeremic B, Picchio M, Schratzenstaller U, Zimmermann FB, Schwaiger M, Molls M. Positron emission tomography for radiation treatment planning. Strahlenther Onkol. 2005;181: 483–99.
3. Nestle U, Weber W, Hentscheland M, Grosu AL. Biological imaging in radiation therapy: role of positron emission tomography. Phys Med Biol. 2009;54:R1–25.
4. Heron DE, Andrade RS, Beriwal S, Smith RP. PET-CT in radiation oncology the impact on diagnosis, treatment planning, and assessment of treatment response. Am J Clin Oncol. 2008;31:352–62.
5. Troost EGC, Schinagl DAX, Bussink J, Boerman OC, van der Kogel AJ, Oyen WJG, Kaanders JHAM.

Innovations in radiotherapy planning of head and neck cancers: role of PET. J Nucl Med. 2010;51:66–76.
6. Madani I, Duthoy W, Derie C, et al. Positron emission tomography-guided, focal dose escalation using intensity-modulated radiotherapy for head and neck cancer. Int J Radiation Oncol Biol Phys. 2007;68(1): 126–35.
7. Vogel WV, Schinagl DAX, van Dalen JA, Kaanders JHAM, Oyen WJG. Validated image fusion of dedicated PET and CT for external beam radiation therapy in the head and neck area. Q J Nucl Med Mol Imaging. 2008;52:74–83.
8. Duprez F, de Neve W, de Gersem W Jr, Lic MC, Madani I. Adaptive dose painting by numbers for head-and-neck cancer. Int J Radation Oncol Biol Phys. 2010 (in press).
9. Grgic A, Nestle U, Schaefer-Schuler A, Kremp S, Kirsch CM, Hellwig D. FDG-PET–based radiotherapy planning in lung cancer: optimum breathing protocol and patient positioning—an individual comparison. Int J Radiation Oncol Biol Phys. 2009;73(1):103–11.
10. Sura S, Greco C, Gelblum D, Yorke ED, Jackson A, Rosenzweig K. ^{18}F-fluorodeoxyglucose positron emission tomography-based assessment of local failure patterns in non-small-cell lung cancer treated with definitive radiotherapy. Int J Radiation Oncol Biol Phys. 2008;70(5):1397–402.
11. Kolodziejczyk M, Kepka L, Dziuk M, Anna Zawadzka A, Szalus N, Gizewska A, Bujko K. Impact of [^{18}F]fluorodeoxyglucose PET-CT staging on treatment planning in radiotherapy incorporating elective nodal irradiation for non-small-cell lung cancer: a prospective study. Int J Radation Oncol Biol Phys. 2010 (in press).
12. Okubo M, Nishimura Y, Nakamatsu K, Okumura M, Shibata T, Kanamori S, Hanaoka K, Hosono M. Radiation treatment planning using positron emission and computed tomography for lung and pharyngeal cancers: a multiple-threshold method for [^{18}F]fluoro-2-deoxyglucose activity. Int J Radiation Oncol Biol Phys. 2010;77(2):350–6.
13. Muijs CT, Beukema JC, Pruim J, Mul VE, Groen H, Plukker JT, Langendijk JA. A systematic review on the role of FDG-PET/CT in tumour delineation and radiotherapy planning in patients with esophageal cancer. Radiother Oncol. 2010;97(2):165–71.
14. Safar V, Dupuis J, Litti E, et al. Interim [^{18}F]fluorodeoxyglucose positron emission tomography scan in diffuse large B-cell lymphoma treated with anthracycline-based chemotherapy plus rituximab. J Clin Oncol. 2012;30(2):184–90.
15. Itti E, Lin C, Dupuis et al. Prognostic value of interim ^{18}F-FDG PET in patients with diffuse large B-Cell lymphoma: SUV-based assessment at 4 cycles of chemotherapy. J Nucl Med. 2009;50(4):527–33.
16. Vahdat S, Oermann EK, Collins SP, Yu X, Abedalthagafi M, DeBrito P, Suy S, Yousefi S, Gutierrez CJ, Chang T, Banovac F, Anderson ED, Esposito G, Collins BT. CyberKnife radiosurgery for inoperable stage IA non-small cell lung cancer: ^{18}F-fluorodeoxyglucose positron emission tomography/computed tomography serial tumor response assessment. J Hematol Oncol. 2010;3:6–11.
17. Devic S, Tomic N, Faria S, Menard S, Lisbona R, Lehnert S. Defining radiotherapy target volumes using ^{18}F-fluoro-deoxy-glucose positron emission tomography/computed tomography: still a Pandora's box? Int J Radiation Oncol Biol Phys. 2010;78(5):1555–62.
18. Hanna GG, Carson KJ, Lynch T, McAleese J, Cosgrove VP, Eakin R, Stewart DP, Zatari A, O'Sullivan JM, Hounsell AR. ^{18}F-fluorodeoxyglucose positron emission tomography/computed tomography–based radiotherapy target volume definition in non–small-cell lung cancer: delineation by radiation oncologists vs. joint outlining with a PET radiologist? Int J Radiation Oncol Biol Phys. 2010;78(4):1040–51.
19. Han D, Yu J, Yu Y, et al. Comparison of ^{18}F-fluorothymidine and ^{18}F-fluorodeoxyglucose PET/CT in delineating gross tumor volume by optimal threshold in patients with squamous cell carcinoma of thoracic esophagus. Int J Radiation Oncol Biol Phys. 2010;76(4):1235–41.
20. Sattler B, Lee JA, Lonsdale M, Coche E. PET/CT (and CT) instrumentation, image reconstruction and data transfer for radiotherapy planning. Radiother Oncol. 2010;96(3):288–97.
21. Yap ML, Vinod SK, Shon IAH, Lin M, Fowler A, Gabriel G, Holloway LC. The registration of diagnostic versus planning fluorodeoxyglucose positron emission tomography/computed tomography in radiotherapy planning for non-small cell lung cancer. Clin Oncol. 2010;22(7):554–60.
22. Zaidi H, El Naqa I. PET-guided delineation of radiation therapy treatment volumes: a survey of image segmentation techniques. Eur J Nucl Med Mol Imaging. 2010;37:2165–87.
23. Choi WS, Lee SW, Park SH, Ryu JS, Oh SJ, Im KC, Choi EK, Kim JH, Jung SH, Kim SK, Ahn SD. Planning study for available dose of hypoxic tumor volume using fluorine-18-labeled fluoromisonidazole positron emission tomography for treatment of the head and neck cancer. Radiother Oncol. 2010;97(2):176–82.
24. Seppälä J, Seppänen M, Arponen E, Lindholm P, Minn H. Carbon-11 acetate PET/CT based dose escalated IMRT in prostate cancer. Radiother Oncol. 2009;93(2):234–40.
25. Chalkidou A, Landau DB, Odell EW, et al. Correlation between Ki-67 immunohistochemistry and ^{18}F-Fluorothymidine uptake in patients with cancer: A systematic review and meta-analysis. Eur J Cancer. 2012 May [Epub ahead of print].
26. Chao KS, Bosch WR, Mutic S, et al. A novel approach to overcome hypoxic tumor resistance: Cu-ATSM-guided intensity-modulated radiation therapy. Int J Radiat Oncol Biol Phys. 2001;49(4):1171–82.
27. Lin Z, Mechalakos J, Nehmeh S et al. The influence of changes in tumor hypoxia on dose-painting treatment plans based on ^{18}F-FMISO positron emission tomography. Int J Radiat Oncol Biol Phys. 2008;70(4):1219–28.
28. Kaanders JH, Bussink J, van der Kogel AJ. ARCON: a novel biology-based approach in radiotherapy. Lancet Oncol. 2002;3(12):728–37.

32 Evidence-Based Positron Emission Tomography

Joon Young Choi

The clinical applications and investigations of positron emission tomography (PET) using F-18 fluoro-2-deoxyglucose (FDG) have been dramatically increasing over the past 10 years. The main cause of this boom is the development of the PET/computed tomography (CT) scanner, which can provide both the metabolic and anatomic information of a cancer. PET/CT has been shown to have a better diagnostic accuracy in tumors than either CT or conventional PET. The individual practitioner makes a clinical decision according to his or her experience. Different chance of exposure to evolving medical technologies makes different behavior for the practitioners to order new modalities. Underutilizing new technology does not offer enough diagnostic information leading to appropriate decision making, and overutilization of technology increases medical cost. The results of PET based on researches can give the appropriate amount of information to practitioners and helps them to make the best medical decisions.

An extensive search of the literature was performed on the use of PET for oncology. In this chapter, current evidence and indications for specific diseases or organs of PET are summarized. Indications were categorized into initial treatment strategy and subsequent treatment strategy. Initial treatment strategy included diagnosis, tumor grading, initial staging, treatment planning, and prognosis prediction. Subsequent treatment strategy included monitoring response to treatment, restaging, diagnosis of recurrence, treatment planning, and prognosis prediction after initial therapy.

The use of FDG PET for initial treatment strategies and subsequent treatment strategies of the discussed cancers is covered by medical insurance in both Korea and in the US.

Head and Neck Cancer

Initial Treatment Strategy

For detection of primary tumor, PET demonstrates high sensitivity of 83–97%, significantly better than that of CT [1–3]. However, it is difficult for PET to determine T stage in head and neck cancer, and PET/CT can be better than CT for T staging. However, further studies are necessary.

For nodal staging, FDG PET showed a good diagnostic efficacy of 67–100% sensitivity and 89–100% specificity for detecting metastatic cervical lymph nodes, which are significantly better than for CT and/or MRI showing a sensitivity of 53–84% and a specificity of 71–95% [1–17]. Recent studies suggest that PET/CT is more accurate than PET for the nodal staging of head and neck cancer [16, 17]. Clinically, in stage N0

J.Y. Choi, M.D., Ph.D. (✉)
Department of Nuclear Medicine, Samsung Medical Center, Sungkyunkwan University Medical School, 50 Irwon-dong, Gangnam-gu, Seoul 135-710, South Korea
e-mail: jynm.choi@samsung.com

E.E. Kim et al. (eds.), *Clinical PET and PET/CT: Principles and Applications*,
DOI 10.1007/978-1-4419-0802-5_32, © Springer Science+Business Media New York 2013

oral squamous cell carcinoma, PET demonstrates a low sensitivity of 33–67%, which supports the need of sentinel lymph node biopsy in such patients [18, 19].

PET or PET/CT can find clinically unexpected distant metastases or second primary cancer in 9–24% of patients with head and neck cancer [1, 13, 14, 20]. The results of PET or PET/CT change the therapeutic plan in 9–31% of patients with head and neck cancer [1, 2, 13–15, 20].

Subsequent Treatment Strategy

For diagnosis of recurrence, FDG PET demonstrates a good diagnostic efficacy of 82–100% sensitivity and 72–100% specificity [21–36]. In several comparative studies, PET (sensitivity, 88–100%; specificity, 78–100%) showed significantly better diagnostic efficacy than CT and/or MRI (sensitivity, 25–96%; specificity, 30–88%) [22, 26, 29, 31, 34, 36].

Radiation therapy and/or chemotherapy following PET are helpful in evaluating the therapeutic response. The sensitivity and specificity of FDG PET for detecting residual viable tumor are 67–100% and 53–95%, respectively [34, 37–44]. For residual viable metastatic lymph node, PET showed a 40–100% of sensitivity and 25–91% of specificity [45–47]. This metabolic response by PET is significantly associated with prognosis of patients [48–52].

Thyroid Cancer

Initial Treatment Strategy

Although FDG PET or PET/CT has been widely used in oncology, there are many reports about clinically unexpected thyroid incidentaloma detected using PET. According to a recent systemic review, the incidence of an unexpected focal abnormality in the thyroid gland found using PET is 1.0% [53]. Overall risk of malignancy in a subgroup of patients undergoing diagnostic confirmations is 33.2% [54–71]. Papillary thyroid carcinoma is the most prevalent thyroid malignancy (82.2%). In eight studies reporting individual maximum standardized uptake values (SUVs), there was a significant difference in maximum SUV between benign lesions (4.6 ± 2.1) and malignant lesions (6.8 ± 4.6; $p<0.001$) with some overlap in values [55, 59, 62, 63, 65, 67, 68, 71] which is compatible with previous PET studies on thyroid nodules [72]. Therefore, the high prevalence of malignancy associated with focal hypermetabolic thyroid nodules found on FDG PET warrants further evaluation when detected. For thyroid nodule evaluation, FDG PET showed an excellent sensitivity and moderate specificity. For initial staging of thyroid cancer, there are few positive results showing the usefulness of PET in addition to conventional staging methods [73]. However, in selected patients suspicious of distant metastasis, FDG PET can be recommended.

Subsequent Treatment Strategy

FDG PET is useful for re-staging and detecting recurrence after total thyroidectomy in patients with differentiate thyroid carcinoma (DTC), which is better than I-131 whole-body scan on Tc-99 m MIBI scan [74]. FDG PET showed a good diagnostic efficacy in the detection of recurrent or metastatic DTC with elevated serum thyroglobulin levels that a radioiodine whole-body scan failed to detect. In a recent meta-analysis, the overall patient-based sensitivity and specificity of FDG PET in such patients are 83.5% and 84.3%, respectively [75]. The pooled lesion-based sensitivity and specificity are 91.6% and 77.5%, respectively [76]. PET/CT showed a better diagnostic efficacy than PET in DTC [77, 78]. In addition, PET/CT changes the management plan in 48–67% of the patients with cancer [77, 78].

In medullary thyroid carcinoma (MTC), FDG PET showed a good diagnostic efficacy for detecting recurrent or residual lesions with elevated serum calcitonin levels [79–81]. The sensitivity of FDG PET for detecting recurrent or residual MTC is 78–96%, which is better than that of the ^{111}In-pentetreotide scan or anatomic imaging modalities.

Lung Cancer

Initial Treatment Strategy

FDG PET is useful for evaluating single pulmonary nodule/mass detected by chest radiography and/or chest CT. According to a meta-analysis including 1,474 patients from 40 studies, PET showed a 97% sensitivity and 78% specificity for differentiating benign from malignant single pulmonary nodule/mass [82]. PET/CT demonstrates a better sensitivity and negative predictive value for characterizing single pulmonary nodule than dynamic chest CT [83]. High sensitivity and negative predictive value of PET help to avoid unnecessary invasive diagnostic procedures in such patients. Cost effectiveness of PET for evaluating single pulmonary nodule was proved in several countries including the US, Japan, Germany, Italy, Australia, and Hungary [84–93].

FDG PET is useful for initial staging of non-small cell lung cancer (NSCLC). According to a meta-analysis including 2,226 patients from 29 studies, PET showed a 79% of sensitivity and 91% of specificity for detecting metastatic mediastinal lymph nodes, which is significantly better than a sensitivity of 60% and a specificity of 77% on chest CT [94]. In another meta-analysis with 1,959 patients from 32 studies, PET showed a sensitivity of 85% and specificity of 90% for detecting metastatic mediastinal lymph nodes, which is significantly better than a sensitivity of 61% and specificity of 79% on chest CT [95]. In a recent meta-analysis with 833 patients from 17 studies, PET showed a sensitivity of 83% and specificity of 92% for detecting metastatic mediastinal lymph nodes, which is significantly better than a sensitivity of 59% and specificity of 78% on chest CT [96]. Because of the whole-body coverage of PET, good results in finding clinically unexpected distant metastasis in 6–11% of patients with NSCLC were demonstrated using PET [97, 98]. For initial staging of NSCLC, PET results contribute to changes in the therapeutic plan such as avoiding unnecessary curative surgery in 11–26% of patients [99, 100]. PET/CT is superior to PET for initial staging of NSCLC [101–103]. The degree of FDG uptake in primary tumor (i.e., SUV) and PET stage are significant prognostic factors in NSCLC [104–109]. Cost effectiveness of PET for initial staging of NSCLC was proved in many countries including the US, France, Germany, Italy, Netherland, Japan, and Australia [87, 92, 110–124].

FDG PET is useful for the initial staging of small cell lung cancer (SCLC) by providing additional information to conventional staging methods [125–131]. The results of PET contribute to the change in therapeutic plan in 8–33% of patients with SCLC [82–87].

Subsequent Treatment Strategy

FDG PET showed good results (sensitivity, 96–100%; specificity, 53–100%) for detecting recurrence of NSCLC after curative treatment, when recurrence is suspicious clinically or radiologically [132–136]. The results of PET contribute to the change in therapeutic plan in 29–63% of patients suspicious of recurrence [134, 135].

FDG PET showed good results for predicting pathologic response of neoadjuvant therapy and restaging in NSCLC. For detecting residual viable primary tumor, PET showed a sensitivity of 81–97% and specificity of 64–100%, which is significantly better than that of chest CT [137–141]. For detecting residual viable metastatic lymph nodes, PET showed a sensitivity of 50–77% and specificity of 83–99%, which is better than that of chest CT [137, 140, 142, 143]. PET response to primary tumor to neoadjuvant therapy is one of the significant prognostic factors in NSCLC [137, 141, 144–146]. PET can help locate clinically unexpected distant metastasis in 17% of patients after neoadjuvant therapy, which helps to avoid unnecessary curative surgery [137].

Although only several studies were reported, FDG PET is useful for therapy response evaluation and re-staging in SCLC because of its superiority to conventional methods [127, 131, 146, 147]. The re-staging results of PET can cause a change in the therapeutic plan in 52% of patients with SCLC. Positive PET results after therapy are associated with poor prognosis [147].

Esophageal Cancer

Initial Treatment Strategy

FDG PET is useful for initial staging of esophageal cancer. For N staging, PET showed a sensitivity of 45–81% and specificity of 69–100%, which is significantly better than 31–60% sensitivity and 71–100% specificity of chest CT [148–157]. For M staging, PET showed a diagnostic accuracy of 43–100%, which is significantly better than 14–64% of chest CT [148, 151, 153, 155, 156]. For comparison with endoscopic ultrasound (EUS), PET demonstrates better or similar results in N staging and better results in M staging [152, 153, 156]. In addition, EUS has a limitation that complete examination is not available in 20–30% of patients because of severe esophageal stenosis [152, 153, 156]. PET can help to locate clinically unexpected M1 disease in 5–20% of patients, which can help in avoiding unnecessary curative surgery [148, 149, 151, 156, 158]. PET findings change the treatment plan in about 40% of patients with esophageal cancer [159, 160]. The SUV of primary tumor, PET stage, and the number of PET-positive lymph nodes are significant prognostic factors in esophageal cancer [151, 154, 159–162]. However, the staging system of esophageal cancer was completely revised in 2010. Therefore, reanalysis or further evaluation is warranted.

Subsequent Treatment Strategy

Although few references are available, FDG PET showed better sensitivity and worse specificity than conventional diagnostic workup for detecting recurrence of esophageal cancer [163, 164].

FDG PET has shown good results for predicting pathologic response of neoadjuvant therapy in esophageal cancer. In a meta-analysis including 691 patients from 24 articles on esophageal cancer, overall accuracy for predicting pathologic response of neoadjuvant therapy was 85% for PET, 54% for CT, and 86% for EUS, respectively [165]. However, to our knowledge, at the time of this meta-analysis, there were no studies dealing with direct comparison of PET with EUS. Subsequent studies reported that PET is better than EUS for predicting pathologic response of neoadjuvant therapy and restaging of esophageal cancer [166, 167].

Gastric Cancer

Initial Treatment Strategy

FDG PET has a complementary role to contrast-enhanced CT for initial staging of adenocarcinoma of the stomach. For lymph node staging, FDG showed a sensitivity of 23–56% and specificity of 92–99%. In comparison with PET, CT demonstrates significantly better sensitivity of 44–78% and worse specificity than in 62–99% [168–173]. In case of signet ring carcinoma that shows low FDG uptake in general, the worst sensitivity for detecting metastatic lymph node is reported [90]. FDG PET showed a better sensitivity for detecting N3 nodes than N1 and N2 nodes, which contributes to treatment strategy changes [169, 174]. For M staging, PET shows favorable results for liver and lung metastasis. On the contrary, PET has a low sensitivity for detecting peritoneal, pleural, and bone metastases [169, 175, 176]. FDG PET can help locate clinically unexpected distant metastasis or second primary cancer in 8% of patients with gastric cancer [171]. Combined use of PET and contrast-enhanced CT improves the staging results in gastric adenocarcinoma [169]. Currently, there are few studies using PET/CT for the initial staging of stomach cancer [173]. Further studies using PET/CT are warranted.

Subsequent Treatment Strategy

FDG PET is useful for detecting recurrence in patients with postoperative gastric cancer. In patients with clinically, endoscopically, or radiologically suspected recurrent gastric cancer, PET showed a sensitivity of 70–81% and specificity of 69–100% [177–179]. In patients without suspicion of recurrence, PET showed a sensitivity of 50% and specificity of 88%, and can find clinically unexpected recurrence in 27% of patients [179, 180]. In known recurrent stomach cancer, PET detects clinically unexpected metastasis in 22 % of patients [181]. PET results had clinical impact, such as change in treatment decision for 17–48% of patients with known or suspected recurrent stomach cancer [179–181].

Metabolic response to chemotherapy measured by PET predicts histopathologic response and survival in gastric cancer, although metabolic response can be evaluated only in FDG-avid tumors [182–186].

Colorectal Cancer

Initial Treatment Strategy

For detecting regional metastatic lymph node of colorectal cancer, FDG PET showed a low sensitivity of 29–37% and high specificity of 83–97%, which are not significantly better than those of CT [187–190].

PET is useful for detecting distant metastasis of colorectal cancer. In a meta-analysis on 61 studies, the sensitivity of PET was 95%, which is better than 60% for nonhelical CT, 65% for helical CT, and 76% for 1.5-T MRI [191]. In advanced colorectal cancer, PET is more sensitive than conventional methods for detecting extrahepatic distant metastasis [192–195]. The results of PET impact the treatment plan in 2–29% of patients with colorectal cancer [188, 192–194].

Subsequent Treatment Strategy

FDG PET is useful for detecting recurrence of colorectal cancer. In a meta-analysis of 11 studies, the sensitivity of PET for diagnosing recurrent colorectal cancer was 97% and specificity was 76% [196]. In another meta-analysis of 32 studies, PET demonstrated a sensitivity of 88% and specificity of 96% for detecting hepatic metastasis, which is better than 83% and 84% for CT, respectively [197]. For detecting recurrent extrahepatic metastasis, PET demonstrates a sensitivity of 92% and specificity of 95%,better than 61% and 91% for CT [197]. For restaging of recurrent colorectal cancer, PET/CT is more accurate than PET [198, 199]. The results of PET impact the treatment plan in 28–61% of patients with recurrent colorectal cancer [196, 197, 199, 200]. In locally advanced rectal cancer, PET is useful in predicting pathologic response to neoadjuvant therapy [201–203].

Uterine Cervical Cancer

Initial Treatment Strategy

FDG PET is useful for detecting lymph node metastasis in uterine cervical cancer. For detecting metastatic pelvic lymph nodes, PET or PET/CT showed a sensitivity of 60–100% (median, 84%) and specificity of 55–100% (median, 84%) [204–209]. For detecting metastatic extrapelvic lymph nodes, PET or PET/CT showed a sensitivity of 50–100% (median, 85%) and specificity of 83–100% (median, 94%) [204, 206, 209–212]. In comparison with CT or MRI, PET showed better results for detecting metastatic lymph nodes [204, 205, 210–214]. Only one study reported that CT and MRI were better than PET for nodal staging [215]. However, PET acquisition protocol was inadequate for obtaining good quality PET images in that study (for example, no attenuation correction). The SUV of primary tumor or para-aortic lymph node, and presence of metastatic extrapelvic lymph nodes on PET are significant prognostic factors in uterine cervical cancer [216–220].

Subsequent Treatment Strategy

FDG PET is useful for detecting recurrence in posttherapy surveillance without symptoms or when recurrence is suspicious [221–231], and is better than CT for detecting recurrence in uterine cervical cancer [229, 231]. FDG PET impacts the therapeutic or management plan in 23–55% of patients with recurrent uterine cervical cancer [230–234]. The findings on posttherapy PET are associated with prognosis of patients with uterine cervical cancer [235, 236].

Ovarian Cancer

Initial Treatment Strategy

There are several reports dealing with the initial staging of FDG PET or PET/CT in ovarian cancer [237–239]. All of the studies suggest that the addition of PET or PET/CT to CT significantly improves the preoperative staging results over CT alone (53% to 69–87%). PET can locate unexpected stage IV disease in 8% of patients (4 of 50), which is not found using CT [238].

Subsequent Treatment Strategy

FDG PET is useful for detecting recurrence and restaging in ovarian cancer. In patients with suspicious recurrence such as elevated serum tumor marker, FDG PET showed better or similar results than CT or MRI [240–246]. Recent studies using PET/CT also report better results than conventional modalities for diagnosing recurrence and restaging [247–249]. FDG PET impacts the therapeutic or management plan in 25–58% of patients with recurrent ovarian cancer [248–251]. PET shows better results for evaluating response to chemotherapy than conventional imaging [252]. Metabolic response to neoadjuvant chemotherapy using PET is predictive of a longer survival compared with non-response [253]. FDG PET is cost effective for detecting recurrence and restaging in ovarian cancer [254, 255].

Cutaneous Malignant Melanoma

Initial Treatment Strategy

FDG PET is useful for the initial staging of patients with cutaneous malignant melanoma. In a recent meta-analysis of 28 published studies, the pooled estimates of PET for the detection of metastasis in the initial staging of cutaneous malignant melanoma had a sensitivity of 83% and specificity of 85%, providing significant additional diagnostic information [257]. PET is more helpful in patients with stage III or IV than with stage I or II, in terms of detecting deep soft-tissue, lymph node, and visceral metastases [256]. The diagnostic performance of PET is low for the detection of small nodal metastases when compared with sentinel lymph nodes biopsy [257]. PET/CT provides additional diagnostic information than PET alone or PET/CT in the initial staging of cutaneous malignant melanoma [256–259]. The findings on FDG PET are associated with disease management changes in 8–64% of patients [256, 260–264].

Subsequent Treatment Strategy

FDG PET is useful for detecting recurrence in cutaneous malignant melanoma which can cause re-staging. In patients with suspicious or known recurrent cutaneous malignant melanoma, PET showed a sensitivity of 74–100% (except comparison studies with sentinel lymph node biopsy) and specificity of 82–100%, which are better than those of conventional imaging methods [257, 262, 265–272]. The results of FDG PET can have an impact on disease management changes in 8–48% of patients [262, 267–272]. A negative effect on patient management using the wrong results of PET is found in 3–20% of patients [268, 271]. Metabolic response to chemotherapy in cutaneous malignant melanoma is associated with patients' good survival [273].

Malignant Lymphoma

Initial Treatment Strategy

FDG PET is useful for the initial staging of patients with malignant lymphoma. In a meta-analysis of 14 studies on the staging of patients including mostly diffuse large B cell lymphoma and Hodgkin lymphoma, with some follicular lymphomas, PET showed the median sensitivity of 90% and the median specificity of 91%, which is better than those of CT [274, 275]. Staging using PET leads to a change of clinical stage in 10–40% of patients [276]. PET/CT is more sensitive and specific than contrast-enhanced full-dose CT for the evaluation of nodal and extranodal lymphomatous involvement [277, 278]. Some histologic types of lymphoma such as marginal zone B cell lymphoma, peripheral T cell lymphoma, and small lymphocytic lymphoma show variable FDG uptake where PET has a limited role in the initial staging [279, 280]. The degree of FDG uptake is associated with prognosis in malignant lymphoma [281].

Subsequent Treatment Strategy

FDG PET is useful in restaging and therapy response evaluation of patients with malignant lymphoma. In a systematic review of 15 published studies, the sensitivity and specificity of PET for detecting active residual disease after chemotherapy were 71–100% and 69–100%, respectively [282]. In contrast, the specificity and positive predictive value of CT was low (4–31% and 19–60%, respectively, except in one study where the positive predictive value was 82%) [282]. A systematic review of 19 published studies showed that the sensitivity and specificity of FDG PET in predicting disease relapse for Hodgkin lymphoma was 50–100% and 67–100%, respectively, and for non-Hodgkin lymphoma it 33–77 % and 82–100 %, respectively [283]. In general, metabolic response to chemotherapy by PET predicts prognosis in malignant lymphoma [284, 285]. In a systematic review of 13 published studies, interim response assessment using PET reflected prognosis with overall sensitivity of 81% and a specificity of 97% for advanced-stage Hodgkin lymphoma, and a sensitivity of 78% and a specificity of 87% for diffuse large B cell lymphoma [286]. The results of FDG PET before high-dose chemotherapy and autologous stem cell transplantation in patients with relapsing/refractory lymphoma are significantly associated with progression-free survival and overall survival on meta-analysis [287]. There is little evidence to support the use of FDG PET for monitoring therapy response of histologic types of lymphomas showing variable FDG uptake.

References

1. Goerres GW, Schmid DT, Gratz KW, et al. Impact of whole body positron emission tomography on initial staging and therapy in patients with squamous cell carcinoma of the oral cavity. Oral Oncol. 2003; 39:547–51.
2. Zanation AM, Sutton DK, Couch ME, et al. Use, accuracy, and implications for patient management of F-18 FDG PET/CT for head and neck tumors. Laryngoscope. 2005;115:1186–90.
3. Burri RJ, Rangaswamy B, Kostakoglu L, et al. Correlation of positron emission tomography standard uptake value and pathologic specimen size in cancer of the head and neck. Int J Radiat Oncol Biol Phys. 2008;17:682–8.
4. Laubenbacher C, Saumweber D, Wagner-Manslau C, et al. Comparison of fluorine-18-fluorodeoxyglucose PET, MRI and endoscopy for staging head and neck squamous-cell carcinomas. J Nucl Med. 1995;36:1747–57.
5. Myers LL, Wax MK, Nabi H, et al. Positron emission tomography in the evaluation of the N0 neck. Laryngoscope. 1998;108:232–6.
6. Adams S, Baum R, Stuckensen T, et al. Prospective comparison of F-18 FDG PET with conventional imaging modalities (CT, MRI, US) in lymph node staging of head and neck. Eur J Nucl Med. 1998;25:1255–60.
7. Hannah A, Scott AM, Tochon-Danguy H, et al. Evaluation of F-18 FDG PET and CT with histopathologic correlation in the initial staging of head and neck cancer. Ann Surg. 2002;236:208–17.
8. Schwartz DL, Ford E, Rajendran J, et al. FDG-PET/CT imaging for preradiotherapy staging of head-and-neck squamous cell carcinoma. Head Neck. 2005;61:129–36.
9. Yen T-C, Chang JT, Ng S-H, et al. Staging of untreated squamous cell carcinoma of buccal mucosa with ^{18}F-FDG PET: comparison with head and neck CT/MRI and histopathology. J Nucl Med. 2005; 46:775–81.
10. Ng S-H, Yen T-C, Liao C-T, et al. F-18 FDG PET and CT/MRI in oral cavity squamous cell carcinoma: a prospective study of 124 patients with histologic correlation. J Nucl Med. 2005;46:1136–43.
11. Chang JT, Chan SC, Yen TC, et al. Nasopharyngeal carcinoma staging by F-18 FDG PET. Head Neck. 2005;62:501–7.
12. Goshen E, Davidson T, Yahalom R, et al. PET/CT in the evaluation of patients with squamous cell cancer of the head and neck. Int J Oral Maxillofac Surg. 2006;35:332–6.

13. Brouwer J, Senft A, de Bree R, et al. Screening for distant metastases in patients with head and neck cancer: is there a role for (^{18}F)FDG-PET? Oral Oncol. 2006;42:275–80.
14. Fleming AJ, Smith SJ, Paul CM, et al. Impact of [^{18}F]-2-fluorodeoxyglucose-positron emission tomography/computed tomography on previously untreated head and neck cancer patients. Laryngoscope. 2007;117:1173–9.
15. Kim MR, Roh JL, Kim JS, et al. Utility of ^{18}F-fluorodeoxyglucose positron emission tomography in the preoperative staging of squamous cell carcinoma of the oropharynx. Eur J Surg Oncol. 2007;33:633–8.
16. Roh JL, Yeo NK, Kim JS, et al. Utility of 2-[^{18}F] fluoro-2-deoxy-D-glucose positron emission tomography and positron emission tomography/computed tomography imaging in the preoperative staging of head and neck squamous cell carcinoma. Oral Oncol. 2007;43:887–93.
17. Jeong H-S, Baek C-H, Son Y-I, et al. Use of integrated ^{18}F-FDG PET/CT to improve the accuracy of initial cervical nodal evaluation in patients with head and neck squamous cell carcinoma. Head Neck. 2007;29:203–10.
18. Wensing BM, Vogel WV, Marres HA, et al. FDG-PET in the clinically negative neck in oral squamous cell carcinoma. Laryngoscope. 2006;116:809–13.
19. Schoder H, Carlson DL, Kraus DH, et al. ^{18}F-FDG PET/CT for detecting nodal metastases in patients with oral cancer staged N0 by clinical examination and CT/MRI. J Nucl Med. 2006;47:755–62.
20. Choi JY, Lee KS, Kwon OJ, et al. Improved detection of second primary cancer using integrated [^{18}F] fluorodeoxyglucose positron emission tomography and computed tomography for initial tumor staging. J Clin Oncol. 2005;23:7654–9.
21. Lapela M, Grenman R, Kurki T, et al. Head and neck cancer: detection of recurrence with PET and 2-[F-18]fluoro-2-deoxy-D-glucose. Radiology. 1995;197:205–11.
22. Anzai Y, Carroll WR, Quint DJ, et al. Recurrence of head and neck cancer after surgery or irradiation: prospective comparison of 2-deoxy-2-[F-18]fluoro-D-glucose PET and MR imaging diagnoses. Radiology. 1996;200:135–41.
23. Kao CH, ChangLai SP, Chieng PU, et al. Detection of recurrent or persistent nasopharyngeal carcinomas after radiotherapy with ^{18}F-fluoro-2-deoxyglucose positron emission tomography and comparison with computed tomography. J Clin Oncol. 1998;16:3550–65.
24. Farber LA, Benard F, Machtay M, et al. Detection of recurrent head and neck squamous cell carcinomas after radiation therapy with 2-^{18}F-fluoro-2-deoxy-D-glucose positron emission tomography. Laryngoscope. 1999;109:970–5.
25. Stokkel MPM, Tehaard CHJ, Hordijk GJ, et al. The detection of local recurrent head and neck cancer with F-18 FDG PET dual-head PET. Eur J Nucl Med. 1999;26:767–73.
26. Kao C, Tsai S, Wang J, et al. Comparing FDG PET with a combination Tc-99 m tetrofosmin SPECT and CT to detect recurrent or persistent nasopharyngeal carcinomas after radiotherapy. Cancer. 2000; 92:434–9.
27. Terhaard CH, Bongers V, van Rijk PP, et al. F-18 FDG PET scanning in detection of local recurrence after radiotherapy for laryngeal/pharyngeal cancer. Head Neck. 2001;23:933–41.
28. Wong RJ, Schoder LH, Patel SG, et al. Diagnostic and prognostic value of F-18 FDG PET for recurrent head and neck squamous cell carcinoma. J Clin Oncol. 2002;20:4199–208.
29. Yen R, Hung R, Pan M, et al. F-18 FDG PET in detecting residual/recurrent nasopharyngeal carcinomas and comparison with MRI. Cancer. 2003;98:283–7.
30. Kunkel M, Forster GJ, Reichert T, et al. Detection of recurrent oral squamous cell carcinoma by F-18 FDG PET. Cancer. 2003;98:2257–65.
31. Kobota K, Yokoyama J, Yamaguchi K, et al. FDG-PET delayed imaging for the detection of head and neck cancer recurrence after radio-chemotherapy: comparison with MRI/CT. Eur J Nucl Med. 2004;31:590–5.
32. Ng S-H, Yen T-C, Liao C-T, et al. Clinical usefulness of F-18 FDG PET in nasopharyngeal carcinoma patients with questionable MRI findings for recurrence. J Nucl Med. 2004;45:1669–76.
33. Ryan WR, Fee WE, Le Q, et al. PET for surveillance of head and neck cancer. Laryngoscope. 2005;115:645–50.
34. Chan SC, Ng SH, Chang JT, et al. Advantages and pitfalls of ^{18}F-fluoro-2-deoxy-D-glucose positron emission tomography in detecting locally residual or recurrent nasopharyngeal carcinoma: comparison with magnetic resonance imaging. Eur J Nucl Med Mol Imaging. 2006;33:1032–40.
35. Halpern BS, Yeom K, Fueger BJ, et al. Evaluation of suspected local recurrence in head and neck cancer: a comparison between PET and PET/CT for biopsy proven lesions. Eur J Radiol. 2007;62:199–204.
36. Lee JC, Kim JS, Lee JH, et al. F-18 FDG-PET as a routine surveillance tool for the detection of recurrent head and neck squamous cell carcinoma. Oral Oncol. 2007;43:686–92.
37. Lowe VJ, Dunphy FR, varvares M, et al. Evaluation of chemotherapy response in patients with advanced head and neck cancer using FDG PET. Head Neck. 1997;19:666–74.
38. McCollum AD, Burrell SC, Haddad RL, et al. PET with F-18 FDG to predict pathologic response after induction chemotherapy and definitive chemoradiotherapy in head and neck cancer. Head Neck. 2004;26:890–6.
39. Nam SY, Lee SW, Im KC, et al. Early evaluation of the response to radiotherapy of patients with

squamous cell carcinoma of the head and neck using F-18 FDG PET. Oral Oncol. 2005;41:390–5.
40. Yao M, Smith RB, Graham MM, et al. The role of FDG PET in management of neck metastasis from head-and-neck cancer after definitive radiation treatment. Int J Radiat Oncol Biol Phys. 2005;1563: 991–9.
41. Andrade RS, Heron DE, Degirmenci B, et al. Posttreatment assessment of response using FDG-PET/CT for patients treated with definitive radiation therapy for head and neck cancers. Int J Radiat Oncol Biol Phys. 2006;165:1315–22.
42. Brkovich VS, Miller FR, Karnad AB, et al. The role of positron emission tomography scans in the management of the N-positive neck in head and neck squamous cell carcinoma after chemoradiotherapy. Laryngoscope. 2006;116:855–8.
43. Kim SY, Lee SW, Nam SY, et al. The feasibility of ^{18}F-FDG PET scans 1 month after completing radiotherapy of squamous cell carcinoma of the head and neck. J Nucl Med. 2007;48:373–8.
44. Ong SC, Schoder H, Lee NY, et al. Clinical utility of ^{18}F-FDG PET/CT in assessing the neck after concurrent chemoradiotherapy for locoregional advanced head and neck cancer. J Nucl Med. 2008;49: 532–40.
45. Gourin CG, Williams HT, Seabolt WN, et al. Utility of positron emission tomography-computed tomography in identification of residual nodal disease after chemoradiation for advanced head and neck cancer. Laryngoscope. 2006;116:705–10.
46. Nayak JV, Walvekar RR, Andrade RS, et al. Deferring planned neck dissection following chemoradiation for stage IV head and neck cancer: the utility of PET-CT. Laryngoscope. 2007;117:2129–34.
47. Yao M, Luo P, Hoffman HT, et al. Pathology and FDG PET correlation of residual lymph nodes in head and neck cancer after radiation treatment. Am J Clin Oncol. 2007;30:264–70.
48. Kitagawa Y, Sadato N, Azuma H, et al. FDG PET to evaluate combined intra-arterial chemotherapy and radiotherapy of head and neck neoplasms. J Nucl Med. 1999;40:1132–7.
49. Brun E, Kjellen E, Tennvall J, et al. FDG PET studies during treatment: prediction of therapy outcome in head and neck squamous cell carcinoma. Head Neck. 2002;24:127–35.
50. Allal AS, Dulguerov P, Allaoua M, et al. Standardized uptake value of FDG in predicting outcome in head and neck carcinomas treated by radiotherapy with or without chemotherapy. J Clin Oncol. 2002;20: 1398–404.
51. Kunkel M, Forster GJ, Reichert T, et al. Radiation response non-invasively imaged by F-18 FDG-PET predicts local tumor control and survival in advanced oral squamous cell carcinoma. Oral Oncol. 2003;29:170–7.
52. Sanghera B, Wong WL, Lodge MA, et al. Potential novel application of dual time point SUV measurements as a predictor of survival in head and neck cancer. Nucl Med Commun. 2005;26:861–7.
53. Shie P, Cardarelli R, Sprawls K, Fulda KG, Taur A. Systematic review: prevalence of malignant incidental thyroid nodules identified on fluorine-18 fluorodeoxyglucose positron emission tomography. Nucl Med Commun. 2009;30:742–8.
54. Agress Jr H, Cooper BZ. Detection of clinically unexpected malignant and premalignant tumors with whole-body FDG-PET: histopathologic comparison. Radiology. 2004;230:417–22.
55. Bogsrud TV, Karantanis D, Nathan MA, et al. The value of quantifying ^{18}F-FDG uptake in thyroid nodules found incidentally on whole-body PET-CT. Nucl Med Commun. 2007;28:373–81.
56. Chen YK, Ding HJ, Chen KT, et al. Prevalence and risk of cancer of focal thyroid incidentaloma identified by ^{18}F-fluorodeoxyglucose positron emission tomography for cancer screening in healthy subjects. Anticancer Res. 2005;25:1421–6.
57. Choi JY, Lee KS, Kim HJ, et al. Focal thyroid lesions incidentally identified by integrated ^{18}F-FDG-PET/CT: clinical significance and improved characterization. J Nucl Med. 2006;47:609–15.
58. Chu QD, Connor MS, Lilien DL, Johnson LW, Turnage RH, Li BD. Positron emission tomography (PET) positive thyroid incidentaloma: the risk of malignancy observed in a tertiary referral center. Am Surg. 2006;72:272–5.
59. Cohen MS, Arslan N, Dehdashti F, et al. Risk of malignancy in thyroid incidentalomas identified by fluorodeoxyglucose-positron emission tomography. Surgery. 2001;130:941–6.
60. Even-Sapir E, Lerman H, Gutman M, et al. The presentation of malignant tumours and pre-malignant lesions incidentally found on PET-CT. Eur J Nucl Med Mol Imaging. 2006;33:541–52.
61. Ishimori T, Patel PV, Wahl RL. Detection of unexpected additional primary malignancies with PET/CT. J Nucl Med. 2005;46:752–7.
62. Kang KW, Kim SK, Kang HS, Lee ES, Sim JS, Lee IG, et al. Prevalence and risk of cancer of focal thyroid incidentaloma identified by ^{18}F-fluorodeoxyglucose positron emission tomography for metastasis evaluation and cancer screening in healthy subjects. J Clin Endocrinol Metab. 2003;88:4100–4.
63. Kim TY, Kim WB, Ryu JS, Gong G, Hong SJ, Shong YK. ^{18}F-fluorodeoxyglucose uptake in thyroid from positron emission tomogram (PET) for evaluation in cancer patients: high prevalence of malignancy in thyroid PET incidentaloma. Laryngoscope. 2005; 115:1074–8.
64. King DL, Stack Jr BC, Spring PM, Walker R, Bodenner DL. Incidence of thyroid carcinoma in fluorodeoxyglucose positron emission tomography positive thyroid incidentalomas. Otolaryngol Head Neck Surg. 2007;137:400–4.

65. Kurata S, Ishibashi M, Hiromatsu Y, et al. Diffuse and diffuse-plus-focal uptake in the thyroid gland identified by using FDG-PET: prevalence of thyroid cancer and Hashimoto's thyroiditis. Ann Nucl Med. 2007;21:325–30.
66. Lardinois D, Weder W, Roudas M, et al. Etiology of solitary extrapulmonary positron emission tomography and computed tomography findings in patients with lung cancer. J Clin Oncol. 2005;23:6846–53.
67. Little SG, Rice TW, Bybel B, et al. Is FDG-PET indicated for superficial esophageal cancer? Eur J Cardiothorac Surg. 2007;31:791–6.
68. Nam SY, Roh JL, Kim JS, Mason DP, Murthy SC, Falk GW, et al. Focal uptake of (18) F-fluorodeoxyglucose by thyroid in patients with nonthyroidal head and neck cancers. Clin Endocrinol (Oxf). 2007;67:135–9.
69. Nishiyama Y, Yamamoto Y, Yokoe K, et al. FDG-PET as a procedure for detecting simultaneous tumours in head and neck cancer patients. Nucl Med Commun. 2005;26:239–44.
70. Van Westreenen HL, Westerterp M, Jager PL, et al. Synchronous primary neoplasms detected on ^{18}F-FDGPET in staging of patients with esophageal cancer. J Nucl Med. 2005;46:1321–5.
71. Yi JG, Marom EM, Munden RF, et al. Focal uptake of fluorodeoxyglucose by the thyroid in patients undergoing initial disease staging with combined PET/CT for non-small cell lung cancer. Radiology. 2005;236:271–5.
72. Kresnik E, Gallowitsch HJ, Mikosch P, et al. Fluorine-18-fluorodeoxyglucose positron emission tomography in the preoperative assessment of thyroid nodules in an endemic goiter area. Surgery. 2003;133:294–9.
73. Jeong H-S, Baek C-H, Son Y-I, et al. Integrated ^{18}F-FDG PET/CT for the initial evaluation of cervical node level of patients with papillary thyroid carcinoma: comparison with ultrasound and contrast-enhanced CT. Clin Endocrinol. 2006;65:402–7.
74. Grunwald F, Kalicke T, Feine U, et al. Fluorine-18 fluorodeoxyglucose positron emission tomography in thyroid cancer: results of a multicentre study. Eur J Nucl Med. 1999;26:1547–52.
75. Dong M-J, Liu Z-F, Zhao K, et al. Value of ^{18}F-FDG-PET/PET-CT in differentiated thyroid carcinoma with radioiodine-negative whole-body scan: a meta-analysis. Nucl Med Commun. 2009;30:639–50.
76. Nahas Z, Goldenberg D, Fakhry C, et al. The role of positron emission tomography/computed tomography in the management of recurrent papillary thyroid carcinoma. Laryngoscope. 2005;115:237–43.
77. Palmedo H, Bucerius J, Joe A, et al. Integrated PET/CT in differentiated thyroid cancer: diagnostic accuracy and impact on patient management. J Nucl Med. 2006;47:616–24.
78. de Groot JW, Links TP, Jager PL, Kahraman T, Plukker JT. Impact of ^{18}F-fluoro-2-deoxy-D-glucose positron emission tomography (FDG-PET) in patients with biochemical evidence of recurrent or residual medullary thyroid cancer. Ann Surg Oncol. 2004;11:786–94.
79. Diehl M, Risse JH, Brandt-Mainz K, et al. Fluorine-18 fluorodeoxyglucose positron emission tomography in medullary thyroid cancer: results of a multicentre study. Eur J Nucl Med. 2001;28:1671–6.
80. Szakall Jr S, Esik O, Bajzik G, et al. ^{18}F-FDG PET detection of lymph node metastases in medullary thyroid carcinoma. J Nucl Med. 2002;43:66–71.
81. Rubello D, Rampin L, Nanni C, et al. The role of ^{18}F-FDG PET/CT in detecting metastatic deposits of recurrent medullary thyroid carcinoma: a prospective study. Eur J Surg Oncol. 2008;34:581–6.
82. Gould MK, Maclean CC, Kuschner WG, Rydzak CE, Owens DK. Accuracy of positron emission tomography for diagnosis of pulmonary nodules and mass lesions: a meta-analysis. JAMA. 2001;285:914–24.
83. Yi CA, Lee KS, Kim B-T, et al. Tissue characterization of solitary pulmonary nodule: comparative study between helical dynamic CT and integrated PET/CT. J Nucl Med. 2006;47:443–50.
84. Gambhir SS, Shepherd JE, Shah BD, et al. Analytical decision model for the cost-effective management of solitary pulmonary nodules. J Clin Oncol. 1998;16:2113–25.
85. Gould MK, Lillington GA. Strategy and cost in investigating solitary pulmonary nodules. Thorax. 1998;53(Suppl 2):S32–7.
86. Gould MK, Sanders GD, Barnett PG, et al. Cost-effectiveness of alternative management strategies for patients with solitary pulmonary nodules. Ann Intern Med. 2003;138:724–35.
87. Kubota K, Yamada S, Fukuda H, et al. Cost effectiveness analysis of FDG-PET in the differential diagnosis and staging of lung cancer in Japan. Kaku Igaku. 1997;34:329–36.
88. Tsushima Y, Aoki J, Endo K. Whether and under what conditions FDG-PET might be cost-effective in evaluating solitary pulmonary nodules depicted on lung cancer screening in Japan. Nippon Igaku Hoshasen Gakkai Zasshi. 2003;63:390–8.
89. Tsushima Y, Endo K. Analysis models to assess cost effectiveness of the four strategies for the work-up of solitary pulmonary nodules. Med Sci Monit. 2004;10:MT65–72.
90. Dietlein M, Moka D, Weber K, Theissen P, Schicha H. Cost-effectiveness of PET in the management algorithms of lung tumors: comparison of health economic data. Nucl Med. 2001;40:122–8.
91. Gugiatti A, Grimaldi A, Rossetti C, et al. Economic analyses on the use of positron emission tomography for the work-up of solitary pulmonary nodules and for staging patients with non-small-cell-lung-cancer in Italy. Q J Nucl Med. 2004;48:49–61.
92. Miles KA. An approach to demonstrating cost-effectiveness of diagnostic imaging modalities in Australia illustrated by positron emission tomography. Australas Radiol. 2001;45:9–18.

93. Kalvin B, Fekeshazy A, Lengyel Z, Szakall Jr S, Agoston P, Lengyel E, et al. Cost-effective PET investigations in oncology. Magy Onkol. 2002;46: 203–23.
94. Dwamena BA, Sonnad SS, Angobaldo JO, Wahl RL. Metastases from non-small cell lung cancer: mediastinal staging in the 1990s–meta-analytic comparison of PET and CT. Radiology. 1999;213:530–6.
95. Gould MK, Kuschner WG, Rydzak CE, et al. Test performance of positron emission tomography and computed tomography for mediastinal staging in patients with non-small-cell lung cancer: a meta-analysis. Ann Intern Med. 2003;139:879–92.
96. Birim O, Kappetein AP, Stijnen T, Bogers AJ. Meta-analysis of positron emission tomographic and computed tomographic imaging in detecting mediastinal lymph node metastases in nonsmall cell lung cancer. Ann Thorac Surg. 2005;79:375–82.
97. Pieterman RM, van Putten JW, Meuzelaar JJ, et al. Preoperative staging of non-small-cell lung cancer with positron-emission tomography. N Engl J Med. 2000;343:254–61.
98. Reed CE, Harpole DH, Posther KE, et al. Results of the American College of Surgeons Oncology Group Z0050 trial: the utility of positron emission tomography in staging potentially operable non-small cell lung cancer. J Thorac Cardiovasc Surg. 2003;126:1943–51.
99. van Tinteren H, Hoekstra OS, Smit EF, et al. Effectiveness of positron emission tomography in the preoperative assessment of patients with suspected non-small-cell lung cancer: the PLUS multicentre randomised trial. Lancet. 2002;359:1388–93.
100. Viney RC, Boyer MJ, King MT, et al. Randomized controlled trial of the role of positron emission tomography in the management of stage I and II non-small-cell lung cancer. J Clin Oncol. 2004;22:2357–62.
101. Lardinois D, Weder W, Hany TF, et al. Staging of non-small-cell lung cancer with integrated positron-emission tomography and computed tomography. N Engl J Med. 2003;348:2500–7.
102. Cerfolio RJ, Ojha B, Bryant AS, Raghuveer V, Mountz JM, Bartolucci AA. The accuracy of integrated PET-CT compared with dedicated PET alone for the staging of patients with nonsmall cell lung cancer. Ann Thorac Surg. 2004;78:1017–23.
103. Shim SS, Lee KS, Kim BT, et al. Non–small cell lung cancer: prospective comparison of integrated FDG PET/CT and CT alone for preoperative staging. Radiology. 2005;236:1011–9.
104. Vansteenkiste JF, Stroobants SG, Dupont PJ, et al. Prognostic importance of the standardized uptake value on 18F-fluoro-2-deoxy-glucose–positron emission tomography scan in non–small-cell lung cancer: an analysis of 125 cases. J Clin Oncol. 1999;17:3201–6.
105. Cerfolio RJ, Bryant AS, Ohja B, Bartolucci AA. The maximum standardized uptake values on positron emission tomography of a non-small cell lung cancer predict stage, recurrence, and survival. J Thorac Cardiovasc Surg. 2005;130:151–9.
106. Sasaki R, Komaki R, Macapinlac H, et al. [18F]fluorodeoxyglucose uptake by positron emission tomography predicts outcome of non-small-cell lung cancer. J Clin Oncol. 2005;23:1136–43.
107. Berghmans T, Dusart M, Paesmans M, et al. Primary tumor standardized uptake value (SUVmax) measured on fluorodeoxyglucose positron emission tomography (FDG-PET) is of prognostic value for survival in non-small cell lung cancer (NSCLC): a systematic review and meta-analysis (MA) by the European Lung Cancer Working Party for the IASLC Lung Cancer Staging Project. J Thorac Oncol. 2008;3:6–12.
108. Hicks RJ, Kalff V, MacManus MP, et al. (18)F-FDG PET provides high-impact and powerful prognostic stratification in staging newly diagnosed non-small cell lung cancer. J Nucl Med. 2001;42:1596–604.
109. Mac Manus MP, Hicks RJ, Ball DL, et al. F-18 fluorodeoxyglucose positron emission tomography staging in radical radiotherapy candidates with nonsmall cell lung carcinoma: powerful correlation with survival and high impact on treatment. Cancer. 2001;92:886–95.
110. Gambhir SS, Hoh CK, Phelps ME, Madar I, Maddahi J. Decision tree sensitivity analysis for cost-effectiveness of FDG-PET in the staging and management of non-small-cell lung carcinoma. J Nucl Med. 1996;37:1428–36.
111. Scott WJ, Shepherd J, Gambhir SS. Cost-effectiveness of FDG-PET for staging non-small cell lung cancer: a decision analysis. Ann Thorac Surg. 1998;66:1876–83.
112. Alzahouri K, Lejeune C, Woronoff-Lemsi MC, Arveux P, Guillemin F. Cost-effectiveness analysis of strategies introducing FDG-PET into the mediastinal staging of non-small-cell lung cancer from the French healthcare system perspective. Clin Radiol. 2005;60:479–92.
113. Dietlein M, Scheidhauer K, Lauterbach KW, Schicha H. Quality criteria for cost-benefit analysis in oncologic nuclear medicine and state of its realization. Z Arztl Fortbild Qualitatssich. 1999;93:49–55.
114. Dietlein M, Weber K, Gandjour A, Moka D, Theissen P, Lauterbach KW, et al. Cost-effectiveness of FDG-PET for the management of potentially operable non-small cell lung cancer: priority for a PET-based strategy after nodal-negative CT results. Eur J Nucl Med. 2000;27:1598–609.
115. Weber WA, Dietlein M, Hellwig D, Kirsch CM, Schicha H, Schwaiger M. PET with (18) F-fluorodeoxyglucose for staging of non-small cell lung cancer. Nucl Med. 2003;42:135–44.
116. van Tinteren H, Hoekstra OS, Smit EF, Verboom P, Boers M, PLUS Study Group. Toward less futile surgery in non-small cell lung cancer? A randomized clinical trial to evaluate the cost-effectiveness of positron emission tomography. Control Clin Trials. 2001;22:89–98.

117. Verboom P, van Tinteren H, Hoekstra OS, Smit EF, van den Bergh JH, Schreurs AJ, et al. Cost-effectiveness of FDG-PET in staging non-small cell lung cancer: the PLUS study. Eur J Nucl Med Mol Imaging. 2003;30:1444–9.
118. Verboom P, Herder GJ, Hoekstra OS, Smit EF, van den Bergh JH, van Velthoven PC, et al. Staging of non-small-cell lung cancer and application of FDG-PET. A cost modeling approach. Int J Technol Assess Health Care. 2002;18:576–85.
119. Sloka JS, Hollett PD, Mathews M. Cost-effectiveness of positron emission tomography for non-small cell lung carcinoma in Canada. Med Sci Monit. 2004; 10:MT73–80.
120. Nguyen VH, Peloquin S, Lacasse Y. Cost-effectiveness of positron emission tomography for the management of potentially operable non-small cell lung cancer in Quebec. Can Respir J. 2005; 12:19–25.
121. Kosuda S, Ichihara K, Watanabe M, Kobayashi H, Kusano S. Decision tree sensitivity analysis for cost-effectiveness of chest FDG-PET in patients with a pulmonary tumor (non-small cell carcinoma). Kaku Igaku. 1998;35:395–404.
122. Kosuda S, Ichihara K, Watanabe M, Kobayashi H, Kusano S. Decision-tree sensitivity analysis for cost-effectiveness of chest 2-fluoro-2-D-[(18) F]fluorodeoxyglucose positron emission tomography in patients with pulmonary nodules (non-small cell lung carcinoma) in Japan. Chest. 2000;117: 346–53.
123. Kosuda S, Ichihara K, Watanabe M, Kobayashi H, Kusano S. Decision-tree sensitivity analysis for cost-effectiveness of whole-body FDG PET in the management of patients with non-small-cell lung carcinoma in Japan. Ann Nucl Med. 2002;16:263–71.
124. Abe K, Kosuda S, Kusano S. Medical economics of whole-body FDG PET in patients suspected of having non-small cell lung carcinoma–reassessment based on the revised Japanese national insurance reimbursement system. Ann Nucl Med. 2003;17:649–55.
125. Schumacher T, Brink I, Mix M, et al. FDG-PET imaging for the staging and follow-up of small cell lung cancer. Eur J Nucl Med. 2001;28:483–8.
126. Shen YY, Shiau YC, Wang JJ, Ho ST, Kao CH. Whole-body 18F-2-deoxyglucose positron emission tomography in primary staging small cell lung cancer. Anticancer Res. 2002;22:1257–64.
127. Blum R, MacManus MP, Rischin D, Michael M, Ball D, Hicks RJ. Impact of positron emission tomography on the management of patients with small-cell lung cancer: preliminary experience. Am J Clin Oncol. 2004;27:164–71.
128. Bradley JD, Dehdashti F, Mintun MA, Govindan R, Trinkaus K, Siegel BA. Positron emission tomography in limited-stage small cell lung cancer: a prospective study. J Clin Oncol. 2004;22: 3248–54.
129. Niho S, Fujii H, Murakami K, et al. Detection of unsuspected distant metastases and/or regional nodes by FDG-PET in LD-SCLC scan in apparent limited-disease small-cell lung cancer. Lung Cancer. 2007; 57:328–33.
130. Fischer BM, Mortensen J, Langer SW, et al. A prospective study of PET/CT in initial staging of small-cell lung cancer: comparison with CT, bone scintigraphy and bone marrow analysis. Ann Oncol. 2007;18:338–45.
131. Kut V, Spies W, Spies S, Gooding W, Argiris A. Staging and monitoring of small cell lung cancer using [^{18}F]fluoro-2-deoxy-D-glucose-positron emission tomography (FDG-PET). Am J Clin Oncol. 2007;30:45–50.
132. Bury T, Corhay JL, Duysinx B, et al. Value of FDG-PET in detecting residual or recurrent nonsmall cell lung cancer. Eur Respir J. 1999;14:1376–80.
133. Patz Jr EF, Lowe VJ, Hoffman JM, Paine SS, Harris LK, Goodman PC. Persistent or recurrent bronchogenic carcinoma: detection with PET and 2-[F-18]-2-deoxy-D-glucose. Radiology. 1994;191:379–82.
134. Hicks RJ, Kalff V, MacManus MP, et al. The utility of (18)F-FDG PET for suspected recurrent non-small cell lung cancer after potentially curative therapy: impact on management and prognostic stratification. J Nucl Med. 2001;42:1605–13.
135. Keidar Z, Haim N, Guralnik L, et al. PET/CT using 18F-FDG in suspected lung cancer recurrence: diagnostic value and impact on patient management. J Nucl Med. 2004;45:1640–6.
136. Vansteenkiste J, Fischer BM, Dooms C, Mortensen J. Positron emission tomography in prognostic and therapeutic assessment of lung cancer: systematic review. Lancet Oncol. 2004;5:531–40.
137. Hellwig D, Graeter TP, Ukena D, Georg T, Kirsch CM, Schafers HJ. Value of F-18-fluorodeoxyglucose positron emission tomography after induction therapy of locally advanced bronchogenic carcinoma. J Thorac Cardiovasc Surg. 2004;128:892–9.
138. Cerfolio RJ, Bryant AS, Winokur TS, Ohja B, Bartolucci AA. Repeat FDG-PET after neoadjuvant therapy is a predictor of pathologic response in patients with non-small cell lung cancer. Ann Thorac Surg. 2004;78:1903–9.
139. Choi NC, Fischman AJ, Niemierko A, et al. Dose–response relationship between probability of pathologic tumor control and glucose metabolic rate measured with FDG PET after preoperative chemoradiotherapy in locally advanced non-small-cell lung cancer. Int J Radiat Oncol Biol Phys. 2002;54: 1024–35.
140. Cerfolio RJ, Ojha B, Mukherjee S, Pask AH, Bass CS, Katholi CR. Positron emission tomography scanning with 2-fluoro-2-deoxy–glucose as a predictor of response of neoadjuvant treatment for non-small cell carcinoma. J Thorac Cardiovasc Surg. 2003;125:938–44.

141. Weber WA, Petersen V, Schmidt B, et al. Positron emission tomography in non-small-cell lung cancer: prediction of response to chemotherapy by quantitative assessment of glucose use. J Clin Oncol. 2003; 21:2651–7.
142. De Leyn P, Stroobants S, De Wever W, et al. Prospective comparative study of integrated positron emission tomography-computed tomography scan compared with remediastinoscopy in the assessment of residual mediastinal lymph node disease after induction chemotherapy for mediastinoscopy-proven stage IIIA-N2 non-small-cell lung cancer: a Leuven Lung Cancer Group Study. J Clin Oncol. 2006;24:3333–9.
143. Cerfolio RJ, Bryant AS, Ojha B. Restaging patients with N2 (stage IIIa) non-small cell lung cancer after neoadjuvant chemoradiotherapy: a prospective study. J Thorac Cardiovasc Surg. 2006;131: 1229–35.
144. Mac Manus MP, Hicks RJ, Matthews JP, et al. Positron emission tomography is superior to computed tomography scanning for response-assessment after radical radiotherapy or chemoradiotherapy in patients with non-small-cell lung cancer. J Clin Oncol. 2003;21:1285–92.
145. Ansteenkiste JF, Stroobants SG, De Leyn PR, Dupont PJ, Verbeken EK. Potential use of FDG-PET scan after induction chemotherapy in surgically staged IIIa-N2 non-small-cell lung cancer: a prospective pilot study. Ann Oncol. 1998;9: 1193–8.
146. Zhao DS, Valdivia AY, Li Y, Blaufox MD. ^{18}F-fluorodeoxyglucose positron emission tomography in small-cell lung cancer. Semin Nucl Med. 2002;32:272–5.
147. Pandit N, Gonen M, Krug L, Larson SM. Prognostic value of [^{18}F]FDG-PET imaging in small cell lung cancer. Eur J Nucl Med Mol Imaging. 2003;30: 78–84.
148. Block MI, Patterson GA, Sundaresan RS, et al. Improvement in staging of esophageal cancer with the addition of positron emission tomography. Ann Thorac Surg. 1997;64:770–6.
149. Flanagan FL, Dehdashti F, Siegel BA, et al. Staging of esophageal cancer with ^{18}F-fluorodeoxyglucose positron emission tomography. AJR. 1997;168: 417–24.
150. Luketich JD, Schauer PR, Meltzer CC, et al. Role of positron emission tomography in staging esophageal cancer. Ann Thorac Surg. 1997;64:765–9.
151. Luketich JD, Friedman DM, Weigel TL, et al. Evaluation of distant metastases in esophageal cancer: 100 consecutive positron emission tomography scans. Ann Thorac Surg. 1999;68:1133–6.
152. Choi JY, Lee KH, Shim YM, et al. Improved detection of individual nodal involvement in squamous cell carcinoma of the esophagus by FDG PET. J Nucl Med. 2000;41:808–15.
153. Flamen P, Lerut A, van Cutsem E, et al. Utility of positron emission tomography for the staging of patients with potentially operable esophageal carcinoma. J Clin Oncol. 2000;18:3202–10.
154. Kato H, Kuwano H, Nakajima M, et al. Comparison between positron emission tomography and computed tomography in the use of the assessment of esophageal carcinoma. Cancer. 2002;94:921–8.
155. Yoon YC, Lee KS, Shim YM, Kim BT, Kim K, Kim TS. Metastasis to regional lymph nodes in patients with esophageal squamous cell carcinoma: CT versus FDG PET for presurgical detection prospective study. Radiology. 2003;227:764–70.
156. Heeren PA, Jager PL, Bongaerts F, van Dullemen H, Sluiter W, Plukker JT. Detection of distant metastases in esophageal cancer with (18)F-FDG PET. J Nucl Med. 2004;45:980–7.
157. Kato H, Miyazaki T, Nakajima M, Takita J, Kimura H, Faried A, et al. The incremental effect of positron emission tomography on diagnostic accuracy in the initial staging of esophageal carcinoma. Cancer. 2005;103:148–56.
158. Meyers BF, Downey RJ, Decker PA, et al. The utility of positron emission tomography in staging of potentially operable carcinoma of the thoracic esophagus: results of the American College of Surgeons Oncology Group Z0060 trial. J Thorac Cardiovasc Surg. 2007;133:738–45.
159. van Westreenen HL, Heeren PA, van Dullemen HM, et al. Positron emission tomography with F-18-fluorodeoxyglucose in a combined staging strategy of esophageal cancer prevents unnecessary surgical explorations. J Gastrointest Surg. 2005;9:54–61.
160. Duong CP, Demitriou H, Weih LA, et al. Significant clinical impact and prognostic stratification provided by FDG-PET in the staging of oesophageal cancer. Eur J Nucl Med Mol Imaging. 2006;33:759–69.
161. Choi JY, Jang HJ, Shim YM, et al. ^{18}F-FDG PET in patients with esophageal squamous cell carcinoma undergoing curative surgery: prognostic implications. J Nucl Med. 2004;45:1843–50.
162. Cerfolio RJ, Bryant AS. Maximum standardized uptake values on positron emission tomography of esophageal cancer predicts stage, tumor biology, and survival. Ann Thorac Surg. 2006;82:391–4.
163. Flamen P, Lerut A, Van Cutsem E, et al. The utility of positron emission tomography for the diagnosis and staging of recurrent esophageal cancer. J Thorac Cardiovasc Surg. 2000;120:1085–92.
164. Kato H, Miyazaki T, Nakajima M, Fukuchi M, Manda R, Kuwano H. Value of positron emission tomography in the diagnosis of recurrent oesophageal carcinoma. Br J Surg. 2004;91:1004–109.
165. Westerterp M, van Westreenen HL, Reitsma JB, et al. Esophageal cancer: CT, endoscopic US, and FDG PET for assessment of response to neoadjuvant therapy-systematic review. Radiology. 2005;236:841–51.
166. Swisher SG, Maish M, Erasmus JJ, et al. Utility of PET, CT, and EUS to identify pathologic responders

in esophageal cancer. Ann Thorac Surg. 2004;78:1152–60.

167. Cerfolio RJ, Bryant AS, Ohja B, Bartolucci AA, Eloubeidi MA. The accuracy of endoscopic ultrasonography with fine-needle aspiration, integrated positron emission tomography with computed tomography, and computed tomography in restaging patients with esophageal cancer after neoadjuvant chemoradiotherapy. J Thorac Cardiovasc Surg. 2006;129:1232–41.
168. Mochiki E, Kuwano H, Katoh H, Asao T, Oriuchi N, Endo K. Evaluation of ^{18}F-2-deoxy-2-fluoro-D-glucose positron emission tomography for gastric cancer. World J Surg. 2004;28:247–53.
169. Chen J, Cheong JH, Yun MJ, et al. Improvement in preoperative staging of gastric adenocarcinoma with positron emission tomography. Cancer. 2005;103: 2383–2290.
170. Yun M, Lim JS, Noh SH, et al. Lymph node staging of gastric cancer using (18)F-FDG PET: a comparison study with CT. J Nucl Med. 2005;46:1582–8.
171. Mukai K, Ishida Y, Okajima K, Isozaki H, Morimoto T, Nishiyama S. Usefulness of preoperative FDG-PET for detection of gastric cancer. Gastric Cancer. 2006;9:192–6.
172. Kim SK, Kang KW, Lee JS, et al. Assessment of lymph node metastases using ^{18}F-FDG PET in patients with advanced gastric cancer. Eur J Nucl Med Mol Imaging. 2006;33:148–55.
173. Yang QM, Kawamura T, Itoh H, et al. Is PET-CT suitable for predicting lymph node status for gastric cancer? Hepatogastroenterol. 2008;55:782–5.
174. Dassen AE, Lips DJ, Hoekstra CJ, Pruijt JFM, Bosscha J. FDG-PET has no definite role in preoperative imaging in gastric cancer. Eur J Surg Oncol. 2009;35:449–55.
175. Yoshioka T, Yamaguchi K, Kubota K, et al. Evaluation of ^{18}F-FDG PET in patients with advanced, metastatic, or recurrent gastric cancer. J Nucl Med. 2003;44:690–9.
176. Lim JS, Yun MJ, Kim MJ, Hyung WJ, Park MS, Choi JY, et al. CT and PET in stomach cancer: preoperative staging and monitoring of response to therapy. Radiographics. 2006;26:143–56.
177. De Potter T, Flamen P, Van Cutsem E, Penninckx F, Filez L, Bormans G, et al. Whole-body PET with FDG for the diagnosis of recurrent gastric cancer. Eur J Nucl Med Mol Imaging. 2002;29:525–9.
178. Park MJ, Lee WJ, Lim HK, Park KW, Choi JY, Kim BT. Detecting recurrence of gastric cancer: the value of FDG PET/CT. Abdom Imaging. 2009;34:441–7.
179. Nakamoto Y, Togashi K, Kaneta T, et al. Clinical value of whole-body FDG-PET for recurrent gastric cancer: a multicenter study. Jpn J Clin Oncol. 2009;39:297–302.
180. Sun L, Su X-H, Guan Y-S, et al. Clinical role of ^{18}F-fluorodeoxyglucose positron emission tomography/computed tomography in post-operative follow up of gastric cancer: initial results. World J Gastroenterol. 2008;14:4627–32.
181. Jadvar H, Tatlidil R, Garcia AA, Conti PS. Evaluation of recurrent gastric malignancy with [F-18]-FDG positron emission tomography. Clin Radiol. 2003;58:215–21.
182. Ott K, Fink U, Becker K, et al. Prediction of response to preoperative chemotherapy in gastric carcinoma by metabolic imaging: results of a prospective trial. J Clin Oncol. 2003;21:4604–10.
183. Stahl A, Ott K, Schwaiger M, Weber WA. Comparison of different SUV-based methods for monitoring cytotoxic therapy with FDG PET. Eur J Nucl Med Mol Imaging. 2004;31:1471–8.
184. Di Fabio F, Pinto C, Rojas Llimpe FL, et al. The predictive value of ^{18}F-FDG-PET early evaluation in patients with metastatic gastric adenocarcinoma treated with chemotherapy plus cetuximab. Gastric Cancer. 2007;10:221–7.
185. Wieder HA, Ott K, Lordick F, et al. Prediction of tumor response by FDG-PET: comparison of the accuracy of single and sequential studies in patients with adenocarcinomas of the esophagogastric junction. Eur J Nucl Med Mol Imaging. 2007;34:1925–32.
186. Ott K, Fink U, Becker K, et al. Prediction of response to preoperative chemotherapy in gastric carcinoma by metabolic imaging: results of a prospective trial. J Clin Oncol. 2003;21:4604–10.
187. Kantorova I, Lipska L, Belohlavek O, Visokai V, Trubac M, Schneiderova M. Routine (18)F-FDG PET preoperative staging of colorectal cancer: comparison with conventional staging and its impact on treatment decision making. J Nucl Med. 2003; 44:1784–8.
188. Furukawa H, Ikuma H, Seki A, et al. Positron emission tomography scanning is not superior to whole body multidetector helical computed tomography in the preoperative staging of colorectal cancer. Gut. 2006;55:1007–11.
189. Abdel-Nabi H, Doerr RJ, Lamonica DM, et al. Staging of primary colorectal carcinomas with fluorine-18 fluorodeoxyglucose whole-body PET: correlation with histopathologic and CT findings. Radiology. 1998;206:755–60.
190. Mukai M, Sadahiro S, Yasuda S, et al. Preoperative evaluation by whole-body ^{18}F-fluorodeoxyglucose positron emission tomography in patients with primary colorectal cancer. Oncol Rep. 2000;7:85–7.
191. Bipat S, van Leeuwen MS, Comans EF, et al. Colorectal liver metastases: CT, MR imaging, and PET for diagnosis–meta-analysis. Radiology. 2005;237:123–31.
192. Lai DT, Fulham M, Stephen MS, et al. The role of whole-body positron emission tomography with [^{18}F]fluorodeoxyglucose in identifying operable colorectal cancer metastases to the liver. Arch Surg. 1996;131:703–7.
193. Fong Y, Saldinger PF, Akhurst T, et al. Utility of ^{18}F-FDG positron emission tomography scanning on selection of patients for resection of hepatic colorectal metastases. Am J Surg. 1999;178:282–7.

194. Truant S, Huglo D, Hebbar M, Ernst O, Steinling M, Pruvot FR. Prospective evaluation of the impact of [18F]fluoro-2-deoxy-D-glucose positron emission tomography of resectable colorectal liver metastases. Br J Surg. 2005;92:362–9.
195. Selzner M, Hany TF, Wildbrett P, McCormack L, Kadry Z, Clavien PA. Does the novel PET/CT imaging modality impact on the treatment of patients with metastatic colorectal cancer of the liver? Ann Surg. 2004;240:1027–34.
196. Huebner RH, Park KC, Shepherd JE, et al. A meta-analysis of the literature for wholebody FDG PET detection of recurrent colorectal cancer. J Nucl Med. 2000;41:1177–89.
197. Wiering B, Krabbe PF, Jager GJ, Oyen WJ, Ruers TJ. The impact of fluor-18-deoxyglucose-positron emission tomography in the management of colorectal liver metastases. Cancer. 2005;104:2658–70.
198. Kim JH, Czernin J, Allen-Auerbach MS, et al. Comparison between 18F-FDG PET, in-line PET/CT, and software fusion for restaging of recurrent colorectal cancer. J Nucl Med. 2005;46:587–95.
199. Votrubova J, Belohlavek O, Jaruskova M, et al. The role of FDG-PET/CT in the detection of recurrent colorectal cancer. Eur J Nucl Med Mol Imaging. 2006;33:779–84.
200. Staib L, Schirrmeister H, Reske SN, Beger HG. Is (18)F-fluorodeoxyglucose positron emission tomography in recurrent colorectal cancer a contribution to surgical decision making? Am J Surg. 2000; 180:1–5.
201. Guillem JG, Puig-La Calle Jr J, et al. Prospective assessment of primary rectal cancer response to preoperative radiation and chemotherapy using 18-fluorodeoxyglucose positron emission tomography. Dis Colon Rectum. 2000;43:18–24.
202. Cascini GL, Avallone A, Delrio P, Guida C, Tatangelo F, Marone P, et al. 18F-FDG PET is an early predictor of pathologic tumor response to preoperative radiochemotherapy in locally advanced rectal cancer. J Nucl Med. 2006;47:1241–8.
203. Capirci C, Rampin L, Erba PA, et al. Sequential FDG-PET/CT reliably predicts response of locally advanced rectal cancer to neo-adjuvant chemo-radiation therapy. Eur J Nucl Med Mol Imaging. 2007;34:1583–93.
204. Rose PG, Adler LP, Rodriguez M, et al. Positron emission tomography for evaluating para-aortic nodal metastasis in locally advanced cervical cancer before surgical staging: a surgicopathologic study. J Clin Oncol. 1999;17:41–5.
205. Narayan K, Hicks RJ, Jobling T, et al. A comparison of MRI and PET scanning in surgically staged loco-regionally advanced cervical cancer: potential impact on treatment. Int J Gynecol Cancer. 2001;11: 263–71.
206. Yen TC, Ng KK, Ma SY, et al. Value of dual-phase 2-fluoro-2-deoxy-D-glucose positron emission tomography in cervical cancer. J Clin Oncol. 2003;23:3651–8.
207. Amit A, Beck D, Lowenstein L, et al. The role of hybrid PET/CT in the evaluation of patients with cervical cancer. Gynecol Oncol. 2006;100:65–9.
208. Choi HJ, Roh JW, Seo SS, et al. Comparison of the accuracy of magnetic resonance imaging and positron emission tomography/computed tomography in the presurgical detection of lymph node metastases in patients with uterine cervical carcinoma. Cancer. 2006;106:914–22.
209. Loft A, Berthelsen AK, Roed H, et al. The diagnostic value of PET/CT scanning in patients with cervical cancer: a prospective study. Gynecol Oncol. 2007;106:29–34.
210. Yeh LS, Hung YC, Shen YY, et al. Detecting para-aortic lymph node metastasis by positron emission tomography of 18F fluorodeoxyglucose in advanced cervical cancer with negative magnetic resonance imaging findings. Oncol Rep. 2002;9:1289–92.
211. Lin WC, Hung YC, Yeh LS, Kao CH, Yen RF, Shen YY. Usefulness of (18)F-fluorodeoxyglucose positron emission tomography to detect para-aortic lymph nodal metastasis in advanced cervical cancer with negative computed tomography findings. Gynecol Oncol. 2003;89:73–6.
212. Yildirim Y, Sehirali S, Avci ME, et al. Integrated PET/CT for the evaluation of para-aortic nodal metastasis in locally advanced cervical cancer patients with negative conventional CT findings. Gynecol Oncol. 2008;108:154–9.
213. Sugawara Y, Eisbruch A, Kosuda S, et al. Evaluation of FDG PET in patients with cervical cancer. J Nucl Med. 1999;40:1125–31.
214. Reinhardt MJ, Ehritt-Braun C, Vogelgesang D, et al. Metastatic lymph nodes in patients with cervical cancer: detection with MR imaging and FDG PET. Radiology. 2001;218:776–82.
215. Williams AD, Cousins C, Soutter WP, et al. Detection of pelvic lymph node metastases in gynecologic malignancy: a comparison of CT, MR imaging, and positron emission tomography. AJR. 2001;177:343–8.
216. Grigsby PW, Siegel BA, Dehdashti F. Lymph node staging by positron emission tomography in patients with carcinoma of the cervix. J Clin Oncol. 2001;1(19):3745–9.
217. Grigsby PW, Dehdashti F, Siegel BA. FDG-PET evaluation of carcinoma of the cervix. Clin Positron Imaging. 1999;2:105–9.
218. Miller TR, Pinkus E, Dehdashti F, et al. Improved prognostic value of 18F-FDG PET using a simple visual analysis of tumor characteristics in patients with cervical cancer. J Nucl Med. 2003;44:192–7.
219. Kidd EA, Siegel BA, Dehdashti F, Grigsby PW. The standardized uptake value for F-18 fluorodeoxyglucose is a sensitive predictive biomarker for cervical cancer treatment response and survival. Cancer. 2007;110:1738–44.

220. Yen TC, See LC, Lai CH, Tsai CS, Chao A, Hsueh S, Hong JH, Chang TC, Ng KK. Standardized uptake value in para-aortic lymph nodes is a significant prognostic factor in patients with primary advanced squamous cervical cancer. Eur J Nucl Med Mol Imaging. 2008;35:493–501.
221. Weber TM, Sostman HD, Spritzer CE, et al. Cervical carcinoma: determination of recurrent tumor extent versus radiation changes with MR imaging. Radiology. 1995;194:135–9.
222. Sun SS, Chen TC, Yen RF, Shen YY, Changlai SP, Kao A. Value of whole body ^{18}F-fluoro-2-deoxyglucose positron emission tomography in the evaluation of recurrent cervical cancer. Anticancer Res. 2001;21:2957–61.
223. Ryu SY, Kim MH, Choi SC, Choi CW, Lee KH. Detection of early recurrence with ^{18}F-FDG PET in patients with cervical cancer. J Nucl Med. 2003;44:347–52.
224. Havrilesky LJ, Wong TZ, Secord AA, Berchuck A, Clarke-Pearson DL, Jones EL. The role of PET scanning in the detection of recurrent cervical cancer. Gynecol Oncol. 2003;90:186–90.
225. Yen TC, See LC, Chang TC, et al. Defining the priority of using ^{18}F-FDG PET for recurrent cervical cancer. J Nucl Med. 2004;45:1632–9.
226. Chang WC, Hung YC, Lin CC, Shen YY, Kao CH. Usefulness of FDG–PET to detect recurrent cervical cancer based on asymptomatically elevated tumor marker serum levels–a preliminary report. Cancer Invest. 2004;22:180–4.
227. Sakurai H, Suzuki Y, Nonaka T, et al. FDG–PET in the detection of recurrence of uterine cervical carcinoma following radiation therapy–tumor volume and FDG uptake value. Gynecol Oncol. 2006;100: 601–7.
228. Chung HH, Kim SK, Kim TH, Lee S, Kang KW, Kim JY, Park SY. Clinical impact of FDG-PET imaging in post-therapy surveillance of uterine cervical cancer: from diagnosis to prognosis. Gynecol Oncol. 2006;103:165–70.
229. Sironi S, Picchio M, Landoni C, Galimberti S, Signorelli M, Bettinardi V, Perego P, Mangioni C, Messa C, Fazio F. Posttherapy surveillance of patients with uterine cancers: value of integrated FDG PET/CT in the detection of recurrence. Eur J Nucl Med Mol Imaging. 2007;34:472–9.
230. Chung HH, Jo H, Kang WJ, Kim JW, Park NH, Song YS, Chung JK, Kang SB, Lee HP. Clinical impact of integrated PET/CT on the management of suspected cervical cancer recurrence. Gynecol Oncol. 2007;104:529–34.
231. Kitajima K, Murakami K, Yamasaki E, Domeki Y, Kaji Y, Sugimura K. Performance of FDG-PET/CT for diagnosis of recurrent uterine cervical cancer. Eur Radiol. 2008;18:2040–7.
232. Belhocine T, Thille A, Fridman V, et al. Contribution of whole-body ^{18}FDG PET imaging in the management of cervical cancer. Gynecol Oncol. 2002;87:90–7.
233. Dizendorf EV, Baumert BG, von Schulthess GK, et al. Impact of whole-body ^{18}F-FDG PET on staging and managing patients for radiation therapy. J Nucl Med. 2003;44:24–9.
234. Lai CH, Huang KG, See LC. Restaging of recurrent cervical carcinoma with dual-phase [^{18}F]fluoro-2-deoxy-D-glucose positron emission tomography. Cancer. 2004;100:544–52.
235. Schwarz JK, Siegel BA, Dehdashti F, Grigsby PW. Association of posttherapy positron emission tomography with tumor response and survival in cervical carcinoma. JAMA. 2007;298:2289–95.
236. Grigsby PW, Siegel BA, Dehdashti F. Posttherapy surveillance monitoring of cervical cancer by FDG-PET. Int J Radiat Oncol Biol Phys. 2004;55: 907–13.
237. Yoshida Y, Kurokawa T, et al. Incremental benefits of FDG positron emission tomography over CT alone for the preoperative staging of ovarian cancer. AJR Am J Roentgenol. 2004;182:227–33.
238. Castellucci P, Perrone AM, Picchio M, et al. Diagnostic accuracy of ^{18}F-FDG PET/CT in characterizing ovarian lesions and staging ovarian cancer: correlation with transvaginal ultrasonography, computed tomography, and histology. Nucl Med Commun. 2007;28:589–95.
239. Kitajima K, Murakami K, Yamasaki E, et al. Diagnostic accuracy of integrated FDG PET/contrast-enhanced CT in staging ovarian cancer: comparison with enhanced CT. Eur J Nucl Med Mol Imaging. 2008;35:1912–20.
240. Hubner KF, McDonald TW, Niethammer JG, et al. Assessment of primary and metastatic ovarian cancer by positron emission tomography (PET) using 2-[^{18}F]deoxyglucose (2-[^{18}F]FDG). Gynecol Oncol. 1993;51:197–204.
241. Jimenez-Bonilla J, Maldonado A, Morales S, et al. Clinical impact of ^{18}F-FDG-PET in the suspicion of recurrent ovarian carcinoma based on elevated tumor marker serum levels. Clin Positron Imaging. 2000;3:231–6.
242. Yen RF, Sun SS, Shen YY, et al. Whole body positron emission tomography with ^{18}F-fluoro-2-deoxyglucose for the detection of recurrent ovarian cancer. Anticancer Res. 2001;21:3691–4.
243. Rose PG, Faulhaber P, Miraldi F, et al. Positive emission tomography for evaluating a complete clinical response in patients with ovarian or peritoneal carcinoma: correlation with second-look laparotomy. Gynecol Oncol. 2001;82:17–21.
244. Torizuka T, Nobezawa S, Kanno T, et al. Ovarian cancer recurrence: role of whole-body positron emission tomography using 2-[fluorine-18]-fluoro-2-deoxy- D-glucose. Eur J Nucl Med Mol Imaging. 2002;29:797–803.
245. Nanni C, Rubello D, Farsad M, et al. (18)F-FDG PET/CT in the evaluation of recurrent ovarian cancer: a prospective study on forty-one patients. Eur J Surg Oncol. 2005;31:792–7.

246. Havrilesky LJ, Kulasingam SL, Matchar DB, et al. FDG-PET for management of cervical and ovarian cancer. Gynecol Oncol. 2005;97:183–91.
247. Mangili G, Picchio M, Sironi S, Viganò R, Rabaiotti E, Bornaghi D, Bettinardi V, Crivellaro C, Messa C, Fazio F. Integrated PET/CT as a first-line re-staging modality in patients with suspected recurrence of ovarian cancer. Eur J Nucl Med Mol Imaging. 2007;34:658–66.
248. Chung HH, Kang WJ, Kim JW, Park NH, Song YS, Chung JK, Kang SB, Lee HP. Role of [18F]FDG PET/CT in the assessment of suspected recurrent ovarian cancer: correlation with clinical or histological findings. Eur J Nucl Med Mol Imaging. 2007;34:480–6.
249. Simcock B, Neesham D, Quinn M, Drummond E, Milner A, Hicks RJ. The impact of PET/CT in the management of recurrent ovarian cancer. Gynecol Oncol. 2006;103:271–6.
250. Nakamoto Y, Saga T, Ishimori T, et al. Clinical value of positron emission tomography with FDG for recurrent ovarian cancer. AJR Am J Roentgenol. 2001;176:1449–54.
251. Soussan M, Wartski M, Cherel P, Fourme E, Goupil A, Le Stanc E, Callet N, Alexandre J, Pecking AP, Alberini JL. Impact of FDG PET-CT imaging on the decision making in the biologic suspicion of ovarian carcinoma recurrence. Gynecol Oncol. 2008;108:160–5.
252. Baum RP, Przetak C. Evaluation of therapy response in breast and ovarian cancer patients by positron emission tomography (PET). Q J Nucl Med. 2001;45:257–68.
253. Avril N, Sassen S, Schmalfeldt B, et al. Prediction of response to neoadjuvant chemotherapy by sequential F-18-fluorodeoxyglucose positron emission tomography in patients with advanced-stage ovarian cancer. J Clin Oncol. 2005;23:7445–53.
254. Smith GT, Hubner KF, McDonald T, et al. Avoiding second-look surgery and reducing costs in managing patients with ovarian cancer by applying F-18-FDG PET. Clin Positron Imaging. 1998;1:263.
255. Smith GT, Hubner KF, McDonald T, et al. Cost analysis of FDG PET for managing patients with ovarian cancer. Clin Positron Imaging. 1999;2:63–70.
256. Krug B, Crott R, Lonneux M, Baurain JF, Pirson AS, Vander Borght T. Role of PET in the initial staging of cutaneous malignant melanoma: systematic review. Radiology. 2008;249:836–44.
257. Mottaghy FM, Sunderkotter C, Schubert R, Wohlfart P, Blumstein NM, Neumaier B, et al. Direct comparison of [18F]FDG PET/CT with PET alone and with side-by-side PET and CT in patients with malignant melanoma. Eur J Nucl Med Mol Imaging. 2007;34:1355–64.
258. Strobel K, Skalsky J, Steinert HC, et al. S-100B and FDG-PET/CT in therapy response assessment of melanoma patients. Dermatology. 2007;215:192–201.
259. Bastiaannet E, Oyen WJ, Meijer S, et al. Impact of [18F]fluorodeoxyglucose positron emission tomography on surgical management of melanoma patients. Br J Surg. 2006;93:243–9.
260. Damian DL, Fulham MJ, Thompson E, Thompson JF. Positron emission tomography in the detection and management of metastatic melanoma. Melanoma Res. 1996;6:325–9.
261. Tyler DS, Onaitis M, Kherani A, et al. Positron emission tomography scanning in malignant melanoma. Cancer. 2000;89:1019–25.
262. Jadvar H, Johnson DL, Segall GM. The effect of fluorine-18 fluorodeoxyglucose positron emission tomography on the management of cutaneous malignant melanoma. Clin Nucl Med. 2000;25:48–51.
263. Gulec SA, Faries MB, Lee CC, et al. The role of fluorine-18 deoxyglucose positron emission tomography in the management of patients with metastatic melanoma: impact on surgical decision making. Clin Nucl Med. 2003;28:961–5.
264. Falk MS, Truitt AK, Coakley FV, Kashani-Sabet M, Hawkins RA, Franc B. Interpretation, accuracy and management implications of FDG PET/CT in cutaneous malignant melanoma. Nucl Med Commun. 2007;28:273–80.
265. Rinne D, Baum RP, Hor G, Kaufmann R. Primary staging and follow-up of high risk melanoma patients with whole-body 18F-fluorodeoxyglucose positron emission tomography: results of a prospective study of 100 patients. Cancer. 1998;82:1664–71.
266. Wagner JD, Schauwecker D, Davidson D, Logan T, Coleman 3rd JJ, Hutchins G, et al. Inefficacy of F-18 fluorodeoxy-D-glucose-positron emission tomography scans for initial evaluation in early-stage cutaneous melanoma. Cancer. 2005;104:570–9.
267. Stas M, Stroobants S, Dupont P, Gysen M, Hoe LV, Garmyn M, et al. 18-FDG PET scan in the staging of recurrent melanoma: additional value and therapeutic impact. Melanoma Res. 2002;12:479–90.
268. Mijnhout GS, Comans EF, Raijmakers P, Hoekstra OS, Teule GJ, Boers M, et al. Reproducibility and clinical value of 18F-fluorodeoxyglucose positron emission tomography in recurrent melanoma. Nucl Med Commun. 2002;23:475–81.
269. Fuster D, Chiang S, Johnson G, Schuchter LM, Zhuang H, Alavi A. Is 18F-FDG PET more accurate than standard diagnostic procedures in the detection of suspected recurrent melanoma? J Nucl Med. 2004;45:1323–7.
270. Reinhardt MJ, Joe AY, Jaeger U, Huber A, Matthies A, Bucerius J, et al. Diagnostic performance of whole body dual modality 18F-FDG PET/CT imaging for N- and M-staging of malignant melanoma: experience with 250 consecutive patients. J Clin Oncol. 2006;24:1178–87.
271. Nguyen NC, Chaar BT, Osman MM. Prevalence and patterns of soft tissue metastasis: detection with true

whole-body F-18 FDG PET/CT. BMC Med Imaging. 2007;7:8.
272. Koskivuo IO, Seppanen MP, Suominen EA, Minn HR. Whole body positron emission tomography in follow-up of high risk melanoma. Acta Oncol. 2007;46:685–90.
273. Hofman MS, Constantinidou A, Acland K, Healy C, Harries M, O'Doherty M. Assessing response to chemotherapy in metastatic melanoma with FDG PET: early experience. Nucl Med Commun. 2007;28:902–6.
274. Isasi CR, Lu P, Blaufox MD. A metaanalysis of ^{18}F-2-deoxy-2-fluoro-D-glucose positron emission tomography in the staging and restaging of patients with lymphoma. Cancer. 2005;104:1066–74.
275. Seam P, Juweid ME, Cheson BD. The role of FDG-PET scans in patients with lymphoma. Blood. 2007;110:3507–16.
276. Schiepers C, Filmont JE, Czernin J. PET for staging of Hodgkin's disease and non-Hodgkin's lymphoma. Eur J Nucl Med Mol Imaging. 2003;30(Suppl 1):S82–8.
277. Raanani P, Shasha Y, Perry C, et al. Is CT scan still necessary for staging in Hodgkin and non-Hodgkin lymphoma patients in the PET/CT era? Ann Oncol. 2006;17:117–22.
278. la Fougère C, Hundt W, Bröckel N, et al. Value of PET/CT versus PET and CT performed as separate investigations in patients with Hodgkin's disease and non-Hodgkin's lymphoma. Eur J Nucl Med Mol Imaging. 2006;33:1417–25.
279. Jerusalem G, Beguin Y, Najjar F, et al. Positron emission tomography (PET) with ^{18}F-fluorodeoxyglucose (^{18}F-FDG) for the staging of low grade non-Hodgkin's lymphoma (NHL). Ann Oncol. 2001;12:825–30.
280. Elstrom R, Guan L, Baker G, et al. Utility of FDG PET scanning in lymphoma by WHO classification. Blood. 2003;101:3875–6.
281. Okada J, Yoshikawa K, Imazeki K, et al. The use of FDG-PET in the detection and management of malignant lymphoma: correlation of uptake with prognosis. J Nucl Med. 1991;32:686–91.
282. Reske SN. PET and restaging of malignant lymphoma including residual masses and relapse. Eur J Nucl Med Mol Imaging. 2003;30(Suppl 1):S89–96.
283. Terasawa T, Nihashi T, Hotta T, Nagai H. ^{18}F-FDG PET for posttherapy assessment of Hodgkin's disease and aggressive non-Hodgkin's lymphoma: a systematic review. J Nucl Med. 2008;49:13–21.
284. Spaepen K, Stroobants S, Verhoef G, Mortelmans L. Positron emission tomography with [^{18}F]FDG for therapy response monitoring in lymphoma patients. Eur J Nucl Med Mol Imaging. 2003;30 (Suppl 1):S97–105.
285. Hutchings M, Barrington SF. PET/CT for therapy response assessment in lymphoma. J Nucl Med. 2009;50(Suppl 1):21S–30.
286. Terasawa T, Lau J, Bardet S, et al. Fluorine-18-fluorodeoxyglucose positron emission tomography for interim response assessment of advanced-stage Hodgkin's lymphoma and diffuse large B-cell lymphoma: a systematic review. J Clin Oncol. 2009;27:1906–14.
287. Poulou LS, Thanos L, Ziakas PD. Unifying the predictive value of pretransplant FDG PET in patients with lymphoma: a review and meta-analysis of published trials. Eur J Nucl Med Mol Imaging. 2010;37:156–62.

PET/MRI

33

Jae Sung Lee and Keon Wook Kang

Necessity of PET/MRI

As described in the previous chapter, combined positron emission tomography (PET)/computed tomography (CT) scanners have several advantages over conventional stand alone PET (PET only) systems. Most importantly, accurately aligned PET and CT images are produced immediately after the PET/CT examination. In addition, the overall PET scan time is significantly reduced by using the CT information for the PET attenuation correction.

In spite of the advantages of PET/CT, do we really need a combined PET/magnetic resonance imaging (MRI) device? Is there any limitation on CT as an anatomic imaging modality for hybrid PET scans? An obvious negative aspect of PET/CT is the radiation exposure during the examination, which is approximately twice that of individual PET or CT. Therefore, PET/MRI will be potentially useful in studies of pediatric patients, and repeated scans for treatment monitoring. In addition, PET/CT is not a truly simultaneous study. Because the same physical principles are involved in the detection of gamma-rays (PET) and x-rays (CT), the crosstalk of x-rays on PET detectors will cause significant artifacts on PET images if the PET and CT data are simultaneously acquired.

In addition to the limitations involved in PET/CT examination, higher soft-tissue contrast on MRI than on CT is another important reason that PET/MRI is gaining attention as a complementary hybrid imaging modality to PET/CT. The advantageous properties of MRI yield superior diagnostic accuracy to CT, particularly in brain studies. MRI would also be useful in local tumor assessment and whole-body staging in where higher soft-tissue contrast on MRI is beneficial.

Potential Clinical Applications

PET has been used for diagnosis, therapeutic monitoring, and management decisions of diseases in the fields of neurology, cardiology, and oncology. Combined PET/CT is helpful in the diagnosis of a disease by exact localization of metabolic activity, especially in patients with cancer. However, MRI has some advantages over CT. Specifically, MRI provides better soft-tissue contrast than CT, especially in the brain, abdominal organs, and the musculoskeletal system. MRI can provide functional and molecular information, such as MR spectroscopy, diffusion imaging, perfusion imaging, and functional MRI.

Hybrid PET/MRI is still in its infancy, thus little clinical experience has accumulated.

J.S. Lee, Ph.D.
Department of Nuclear Medicine, Seoul National University Hospital, Seoul, South Korea

K.W. Kang, M.D., Ph.D. (✉)
Department of Nuclear Medicine, College of Medicine, Seoul National University, Seoul 110-744, South Korea
e-mail: kangkw@snu.ac.kr

E.E. Kim et al. (eds.), *Clinical PET and PET/CT: Principles and Applications*,
DOI 10.1007/978-1-4419-0802-5_33, © Springer Science+Business Media New York 2013

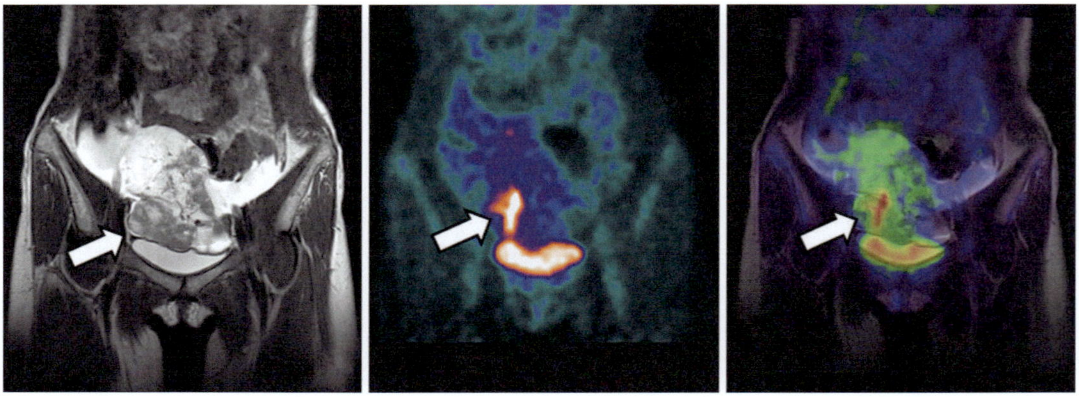

Fig. 33.1 Co-registration of MR (**a**) and PET (**b**) images that were taken on different machines at different time points using Syngo MultiModality Workplace software (Siemens Medical Solutions) in a patient with a Krukenberg tumor. The combined image (**c**) showed a mismatch of PET and MR images of the right ovarian mass because the mass was tilted in both studies

According to a report from a pilot study involving 10 patients with intracranial masses who were scanned with a prototype of a clinical hybrid PET/MRI system that consisted of a MRI-compatible PET system (BrainPET; Siemens Healthcare) inserted into a slightly modified 3-T whole-body MRI scanner (Magnetom Tim Trio; Siemens Healthcare), methionine or DOTATOC PET images from the PET/MRI system showed similar diagnostic image quality to those from the PET/CT studies [1]. From the PET/MR images of a patient with a meningioma, a small satellite lesion is clearly visible in the dorsal area of the frontal sinus. PET/MRI will be helpful in diagnosing small or suspected lesions in the brain by co-localizing PET and MR images, while CT images from PET/CT are not helpful in delineating brain lesions.

The brain is surrounded by the skull, thus rendering an exact combining of PET and MRI that is not collected at the same time, by using registration algorithms with rigid body transformation. However, the whole body is not rigid and combining PET and MR images obtained from different time points leads to errors in co-registration (Fig. 33.1). Simultaneous acquisition of PET and MRI data reduces motion artifacts that particularly affect small lesions. The clinical utility of whole-body hybrid PET/MRI will be better than that of PET/CT in cancers in which the tissues have high soft-tissue contrast on MRI, including musculoskeletal, head and neck, breast, liver, and intracranial tumors. Lung cancer is prone to distant metastasis [2]. Although CT is better in detecting pulmonary lesions than MRI, whole-body MRI is better in detecting brain, adrenal, and bone marrow lesions than CT. Therefore, M staging using whole-body PET/MRI will be superior to PET/CT.

Because both PET and MRI are applicable for visualizing molecular targets or processes of cells in the tissues and body, combining the two modalities will overcome the weakness of each modality. PET has a high sensitivity, but poor spatial resolution, and a limited follow-up time of molecular probes because the radioactivities from PET probes decay in a short period of time. MRI has high spatial resolution, but the sensitivity of molecular probes is approximately 1,000 times less than that of PET. Molecular imaging has two components (molecular probes for targeting specific biomarkers and sensors to detect the signals from those probes). MRI can detect signals from gadolinium or ion-oxide nanoparticles as a molecular probe. Radiolabeled ion-oxide nanoparticles can be detected using both PET and MRI. When PEGylated magnetic silica nanoparticles containing near-infrared fluorescent dye

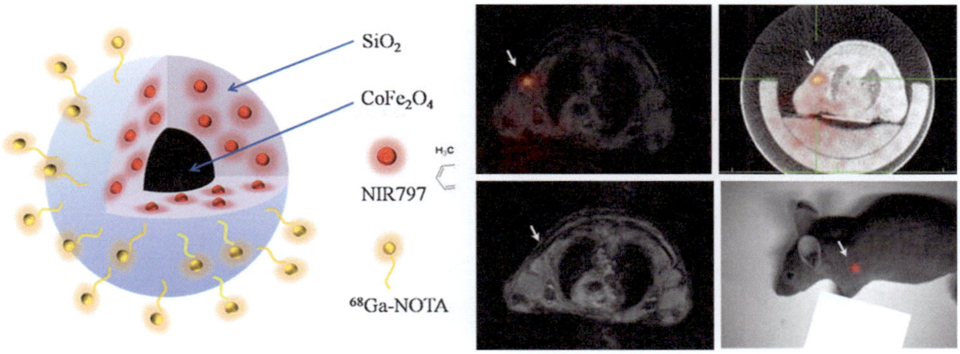

Fig. 33.2 A multimodal probe containing radioisotope, ion-oxide, and fluorescent dye (**a**), PET/CT (**c**), MRI (**d**), and optical images (**e**) of the sentinel lymph node in a mouse. PET/MRI combined image (**b**) shows a hot spot in the left axillary lymph node

(NIR-797 isothiocyanate and iron oxide core conjugated with Ga-68 NOTA) was injected subcutaneously into the foot pads of mice, the nanoparticles localized sentinel lymph nodes by triple modal imaging using animal PET/CT, animal MRI, and an in vivo optical imaging system (Fig. 33.2) [3]. PET is sensitive and makes it easy to localize the distribution of the probe. The injected dose of the probe that is delivered is quantifiable. Although MRI probes are less sensitive than PET probes, MRI probes can be monitored longer than PET probes because MRI probes are not affected by the physical half-life of radioisotopes. If T-cells or stem cells labeled with multimodal probes are injected into the body for therapeutic purposes, the distribution of T-cells or stem cells can be effectively monitored using combined whole-body PET/MRI.

Technical Issues Of PET/MRI

Hardware Systems

To understand the technical issues of PET/MRI hardware, we need to review the principles of gamma-ray detectors used in PET scanners. Common PET detectors consist of scintillation crystals and photosensors. The energy of gamma-rays is absorbed by the scintillation crystal that emits the visible light photons. Therefore, photosensors are required to measure the light output from the scintillation crystals.

Most common photosensors used in PET scanners are photomultiplier tubes (PMTs). PMTs have excellent gain of signal amplification (~10^6) and stability in operation. However, the PMT is sensitive to the external magnetic field because the signal amplification in the PMT relies on the acceleration of electrons that travel over cascade dynodes (Fig. 33.3). Within the PMT located in the strong magnetic field, the trajectories of electrons are changed by Lorenz forces, leading to the distortion of PMT output signals (Figs. 33.4 and 33.5).

Therefore, if the conventional PMT-based PET detector in which the scintillation crystals and PMTs are coupled directly or via a short light guide is used in the back-to-back or serial combination of PET and MRI similar to PET/CT, severe shielding of the PET detectors and gantry is necessary. In addition, PET and MRI scanners should be separated by a certain distance to avoid the direct exposure of PMT-based detectors to the strong magnetic field generated by the MRI coils. In this case, because only sequential PET and MRI scans are permitted, a long total scan time and possible patient movement between the PET and MRI scans are concerns.

Because both the PET and MRI examinations are time-consuming procedures, truly simultaneous PET/MRI is most desired and

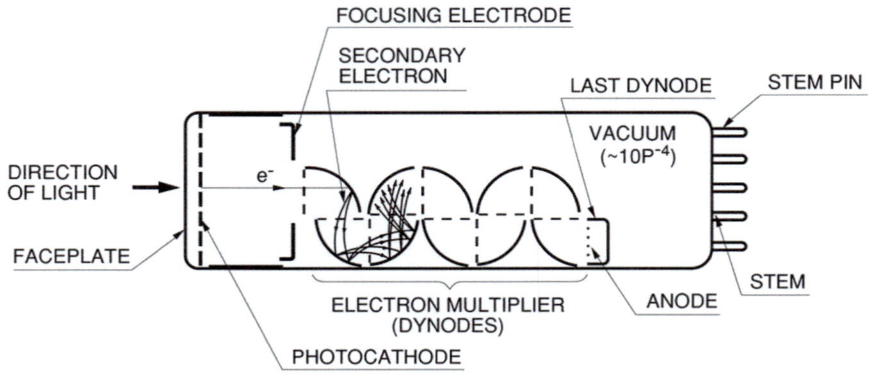

Fig. 33.3 Structure and principle of PMT (Courtesy of Hamamatsu Photonics)

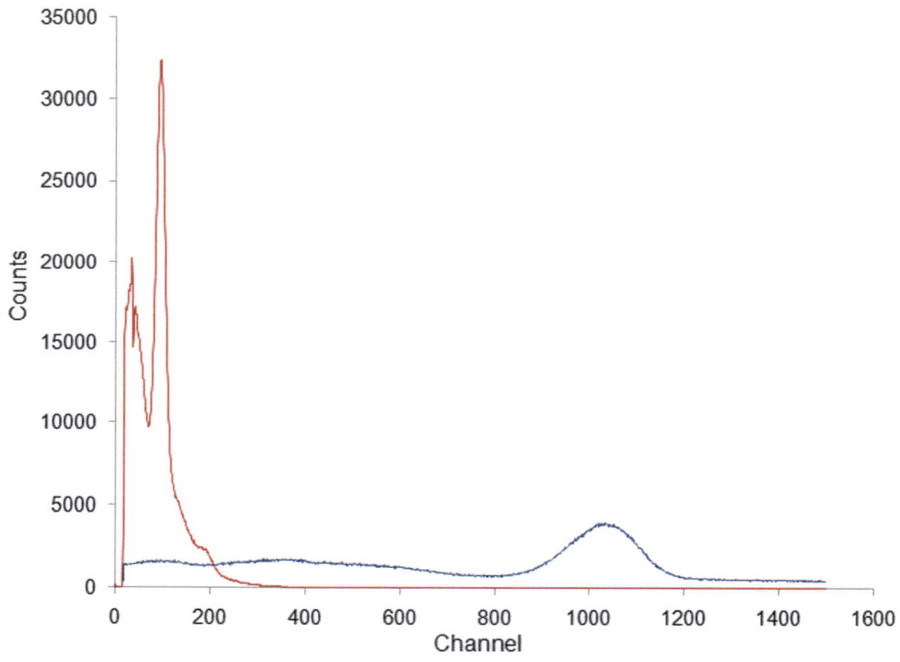

Fig. 33.4 Distortion of energy spectrum of PMT-based scintillation detector (*blue*: B = 0, *red*: B ≠ 0)

several approaches are actively being pursued to achieve this ultimate technical goal of PET/MRI system development. Use of an optical fiber bundle and semiconductor photosensors are two main approaches for simultaneous PET/MRI data acquisition.

The optical fiber bundles are useful in transferring the light signal from the scintillation crystals to PMTs located outside of the fringe magnetic field because the signal traveling along the optical fiber is immune to electromagnetic interference (Fig. 33.6) [5]). Minimization of light loss during the optical signal transfer is the most important technical issue in this approach because the light loss destroys most physical properties of PET detectors.

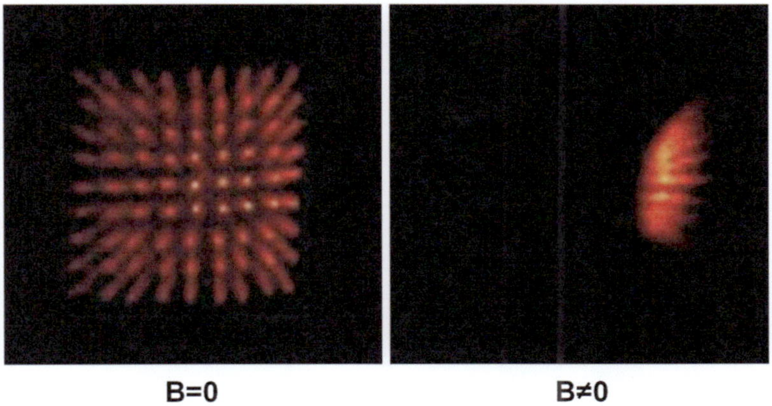

Fig. 33.5 Distortion of the crystal map of a PMT-based block detector by the magnetic field (Reprinted from [4] with permission)

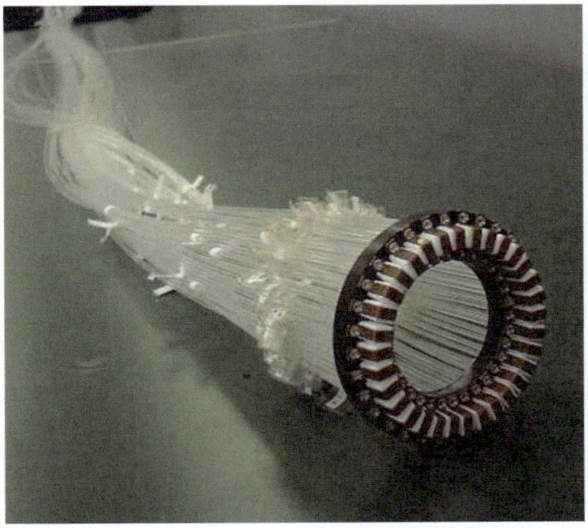

Fig. 33.6 Optical fibers to transfer light signal from scintillation crystal for simultaneous PET/MRI (Reprinted from [5] with permission)

Semiconductor photosensors are not susceptible to electromagnetic interference because the electric signal pathways in these devices are much shorter than in PMTs (Fig. 33.7). The most investigated semiconductor photosensor for MRI-compatible PET detectors is the avalanche photodiode (APD). The APD device has a similar structure to regular photodiodes, but a much higher signal amplification gain (~10^3) because of the avalanche multiplication of photo-generated electron and hole pairs. Another semiconductor photosensor that is attracting attention in PET/MRI is the silicon photomultiplier (SiPM), which is also referred to as Geiger-mode APD, solid-state photomultiplier, and multipixel photon counter. Although SiPM is not a mature technology yet, it is promising for PET/MRI systems because it is insensitive to the magnetic field and has comparative internal gain and timing properties with the PMT [6, 7].

Attenuation Correction

Attenuation and scatter corrections are essential in PET studies because the photon attenuation and Compton scattering are the most dominant physical factors that degrade the quantitative accuracy of PET data. It is difficult to use the conventional rotating gamma- or x-ray transmission sources with PET/MRI to obtain the attenuation maps for 511 keV gamma-rays used in these physical corrections. This is because there is a space constraint in placing the external radiation sources within the MRI scanner, and mechanical movement of radiation sources within the MRI scanner can cause the artifact. Furthermore, the use of these radiation sources in PET/MRI will diminish the advantage of the PET/MRI examination by increasing radiation exposure.

It is therefore necessary to obtain the PET attenuation map from PET data or anatomic MR images. However, no information about the

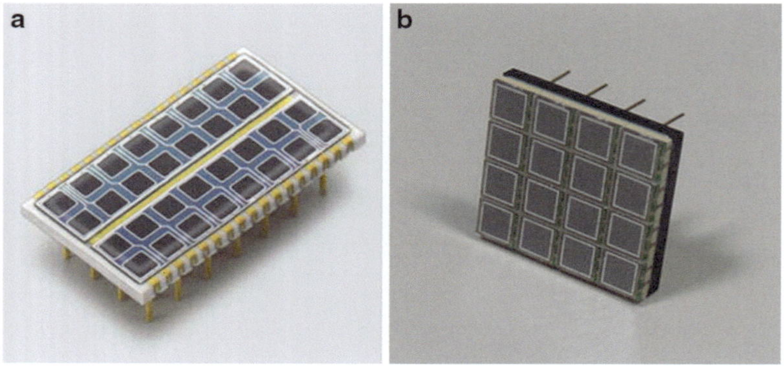

Fig. 33.7 Semiconductor photosensors. (**a**) APD (Courtesy of Hamamatsu Photonics). (**b**) SiPM

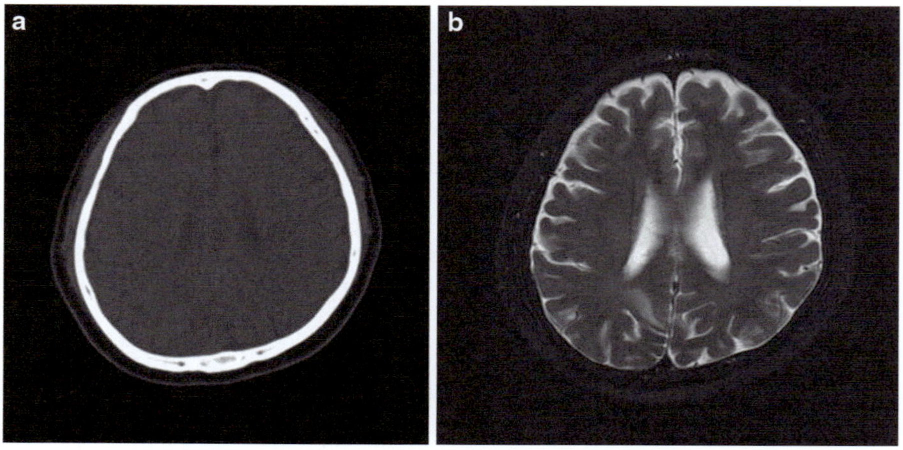

Fig. 33.8 Comparison of x-ray CT (**a**) and MRI (**b**) in the brain

gamma-ray attenuation is intrinsically obtained using MRI, which dominantly provides the information associated with proton distribution (Fig. 33.8). The truncation of extremities frequently shown on MR images as a result of field-of-view limitation is another challenging problem in obtaining the accurate PET attenuation map from MR images (Fig. 33.9; [8, 9]).

A calculated attenuation correction algorithm that is based only on PET data would be a possible choice for imaging the brain because of its simplicity and robustness. In this approach, the head boundary is outlined automatically using an edge detection algorithm on the emission sinogram. Uniform skull thickness is assumed to surround the soft tissue, and uniform attenuation coefficients are assigned to the skull and soft tissues [10, 11]. Although the calculated attenuation correction algorithm can be easily used for brain PET data, this method has limited accuracy in the parietooccipital region due to the assumption of uniform skull thickness and lower frontal region because of the ignorance of air cavities such as the frontal sinuses (Fig. 33.10) [12]).

Another approach is template-guided (atlas-guided or atlas-based) attenuation correction (Figs. 33.11 and 33.12), in which nonrigid image

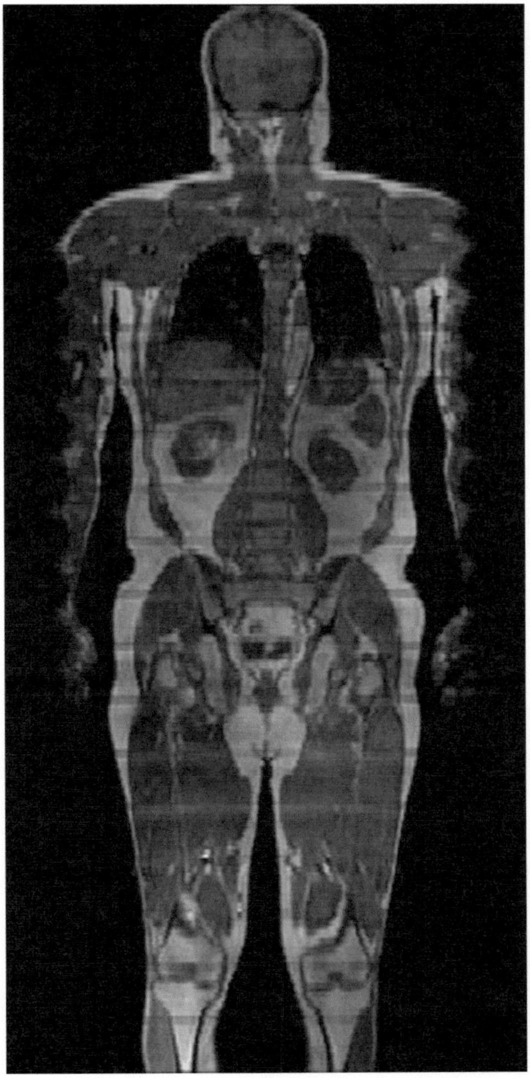

Fig. 33.9 Truncation of extremities frequently shown on MR images (Reprinted from [8] with permission)

registration is performed to obtain the deformation field between the individual MR image or PET image and standard template [13, 14]. The template of the PET attenuation map generated by averaging measured attenuation maps of several subjects after spatial normalization is then transformed using the same deformation field to yield the patient-specific attenuation map. Because the anatomic information of each individual is incorporated into the attenuation map through the spatial normalization procedure, this method has better quantitative accuracy than the calculated attenuation correction method [15]. The accuracy of this method has been validated in human and animal brain PET studies [15–17]. The easy incorporation of bone information into the attenuation map is an advantage of this method over the MRI-segmentation approaches.

A combination of a template-guided approach and pattern recognition was also suggested to predict the attenuation map from the MR image and a set of aligned MRI and CT datasets [18].

Although the template-guided attenuation correction method performs well for the brain PET data, the feasibility of this method in whole-body PET/MRI studies is questionable. Nonrigid image registration in the thorax and abdomen is more technically challenging than in the brain because of the higher intersubject anatomic variability and nonrigidity of the anatomic structures. Furthermore, it would be difficult to fully compensate for the large anatomic variations using a template-guided approach which are especially common in cancer patients after removal of the tumor and affected body areas.

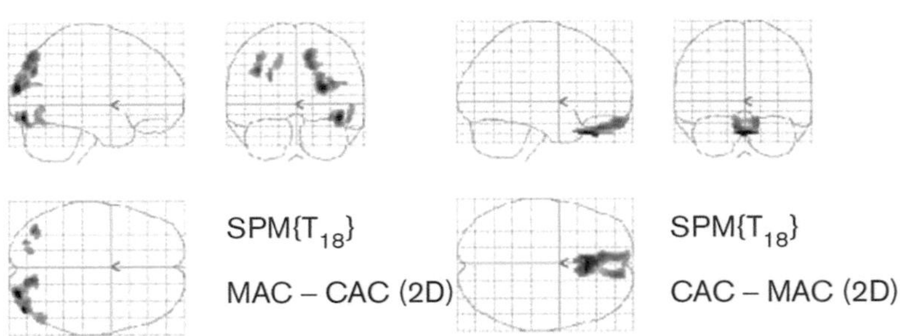

Fig. 33.10 Limitation of calculated attenuation correction (CAC) in brain FDG PET. Comparison with measured attenuation correction (MAC) using $^{68}Ge/^{68}Ga$ transmission sources (Reprinted from [12] with permission)

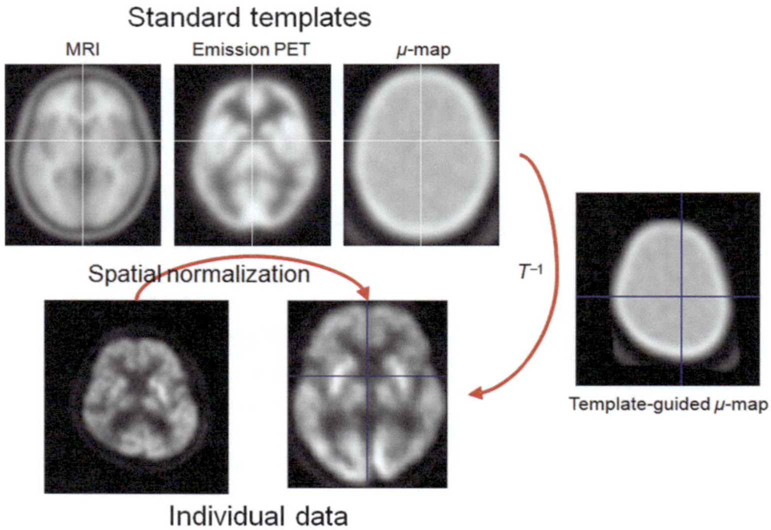

Fig. 33.11 Concept of template-guided (atlas-guided or atlas-based) attenuation correction. Nonrigid image registration is performed to obtain the deformation field (T) between the individual MR (or emission PET) image and standard template, and the template of the attenuation map (μ*-map*) is transformed into an individual space using the same deformation map

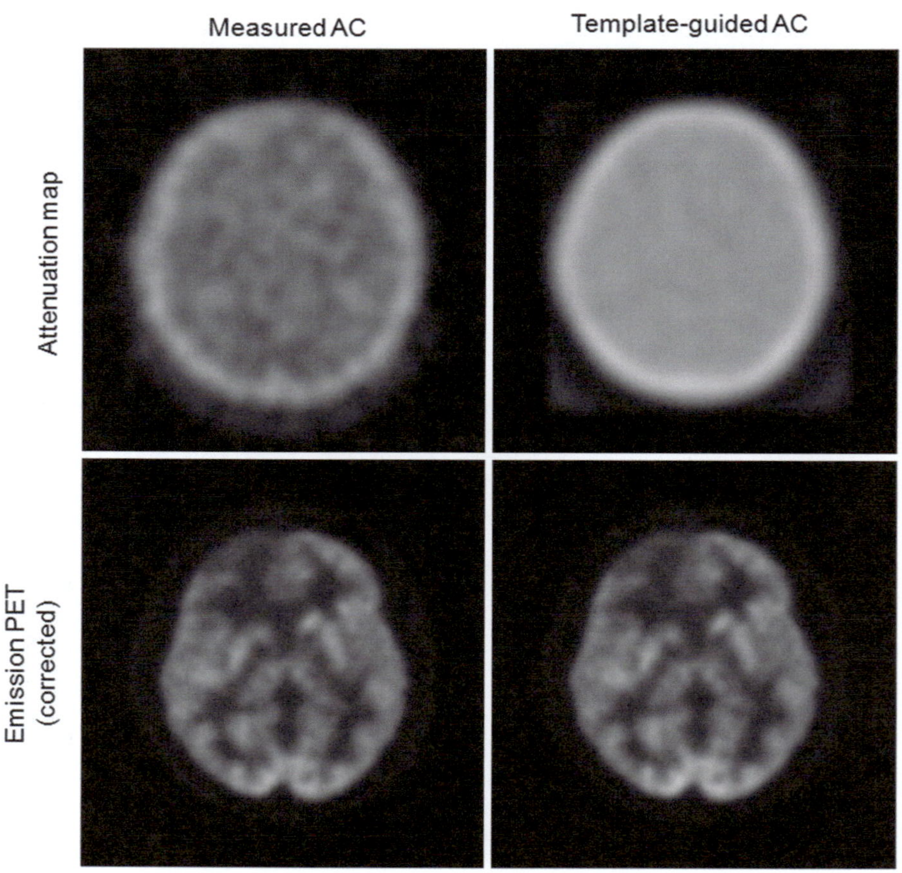

Fig. 33.12 Comparison of template-guided versus measured attenuation corrections

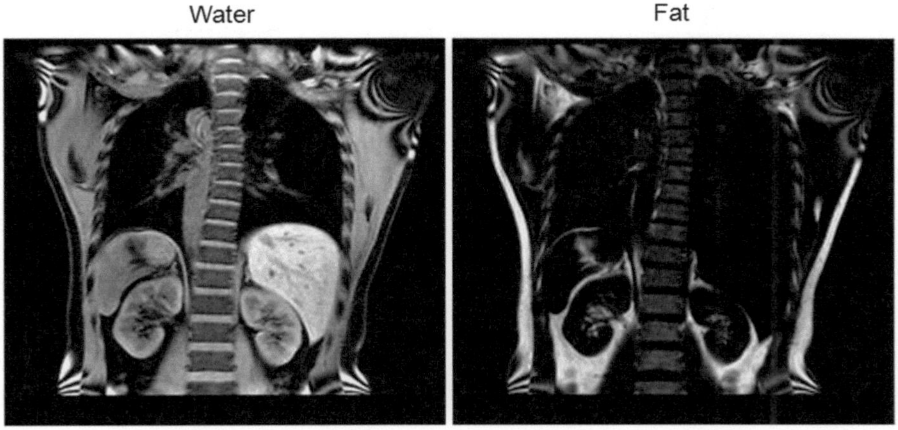

Fig. 33.13 Water-fat separation using two-point Dixon sequence (Courtesy of Prof. IC Song in Seoul National University Hospital)

An alternative approach is the segmented MRI-based attenuation correction method, in which approach MR images are segmented into several tissue classes (i.e., bone, soft tissue, and air) and voxels belonging to these classes are assigned the corresponding known linear attenuation coefficients. The feasibility of this approach in the brain using T1 MRI has been suggested by several authors who have also noted underestimation of the skull thickness associated with the difficulty in delineation of bone tissue on T1 MRI [19].

For whole-body studies, Martinez-Möller et al. [20] suggested segmentation of the attenuation map into four classes (background, lungs, fat, and soft tissue). The authors also proposed that the two-point Dixon MRI sequence is particularly well-suited for the segmentation because it provides separate water and fat images (Fig. 33.13). When this method was applied to CT-based attenuation maps from [^{18}F] fluorodeoxyglucose (FDG) oncologic PET/CT studies, there were no differences in the clinical interpretations made by the experienced observer with nonsegmented and segmented attenuation maps (Fig. 33.14). Although negligible differences in standardized uptake value (SUV) were found in nonosseous lesions, the most osseous lesions showed decreased SUV (average, 8.0%; maximum, 13.1%). Hofmann et al. [21] reported a similar effect of ignoring cortical bone in the attenuation map (Fig. 33.15). Therefore, a possible bias on the SUV estimation in bone metastasis should be considered when this approach is applied.

Because of the short relaxation time and low proton density in bone, it is difficult to extract bone structures from images acquired using conventional MRI sequences. On conventional MR images, the intensity of bone structures cannot be distinguished from that of air and robust segmentation of bone structures is regarded as a difficult task (especially in torso images). Keereman et al. [22] have proposed the use of MR images acquired with an ultrashort echo time (UTE) sequence for a three-class segmented attenuation map (bone, soft tissue, or air). In this approach, the map of R2 (the inverse of the spin–spin relaxation time T2) was calculated from the images (I_1 and I_2) acquired at two different TEs (TE_1=0.14 ms; TE_2=1.80 ms for human head data) using the following equation: $R2=(\ln I_1-\ln I_2)/(TE_2-TE_1)$. Because the signal intensity difference between I_1 and I_2 is greater in the cortical bone region (medium-to-high in I_1 and much lower in I_2) than soft tissue (medium-to-high in

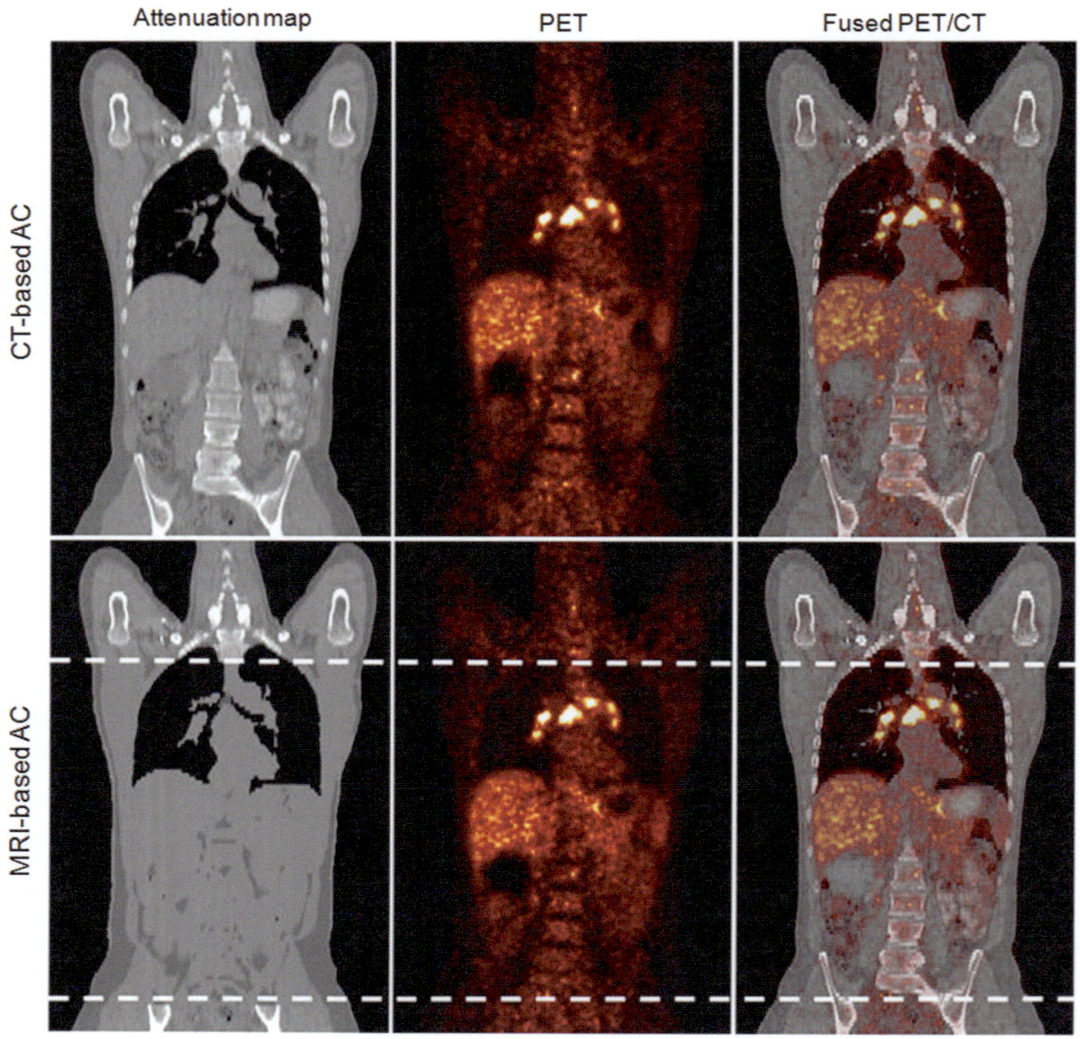

Fig. 33.14 Attenuation correction (AC) of whole-body PET images using MRI segmentation based on two-point Dixon sequence (Reprinted from [20] with permission)

both images) and air (low in both images), the R2 map provides useful information for straightforward segmentation of those regions. Minimizing the acquisition time and overcoming the potential image artifacts introduced by patient motion, Catana et al. [23] recently proposed the use of dual UTE sequence in which the signals from both TEs were collected during the same acquisition (Fig. 33.16). The applicability of this approach in whole-body examinations is currently under investigation.

Current Status of PET/MRI Scanners

PMT-Based PET/MRI (Optical Fiber)

Since the first attempt of acquiring simultaneous PET/MRI scans by the UCLA group, several groups have developed the MRI-compatible PET detectors using optical fiber and PMT, mostly for small animal studies [5, 24–29]. One of the limitations in the early stage of these investigations was the small number of crystal rings because the

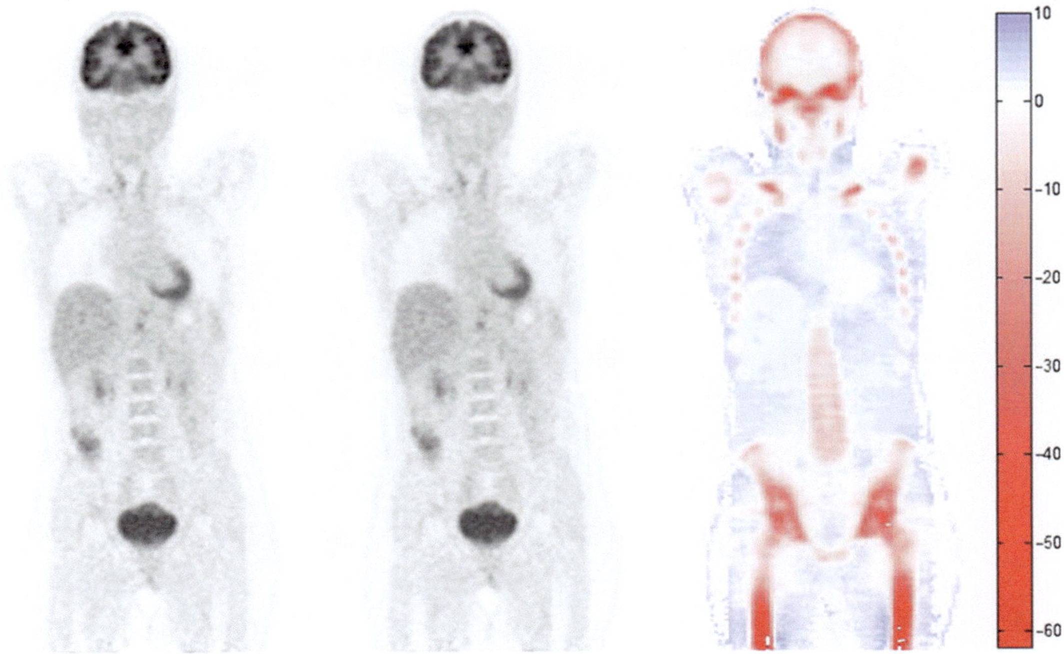

Fig. 33.15 Effects of ignoring bone in attenuation map. (**a**) Corrected on original CT. (**b**) Corrected on CT with all bone structures set to soft tissue. (**c**) Relative difference (%) between (a) and (b) (Reprinted from [21] with permission)

scintillation light was read out by the optical fiber from the side surfaces of the crystals [24–26]. Coupling of 90° bending optical fiber bundles or slanted light guides to the back of crystal array [27, 29] were suggested to overcome this limitation (Fig. 33.17).

The University of Cambridge group suggested a design that combines the optical fiber-based PET detectors with split MRI. In their approach, PMTs are located in regions of low magnetic field and connected by 1.2-m-long fibers to the crystal block placed right in the center of the magnetic field [30].

PMT-Based PET/MRI (Separate Scanners)

In the approach where a conventional PMT-based PET scanner is used, PET and MRI scanners are arranged in parallel, as in the current PET/CT configuration [31]. The combined time-of-flight (TOF) whole-body PET and self-shielded 3T MRI scanners by Philips Healthcare are accommodated in the same scan room, with a patient table between the two scanners (Fig. 33.18). The PET gantry was recrafted to provide magnetic shielding for PMTs so that they operate in nominal magnetic flux levels, and all electronics from the PET gantry were moved to the equipment room so as to satisfy the strict noise requirements of MRI. In a typical clinical environment, an MR image is first acquired for PET attenuation correction and then the patient is moved to the PET scanner for scanning. The patient will then be moved back to the MRI scanner for diagnostic MRI/spectroscopy as required by the clinical indication [8].

APD-Based PET/MRI (Small Animal)

As previously mentioned, APD is the mostly investigated MRI-compatible semiconductor

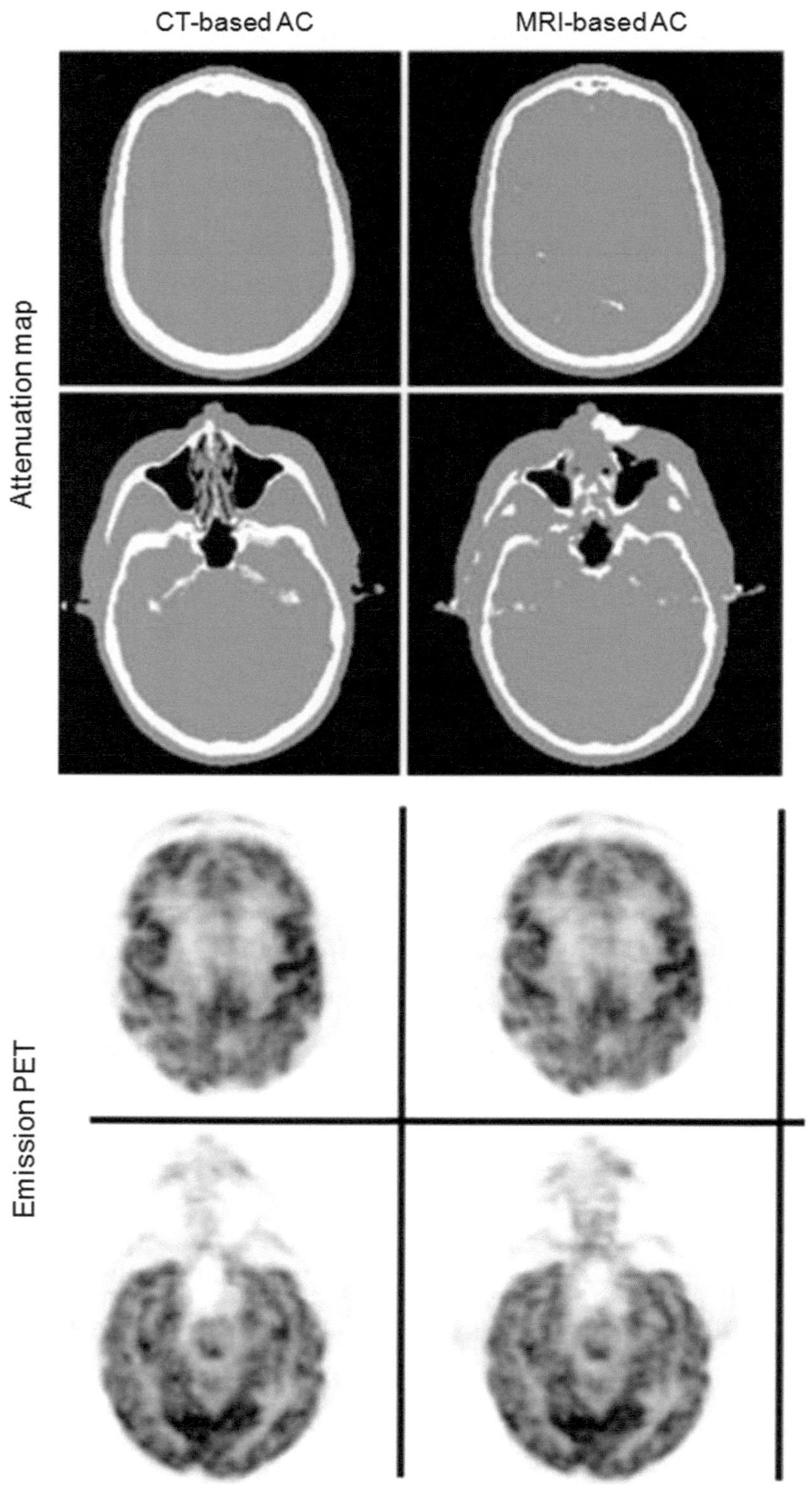

Fig. 33.16 Attenuation correction using MR images acquired using UTE sequence (Reprinted from [23] with permission)

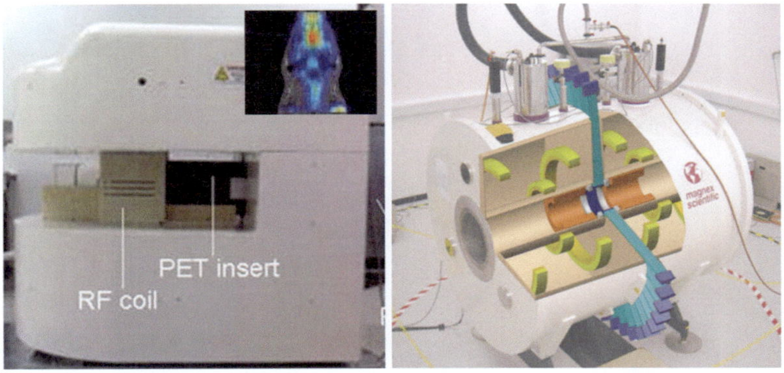

Fig. 33.17 PMT-based PET/MRI using optical fibers. (**a**) PET/MRI using slanted light guides and optical fiber. (**b**) PET/MRI using split magnet and optical fiber (Reprinted from [29] and [28] with permission)

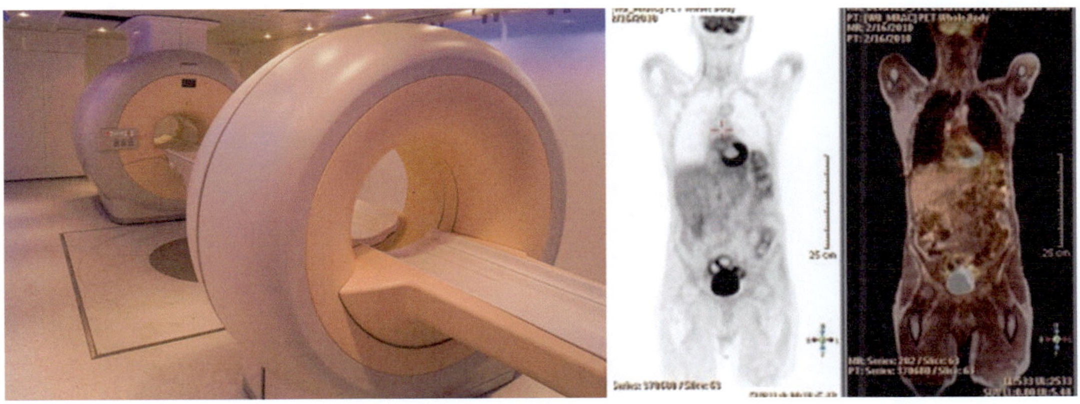

Fig. 33.18 PMT-based PET/MRI using parallel scanners (Courtesy of Philips Healthcare)

photosensor for simultaneous PET/MRI. The feasibility of the APD-based PET detectors has been shown by several groups, and a commercial animal PET system using APD (LabPET™; GE Healthcare) is also available. The APD has several attractive characteristics to be used in the PET detectors closely combined with MRI coil systems for simultaneous PET/MRI, such as its relatively compact size and insensitivity to magnetic fields.

Figures 33.19 through 33.21 show MRI-compatible PET insert systems using the APD that has been developed by several research groups for small animal imaging studies. The PET/MR images acquired using PET insert developed by the University of Tubingen group is shown in Figure 33.19, which consists of 10 APD PET detector modules and is built into 7-T MRI. In each detector module which was built into a MRI-compatible copper shielding, an lutetium oxyorthosilicate (LSO) scintillation crystal array (12 × 12) block is coupled with the APD array [32, 35, 36].

Brookhaven National Lab has also developed an APD-based PET insert for simultaneous PET/MRI acquisition of the rat brain in a 9.4-T animal MRI scanner (Fig. 33.20). The system is modified from the RatCAP (Rat Conscious Animal PET) scanner from the same group, and is capable of imaging an awake rat brain. To minimize the interference between PET and MRI, the nonmagnetic version APD array was used and the detector housing material was changed from aluminum

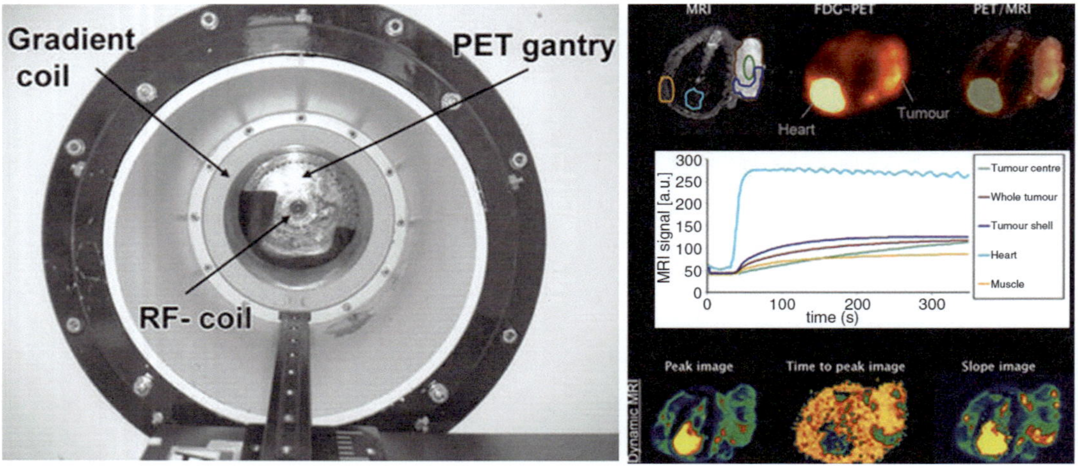

Fig. 33.19 Simultaneously acquired PET/MR images using APD-based MRI-compatible PET insert (Reprinted from [32] with permission)

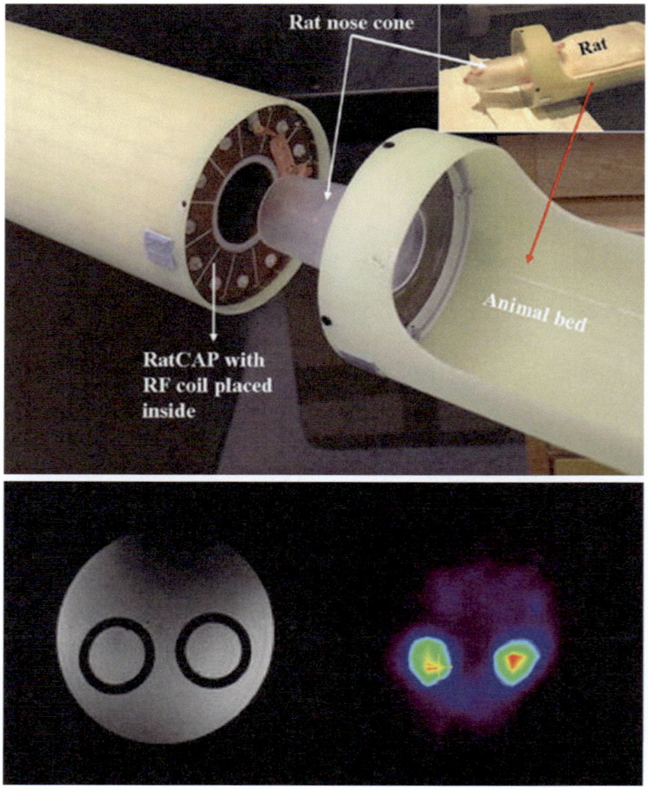

Fig. 33.20 PET/MR images acquired using MRI-compatible RatCAP scanner (Reprinted from [37] with permission)

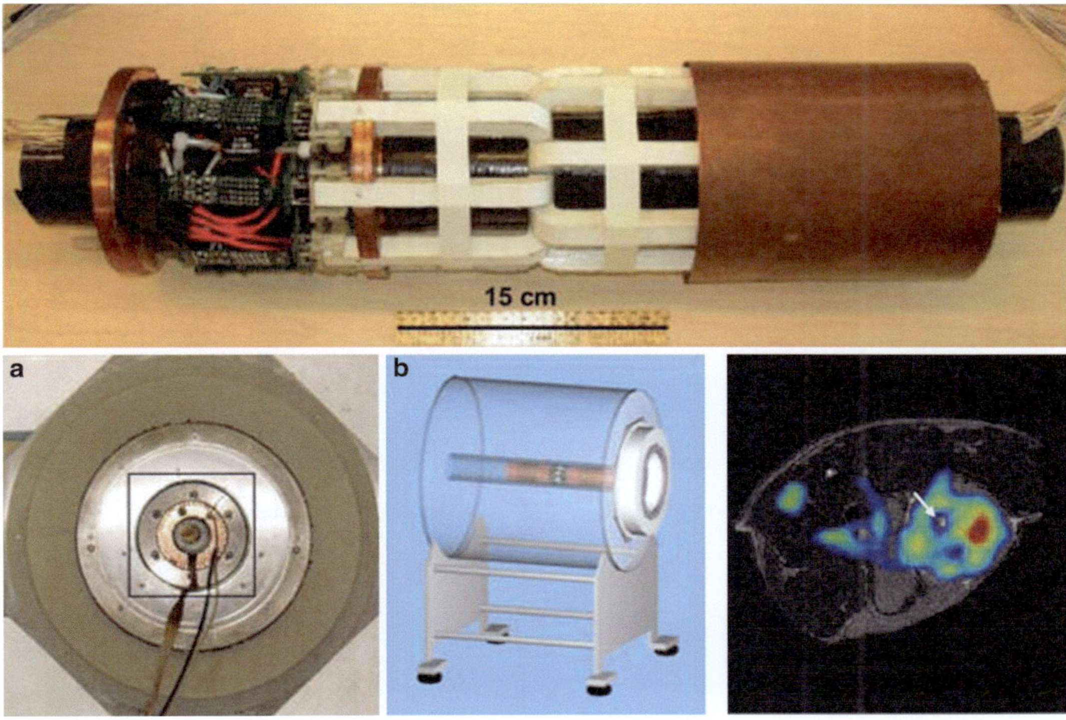

Fig. 33.21 Combined approach with optical fiber and APD technologies (Reprinted from [33] and [34] with permission)

to copper [37]. Extension of this system for breast PET/MRI is currently in progress [38].

The University of California at Davis group combined the optical fiber and APD technologies to develop a similar MRI-compatible PET insert, as shown in Fig. 33.21. In their approach, the LSO crystal array is coupled to a position-sensitive APD (PSAPD) via short 90° bending optical fibers. By use of the optical fibers, the PSAPD and front-end electronics can be placed outside of the MRI field-of-view so that they are less likely to interfere with the MRI system [33, 34].

APD-Based PET/MRI (Clinical)

An APD PET insert for simultaneous human brain PET/MRI was developed by Siemens Healthcare and has been in use for the last several years by several research groups. The insert consists of 192 LSO-APD PET detector modules, has an inner diameter of 35 cm, and was built into a 3-T clinical MRI scanner (Fig. 33.22). Their system has provided useful data to demonstrate the feasibility of simultaneous PET/MRI in human brain studies and to develop MRI-based attenuation and motion corrections [1, 23, 40, 41].

Recently, Siemens Healthcare announced the fully integrated PET/MRI scanner (Biograph mMR) based on the same detector technology. In this system, the LSO-APD PET detector modules were inserted between radiofrequency and gradient coils of large-bore 3-T MRI, yielding a 60-cm bore size for a simultaneous whole body PET/MRI scan with a common axial center (Fig. 33.23).

SiPM-Based PET/MRI

SiPM is a promising alternative semiconductor photosensor for PET/MRI applications. SiPM is composed of an array of micro-APDs operated in

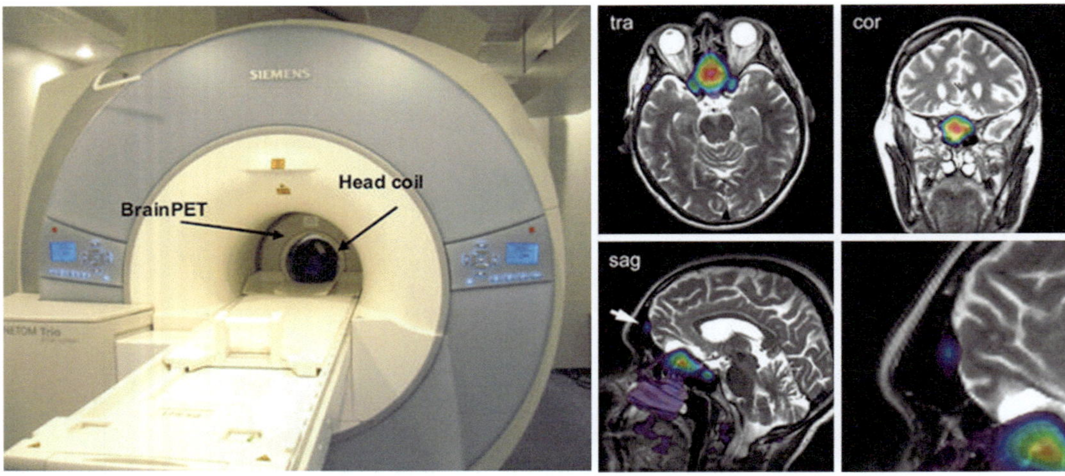

Fig. 33.22 APD PET inserts for brain PET/MRI (Reprinted from [39] and [1] with permission)

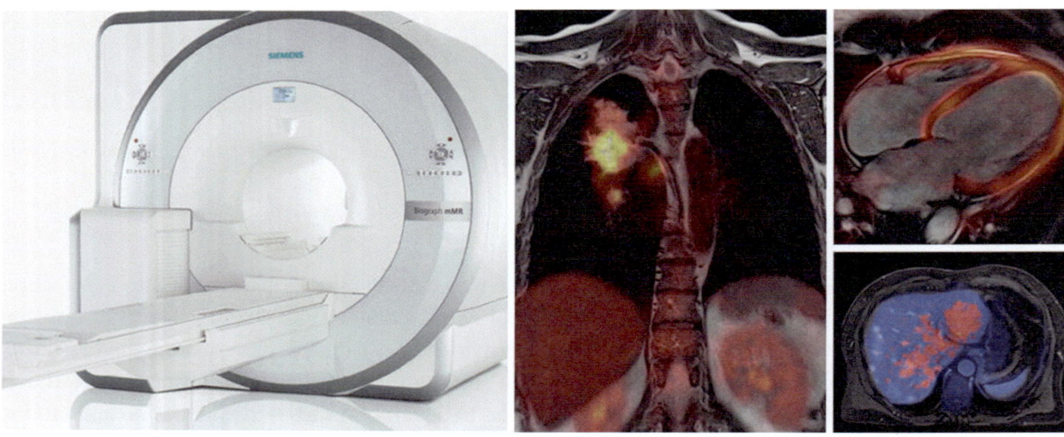

Fig. 33.23 Fully integrated whole-body PET/MRI using APD PET detectors (Courtesy of Siemens Healthcare)

Geiger mode. Because SiPMs operate in Geiger mode rather than in proportional mode, SiPMs provide greater gain than conventional APDs [7]. SiPMs are also relatively compact and inexpensive. Several studies have shown that SiPM-based PET detectors are MRI-compatible and provide excellent coincidence timing resolution sufficient for TOF PET data acquisition [42, 43]. PET/MRI scanners with TOF measurement capability will have the same advantages as TOF PET/CT, including an improvement in image quality [44].

Seoul National University in South Korea reported the first PET prototype based on a 2×6 SiPM array with individual diodes with an active surface of 4.4 mm^2, and showed that this system is feasible for small animal PET imaging studies [45]. Recently, the second SiPM PET of this group was been developed in which the array-type SiPM was used and every aspect of the physical characteristics of the system have been significantly improved from the first version. Figure 33.24 shows the simultaneously acquired PET/MR image using the second SiPM PET system that was combined with a loop radiofrequency coil and 3-T clinical MRI [46, 47].

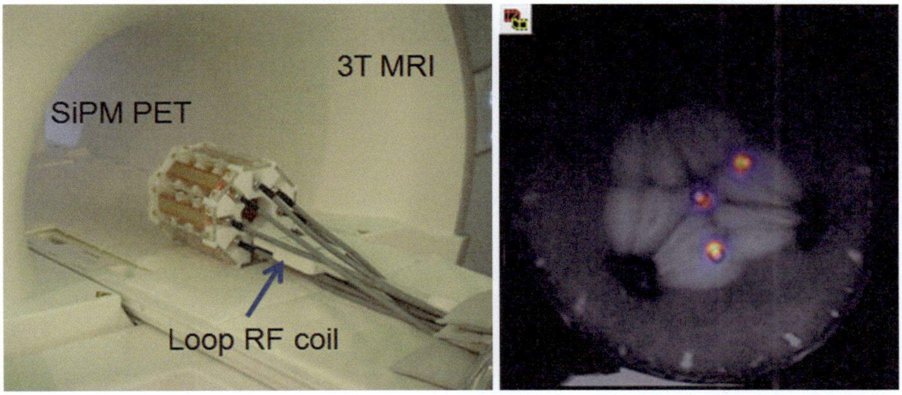

Fig. 33.24 SiPM-based MRI-compatible PET for simultaneous PET/MRI (Reprinted from [46] with permission)

References

1. Boss A, Bisdas S, Kolb A, Hofmann M, Ernemann U, Claussen CD, et al. Hybrid PET/MRI of intracranial masses: initial experiences and comparison to PET/CT. J Nucl Med. 2010;51(8):1198–205.
2. Antoch G, Bockisch A. Combined PET/MRI: a new dimension in whole-body oncology imaging? Eur J Nucl Med Mol Imaging. 2009;36(Suppl 1):S113–20.
3. Kang KW. Preliminary pre-clinical results and overview on PET/MRI/fluorescent molecular imaging. Open Nucl Med J. 2010;2:153–6.
4. Pichler BJ, Wehrl HF, Kolb A, Judenhofer MS. Positron emission tomography/magnetic resonance imaging: the next generation of multimodality imaging? Semin Nucl Med. 2008;38(3):199–208.
5. Yamamoto S, Hatazawa J, Imaizumi M, Shimosegawa E, Aoki M, Sugiyama E, et al. A multi-slice dual layer MR-compatible animal PET system. IEEE Trans Nucl Sci. 2009;56(5):2706–13.
6. Hong SJ, Song IC, Ito M, Kwon SI, Lee GS, Sim KS, et al. An investigation into the use of Geiger-mode solid-state photomultipliers for simultaneous PET and MRI acquisition. IEEE Trans Nucl Sci. 2008;55(3):882–8.
7. Lee JS, Hong SJ. Geiger-mode avalanche photodiodes for PET/MRI. In: Iniewski K, editor. Electronic circuits for radiation detection. Boca Raton: CRC Press; 2010. p. 179–200.
8. Hu Z, Ojha N, Renisch S, Schulz V, Torres I, Buhl A, et al. MR-based attenuation correction for a whole-body sequential PET/MR system. IEEE Nucl Sci Symp Conf Rec. 2009:3508–12.
9. Delso G, Martinez-Moller A, Bundschuh RA, Nekolla SG, Ziegler SI. The effect of limited MR field of view in MR/PET attenuation correction. Med Phys. 2010;37(6):2804–12.
10. Bergstrom M, Litton J, Eriksson L, Bohm C, Blomqvist G. Determination of object contour from projections for attenuation correction in cranial positron emission tomography. J Comput Assist Tomogr. 1982;6(2):365–72.
11. Siegel S, Dahlbom M. Implementation and evaluation of a calculated attenuation correction for PET. IEEE Trans Nucl Sci. 1992;39(4):1117–21.
12. Kaneko K, Kuwabara Y, Sasaki M, Koga H, Abe K, Baba S, et al. Validation of quantitative accuracy of the post-injection transmission-based and transmissionless attenuation correction techniques in neurological FDG-PET. Nucl Med Commun. 2004;25(11):1095–102.
13. Stodilka RZ, Kemp BJ, Prato FS, Kertesz A, Kuhl D, Nicholson RL. Scatter and attenuation correction for brain SPECT using attenuation distributions inferred from a head atlas. J Nucl Med. 2000;41(9):1569–78.
14. Montandon ML, Zaidi H. Atlas-guided non-uniform attenuation correction in cerebral 3D PET imaging. Neuroimage. 2005;25(1):278–86.
15. Kim JS, Lee JS, Park MH, Kim KM, Oh SH, Cheon GJ, et al. Feasibility of template-guided attenuation correction in cat brain PET imaging. Mol Imaging Biol. 2010;12(3):250–8.
16. Montandon ML, Zaidi H. Quantitative analysis of template-based attenuation compensation in 3D brain PET. Comput Med Imaging Graph. 2007;31(1):28–38.
17. Kops ER, Herzog H. Template based attenuation correction for PET in MR-PET scanners. IEEE Nucl Sci Symp Conf Rec. 2008;3786–9.
18. Hofmann M, Steinke F, Scheel V, Charpiat G, Farquhar J, Aschoff P, et al. MRI-based attenuation correction for PET/MRI: a novel approach combining pattern recognition and atlas registration. J Nucl Med. 2008;49(11):1875–83.
19. Zaidi H, Montandon ML, Slosman DO. Magnetic resonance imaging-guided attenuation and scatter corrections in three-dimensional brain positron emission tomography. Med Phys. 2003;30(5):937–48.

20. Martinez-Möller A, Souvatzoglou M, Delso G, Bundschuh RA, Chefd'hotel C, Ziegler SI, et al. Tissue classification as a potential approach for attenuation correction in whole-body PET/MRI: evaluation with PET/CT data. J Nucl Med. 2009;50(4):520–6.
21. Hofmann M, Pichler B, Scholkopf B, Beyer T. Towards quantitative PET/MRI: a review of MR-based attenuation correction techniques. Eur J Nucl Med Mol Imaging. 2009;36(Suppl 1):S93–104.
22. Keereman V, Fierens Y, Broux T, De Deene Y, Lonneux M, Vandenberghe S. MRI-based attenuation correction for PET/MRI using ultrashort echo time sequences. J Nucl Med. 2010;51(5):812–8.
23. Catana C, van der Kouwe A, Benner T, Michel CJ, Hamm M, Fenchel M, et al. Toward implementing an MRI-based PET attenuation-correction method for neurologic studies on the MR-PET brain prototype. J Nucl Med. 2010;51(9):1431–8.
24. Shao Y, Cherry SR, Farahani K, Meadors K, Siegel S, Silverman RW, et al. Simultaneous PET and MR imaging. Phys Med Biol. 1997;42(10):1965–70.
25. Marsden PK, Strul D, Keevil SF, Williams SCR, Cash D. Simultaneous PET and NMR. Br J Radiol. 2002;75:S53–9.
26. Yamamoto S, Takamatsu S, Murayama H, Minato K. A block detector for a multislice, depth-of-interaction MR-compatible PET. IEEE Trans Nucl Sci. 2005; 52(1):33–7.
27. Raylman RR, Majewski S, Lemieux SK, Velan SS, Kross B, Popov V, et al. Simultaneous MRI and PET imaging of a rat brain. Phys Med Biol. 2006;51(24): 6371–9.
28. Lucas AJ, Hawkes RC, Guerra P, Ansorge RE, Nutt RE, Clark JC, et al., editors. Development of a combined microPET®-MR system. IEEE Nucl Sci Symp Conf Rec. 2006;2345–8.
29. Yamamoto S, Imaizumi M, Kanai Y, Tatsumi M, Aoki M, Sugiyama E, et al. Design and performance from an integrated PET/MRI system for small animals. Ann Nucl Med. 2010;24(2):89–8.
30. Hawkes RC, Fryer TD, Siegel S, Ansorge RE, Carpenter TA. Preliminary evaluation of a combined microPET-MR system. Technol Cancer Res Treat. 2010;9(1):53–60.
31. Cho ZH, Son YD, Kim HK, Kim KN, Oh SH, Han JY, et al. A fusion PET-MRI system with a high-resolution research tomograph-PET and ultra-high field 7.0T-MRI for the molecular-genetic imaging of the brain. Proteomics. 2008;8(6):1302–23.
32. Wehrl HF, Judenhofer MS, Wiehr S, Pichler BJ. Pre-clinical PET/MR: technological advances and new perspectives in biomedical research. Eur J Nucl Med Mol Imaging. 2009;36(Suppl 1):S56–68.
33. Catana C, Wu Y, Judenhofer MS, Qi J, Pichler BJ, Cherry SR. Simultaneous acquisition of multislice PET and MR images: initial results with a MR-compatible PET scanner. J Nucl Med. 2006;47(12):1968–76.
34. Catana C, Procissi D, Wu Y, Judenhofer MS, Qi J, Pichler BJ, et al. Simultaneous in vivo positron emission tomography and magnetic resonance imaging. Proc Natl Acad Sci USA. 2008;105(10):3705–10.
35. Judenhofer MS, Catana C, Swann BK, Siegel SB, Jung WI, Nutt RE, et al. PET/MR images acquired with a compact MR-compatible PET detector in a 7-T magnet. Radiology. 2007;244(3):807–14.
36. Judenhofer MS, Wehrl HF, Newport DF, Catana C, Siegel SB, Becker M, et al. Simultaneous PET-MRI: a new approach for functional and morphological imaging. Nat Med. 2008;14(4):459–65.
37. Maramraju SH, Junnarkar S, Ravindranath B, Southekal S, Stoll S, Smith SD. An MR compatible PET scanner based on RatCAP for small animal imaging at 9.4T. IEEE Nucl Sci Symp Conf Rec. 2008;2679–82.
38. Ravindranath B, Maramraju SH, Junnarkar SS, Southekal SS, Stoll SP, Pratte JF, et al., editors. A simultaneous PET/MRI breast scanner based on the RatCAP. IEEE Nucl Sci Symp Conf Rec. 2008;4650–4655.
39. Herzog H, Pietrzyk U, Shah NJ, Ziemons K. The current state, challenges and perspectives of MR-PET. Neuroimage. 2010;49(3):2072–82.
40. Schlemmer HPW, Pichler BJ, Schmand M, Burbar Z, Michel C, Ladebeck R, et al. Simultaneous MR/PET imaging of the human brain: feasibility study. Radiology. 2008;248(3):1028–35.
41. Catana C, Benner T, van der Kouwe A, Byars L, Hamm M, Chonde DB, et al. MRI-Assisted PET motion correction for neurologic studies in an integrated MR-PET scanner. J Nucl Med. 2011;52(1):154–61.
42. Kim CL, Wang GC, Dolinsky S. Multi-pixel photon counters for TOF PET detector and its challenges. IEEE Trans Nucl Sci. 2009;56(5):2580–5.
43. Degenhardt C, Prescher G, Frach T, et al. The digital silicon photomultiplier – a novel sensor for the detection of scintillation light. IEEE Nucl Sci Symp Conf Rec. 2009;2383–6.
44. Lee JS. Technical advances in current PET and hybrid imaging systems. Open Nucl Med J. 2010;2:192–208.
45. Kwon SI, Lee JS, Yoon HS, Ito M, Ko GB, Choi JY, et al. Development of small animal PET prototype using silicon photomultiplier (SiPM): initial results of phantom and animal imaging studies. J Nucl Med. 2011;52(4):572–9.
46. Ko GB, Yoon HS, Kwon SI, Hong SJ, Lee DS, Lee JS. Development of FPGA-based coincidence units with veto function. Biomed Eng Lett. 2011;1(1):27–31.
47. Yoon HS, Ko GB, Kwon SI, Lee CM, Ito M, Chan Song I, et al. Initial results of simultaneous PET/MRI experiments with an MRI-compatible silicon photomultiplier PET scanner. J Nucl Med. 2012;53(4):608–14.

Index

E.E. Kim et al. (eds.), *Clinical PET and PET/CT: Principles and Applications*,
DOI 10.1007/978-1-4419-0802-5, © Springer Science+Business Media New York 2013

C

D

MIX
Papier aus verantwortungsvollen Quellen
Paper from responsible sources
FSC® C105338

If you have any concerns about our products,
you can contact us on
ProductSafety@springernature.com

In case Publisher is established outside the EU,
the EU authorized representative is:
Springer Nature Customer Service Center GmbH
Europaplatz 3, 69115 Heidelberg, Germany

Printed by Libri Plureos GmbH
in Hamburg, Germany